THE NE[...]
HEALING
HERBS

THE NEW
HEALING
HERBS

THE **ESSENTIAL GUIDE** TO MORE THAN **125** OF
NATURE'S MOST POTENT HERBAL REMEDIES

MICHAEL CASTLEMAN

RODALE®

© 2009 by Rodale Inc.

Printed in the United States of America

Rodale Inc. makes every effort to use acid-free ♾, recycled paper ♻.

Illustrations on pages 63, 73, 75, 78, 84, 95, 112, 115, 124, 127, 176, 186, 196, 201, 226, 271, 297, 314, 316, 337, 345, 361, 363, 373, 379, 381, 395, 397, 425, 434, and 487 by Michael Gellatly; all others by Wayne Michaud

Book design by Christina Gaugler

Library of Congress Cataloging-in-Publication Data

Castleman, Michael.
    The new healing herbs : the essential guide to more than 125 of nature's most potent herbal remedies / Michael Castleman.
        p.   cm.
    Includes bibliographical references and index.
    ISBN-13 978–1–60529–888–7 hardcover
    ISBN-10 1–60529–888–3 hardcover
    ISBN-13 978–1–60529–889–4 paperback
    ISBN-10 1–60529–889–1 paperback
    1. Herbs—Therapeutic use.   2. Medicinal plants.   I. Title.
RM666.H33C393 2009
615'.321—dc22   2009014988

2 4 6 8 10 9 7 5 3 1 hardcover
2 4 6 8 10 9 7 5 3 1 paperback

We inspire and enable people to improve their lives and the world around them

For more of our products visit **rodalestore.com** or call 800-848-4735

Contents

◆

PART I

CHAPTER 1

5,000 Years of Herbal Healing

CHAPTER 2

Are Healing Herbs Safe?

CHAPTER 3

Getting the Most from Nature's Medicines

CHAPTER 4

The Best Sources Are Close at Hand

◆

PART II

CHAPTER 5

The Cream of the Herbal Crop

CHAPTER 6

Introduction

Twenty years ago, when I wrote the first edition of *The Healing Herbs*, it was clear that herbal medicine was becoming increasingly popular. But no one involved with herbal healing in the late 1980s had any inkling of the explosion in popularity that herbal medicine would enjoy as the 20th century turned into the 21st. And in my wildest dreams, I could not have imagined how popular *The Healing Herbs* would become—now more than one million copies sold in English, Spanish, French, Italian, and other languages.

Herbal medicine is now an industry worth more than $4 billion a year, about five times the size it was when the original edition of this book was published in 1991. According to a national survey conducted for *Prevention* magazine, 49 percent of American adults—more than 100 million people—use an herbal medicine each year, and 24 percent—some 25 million people—call themselves "regular users." And a study published in 2005 in *Archives of Internal Medicine* shows that in adults over the age of 18, 16 percent of men and 19 percent of women use a medicinal herb every week.

This third edition has been expanded from 100 herbs to 130. The new herbs—including andrographis, butterbur, cat's claw, elderberry, and maitake mushrooms—are not "new" in the sense of newly discovered. These plants have been well known for centuries, and in the case of elderberry, since ancient times. But only during the past decade have studies clearly shown how medicinally valuable they are.

Twenty years ago, the medical profession was, at best, skeptical of herbal medicine. No longer. Today, it's not at all unusual for physicians to recommend echinacea for the common cold, ginger to prevent motion sickness and morning sickness, black cohosh for menopausal discomforts, cranberry to prevent urinary tract infections, St. John's wort to treat depression, or elderberry to treat flu.

Doctors have become more open to herbal medicine in part because their friends and family members have reported success with it. But in addition, mainstream American medical journals have changed their position on herbs. Twenty years ago, major journals were quick to publish reports of medicinal herbs' hazardous side effects (including several reports that turned out to be erroneous), but only rarely did they publish information about herbs' benefits. Today, these same journals publish a steady stream of studies in support of herbal healing. A report in the *British Medical Journal* (now *BMJ*) was largely responsible for popularizing St. John's wort as an antidepressant. A review in the *Journal of Family Practice* concluded that echinacea is an effective cold treatment. Studies published in *Lancet* have demonstrated the effectiveness of feverfew in migraine prevention. A study in the *New England Journal of Medicine*, once openly hostile to herbs, showed that cranberry juice helps prevent urinary tract infections. And reports in the *Journal of the American Medical Association*, another traditional herb-basher, have supported ginkgo as a treatment for Alzheimer's disease and saw palmetto for benign prostate enlargement. (All of these studies and many more are summarized throughout this revised edition.)

In other words, herbal medicine is more mainstream in the United States today than it's been in 100 years. It's still not as medically accepted in this country as it is in some other countries, notably Germany, nor as mainstream as it was in 19th-century America, before the pharmaceutical industry took medicine out of the herb garden and moved it into the laboratory. But herbal medicine is no longer the fringe practice that it was when the first edition of this book appeared in 1991.

Medicinal herb products have also come a long way in the last 20 years. Not only are there many more of them, but they are much more widely available, now stocked by many pharmacies and even some supermarkets. And they have become more reliable with the advent of "stan-dardized extracts," preparations from plants bred to contain a certain concentration of pharmacologically active compounds, and then grown, harvested, stored, and prepared under controlled conditions to produce reasonably reliable dose uniformity. Standardized extracts are not quite as dose-controlled as laboratory-synthesized pharmaceuticals, but they're close, and considerably more dose-controlled than bulk herbs.

Unfortunately, the past decade has also witnessed a few serious safety problems with herbs, two in particular. In one, an estimated 30 young adults died after taking mega-overdoses of Chinese ephedra (ma huang). They were not using this herb medicinally, but rather to experience amphetamine-like intoxication. They took hundreds of times the dose that responsible herbalists would recommend. In addition, 82 people worldwide suffered liver damage—and nine died—while using kava, the South Pacific herbal tranquilizer. It turned out that kava's meteoric rise to popularity led to adulteration of the root with aerial parts of the plant that contain compounds toxic to the liver. Because of the scandal, kava's popularity plummeted, adulteration ceased, and so did reports of liver damage.

But despite occasionally scary headlines, herbal medicines have an admirable safety record overall. With more Americans using more medicinal herbs than at any time in the past century, there have been few serious mishaps, especially when compared with the side effects—and deaths—from pharmaceuticals. (For more on this, see Chapter 2.)

Nonetheless, safety concerns seem destined to remain the most pressing issue in herbal medicine, largely because the Food and Drug Administration has to date refused to reopen its review process for over-the-counter drugs to include evaluation of herbs. (For more on this, see Chapter 1.) But for the first time, considerable numbers of FDA staff support the use of healing herbs. I'm cautiously optimistic that over the next decade, the FDA will adopt medicinal herb labeling regulations that are more appropriate to Americans' needs.

Meanwhile, *The New Healing Herbs*—completely revised, updated, and expanded—should help you use medicinal herbs confidently, effectively, and above all, safely.

How to Use This Book

Some people become so enamored of herbal healing that they reject mainstream medicine entirely. This is a serious mistake. Herbal healing can make an important contribution to human well-being, but it also has its limits. Responsible herbalists consult physicians and use pharmaceuticals appropriately. In general, if a minor ailment does not respond to herbal self-treatment within 2 weeks, consult a physician.

For some conditions, all you need is an herbal remedy: aloe for minor burns, dill for infant colic, or clove oil for fast, temporary toothache relief.

For others, you can mix and match several approaches. Consider upset stomach. You might change what you eat: fewer hard-to-digest fats and more easily digestible fresh fruits and veg-etables. You might change how you eat: more slowly, in a relaxed setting, chewing more thoroughly. You might take a pharmaceutical antacid. Or you might try one of the many herbs that help soothe the stomach, such as fennel, caraway, peppermint, or ginger.

Of course, many conditions require professional care, such as high blood pressure, diabetes, heart disease, and congestive heart failure. But healing herbs can still play an important role in your overall treatment plan as complements to standard therapies and in consultation with your physician.

Before you start using healing herbs:

❦ Read Chapter 2 to gain a basic understanding of herbal safety issues. All the herbs discussed in this book can be used safely if they are used responsibly. However, when used improperly, some may cause harm.

❦ Before you ingest any healing herb, read Chapters 3 and 4 to make sure you understand how to obtain and prepare it. For example, an infusion is not a tea.

❦ Before using any herb discussed in Chapter 5, pay special attention to the sections titled "Rx Recommendations" and "The Safety Factor."

❦ Finally, if you'd like to use herbs for any condition requiring professional treatment, take this book with you the next time you consult your physician.

PART I

There is nothing in the most advanced contemporary medicine whose

embryo cannot be found in the medicine of the past.

—Maximilien E. P. Littre, French lexicographer

Chapter 1

FROM MAGIC TO MEDICINE

5,000 Years of Herbal Healing

In 1991, on a glacier in the Italian Alps that had melted back to an unusual extent, hikers stumbled on a dead body. It turned out to be the naturally mummified body of a prehistoric man who had frozen to death some 5,300 years before and whose remains had been preserved in the ice.

Dubbed the Iceman, he's been studied by Italian anthropologists ever since. He wore straw-lined leather shoes, leather clothing, a thick coat made from woven grass, and a bearskin cap. He carried a wooden bow, a leather quiver filled with stone-tipped arrows, a flint-bladed knife, a wood-handled ax with a copper blade, and a food pouch that still contained dried deer meat and a prune.

The Iceman's pouch also contained two mysterious corklike lumps about the size of walnuts that were pierced through and strung together on a leather thong, indicating that they were of value. The lumps turned out to be bracket fungus (*Piptoporus betulinus*), one of many mushrooms that grow in shelflike plates on tree trunks. This species of fungus contains agaric acid, a potent laxative, and an oily resin that is toxic to some bacteria and intestinal parasites.

The scientists studying the Iceman had no idea why he would have carried bracket fungus until, in 1998, a painstaking autopsy of his digestive tract turned up the eggs of an intestinal parasite (*Trichuris trichiura*).

It now appears that the Iceman knew he had a medical problem and was using bits of bracket fungus to treat his condition. Given its laxative and antiparasitic action, the fungus probably provided some benefit.

This discovery ranks as the world's oldest documented example of the practice of medicine, and it suggests that prehistoric humanity was more medically sophisticated than previously believed. After all, the Iceman or someone else had diagnosed his malady correctly and had recommended a reasonably appropriate treatment—an herbal treatment—around 3300 B.C.

Animal Attractions

Just what is a healing herb? The word *herb* comes from the Latin for "grass." Technically, herbs are plants that wither each autumn, plants other than shrubs or trees. But many woody perennials such as slippery elm, tea tree, and white willow are also used in herbal healing. To an herbalist, the phrase "healing herbs" applies to every plant with medicinal value.

Prehistoric sites show that the Neanderthals used yarrow, marshmallow, and other herbs some 60,000 years ago. What attracted them to these plants?

Animals played a key role. Prehistoric humans were keen observers of the world around them. No doubt our ancestors noticed that when animals appeared ill, they sometimes ate plants that they ordinarily ignored. Humans sampled these plants, in many cases noticing curious effects—wakefulness, sleepiness, laxative action, increased urination, and so on. The herbs that caused these effects were incorporated into prehistoric shamanism, and later into medicine.

Animal-inspired herbalism has continued into modern times. The controversial herbal cancer therapy marketed in the 1940s by Harry Hoxsey was reportedly inspired by a cancer-stricken horse that ate unusual herbs (more on this later).

Aromatic Magic

Early humans were also attracted to healing herbs' aromas. They rubbed strong-smelling herbs on their bodies to repel insects and to hide their human scent from animals that they feared or hunted. They also adorned themselves with sweet-smelling herbs to please their mates.

Fragrant herbs evolved into the first perfumes and embalming mixtures. Demand for them spurred ancient trade. During the Middle Ages, when Europeans believed that bathing was unhealthy and farm animals often shared human living quarters, homemakers spread aromatic "strewing herbs" to freshen the air. Herbalists still prepare scent baskets (known as potpourris) today, and the perfume industry still creates most of its fragrances from herbal essences.

But foul odors, not fragrant ones, were key to the development of herbal healing. Early humans used plants such as rosemary, thyme, dill, and virtually all of today's culinary spices to mask the stench of rotting food, especially meats. Today, we use culinary herbs and spices only as flavor enhancers, but to prehistoric humanity, flavor enhancement was incidental to food preservation.

Prehistoric humanity had no refrigeration, and food spoiled quickly. Spoilage destroyed precious reserves, and early humans learned the hard way that eating rotten food caused illness and sometimes death. No doubt some prehistoric homemaker happened to lay some rotting food on a bed of wild mint, sage, basil, or some other aromatic herb, hoping the herb's fragrance would mask the item's malodorousness. It did, and as a bonus, the food didn't spoil as quickly.

Our ancestors began wrapping foods, especially meats, in aromatic herbs to preserve them, which led to other astonishing discoveries. Those who ate preservative herbs along with the food suffered less illness. As an added benefit, the food tasted better.

Surely, our ancestors must have decided, aromatic herbs were magic. As time passed and magic was incorporated into religion, ancient civilizations came to view aromatic herbs as gifts from the gods. This is why many herbs figure prominently in ancient myths and religions.

Thanks to modern science, we know that the oils that give aromatic herbs their fragrance and flavor contain antimicrobial compounds that kill many food-spoiling, disease-causing microorganisms. In fact, both rosemary and sage have food-preservative action comparable to that of the commercial preservatives BHA and BHT.

Trial and Error

Our ancestors also discovered many healing herbs simply by trial and error. They learned through experience that some plants healed, while others harmed. They had little control over their world or their bodies. Their average life expectancy was barely 30 years. Because their lives were so full of threatening, often fatal, surprises, anything that made life more predictable acquired an aura of magic and healing.

It's no coincidence that shamans from prehistoric times down to the present day have relied heavily on herbs, such as ipecac, buckthorn, and wormwood, that cause vomiting, purging, and hallucinations. Any predictable effect was better than none, and the ability to induce vomiting, purging, or visions made shamans/herbalists appear to possess magic powers.

The allure of predictable action remained central to medicine for thousands of years. Herbs that induced vomiting (emetics) or had powerful laxative action were used routinely in medicine until well into the 19th century.

Major effects made big impressions, but early humans also recognized herbs' more subtle benefits. We'll never know what possessed some ancient Chinese peasant to brew a tea from the small, ungainly stalks of ma huang (Chinese ephedra), but several thousand years ago,

someone did. In the process, that person stumbled upon one of the world's oldest medicines, a decongestant whose laboratory analog, pseudoephedrine, is still an ingredient in today's cold formulas, such as Sudafed.

Similarly, we'll never know how many roots ancient Asians dug up before they discovered ginger. Or why Native Americans had a hunch that black cohosh might be useful in gynecology. All over the world, however, ancient peoples dug, dried, chewed, pounded, rubbed, and brewed the plants around them. In this way, they discovered the vast majority of healing herbs still in use today.

Isolated Cultures, Similar Herbs

Herbal trial and error becomes even more remarkable when we consider that cultures separated by thousands of miles arrived at similar uses for many healing herbs. What's more, they almost certainly did so independently of one another.

There are four major herbal traditions: Chinese, Ayurvedic (in India), European (including Egyptian), and Native American. The ancient spice trade clearly introduced Asian herbs such as garlic, ginger, and cinnamon into Europe thousands of years ago. And a few ancient herbalists, notably the 1st-century Greek Dioscorides, traveled extensively, learning the herbal wisdom of many cultures around the ancient world.

Nonetheless, early Asian and European herbalists were largely isolated from one another. In modern times, it's difficult to comprehend just how isolated they were. Until the 1st century A.D., it took 2 years for spice traders to make the round trip from Greece to India's black-pepper-producing region.

Even in this age of instant global communication, different healing systems still operate relatively independently of one another. During the 1970s and early 1980s, ginkgo became an important medicine in France and Germany for aging-related ailments, with sales topping $500 million a year. Most U.S. medical school libraries stocked the German and French journals showing ginkgo's remarkable effectiveness, yet American physicians virtually ignored ginkgo well into the 1990s. How connected could the ancient herbalists have been?

Even granting a nearly impossible level of herbal cross-fertilization between Asia and Europe, the land bridge between Asia and North America became the Bering Sea about 10,000 years ago. Until the 15th century, Old World cultures were almost entirely isolated from the Americas. Nonetheless, Old and New World herbalists used many herbs similarly.

- Angelica and licorice: Asians, Europeans, and Native Americans relied on these herbs as treatments for respiratory ailments.

- Hop and the mints: All of the ancient herbal traditions used these herbs as stomach soothers.

- Blackberry and raspberry: Around the world, these herbs played a role in treating diarrhea.

- Uva-ursi: Asians, Europeans, and Native Americans all discovered this herb's diuretic properties.

- White willow: All of the herbal healing disciplines used this herb to treat pain and inflammation.

During the 19th century, chemists used this "herbal convergence" to point them to the plants whose extracts became the first pharmaceuticals. According to a report in the journal *Science*, about 75 percent of the pharmaceuticals derived from plants came to the attention of drug companies because of their use in traditional herbal medicine.

Homage to the "Wise Women"

Most medical histories chronicle great achievements by great men: Hippocrates, the father of medicine; Galen, Rome's leading physician; William Harvey's explanation of blood circulation; Edward Jenner's inoculations against smallpox; Louis Pasteur's Germ Theory; Alexander Fleming's discovery of penicillin.

The contributions of these men unquestionably changed the world. But from ancient times down to the present day, a relatively small number of male physicians made the great discoveries and ministered to the rich and royal while an enormous number of unsung women herbalists took care of everyone else.

Women healers have gone by many names: midwives, wise women, green women, witches, old wives, and nurses. Most physicians have never taken women's folk healing very seriously, and scientists often dismiss folk wisdom as "old wives' tales."

Yet the truth is that medically untrained women, who learn at the feet of other women, still provide most of the world's primary care. Even in the United States, most people view physicians as the health care choice of last resort. The medical profession promotes the idea that family doctors are our primary providers, but studies show that before people call health professionals, about 90 percent consult a friend or family member. These informal heath advisors are overwhelmingly women.

Ancient physicians officially recognized women's leading role in obstetrics and gynecology more than 2,000 years ago in the Hippocratic Oath, which many graduating medical students still recite today: "I will prescribe no . . . pessary [contraceptive device] to produce abortion." Anti-abortion activists have seized on this statement as a condemnation of abortion. In fact, it withdrew male doctors from gynecology and gave the field—including abortion, which was widely practiced in the ancient world—to the midwives.

Whatever your personal opinion of abortion, there's no doubt that women have always sought to control their fertility. After all, until about 150 years ago, childbirth was a leading cause of death among women.

Midwives completely dominated obstetrics and gynecology until the late 19th century. It's no coincidence that many herbs were traditionally used to calm the womb, trigger menstruation, induce abortion, promote or dry up mothers' milk, and treat infant colic and infectious diarrhea (still a leading cause of infant death in Third World nations). These were the daily concerns that women patients presented to the women who were their herbal healers.

Sometimes medically unschooled women herbalists introduced university-trained physicians to powerful medicines, such as the heart drug digitalis from foxglove. But by and large, male physicians dismissed female folk healers as ignorant practitioners of medicine that was, at best, inferior, and at worst, worthless.

Nonetheless, women herbalists have played a key—and largely undocumented—role in medical history. Just as herbs are the forgotten sources of many medicines, the "wise women" represent the forgotten healers whose thousands

of years of collective experience taught us how to use herbs safely and effectively.

The wise women were particularly adept at contraception. Around 700 B.C, an oracle sent Greek colonists to the coast of what is now Libya to found a colony, Cyrene. It was located in a dry, desolate, inhospitable place, but the colonists soon discovered a local plant that made them wealthy, silphion (in Latin, *silphium*), a species of fennel.

Silphium was a remarkably effective contraceptive. When women ate it, they did not conceive. The herb quickly became the contraceptive of choice around the Mediterranean. Cyrenian coins depicted the plant, often held by a woman. Poets wrote of its powers. Unfortunately, overharvesting eventually wiped it out.

Shen Nung and *The Classic of Herbs*

The origins of Chinese herbalism are lost in the mists of time. Legend has it that around 3400 B.C. (the time of the Iceman), "the divine farmer," mythical emperor-sage Shen Nung, invented agriculture and discovered that many plants have medicinal value. He tested herbs on himself and recorded their effects—only to die after consuming too much of one that turned out to be poisonous.

Chinese herbalists credit Shen Nung as the author of China's first great herb guide, or "herbal," the *Pen Tsao Ching* (*Classic of Herbs*), which listed 237 herbal prescriptions using dozens of herbs, including ephedra, rhubarb, and opium poppy. Most authorities agree, however, that the *Pen Tsao Ching* was not written down until the Han dynasty, around A.D. 100. It chronicles not the discoveries of one mythical emperor but rather the collected insights of generations of Chinese herbalists.

Chinese herbalists discovered many medicinal plants, notably ginseng, tea, sesame, garlic, and cinnamon. Starting around A.D. 500, it became customary for Chinese emperors to commission updates of Shen Nung's herb guide. Over the centuries, these became increasingly elaborate—and contradictory. By 1590, when Li Shih-Chen published his landmark 52-volume *Pen Tsao Kang Mu* (*Catalogue of Medicinal Herbs*), he included 1,094 medicinal plants and an astounding 11,000 herbal formulas.

Practitioners of Chinese herbalism still study Li's work, but they have simplified his art. Today, Chinese medicine employs about 300 herbs, 150 of which are considered indispensable. These include Chinese angelica (dang gui), burdock, chrysanthemum, cinnamon, dandelion, garlic, gentian, ginger, ginseng, hawthorn, licorice, lotus, mint, rhubarb, scullcap, senna, and tea.

Starting in the mid-19th century, European colonialists introduced Western medicine into China, dismissing traditional Chinese herbalism and acupuncture as nonsense. The Chinese felt the same way about the "foreign devils'" medicine, and the two systems seemed irreconcilable.

Shortly after the establishment of the People's Republic in 1949, however, the Chinese government decided that China's huge, medically underserved population could benefit from the integration of Western and Chinese medicine. Today, in many places in China, Western-trained physicians practice alongside traditional herbalists and acupuncturists. Chinese and Western physicians examine the same patients, confer with each other, and often coordinate their recommendations.

A turning point in American acceptance of Chinese medicine occurred in 1972, when President Richard Nixon first visited China. During his visit, the Americans were taken to a hospital. Network news broadcast astonishing footage of a woman having abdominal surgery while fully conscious, her only anesthesia being a few acupuncture needles in her earlobes and feet.

While accompanying President Nixon to China, *New York Times* columnist James Reston developed appendicitis and had to have surgery. Afterward, he decided to try acupuncture for postsurgical pain control. He was so pleased with the results that he wrote a testimonial column in the nation's most influential newspaper; his account helped open the United States to acupuncture and Chinese herbalism.

Jivaka and the Vedas

According to legend, around the time of the Hebrew exodus from Egypt (1200 B.C.), a poor Indian boy named Jivaka went to study medicine under the great Punarvasu Atreya, founder of India's first medical school at the University of Taxila in the Punjab. Having no money, the lad offered to become Atreya's servant in exchange for training.

After 7 years, Jivaka asked his teacher when his studies would be completed. Instead of answering, Atreya challenged him to scour the countryside and collect all the plants that he considered medically useless. Jivaka searched for many days. When he finally returned, he was sullen and empty-handed. He told his mentor that he was unable to find a single plant without healing power. Atreya replied, "Go! You now have the knowledge to be a physician."

Centered in the Indus Valley near the present India-Pakistan border, ancient Indian civilization was quite advanced. Excavations at Harappa and Mohenjo Daro dating to about 2500 B.C. have revealed municipal water and sewerage systems more advanced than the ones the Romans developed 2,000 years later.

Ancient Indians called their medicine Ayurveda, from two Sanskrit words: *ayur*, life, and *veda*, knowledge. Ayurvedic medicine developed from the *Vedas*, India's four books of classic wisdom.

The oldest, the 4,500-year-old *Rig Veda*, is a collection of 1,028 Hindu hymns, recited orally starting around 2500 B.C. and written down 1,000 years later. The *Rig Veda* contains astonishingly detailed descriptions of eye surgery, limb amputation, and formulas for medicines using 67 medicinal herbs, including ginger, cinnamon, and senna. The 3,200-year-old *Atharva Veda* also discusses many healing herbs.

Around 700 B.C. (4 centuries before Hippocrates), Charaka, a professor at the University of Taxila, wrote Ayurvedic medicine's first medical encyclopedia. Called the *Charaka Samhita*, it listed 500 herbal formulas. A century later, another famous Ayurvedic, Susruta, wrote the *Susruta Samhita*, which also emphasized herbal healing.

In 250 B.C., India's King Asoka converted to Buddhism and launched a 1,000-year golden age of Ayurvedic medicine. Asoka sent Buddhist monk-physicians around the country to heal the sick and convert them to Buddhism. As the centuries passed, pilgrims came from as far away as China and Persia to receive Ayurvedic treatment.

One herb that Ayurvedic healers introduced was *Rauwolfia serpentina*. It's the source of resperine, which was used in Western medicine until after World War II to manage high blood pressure.

After A.D. 600, Ayurvedic healing influenced Arab medicine, which combined Greco-Roman, Middle Eastern, and Asian therapies. Arab physicians in turn introduced some Ayurvedic practices into Europe.

During the 19th century, the British introduced Western medicine into India, but a majority of Indians and Pakistanis still rely on Ayurvedic medicine or homeopathy, both of which emphasize medicinal herbs instead of drugs.

10,000 Healing Herbs

The land between the Tigris and Euphrates rivers in present-day Iraq was at one time home to the Sumerians, Assyrians, Babylonians, and Persians. The earliest Sumerians had no physicians. Sick people congregated in public squares, and passersby gave them advice.

As Sumerian culture developed, so did its medicine. In late Sumerian mythology, the gods give Sumeria's original healer, Thrita, a golden knife, 10,000 healing herbs, and the medical wisdom to use them. One of the world's oldest surviving prescriptions is a Sumerian clay tablet from around 2100 B.C. that mentions several herbs, including myrrh, cypress, and opium poppy.

By 1000 B.C., the Assyrians had three kinds of healers: herb doctors (internists), knife doctors (surgeons), and word doctors (psychiatrists). Herb doctors were the most numerous and prominent, in part because Assyria was strategically placed along the ancient Spice Route (also known as the Silk Route) from Asia to Egypt. Archeologists have unearthed the remains of an Assyrian pharmacy that stocked 230 herbs, including almond, anise, caraway, coriander, juniper, saffron, sesame, turmeric, and willow.

The Assyrians, and later the Babylonians and Persians, played a major role in the ancient spice trade, one of the world's oldest forms of commerce. Spices had many advantages over other trade goods. Great demand made them high-profit items. When properly dried and stored, spices could travel great distances without spoiling. They didn't have to be fed like cattle and slaves. And they took up little space, which meant they could be transported easily— and hidden from thieves.

No wonder that in the Biblical story, when Joseph's jealous brothers sold him into slavery, he was purchased by "a caravan . . . coming from Gilead [Jordan], their camels bearing gum, balm, and myrrh on their way to carry it down to Egypt" (Genesis 37:25).

Imhotep and the "Stinking Ones" of the Nile

In 1874, in the Valley of the Tombs near Luxor, the German Egyptologist Georg Ebers discovered the world's oldest surviving medical text, a 65-foot papyrus dating from shortly after the time of Joseph, around 1500 B.C. The *Ebers Papyrus* listed 876 herbal formulas from more than 500 plants, including aloe, caraway, cardamom, castor, chamomile, cinnamon, coriander, fennel, fenugreek, garlic, gentian, ginger, juniper, mint, myrrh, onion, opium poppy, saffron, sage, sesame, and thyme. This represents about one-third of the herbs in today's Western herbal pharmacopoeia.

Some Ebers formulas strike the modern reader as bizarre, such as a shampoo made from a dog's paw, decayed palm leaves, and a donkey hoof, all boiled in oil and then rubbed on the head. Others sound surprisingly contemporary, such as the recommendation to bandage moldy bread over wounds to prevent infection. Modern antibiotics were originally derived from molds.

In Egyptian mythology, medicine was created by Thoth, the god of knowledge. Thoth also invented writing and the arts and sciences. The most notable Egyptian physician was Imhotep, who was also the architect to Pharaoh Zoser (3000 B.C.).

Imhotep is credited with designing one of the first pyramids, but as time passed, he was remembered mostly as a healer. Imhotep became deified, and around 700 B.C., Egypt's medical school at Memphis was dedicated to him, as was a nearby school for midwives.

The Egyptians imported enormous quantities of herbs for perfumes, embalming mixtures, and medicines. They also considered plants important spoils of war. In 1475 B.C., when Pharaoh Thutmose III conquered what is now Syria, he demanded as tribute specimens of all Syrian plants not found in Egypt.

The Egyptians loved aromatic herbs. The ancient kingdom's access to both the Mediterranean and Arabian seas allowed them to import aromatics from as far away as Spain to the west and the Spice Islands (Indonesia) to the east.

However, the Egyptians' affection for fragrant herbs paled next to their obsession with two herbs that many ancients considered foulsmelling: garlic and onion. The Egyptians believed that garlic and onion strengthened the body and prevented disease (a view supported by modern science). They ate so much that the Greek historian Herodotus called them "the stinking ones." Six cloves of garlic were found in the tomb of King Tut.

The Egyptians also gave their slaves daily rations of garlic and onions to keep them strong and healthy. In 450 B.C., Herodotus wrote of an inscription inside the Cheops Pyramid at Giza (built in 2900 B.C.) that said "1,600 talents of silver" (about $4 million) had been spent on garlic and onions for its builders.

According to legend, a garlic shortage once forced the Egyptians to cut their slaves' rations. The slaves were so incensed that they refused to work. If this story is true, it would be the world's earliest recorded strike.

Egyptian farmers could not satisfy the demand for garlic and onions, so the Egyptians turned to the Philistines, who lived in nearby Canaan (Israel). The Philistine city of Askelon, in Gaza, became a major garlic and onion trading center, not only for the Egyptians but also for the Greeks and Romans. The Romans favored the Philistines' small green onions, calling them *ascalonia* after Askelon. The word evolved into *escallon*, and finally into our *scallion*.

Middle Eastern herbalists also used opium. Recent excavations of ancient tombs in Israel dating to 1400 B.C. have turned up distinctive pottery vessels shaped like opium poppy pods and containing residues of opium, the narcotic that's still used today, typically as morphine.

By about 500 B.C., Egyptian herbalists were considered the finest in the Mediterranean, and rulers from Rome to Babylon recruited them as court physicians. Aspiring physicians—Rome's Galen among them—went to Egypt to study with the medical masters of the Nile.

From Aesculapius to Hippocrates

The early Greeks viewed illness as a divine curse and prayed to Apollo, god of medicine, for recovery. In Greek mythology, Apollo had a son, Aesculapius, a physician-god like Imhotep, who treated the sick with help from his daughters, Hygeia and Panacea. Hygeia, the source of our word *hygiene*, represented healthy living, while Panacea, whose name means cure-all, treated disease.

When ill, early Greeks visited temples dedicated to Aesculapius, where physician-priests treated them with baths, exercise, massage, fasting, prayer, herbs, and counseling. Treatment culminated in animal sacrifices to entice Aesculapius's spirit into patients' dreams to tell them how to get well. The program was similar to the regimens at many of today's health spas, except for the sacrifices—and the snakes.

Snakes were sacred to Aesculapius, and they slithered freely around his temple grounds. One omen of imminent recovery was to have a snake lick a patient's wounds. Snakes' tongues thus became symbols of healing, and they remained ingredients in medicinal potions well into the Middle Ages.

An echo of the snake-as-healer belief survives today. Aesculapius was often pictured carrying a staff with a snake wrapped around it. The snake-staff combination became the caduceus, the symbol of medicine.

The Aesculapian priesthood was a family affair, with sons following their fathers into the healing temples. On the island of Kos, off the coast of Turkey, one Aesculapian family produced Hippocrates (460–377 B.C.), the father of Western medicine. Hippocrates rebelled against Aesculapius, however, by secularizing Greek medicine. He believed that diseases came not from the gods but from natural causes: the environment, climate, and diet.

Homer wrote in the *Iliad* that Greek medicine came from Egypt. Kos is located only a short voyage from the land of Imhotep. But Hippocrates clearly elaborated on Egyptian practices. From his seat under a plane tree (of the sycamore family), he was the first physician to examine patients closely and the first to use case studies in medical training, a method that medical schools still employ today.

Hippocrates never wrote a word, but his students compiled the 72-volume *Corpus Hippocraticum*. It mentions 350 medicinal plants, including mint, rosemary, thyme, anise, clove, cinnamon, and burdock.

Hippocrates taught that health depended on a balance among the body's four fluids, or "humors": blood, phlegm, yellow bile, and black bile. Hippocrates' Humoral Theory of illness remained a cornerstone of European medicine until the mid-19th century, when Pasteur's Germ Theory supplanted it.

The humors had four qualities: hot, cold, dry, and wet. Hippocrates prescribed warming herbs such as ginger for diseases that he believed were caused by cold, and cooling herbs such as mint for ailments brought on by heat. All of the classic herbals assigned Hippocratic qualities to healing herbs—warming, cooling, and so on, and listed the "foul humors" that they supposedly relieved.

Aesculapian priests and later Greek physicians grew and gathered many herbs. They also bought medicinal plants from herbalists known as root gatherers or rhizomists. (In botany, a rhizome is an underground stem.) The rhizo-mists were peasant herbalists who sold medicinal plants in market towns.

Hippocrates had no women students, but many midwives were also rhizomists. Homer mentions one named Agamede, who was famous for her knowledge of healing herbs.

Shortly before Hippocrates' death, Theophrastus (372–285 B.C.), the father of botany, was born. He wrote *Historia Plantarum* (*An Inquiry into Plants*) and *De Causis Plantarum* (*The Growth of Plants*), which remained standard references for more than 1,000 years. Many of the 550 plants that Theophrastus discussed were used in healing. Theophrastus owned a prominent herb shop in Athens. He was also a friend of Aristotle. When the noted philosopher died, he bequeathed Theophrastus his garden.

Roman Herbalists: Dioscorides, Pliny, and Galen

The first true medical botanist was Pedanius Dioscorides (A.D. 40–90). Born in Turkey, he was Greek, but he served as a physician with the Roman legions of Emperor Nero.

Dioscorides traveled from Germany to the Middle East with the army. In A.D. 78, he published *De Materia Medica* (*On Medicines*), Europe's first real herbal. It discussed 600 plants, including aloe, anise, chamomile, cinnamon, dill, marjoram, poppy, rhubarb, and thyme.

As an army physician, Dioscorides concentrated on soldiers' medicine, particularly treatment of wounds. But *De Materia Medica* also included a great deal of herbal folk wisdom, so it's clear that he sought out herbalists during his travels.

De Materia Medica remained a standard medical reference for 1,500 years. Virtually every herbal published through the 17th century referred to it. After the invention of printing in the 1450s, *De Materia Medica* was one of the first books published. The oldest copy in the United States, from 1547, is in the Lloyd Library collection in Cincinnati (more on the Lloyd brothers later).

It's fitting that Rome's legions produced a great herbalist, because part of their mission was to protect the Roman spice trade with Asia from barbarian incursions and provincial revolts. By the 1st century A.D., the herb and spice trade was a cornerstone of Roman commerce. Roman demand for medicinal, culinary, and perfume herbs was almost insatiable.

Shortly before the publication of *De Materia Medica*, Greek merchants discovered the secret of the Indian Ocean's shifting monsoon winds, which blew toward India part of the year and toward Egypt the rest. Capitalizing on this new insight, spice merchants were able to reduce by half—from 2 years to 1—the round trip from Rome to the region in India where black pepper grew. As a result, the price of black pepper and many other herbs came down to the modern equivalent of about $100 per ounce.

While Dioscorides traveled the Empire, back in Rome, Caius Plinius Secundus, or Pliny the Elder (A.D. 23–79), was busy compiling ancient scientific knowledge into his 37-volume *Historia Naturalis* (*Natural History*). Volumes 12 through 19 dealt with botany, and 20 through 27 specifically addressed herbal medicine.

Pliny made some wild assertions. For colds, he advised "kissing the hairy muzzle of a mouse." But many of his herbal recommenda-

tions were more plausible and guided physicians for centuries.

In August of A.D. 79, Pliny traveled to Pompeii upon learning that Mount Vesuvius was rumbling. When the volcano exploded on August 24, Pliny was perched on a nearby hill, taking notes. He died of asphyxiation.

Fifty years after Pliny, Claudius Galenus, better known as Galen (A.D. 131–200), became Rome's leading physician. Born into a wealthy family in Pergamum (now Bergama), Turkey, Galen studied medicine in Greece and Alexandria, then worked for several years as a physician to Pergamum's gladiators. At age 30, he moved to Rome, and eventually he became the physician to Emperor Marcus Aurelius.

Galen was notoriously arrogant, boastful, and dogmatic. He rebelled against the Hippocratic idea of examining patients and practiced a highly theoretical form of medicine that dominated physician training in Europe for more than 1,000 years.

At a time when midwife-herbalists used single herbs or formulas with only a few ingredients, Galen insisted on "polypharmacy"—complex concoctions of herbs, animal parts, and minerals called galenicals. Galen's wealthy patients liked galenicals because they were expensive and therefore exclusive. As the centuries passed, Europe's nobility came to favor costly galenicals, while the peasantry stuck with single herbs or simple formulas, which became known as simples.

Roman rhizomists—*herbarii*, in Latin—congregated around Capitoline Hill. They were a motley crew. Physicians accused them of mislabeling and adulterating their herbs. Pliny and Galen boycotted them and urged physicians to grow and gather their own medicinal plants. The *herbarii* grew so troublesome that several emperors attempted to control them with a licensing system, but it failed.

Roman Assassins: From Mithridates to *Theriaca*

Roman herbalists were as likely to be killers as healers. The Imperial court seethed with murderous intrigue. Among the available assassination methods—knifing, "accidents," and poisoning—the herbal approach was most popular.

Political notables were typically surrounded by bodyguards, making knifings and accidents difficult to arrange. Physical assault also involved considerable risk of capture. By comparison, poisoning could be carried out from a safe distance. Death occurred some time after the deed, allowing for escape or alibi. And in an age before autopsy, when apparently healthy people often sickened and died suddenly, wily poisoners might remain above suspicion.

As a result, rulers throughout the Roman empire became obsessed with the identification of herbal poisons and the development of antidotes, known in Latin as *theriaca* (in English, "theriacs"). The word comes from the Greek *theriakon*, meaning remedies for venomous bites.

The ancient world's most poison-paranoid ruler was Mithridates Eupator (120–66 B.C.), king of Pontus, on the Black Sea. Mithridates governed by terror and was convinced (probably rightly) that he was destined to be poisoned. As a result, he delved into botany, believing that familiarity with both poisonous and medicinal plants was his best defense. His botanical expertise is commemorated in the genus name of boneset (page 109), *Eupatorium*.

In addition to formulating dozens of theriacs, Mithridates supposedly ordered his court physician, Krateus, to concoct the ultimate herbal poison. The ancient king took increasing doses to develop a tolerance and make himself immune.

Then, in 66 B.C., the Romans attacked. Facing capture and execution, Mithridates tried to poison himself. But according to legend, he'd become so tolerant that no poison could kill him. Finally, he ordered a slave to stab him to death. To this day, the word *mithridatism* means an acquired tolerance to poisons.

Mithridates made a big impression in Rome, where the nobility offered to pay enormous sums for any antidotes attributed to the king of Pontus. Needless to say, Rome's unscrupulous *herbarii* were only too happy to peddle bogus mixtures as "Mithridates' Theriac."

A century after the unpoisonable king's death, Emperor Nero became nearly insane with fear of poisoning, in part because he'd gained the throne by poisoning his stepbrother. Nero ordered his physician, Andromachus of Crete, to improve on Mithridates' Theriac. Andromachus mixed 78 herbal, animal, and mineral ingredients—including opium, a lizard, and snake flesh (in homage to Aesculapius)—to create Andromachus's Theriac. The antidote became popular with the wealthy throughout Rome.

Slave midwife-herbalists were highly valued as poisoners. They could often be placed as concubines in the bedrooms of their intended victims, beyond the reach of bodyguards and tasters, who sampled rulers' food and drink before they ate, just in case. The slave herbalist Locusta became famous for her skill as a poisoner. After one important murder, she received her freedom and a gift of land.

Not to be outdone by Andromachus, Galen

wrote a book containing more than 100 theriac recipes. He also developed his own, Galene, a polypharmaceutical brew of 70 ingredients, including dozens of herbs, honey, wine, minerals, and animal parts. It took 40 days to prepare.

When Rome fell, the barbarians seized not only Rome's lands and wealth but also its vast stores of herbs and spices. During one attack, the barbarians demanded horses, money—and 3,000 pounds of black pepper.

Theriaca eventually evolved into the Elizabethan English word *treacle*. The Elizabethan peasantry used garlic as an all-purpose medicine and antidote, and it became known as the poor man's treacle.

Avicenna and the Invention of Pharmacy

As Rome collapsed, Arab civilization filled the intellectual vacuum. From A.D. 600 to 800, Islamic armies forged an empire stretching from Spain across Northern Africa to India. Unlike the barbarians who seized Roman Europe, the Arabs venerated Greco-Roman culture and learning. Along with the spoils of conquest, they sent tens of thousands of Greco-Roman books to Baghdad, where they were translated into Arabic and studied.

Ibn-Sina, or Avicenna (A.D. 980–1037), was the leading Arab physician. While still quite young, he cured an Arab prince of a serious illness. Afterward, his services were in great demand. A follower of Galen, he wrote the *Canon of Medicine*, the West's medical bible for 600 years. Book Two discussed healing herbs, including nutmeg, senna, sandalwood, rhubarb, myrrh, cinnamon, clove, and rosewater.

The Arabs revered Galen but were not ruled by polypharmacy. They simplified Galen's formulas and developed pharmacy as a field distinct from medicine. The first pharmacies appeared in Baghdad in the 9th century.

Arab pharmacists replaced galenicals with syrups, ointments, and tinctures (alcohol extracts). They were the first to distill pure alcohol, whose name is derived from the Arabic *al-kohl*, or "quintessence." Arab medicine also gave us the terms *alkalai*, from *al-qali*, or "ashes," and *sugar*, from *sukkar*, meaning "grain or pebble."

From A.D. 800 until it was recaptured by the Christians in the 1400s, Spain rivaled Baghdad as a center of Arab herbalism. One influential herbalist was Abul-Kasim Khalef ibn Abbas, in Spanish, Abulcasis (A.D. 936–1013). He lived in Cordoba and wrote *Liber Servitoris* (*The Book of Simples*), an important source for later European herbals.

The other prominent herbalist was Ibn al-Baitar (A.D. 1197–1248), a botanist from Malaga who collected 1,500 plants from Spain to Syria. He also wrote the most complete Arab herbal, the *Corpus of Simples*. It introduced 200 new healing herbs (and poisons), including tamarind, aconite, and nux vomica (strychnine).

Monasteries and Liqueurs

After the fall of Rome, European medicine was dominated by the Catholic Church, which adopted the pre-Hippocratic Greek belief that illness was a punishment from God and was treatable only by prayer and penance. But Catholic monks preserved Greco-Roman herbalism by copying the ancient texts.

Among the monastic orders, the Benedictines were the most avid herbalists. They were the first Europeans to adopt the Arab practice of making tinctures. They flavored wine with digestion-promoting herbs and created the fore-runners of today's liqueurs. One is still called Benedictine.

Charlemagne (A.D. 742–814) was so impressed by the Benedictines' herb gardens that he ordered all of the monasteries in his vast realm to plant "physic gardens" to ensure an adequate supply of healing herbs. Charlemagne described herbs as "friends of the physician and cook."

Around A.D. 820, the Benedictines designed their ideal monastery, known as the Plan of St. Gall. In one corner was a medical area that included an infirmary, bath, doctor's room, and bloodletting room. It also featured a 1,000-square-foot physic garden that contained two dozen herbs, among them cumin, fennel, fenu-greek, mint, pennyroyal, rose, rosemary, rue, sage, savory, and watercress.

In another corner was a kitchen garden that also contained many herbs. Among them was dill, which was commonly mixed with salt water to preserve vegetables, particularly cucumbers. We enjoy them today as dill pickles.

The most notable Benedictine herbalist was Hildegard of Bingen (1098–1179), abbess of the Rupertsburg convent in the German Rhineland. Hildegard was a Renaissance woman centuries before the Renaissance; she was a nun, adminis-trator, composer, writer, and herbalist. She wrote religious music that is still performed today.

Hildegard claimed that visions of God com-manded her to treat the sick and compile herbal formulas. Her book, *Hildegard's Medicine*, com-bined mystical Catholicism and early German folk medicine, along with the author's own exten-sive herbal experience. Hildegard's favorite herbs included aloe, apple, basil, bay, blackberry, caraway, celery, clove, dill, fennel, garlic, hyssop, licorice, marjoram, myrrh, nettle, nutmeg, onion, oregano, parsley, raspberry, rosemary, rue, thyme, and watercress.

Hildegard's herbal is unique. She wrote an original medical work based on her own experi-ence at a time when the few literate Euro-peans—mostly monks—were content to copy the Greeks, Romans, and Avicenna. What's more, she was the only medieval woman who left any account of "wise women" healing practices.

Some of Hildegard's advice sounds silly. For poor vision, she advocated rubbing the eyes with a topaz soaked in wine. However, many of her recommendations were quite sen-sible. She advocated eating a balanced diet and brushing the teeth with aloe and myrrh, which have antibacterial, decay-preventive properties.

While Hildegard relied on simples, galenicals continued to be valued, largely by the nobility, who had access to galenically inclined physi-cians and the wealth to afford all the ingredi-ents that Galen's polypharmaceuticals required. The men who mixed medieval galenicals were the first alchemists.

Around the time that the Benedictines invented liqueur, Germanic Angles and Saxons were settling England. They brought European herbalism with them, and they learned how the native Celts and their priests, the Druids, used healing herbs.

Around A.D. 950, a nobleman named Bald persuaded England's King Alfred to commission the first British herbal. The book combined Anglo-Saxon and Celtic herbalism with Greco-Roman and Arab practices sent by the Patriarch of Jerusalem. It was called the *Leech Book of Bald*. (*Leech* comes from *laece*, the Anglo-Saxon term for doctor.) It discussed 500 plants, including vervain and mistletoe, both sacred to the Druids. A surviving copy is on display at the British Museum in London.

With the Renaissance, European medicine took a secular turn. After the invention of printing, monks stopped copying the ancient herbals, but they continued to tend their gardens. In 1868, an Austrian monk, Gregor Mendel, published *Plant Hybridization*, an account of his experiments with peas. It launched the modern science of genetics.

Wise Women: From Healers to Witches

Hildegard of Bingen was lucky to have lived in the 12th century. Had she practiced herbalism from 1300 to 1650, she probably would have been burned as a witch.

It's not clear what led to Europe's 350 years of witch hunts. Feminists link the practice to the rise of secular medicine as a male-dominated profession. Others blame the hysteria on bubonic plague (the Black Death), which swept Europe in waves and killed half of its population.

A more recent theory holds that European rulers and the Catholic Church became alarmed by a decline in population, which they blamed on the contraceptive herbalism of the wise women. The leading medieval contraceptive herbs were all abortifacients, or "morning-after" plants, in modern parlance. The most popular were pennyroyal, artemesia, and rue. Modern research shows that all three stimulate uterine contractions and abortion.

Whatever the cause of the witch hunts, after 1300 the image of the folk herbalist changed from helpful wise woman to evil witch. Witch hunts started in Germany and eventually reached all of Europe. Accusations of "sexual intercourse with the Devil" were typically accompanied by testimony that the alleged witch practiced herbal medicine and made healing mixtures, cosmetics, love potions, aphrodisiacs, abortifacients, and poisons.

Accusations of poisoning were particularly damning. It's quite possible that some women herbalists continued the Roman tradition of herbal assassination, but this was before the discovery of the dose-response relationship: the idea that the greater the dose, the greater the effect. Many so-called witches' plants, poisonous in large amounts, caused no harm in therapeutic or cosmetic amounts. Nonetheless, the witch hunters considered them poisons.

One plant associated with witchcraft was called devil's herb. Large amounts are lethal when taken internally. When placed in the eyes, the juice causes the pupils to dilate, and medieval women used devil's herb cosmetically. Eventually, the plant was renamed belladonna, or "beautiful woman."

Then there was witch's bells. Large amounts are poisonous, but small amounts stimulate the heart. After the witch-hunt era, the plant's name was changed to foxglove, source of the heart drug digitalis.

Conviction of witchcraft meant death. At the height of the witch hunts, as many as 600 women a year—about two a day—were executed in parts of Germany. At Toulouse, France, 400 were put to death in a single day.

North America did not escape the hysteria. The Salem witch trials in Massachusetts (1692) resulted in 20 women being executed.

Records suggest that they, too, were wise women herbalists.

After the witch hunts, the saintly Hildegard was forgotten, replaced by the witches of Shakespeare's *Macbeth*, who threw mandrake, belladonna, and other evil herbs into their bubbling cauldron. Witches were also vilified in the stories that have become today's fairy tales. In "Snow White," for example, the evil queen-witch concocts an herbal poison, coats an apple with it, and slips it to Snow White, who falls into a coma, thus following a tradition of herbal poisoning dating back to the Romans.

The witch hunts failed to eradicate women's herbalism, but they succeeded in driving it underground. More than a century after the last witch hunts, the "old woman" who helped popularize foxglove said that it was a "secret family recipe." (More on this later.) Her forebears had good reason to keep their use of witch's bells a secret.

A World Hungry for Spices

The fall of Rome devastated the spice trade. Arab merchants continued to import Asian herbs into Europe, but the commerce declined and prices soared. During the Middle Ages, a pound of ginger could buy a fat sheep. Black pepper was counted out corn by corn and used to pay rents, taxes, and dowries. One pound of pepper could buy a serf his freedom.

Then came the Crusades. From 1095 until 1291, European armies attempted to wrest the Holy Land from Islamic control. Their efforts failed militarily, but while in the Middle East, the Crusaders tasted Asian spices and returned home craving more.

The 1296 publication of Marco Polo's travelogue heightened European fascination with the Orient and its herbs. Polo's father and uncle were merchants who set out from Venice to China in 1271, taking the 17-year-old Marco with them. The young Italian became a favorite of Kublai Kahn, and when he returned in 1295, his famous memoir was filled with mouthwatering accounts of Asia's wonderful spices.

The ancient Spice Routes slowly reopened. Around 1300, British spice dealers obtained a royal charter to become the Guild of Pepperers. They bought black pepper and other herbs from brokers in Venice, who traded with Arab importers. By 1400, Venice alone imported 2,500 tons of ginger and black pepper a year. European demand seemed limitless.

Then something terrible happened. During the 1400s, the Mongols, who supported trade with Europe, lost Western Asia to the Ottoman Turks, who closed the trade routes. In Venice and Genoa, cities enriched by the spice trade, Italian merchants grew desperate for new avenues to the East. If the world was round, as some claimed, it might be possible to sail west across the Atlantic and reach the Indies.

It was no coincidence that Christopher Columbus hailed from Genoa. He never reached the East Indies, but he returned from the New World with allspice and red pepper, which the Caribbean Indians called *kian*, or "cayenne."

In 1498, when the Portuguese explorer Vasco da Gama succeeded in sailing around Africa to India, his first words in Calcutta were, "We come in search of Christians and spices."

The Portuguese and Dutch took an early lead in world exploration. They monopolized the sea route around Africa to India and the Spice Islands (Indonesia), as well as the trade in cinnamon, cloves, tea, and black pepper.

The Spanish concentrated on the New World and its gold. Sometimes they found the precious metal, sometimes other valuables. In 1519, Hernando Cortez watched as Mexico's Aztec ruler, Montezuma, toasted his arrival by sipping from a golden goblet. Cortez coveted the goblet—but the herbal beverage that it contained, *chocolatl* or "chocolate," eventually became more important than the Aztec's gold.

In addition to chocolate, Spanish conquistadors returned home with corn, tobacco, potatoes, carrots, strawberries, lima beans, tomatoes, sarsaparilla, passionflower, and the most important new healing herb of all, cinchona (Jesuit or Peruvian bark). Cinchona was the first effective treatment for malaria (also known as ague, intermittent fever, and swamp fever), which had plagued the Mediterranean area and Europe since ancient times. Centuries later, cinchona became the source of the antimalarial drug quinine.

The Spanish may also have returned from the New World with something else: syphilis. A doctor in Seville claimed that he had treated Columbus's crew in 1493. It's possible that they became infected in Haiti. Or perhaps increased trade spread a disease that had existed for ages in isolated pockets around the Mediterranean.

In any event, an epidemic of unusually virulent syphilis swept through Europe in 1494, killing thousands. Europeans considered the disease an import from the New World and looked across the Atlantic for a cure. They focused on sarsaparilla, which was widely used until well into the 19th century. The herb turned out to be ineffective against the disease.

Another syphilis treatment was mercury. It played a key role in the schism that developed in the early 19th century between pro-mercury "regular" physicians and anti-mercury herbal "Eclectics."

Spain kept chocolate, cinchona, and other New World plants secret for years. Eventually, they were revealed in a book by Spanish physician-botanist Nicolas Monardes. The book became a huge bestseller. It was published in English in 1577, with the title *Joyful Newes out of the Newe Founde Worlde*.

Twenty years after *Joyful Newes*, the British still played a minor role in world exploration. That changed in 1599, when the Dutch suddenly tripled the price of black pepper. The British were outraged. Eighty London merchants pooled their capital and established the British East India Company, which began importing pepper and other herbs directly from India.

The British eventually took control of the subcontinent and Ceylon (Sri Lanka). The East India Company also imported Chinese tea, which quickly became as British as the Union Jack.

The East India Company's tea was very popular in England's North American colonies. In 1773, when Parliament tried to tax it, New England tea lovers dumped several tons into Boston Harbor in protest. The Boston Tea Party helped ignite the American Revolution.

Paracelsus and the Doctrine of Signatures

Around 1500, Italian mathematician Giambattista della Porta of Naples conceived the first new medical philosophy since Galen. Called the Doctrine of Signatures, it claimed that a plant's physical appearance revealed its healing value. As British herbalist William Coles explained in his *Art of Simpling* (1656), God had not only "stamped upon plants . . . a distinct forme but also given them particular signatures whereby a Man may read the use of them."

According to Coles, "Wall-nuts [walnuts] have the perfect signature of the Head. The outer husk represents the Pericranium or outward skin of the skull, whereon the hair groweth, and therefore those husks are exceedingly good for wounds in the head. The inner woody shell hath the Signature of the Skull . . . and the Kernel hath the very figure of the Brain. If the Kernel be bruised, moistened with wine, and laid upon the Head, it comforts the head and brain mightily." Some herbals still suggest walnuts for headache.

The most vocal champion of the Doctrine of Signatures was Phillippus Aureolus Theophrastus Bombastus von Hohenheim (1493–1541), the son of a Swiss alchemist/physician. A brilliant, arrogant student of medicine, he lived up to his name, Bombastus. But he changed it to Paracelsus ("greater than Celsus"), convinced that he was more brilliant than the Roman physician Celsus (53 B.C.–A.D. 7), then considered on a par with Galen.

Paracelsus taught at the University of Basel in Switzerland in the 1520s. At a time when medical students studied only Hippocrates, Galen, Celsus, and Avicenna, Paracelsus publicly burned their books to symbolize his rejection of Galenic dogma. He also replaced the ancient Humoral Theory of illness with the Doctrine of Signatures.

Strange as it sounds today, the doctrine was based on experience with healing herbs, though it overgeneralized that experience badly. For instance, the stems of dandelion are hollow, allowing air to pass through them. Based on this characteristic, the doctrine declared dandelion a respiratory remedy.

The Doctrine of Signatures quickly became the new medical dogma. Bile has a yellowish tinge, and jaundice, a liver problem, turns the skin yellow. Under the doctrine, any yellow flower or root was considered a liver medicine. Similarly, any plant with long, snaking roots was used to treat snakebite. Plants with heart-shaped leaves were considered heart remedies. Juicy plants were used as diuretics and lactation promoters.

In addition to promoting the insurgent medical philosophy, Paracelsus further offended the professional medical community by writing in the vernacular instead of in Latin, thus opening medicine to those unschooled in the language of the universities. He correctly predicted the discovery of "active principles" in plants and pioneered the chemical extraction of plant oils.

Paracelsus also discovered the dose-response relationship. "It depends only on the dose," he wrote, "whether a poison is a poison or not." This insight came too late to save thousands of alleged witches executed in part for possession of alleged poisons, but it allowed Paracelsus to introduce many potentially toxic minerals into medicine in very small doses. He used arsenic, sulfur, lead, antimony, and particularly mercury, not just for syphilis but also for many other diseases. In time, physicians came to view mercury as a panacea.

The Age of the Herbals

With the invention of printing in the 1450s, herbals proliferated, and England's university-trained physicians began to fear the loss of their medical monopoly. Emboldened by the witch hunts, they lobbied their influential patients in the British Court to restrict the practice of medicine to them, outlawing it to "rogues, horse-gelders, rat catchers, idiots, and witches."

In a 1511 decree, Henry VIII reserved the practice of medicine for university-trained physicians and barber-surgeons who had completed apprenticeships. Anyone else had to pass a test administered in Latin by the Bishop of London and a committee of prominent doctors.

Of course, folk herbalists could not read Latin. Most didn't read English. Some stopped practicing. Many became "green men and women," latter-day rhizomists who supplied herbs to the physicians and the early pharmacists, or apothecaries, often while continuing to practice herbal healing stealthily and illegally.

In time, England's herbalists rebelled against the suppression of folk medicine by publishing two anonymous herbals. *Bancke's Herball* (1525), a compilation of English herb lore, was the first herbal printed in English. The *Grete Herball* (1526) was a translation of amalgamated French and German books.

Henry VIII's edict eventually led to a major shortage of doctors. In 1543, he rescinded it with the Herbalists' Charter: "From henceforth, it shall be lawful for every . . . King's subject, having knowledge and experience of . . . Herbs and Roots . . . to practice, use, and minister to any Sore, Wound, Swelling, or Disease any Herbs, Ointments, Baths, Pulsters (poultices) and Emplaisters (plasters), according to their Cunning, Experience, and Knowledge . . . without Suit, Vexation, Trouble, Penalty, or Loss of their Goods."

The Herbalists' Charter came just 1 year after German botanist Leonhard Fuchs (1501–1566) published *De Historia Stirpium* (*On Plants*), the first original book of medical botany since Dioscorides' treatise almost 1,500 years earlier. Illustrated with detailed woodcuts, it discussed 500 healing herbs, including 100 from the New World.

In 1546, the University of Padua in Italy planted the first academic botanical garden, which helped launch the modern science of botany. In time, most major universities and many physicians and apothecaries planted their own physic gardens.

William Turner, the father of British botany, published his *New Herball* in 1551. Turner supported both Paracelsus's Doctrine of Signatures, still an insurgent philosophy at the time, and his dose-response concept. He advised against taking large amounts of healing herbs.

In 1554, the Belgian physician-botanist Rembert Dodoens (1517–1585) published a Dutch herbal, which was revised and re-released in Latin in 1583. A London publisher commissioned Dr. Robert Priest to translate the herbal into English, but Dr. Priest died before completing the project, and his translation disappeared.

Enter John Gerard (1545–1612), who had apprenticed as a barber-surgeon but loved horticulture. He established a noted physic garden in Fetter Lane, London, that contained more than 1,000 species, including England's first potatoes. In 1586, Gerard was appointed curator of the College of Physicians' Physic Garden, and soon after, he became herbalist to King James I.

In 1597, Gerard published his *Herball or Generall Historie of Plantes*, in which he displayed the College of Physicians' characteristic contempt for "overbold apothecaries, and foolish women." However, Gerard apparently had nothing against plagiarism. He obliquely acknowledged Dr. Priest, leading to accusations that he'd obtained Priest's lost translation of Dodoens's herbal and published it as his own.

Although Gerard denied any wrongdoing, and his herbal contained a good deal of original information on herb gardening, most authorities believe that he stole Priest's work.

John Parkinson (1567–1650) was another pioneering British herbalist. In 1640, he published *Theatrum Botanicum* (*The Theater of Plants*), subtitled *The Universall and Complete Herball*. It was no understatement. The 1,800-page book discussed 3,800 plants, which Parkinson organized into 17 "Classes or Tribes," including "Venomous, Sleepy, and Hurtfull Plants, and Their Counter Poysons"; "Hot and Sharpe Biting Plantes"; and "Strange and Outlandish Plants."

Parkinson's classification system appears quaint today, but during the 17th century, it was taken quite seriously. Many scientists proposed similar systems, but none stuck until 1737. That's when Swedish naturalist Carl Linne, also known as Carolus Linnaeus (1707–1778), developed his Latin binomial genus-and-species system based on reproductive characteristics. After Darwin, scientists added evolutionary criteria, but to this day, plants and animals are still named using Linnaeus's binomial formula.

As university medicine slowly became more scientific, leading physicians stopped growing their own herbs. They turned instead to the increasing number of apothecaries, who used mortars and pestles to powder healing herbs. The mortar and pestle remain symbols of pharmacy today.

In 1673, London's apothecaries established Britain's finest medicinal herb garden, the 3.8-acre Chelsea Physic Garden. Today, it contains 5,000 species of herbs from around the world. Located 2 miles west of Picadilly Circus, it is open to the public.

Nicholas Culpeper: England's Herbal Robin Hood

Nicholas Culpeper was by far England's most influential herbalist. His *Complete Herbal and English Physician*, first published in 1652, has been in print ever since. It has appeared in more than 100 editions, a record surpassed by only the Bible and Shakespeare. A century after Culpeper's death, literary lion Dr. Samuel Johnson wrote, "Culpeper . . . undoubtedly merits the gratitude of posterity."

Culpeper was—and still is—loathed as well as loved. His herbalist contemporary, William Coles, denounced him as "a man very ignorant in simples." More than 250 years later, in *The Old English Herbals* (1922), Elinour Rohde wrote, "The infamous Nicholas Culpeper was a false prophet of herbalism . . . [author of] an absurd book." And today, scientists scoff at Culpeper's devotion to astrology and most of his prescriptions.

Egotistical and brash, Culpeper came of age during the English Civil War (1642–1648), which pitted King Charles I and the monarchist aristocracy against Oliver Cromwell and the Puritan Parliament. The Puritans won, abolished the monarchy, and executed Charles.

Culpeper came from an aristocratic family, but he was a Puritan and fought for Cromwell. He took a musket ball in the chest, which left him in poor health for the rest of his life and influenced his decision to study medicine.

As an aristocrat, Culpeper attended Cambridge, where he fell in love and planned to elope. But his fiancée was killed when lightning struck her carriage on her way to their secret rendezvous. Beside himself with grief, Culpeper left Cambridge and became an apothecary's apprentice, a major social step downward for anyone who had attended the university.

Culpeper was an anomaly. Trained at Cambridge, he could read Greek and Latin as well as the physicians. He resented the snobbery of former classmates who became doctors and looked down on apothecaries. Furthermore, as a Puritan, he was outraged that the monarchist College of Physicians ignored the medical needs of the largely Puritan lower classes. Culpeper's solution was to become England's medical Robin Hood.

In 1649, Culpeper translated the College of Physicians' Latin manual, the *Pharmacopoiea Londinensis*, into English, calling it *The London Dispensatory and Physical Directory*. It gave apothecaries and others illiterate in Latin their first look at the 1,600 simples and 1,100 other formulas that constituted the state of the art in 17th-century British medicine.

Culpeper's audacity earned him the physicians' undying hatred. Apothecaries, midwives, and the common people, however, lionized him for giving them access to professional medical information.

Culpeper's apothecary shop in Spitalfields, near London, became wildly popular. He often treated the poor for free. The College of Physicians attacked him relentlessly, and in response, he became increasingly combative.

Culpeper wrote a series of essays, "The Epistles," in which he accused the physicians of greed for their high fees and stupidity for their outdated devotion to Galen and Avicenna: "[We have] a company of proud, domineering doctors whose wits were born 500 years before themselves. . . . College, College, thou art Diseased, and I will tell thee the Cause. The Cause is Mammon [greed]. The Cure: Fear God. Love the Saints. Be Studious. Hate Covetousness. Regard the Poor."

To make herbal medicine even more accessible, Culpeper published his own herbal in 1652. It was revolutionary because it gave equal weight to the official herbalism of the ancient masters and the homegrown folk wisdom of England's country people.

Today, critics dismiss Culpeper because of his devotion to astrology. In his herbal, Mars owned garlic, lavender was under Mercury, and the sun claimed rosemary under the celestial Ram. But astrology was considered a legitimate science in Culpeper's day. All the universities taught it, and the College of Physicians routinely factored it into diagnosis and treatment decisions. In fact, one reason that the college hated Culpeper was that he accused them of making astrological errors.

Culpeper's real problem was that he rarely met an herb he didn't consider a panacea. He touted dozens of herbs "to heal all inward and outward hurts." He called about a third of the herbs in his herbal sure cures for "the bites and stings of venomous creatures." He also promoted scores of herbs to "bring down women's courses" (promote menstruation), many more than midwives of that era considered abortifacient.

Perhaps Culpeper can be forgiven his exaggerations. In the 1650s, very little was known about the body, and statements that seem to be gross misrepresentations today may not have been all that far-fetched back then.

Physicians call most medical problems "self-limiting"—that is, if you wait long enough, they go away by themselves. Take almost any herb for "inward or outward hurts," and most clear up, with or without all the herbs Culpeper recommended. The same goes for attacks by "venomous creatures." Few bites and stings are fatal. Most eventually resolve on their own.

Unfortunately, Culpeper's promotion of every herb for every ill has haunted herbalism ever since. Well into the 1970s, some herbals touted Culpeper-style hyperbole as truth, providing easy—and legitimate—targets for attacks by herb skeptics. Nicholas Culpeper was a seminal figure in botanical medicine, but his herbal should be viewed as history and nothing more.

Dr. Withering's Wise Woman

In 1767, 26-year-old William Withering had barely begun practicing medicine in Stafford, England, when he was called to treat 17-year-old Helena Cookes. She was bedridden with a lingering illness that kept her from her favorite pastime, painting watercolors of wildflowers.

Like every other medical student, Withering had studied botany. He hated it. Still, he was quite taken with the young Miss Cookes. He gathered wildflowers for his patient to paint while in bed, and 5 years later, married her. Along the way, he developed a passion for medical botany.

"In the year 1775," he later wrote, "my opinion was asked concerning a recipe for the cure of dropsy [congestive heart failure]. I was told it had been a family secret of an old woman in Shropshire, who sometimes made cures after regular practitioners had failed." The old woman's recipe contained 20 herbs, but Withering

quickly decided that the heart stimulator was foxglove. Withering began using foxglove himself and gained a reputation for treating the heart problem.

In 1776, Dr. Erasmus Darwin (Charles's grandfather) asked Withering to treat a woman with dropsy. Withering gave her foxglove, and she improved. Darwin submitted a report to a British medical journal claiming that he himself had cured the woman using foxglove. He did not mention Withering.

Furious, Withering published his *Account of the Foxglove and Its Medical Uses*, which summarized his results in 163 cases. The drug derived from foxglove, digitalis, was considered a state-of-the-art treatment for congestive heart failure well into the 20th century.

Sickly Colonists, Robust Indians

Europeans considered Indians "ignorant savages"—except when it came to health and healing. Explorers and colonists were all too familiar with the plagues, pestilence, and suffering back in Europe. They marveled at the Indians' good health, physical stamina, and fine, unrotted teeth. Not surprisingly, many became eager students of Indian herbal medicine.

Each tribe had its own medical mythology, but this Cherokee tale is typical. Long ago, humanity grew too numerous. Hunters killed so much game that the animals feared for their survival. The bears, deer, birds, and other creatures decided to unleash diseases to reduce hunting. But the plants decided that the animals had acted unfairly. The trees, shrubs, grasses, and flowers showed humanity how they could cure the diseases that the animals had unleashed.

One of the first Europeans to appreciate Indian medicine was Jacques Cartier, the French explorer who discovered Canada's St. Lawrence River. In 1536, he sailed to the site of present-day Quebec, where he and his crew dug in for the winter. Within a few months, 25 of his 100 men had died of "sailors' disease" (scurvy), and most of the rest were gravely ill.

Scurvy was a terrible scourge during the Age of Exploration. On his famous voyage around Africa, Vasco da Gama lost 100 of his 160 crew members to it. During the 16th and 17th centuries, ships were sometimes sighted adrift on the high seas, their entire crews dead from scurvy.

Fortunately for Cartier, an Indian gave the sickly explorers a tea brewed from yellow cedar bark and leaves. Everyone recovered. Later, the tea was shown to contain vitamin C, which prevents and cures scurvy.

In Boston, Puritan minister-physician Cotton Mather (1663–1728) wrote that Indian healers produced "many cures that are truly stupendous." And when John Wesley (1703–1791), founder of Methodism, visited America in the 1730s, he wrote that the Indians had "exceedingly few" diseases and that their medicines were "quick and generally infallible."

Later, even ardent Indian haters in the U.S. Army marveled at the effectiveness of Indian wound treatments. Also, many early American physicians touted their apprenticeships to Indian herbalists.

Of course, Indian healers also had their critics, mostly among university-trained physicians. Philadelphia doctor Benjamin Rush (1745–1813), a signer of the Declaration of Independence, declared, "We have no discoveries in the materia medica . . . from the Indians. It would be a reproach to our schools of physic if modern physicians were not more successful than Indians."

How wrong Dr. Rush was. The Indians introduced white settlers to many valuable healing herbs, such as black cohosh, black haw, boneset, cascara sagrada, chaparral, echinacea, goldenseal, lobelia, Oregon grape, sarsaparilla, slippery elm, and witch hazel.

Healing Herbs in Early America

In their "kitchen gardens," American colonists grew both culinary and medicinal herbs, including balm, basil, caraway, chamomile, comfrey, dill, fennel, garlic, hyssop, lavender, licorice, marjoram, mints, mustard, parsley, rosemary, rue, saffron, sage, savory, shallots, tarragon, and thyme.

Thomas Jefferson was a typical herb grower. His 1,000-square-foot garden at Monticello contained 26 herbs. As president, while negotiating the Louisiana Purchase from the French, he went to great lengths to obtain some French tarragon for his garden.

Nurse/midwives also grew or purchased many medicinal herbs. One was Martha Ballard, who lived in Maine and kept a diary (1785–1812) that chronicled her life, including her practice of midwifery and herbal medicine. She used 52 herbs grown in the area around her home on the Kennebec River, northeast of Portland, including anise, balm, buckthorn, burdock, catnip, chamomile, comfrey, feverfew, hop, hyssop, mullein, mustard, onion, pennyroyal, rhubarb, rue, sage, shepherd's purse, and yarrow. She also purchased 24 herbs imported from elsewhere, among them aloe, licorice, myrrh, pepper, and senna.

Herbs were prized imports into early America. In addition to Chinese tea, black pepper was very popular. New England shipping magnate Elias Hasskett Derby, one of early America's first homegrown millionaires, made much of his money importing black pepper from Sumatra.

Herbs were also a major colonial export. Furs, tobacco, and cotton generated the most money, but pound for pound, nothing beat ginseng, the herb prized in Asia as the ultimate tonic.

French Jesuits began shipping Canadian ginseng to China in the early 1700s, where it brought the then-astounding price of $5 a pound. By the 1740s, news of the unassuming plant's value in the Orient spread south to the 13 colonies. Shipping agents bought it for $1 a pound, more than the wholesale value of the rarest furs. Foragers scoured the countryside, and frontier scouts, surveyors, and trappers collected ginseng as a sideline to their other work.

By the 1770s, rapacious collection had wiped out ginseng east of the Appalachians, forcing collectors into the western wilderness. The search for ginseng played a key role in the exploration of western Pennsylvania, West Virginia, Kentucky, and Tennessee. One noted ginseng collector was Daniel Boone, who, according to one account, lost 12 tons of wild ginseng when his boat capsized in the Ohio River.

The American Revolution gave the new nation not only its independence but also its first herbal, *Materia Medica Americana* (1787), by Dr. Johann David Schopf (1752–1800). Ironically, Dr. Schopf came to America in 1777 as a doctor for the Hessian mercenaries who fought for the British. After the war, he stayed long enough to compile his book on medicinal plants.

America's first resident medical botanist was Constantine S. Rafinesque (1784–1841). Born in Europe, he came to the United States as a young man and studied the herbs of the Mississippi Valley with Native American healers. In 1819, Rafinesque became a professor of botany at a college in Kentucky, where he wrote *Medical Flora* (1828).

Rafinesque coined the term *Eclectic* to describe the kind of medicine that he advocated, a combination of European, Asian, Indian, and slave herbalism. Shortly after his death, 19th-century America's most scientific herbalists decided to call themselves the Eclectics.

The Shakers: America's Premier Healing Herb Growers

Today, most Americans associate the word *Shaker* with simple but high-quality furniture. Throughout the 19th century, however, the Shakers were better known for the high quality of their medicinal herbs.

An English Quaker, Ann Lee, founded the sect in Manchester, England, in the early 1770s. She believed in worshipping God with singing and dancing called shaking, hence the name Shaking Quakers, then Shakers. Not surprisingly, Lee was imprisoned for a time as a witch.

In 1774, Lee and eight Shakers arrived in New York and founded their first community near Albany. The Shakers practiced strict pacifism as well as gender equality and segregation. Marriage and sex were banned. Member families were broken up. Meals were eaten in silence.

Eventually, the Shakers established 24 communities, from Maine to Indiana to Florida.

Eight lasted through World War I. One still exists: Sabbathday Lake in New Gloucester, Maine.

Ann Lee's motto was "Hands to work, hearts to God." Her industrious followers launched the American medicinal herb industry in 1799, first collecting healing herbs from the wild, then growing them. The herb business prospered, and in 1824, the Sabbathday Lake community built a large herb building for drying and processing. It still stands today.

The Shakers sold their herbs through a nationally distributed catalog. The first one (1831) was headlined: "Why send to Europe's bloody shore for plants that grow by our own door?" It offered 142 herbs, roots, barks, and seeds, including angelica, basil, bayberry, belladonna, black and blue cohosh, boneset, cannabis (marijuana), catnip, chamomile, coltsfoot, comfrey, elecampane, gentian, hop, hyssop, jimson weed, juniper, lady's slipper, licorice, lobelia, marshmallow, motherwort, mullein, nux vomica, opium poppy, pennyroyal, peppermint, rosemary, saffron, senna, slippery elm, valerian, walnut, white oak, and wild cherry. The Shakers also sold a few culinary "sweet" herbs: sage, marjoram, savory, and thyme.

Unlike Rome's *herbarii*, the Shakers developed a reputation for honesty and herbal purity. In 1851, Rafinesque said that they had "the best medicinal gardens in the U.S. They cultivate a great variety and sell them cheap, fresh, and genuine."

Pacifism did not prevent the Shakers from selling medicinal herbs to the Union Army during the Civil War. They supplied much of the Union's opium. After the war, the Shakers sold medicinal herbs directly to hospitals and the embryonic pharmaceutical industry.

The Shakers also invented the modern pill. Before pills, powdered herbs were sold loose in envelopes, which were inconvenient to ship. Shaker craftsmen drilled holes in simple wood frames to create the first pill molds. The herbalists poured in measured amounts of herbal powders, then hammered pegs into the holes to press the powders into pills.

When patent medicines became popular after the Civil War, the Shakers marketed several. Their biggest seller was Dr. Corbett's Shaker Sarsaparilla Syrup, with sarsaparilla, dandelion, black cohosh, yellow dock, juniper, and several other herbs. The Shakers touted it for arthritis, insomnia, syphilis, anxiety, stomach distress, gynecological complaints, and diseases of the blood, kidneys, liver, heart, and lungs. Two other popular items were Pain King, with opium, and Tamar Laxative, with dried prunes and senna.

The Shaker herb business died after World War II, but the Sabbathday Lake community revived it in the 1960s. The community's herb garden, herb building, and museum are open to the public.

Thomson's Botanic Medicine

Early America's leading herbalist was Samuel Thomson (1760–1843). Born in Alstead, New Hampshire, he studied with a midwife and Indian healers. Around 1800, Thomson's daughter became seriously ill. Unsure of his skills, he called a physician, who pronounced her incurable. Then, as the story goes, Thomson cured her with herbs and hot baths. Soon after, he declared himself a "doctor."

Thomson detested the regular physicians of his day, who relied on bloodletting, violent laxatives (cathartics), and mercury. These treatments were called heroic medicine, but the heroism was entirely on the part of the patients.

Consider the case of George Washington. One day in 1799, the elderly but generally healthy father of our country developed a sore throat with a fever and chills. Chances are, he had strep throat or some other minor infection, which probably would have cleared up with rest, hot liquids, and herbal antibiotics such as garlic and onion.

Instead, Washington's heroic physicians bled him of 4 pints of blood, leaving him anemic and weak. Then they gave him cathartics and mercury. He was dead within 24 hours.

Thomson developed a medical system based on herbs and hot baths, inspired by European herbalism and mineral baths and Indian herbalism and sweat lodges. His favorite herb was lobelia or Indian tobacco, which in large amounts causes vomiting, hence its names emetic herb and puke weed.

In 1809, Thomson was arrested for murder after allegedly administering a fatal dose of lobelia. He was acquitted due to a lack of evidence that lobelia was poisonous.

Samuel Thomson may not have been the nation's greatest herbalist, but he was our first medical marketing genius. In 1813, he obtained a patent for Thomson's Improved System of Botanic Practice of Medicine, which allowed him to sell his Indian-inspired herbalism nationwide while still retaining its ownership. Thomson sold "family rights" to his medical system for $20. Starting in 1822, he charged another $2 for his book, *The New Guide to Health, or the Botanic Family Physician.*

Thomson's motto was "Every man his own physician," but the vast majority of his "family rights" were purchased by women. Many of them welcomed the opportunity to add some semblance of legitimacy to the word-of-mouth herbalism that they had learned from their mothers and other women.

In 1839, at the height of his popularity, Thomson claimed 3 million adherents. This was no doubt an exaggeration, but Thomsonian herbalism was very popular. Thomson boasted that half of Ohio practiced his herbal healing. His critics said it was only one-third.

Initially, Thomsonian herbalists used 65 herbs, all available from the Shakers. Thomson soon realized that he could make more money by selling prepackaged herbal formulas. He organized his family members into Friendly Botanic Societies, cooperatives that bought his formulas and distributed them around the country. Because Thomson's formulas were part of his patented medical system, they became known as patent medicines.

As time passed, patent medicines became a major industry. Some were quality products, but many were worthless concoctions of alcohol, opium, and cocaine sold by hucksters whose outrageous claims eventually spurred Congress to create the Food and Drug Administration (FDA).

After Thomson's death in 1843, his medical system fell from fashion. But some practitioners preserved it. One was Dr. John Kellogg of Battle Creek, Michigan, who invented the nation's first health food, the cornflake, and founded Kellogg's cereal company. For the most part, though, Thomsonian medicine was replaced by homeopathy and Eclectic herbalism.

Homeopathy: Herbal Microdoses

From 1830 through World War I, the main competition for regular American physicians came from homeopathy, the herbally inclined medical system created by a disillusioned German physician, Dr. Samuel Hahnemann (1755–1843). Trained in heroic medicine, Dr. Hahnemann decided that bloodletting, cathartics, and mercury did more harm than good.

Dr. Hahnemann did not reject all heroic treatments. On the contrary, he was impressed with several. One was cinchona bark, the antimalarial. Another was the cowpox inoculation, initiated by Edward Jenner in 1796. It was the first effective preventive for another age-old scourge, smallpox.

In healthy people, both of these treatments produce low-level symptoms of the diseases that they are used to prevent. Dr. Hahnemann called the phenomenon homeopathy, from the Greek for "treatment by similars."

Dr. Hahnemann tested hundreds of herbs and other substances on himself, carefully cataloging their effects. Eventually, he began using them to treat illnesses with similar symptoms. His approach was less drastic than heroic medicine's, and he enjoyed considerable success. He also attracted a large following.

Homeopathy came to the United States in the 1830s. It quickly won many supporters who were fed up with heroic medicine, including Mark Twain, Daniel Webster, and John D. Rockefeller. Homeopaths popularized several drugs that are used today, including ergot derivatives for migraines and nitroglycerin for the chest pain of angina.

By the early 20th century, however, homeopathy fell from U.S. medical fashion. One reason was the decline of heroic medicine. As regular physicians stopped opening veins and using mercury, their critics had less to criticize. Another reason was the unrelenting hostility of the American Medical Association (AMA). Around 1900, an estimated 25 percent of regular physicians also prescribed some homeopathic medicines. The AMA decreed that any physician caught using homeopathy would be drummed out of the organization.

The major reason for homeopathy's decline, though, was its Law of Potentization, Dr. Hahnemann's assertion that his medicines grew *stronger* as they became more *dilute*. The Law of Potentization violated Paracelsus's dose-response relationship, a cornerstone of pharmacology. Critics charged that medicines homeopaths considered extremely powerful were so dilute that they did not contain even a single molecule of the active ingredient. As a result, American scientists dismissed homeopathy—and its largely herbal medicines—as nonsense. By the 1950s, homeopathy was just about dead in this country.

Homeopaths can't explain the Law of Potentization, but they insist that more than 150 years of clinical experience show that it works. They have a point. In recent years, rigorous scientific trials have found that homeopathic medicines (most of them herbal) effectively treat colds, flu, hay fever, asthma, fibromyalgia, mosquito bites, rheumatoid arthritis, and infectious diarrhea.

In 1991, nonhomeopathic Dutch epidemiologists at the University of Maastricht published an analysis of 105 studies of homeopathic medicines from 1966 to 1990, most taken from French and German medical journals not usually translated into English. Of the 105 studies, 81 showed significant benefits from homeopathic treatment, while 24 showed no benefit. Some of the studies involved few subjects, however, and most were not double-blind, meaning that researcher bias may have played a role in the results.

Because of those possibilities, the Dutch investigators selected the 21 most scientifically rigorous studies and analyzed the results. Fifteen (71 percent) showed significant benefits from homeopathic treatment. While many questions remain about how homeopathy works, the researchers concluded that "the evidence presented in this review would probably be sufficient for establishing homeopathy as a regular treatment for certain conditions."

Since its founding, homeopathy has been popular in Europe. Today, the physician to the British royal family is a homeopath. Surveys show that many British, French, and German M.D.s prescribe some homeopathic medicines in their practices.

During the last 30 years, America has witnessed a modest homeopathic renaissance. Today, about 9 percent of U.S. doctors—some 5,000 M.D.s—incorporate homeopathic medicines into their practices. Several thousand other health professionals—dentists, podiatrists, veterinarians, nurses, and chiropractors—also use homeopathy.

A study by Harvard researchers suggested that more than 2.5 million Americans have tried homeopathy. Sales of homeopathic medicines now total more than $250 million a year, thanks in part to the fact that increasingly, they are carried by major drugstore chains. What's more, several celebrities—including singer Tina Turner, hairstylist Vidal Sassoon, musicians Yehudi Menuhin and Dizzy Gillespie, and actors Jane Fonda, Cher, Angelica Huston, and Elizabeth Taylor—have gone public with their support for homeopathy.

The Eclectics: America's Scientific Herbalists

Despite the regular physicians' reliance on bloodletting, cathartics, and mercury, most 19th-century medicines were herbal. In 1820, two-thirds of the treatments in the *U.S. Pharmacopoeia* were botanical. By 1880, the figure was almost three-quarters.

In the 1820s, a group of anti-heroic practitioners—Thomsonians, Indian-trained herbalists, and disillusioned regulars—created the Reformed Medical Society to promote nonheroic, largely herbal healing. In 1830, the society met in New York to found a Reformed medical school. The reformers were mostly Easterners, but the East's cities were strongholds of regular medicine.

The Reformers decided to locate their school on the free-thinking western frontier, then located at the Mississippi River. Thomsonian medicine was very popular in Ohio, so the reformers established their school in Cincinnati. They adopted Rafinesque's term, *Eclectic*, to describe their herb-based approach, which combined European, Asian, Indian, and slave herbalism. They called their school the Eclectic Medical Institute.

The institute was the nation's first medical school to admit women, many of whom were Thomsonian herbalists interested in more training. In 1877, however, the Eclectics "yielded to the prejudices of the profession," according to Eclectic historian Henry Felter, and barred women.

The Eclectics were scientific herbalists. They experimented with herbs, performing chemical analyses and extracting active constituents. They published their findings in the scientific journals of the day and were prominent in the early pharmaceutical industry.

The two most important Eclectics were John King and John Uri Lloyd, both of whom taught at the Eclectic Medical Institute. King (1813–1893) was a botanical pharmacologist who introduced physicians to podophyllin, a plant resin still used today to treat warts. In 1855, he published the first edition of his *King's American Dispensatory*, 19th-century America's most comprehensive scientific herbal. The 18th edition (1898) remains in print today.

Lloyd (1849–1936) began his career at age 14 as a Cincinnati pharmacist's apprentice. He loved pharmacy so much that he brought his brothers, Nelson Ashley Lloyd (1851–1925) and Curtis Gates Lloyd (1859–1926), into the field. Eventually, they established Lloyd Brothers Pharmacists, Inc.

John Lloyd specialized in plant chemistry and developed most of the company's products. He was also one of the first presidents of the American Pharmaceutical Association (1887–1888). In his spare time, he wrote eight novels.

Nelson Lloyd managed the business side of Lloyd Brothers. His other love was baseball. He owned the Cincinnati team that eventually became the Reds, and later, he invested in the New York Giants.

Curtis Lloyd specialized in mushrooms. He also managed the brothers' large collection of botany books.

Eventually, the collection outgrew the brothers' homes, so they established the Lloyd Library. Today, the library houses the world's largest private collection of botanical information: 300,000 books and pamphlets as well as 500 journals. For years, the Lloyd Library also published a botanical journal, *Lloydia*, now called the *Journal of Natural Products*. The Lloyd Library in Cincinnati is open to the public.

The years 1880 to 1900 marked the heyday of Eclectic medicine. Its practitioners numbered about 8,000. But with the dawn of the 20th century, Eclectic medicine's popularity declined as herbal medicines were largely replaced by pharmaceutical drugs. The Eclectic Medical Institute graduated its last class in 1939, and American scientific herbalism almost died.

Almost, but not quite. A handful of Eclectic-inspired physicians hung on, particularly in the Pacific Northwest. They called themselves naturopaths, and among them was John Bastyr, N.D. (1912–1995), of Seattle. He was affiliated with the National College of Naturopathic Medicine in Portland, Oregon, the sole surviving medical school that embraced Eclectic herbalism.

In 1978, a group of Bastyr's former students founded the John Bastyr College of Naturopathic Medicine in Seattle, now Bastyr University in nearby Kenmore. Since then, three other naturopathic medical schools have been established: the Southwest College of Naturopathic Medicine in Scottsdale, Arizona; the College of Naturopathic Medicine at the University of Bridgeport, Connecticut; and the Canadian College of Naturopathic Medicine in Etobicoke, Ontario.

Naturopaths are currently licensed to practice in 14 states: Alaska, Arizona, California, Connecticut, Hawaii, Idaho, Kansas, Maine, Montana, New Hampshire, Oregon, Utah, Vermont, and Washington. Washington, D.C.,

Puerto Rico, and the U.S. Virgin Islands also have licensing laws for naturopathic doctors. Four Canadian provinces also license naturopaths: British Columbia, Manitoba, Ontario, and Saskatchewan. Elsewhere, naturopaths practice under other medical credentials, typically as acupuncturists, chiropractors, or clinical nutritionists.

To be admitted to Bastyr University, students must complete standard, college-level premedical requirements. The first 2 years at Bastyr combine a mainstream medical education—courses in anatomy, physiology, human dissection, biochemistry, pathology, microbiology, pharmacology, public health, and physical examination and diagnosis—with courses on naturopathic philosophy, clinical nutrition, homeopathy, and Western, Chinese, and Ayurvedic herbal medicine.

Third- and fourth-year students apprentice with mentor naturopaths, often at Bastyr's clinic in Seattle, which treats more than 25,000 patients a year. At first glance, the clinic looks like a mainstream medical facility. Closer examination reveals, however, that its large in-house pharmacy stocks very few pharmaceuticals and mostly herbal preparations, homeopathic medicines, and nutritional supplements.

The Collapse of Professional Herbal Medicine

In 1805, a German chemist extracted the first drug from an herbal source, morphine from the opium poppy. In 1820, another German chemist achieved another first, the synthesis of an organic compound (urea) from inorganic chemicals. Modern pharmacology was born.

Early pharmacologists developed drugs largely by modifying chemicals extracted from medicinal plants. In addition to morphine, they isolated aspirin from willow bark, quinine from cinchona, caffeine from coffee, menthol from peppermint, and ephedrine (a decongestant) from Chinese ephedra, among many others.

After the Civil War, aspiring American doctors had two basic choices for medical education: apprenticeship to practicing physicians or training at medical schools in the United States or Germany. Compared with the programs in the United States, a German medical education was more scientific and rigorous and took longer, and the medical schools were affiliated with hospitals, where intensive clinical training took place.

German-trained American doctors were harsh critics of U.S. medical education. They urged medical schools to reorganize along German lines. Harvard was one of the first to do so (in 1870), after university president Charles Eliot wrote, "The ignorance and incompetency of the average graduate of American medical schools . . . is horrible to contemplate."

In 1873, a $7 million bequest led to the creation of a German-style medical school and hospital in Baltimore, Johns Hopkins University. When it opened in 1893, Johns Hopkins took the unprecedented step of refusing to admit medical students without college degrees. Harvard quickly followed, making medical training a graduate program.

Other medical schools adopted the Harvard–Johns Hopkins model. They dropped botany in favor of pharmacology. Heroic measures fell from fashion, but so did herbal preparations, replaced by the drugs of the new pharmaceutical industry.

Laboratories and teaching hospitals were

costly, so financing became critical. Harvard, Johns Hopkins, and other well-endowed medical schools spent enormous sums on their facilities. More modestly endowed homeopathic and Eclectic schools could not keep up. As a result, students trained under the Harvard–Johns Hopkins model were considered better doctors, and state licensing boards began requiring the Harvard–Johns Hopkins curriculum. The other medical schools began to close.

Then the influential Carnegie Foundation commissioned Abraham Flexner to survey the quality of the nation's medical schools. His report, released in 1910, praised the Harvard–Johns Hopkins model and condemned all others. Carnegie and other wealthy foundations supported the Harvard–Johns Hopkins-type schools and no others.

By 1940, every surviving U.S. medical school offered only graduate training on the Harvard–Johns Hopkins model. None provided training in herbal healing.

Hoxsey's Herbal Cancer Treatment

The period from 1920 through the 1960s might be called the lost decades of American herbal healing. U.S. medical schools ignored herbs. Pharmaceutical pills and capsules replaced tinctures in the nation's pharmacies. Even many culinary herbs fell from popularity.

Nevertheless, herbal healing didn't die. It simply reverted to what it had been for most of its history—folk medicine practiced mostly by women who grew and gathered their own herbs and prescribed them as the classic herbals recommended.

A few diehards continued to promote herbal healing. Dr. Benedict Lust (1869–1945), the father of modern naturopathy, came to the United States from Germany in 1895. He opened the nation's first health food store and established sanitariums in New Jersey and Florida based on healing baths and herbal medicines. His nephew, John Lust, wrote an influential herbal, *The Herb Book*.

Jethro Kloss (1863–1946), a sanitarium manager and health food pioneer, published *Back to Eden* in 1939. Subtitled "A Story of the Restoration to Be Found in Herb, Root, and Bark," the book helped preserve herbal approaches to healing.

In England, C. F. (Hilda) Leyel (?–1957) almost single-handedly revived British herbalism when she opened the first of her Culpeper shops in 1927. In 1940, she successfully lobbied Parliament not to repeat Henry VIII's mistake of outlawing herbal medicine.

The most flamboyant and controversial herbalist of the mid-20th century, however, was Harry Hoxsey (1901–1974), who loudly proclaimed that his herbal formula cured cancer. A former Appalachian coal miner, Hoxsey graduated from high school but did not attend college and had no formal medical training. He attributed his Hoxsey Cancer Formula to his great-grandfather, who, he claimed, had witnessed a cancer-stricken horse's recovery after eating an odd combination of herbs. Hoxsey started selling the family formula in the 1930s. By the 1950s, his Dallas clinic was the world's largest privately owned cancer center, with branches in 17 states.

Hoxsey's claims outraged Texas medical authorities, and in the 1930s, a Dallas prosecutor arrested him for fraud more than 100 times. The Hoxsey formula didn't work for everyone, but the prosecutor could not find any patients who felt that they had been defrauded. What's more, Hoxsey presented hundreds who swore that his formula had cured their cancers.

The Texas courts ruled in favor of the cancer maverick. Then the prosecutor's brother developed cancer and secretly took the Hoxsey formula. When he recovered, Hoxsey's former prosecutor became his defense attorney.

Hoxsey was also attacked by the AMA. He fought back in court. When AMA officials conceded that the Hoxsey formula had merit as a treatment for skin cancer, the cancer maverick became the first person ever to win a libel suit against the AMA. The FDA eventually closed Hoxsey's clinics for violating federal drug-labeling regulations. His herbal ingredients were not FDA-approved cancer treatments.

Ironically, Hoxsey died of prostate cancer. He took his formula, but it didn't work for him.

The Hoxsey formula is available today at the Bio-Medical Center in Tijuana, Mexico. Studies have found that nine of the formula's herbal ingredients have anti-tumor action: barberry, buckthorn, burdock, cascara sagrada, red clover, licorice, poke, prickly ash, and bloodroot.

The Herbal Renaissance

Starting in the late 1960s, many Americans began changing their attitudes about health and healing. They decided to invest their energy in preventing illness rather than in treating it after the fact.

One step in that direction was a retreat from salt as the nation's main seasoning because of research linking it to high blood pressure, heart disease, and stroke. Many Americans retired their salt shakers and began rediscovering culinary herbs and spices. Many also rediscovered the therapeutic benefits of these plants. By the turn of the 21st century, U.S. medicinal herb sales totaled about $4 billion a year.

The renewed interest in herbal healing has been a result of the convergence of several trends:

- Growing interest in self-care. Mainstream medicine has produced miracles, but it has also become impersonal and often prohibitively expensive. To save time and money and limit their dependence on doctors, many Americans have turned to prevention and self-care. Healing herbs fit neatly into lifestyles focused on sound nutrition, fitness, and stress management.

- Enthusiasm for alternative healing arts. Homeopathy, naturopathy, and Chinese and Ayurvedic medicine have become increasingly popular in recent years. These healing arts make extensive use of herbal medicines.

- Backlash against advanced technology. The very wizardry of high technology creates a yearning for more down-to-earth approaches to human problems. When there's a choice, many Americans prefer healing herbs to the pharmaceuticals often derived from them.

- Environmental awareness. As climate change and the destruction of tropical rainforests have become worldwide political issues, interest has grown in rainforest plants, some of which are herbal medicines and many of which have not been screened for potential medicinal uses. The National Cancer Institute and government agencies around the world have launched testing programs, hoping to identify the therapeutic properties of these plants and others threatened with habitat destruction.

❧ Advocacy by the United Nations. A 1974 World Health Organization report concluded that adequate worldwide health care could not be achieved unless nonindustrialized nations were encouraged to nurture traditional herbal healing. Since then, the United Nations has encouraged the use of traditional medicine alongside Western medicine.

❧ Increasing mainstream medical acceptance. From the 1960s through the 1980s, no mainstream medical schools taught courses on alternative medicine. Today, about 80 do, including Harvard, Johns Hopkins, and Stanford.

Until the 1990s, the only coverage given to herbal medicine by mainstream medical journals was warnings, often overblown, about the alleged dire risks of using herbs. Today, leading journals—including the *Journal of the American Medical Association, the New England Journal of Medicine,* and *the British Medical Journal*— publish articles demonstrating the benefits of healing herbs. A survey of 31,000 adults by Harvard researchers shows that use of herbal medicines has increased steadily in the last decade. In 1997, 12 percent of American adults had used an herbal medicine at least once. Today, the figure is 20 percent.

What's more, mainstream doctors have become increasingly willing to recommend herbs for some conditions. Some physicians suggest echinacea for colds, ginger for motion sickness, and St. John's wort for depression.

The FDA vs. Healing Herbs

Unfortunately, the Food and Drug Administration, the federal agency that regulates medicinal herbs, has been very slow to embrace the herbal renaissance. Critics of herbs are quick to cry "hucksterism" when herb marketers sell their products as dietary supplements with vague labeling. This sorry state of affairs is a direct result of current FDA regulations.

Back in the 19th century, patent medicines laced with alcohol, cocaine, and even heroin raised cries for national drug regulation. But it took *The Jungle,* Upton Sinclair's exposé of the meat-packing industry, to finally convince Congress to prohibit the adulteration and mislabeling of foods and drugs.

Congress established the FDA in 1928, but the agency had little authority. Then in 1937, an antibiotic, elixir of sulfanilamide, killed 107 people because it contained a toxic ingredient. The following year, Congress passed the Food, Drug, and Cosmetic Act, which led to the first U.S. drug regulations.

The FDA remained pretty lax about enforcement until 1959. That's when about 8,000 European babies were born with terrible birth defects because their mothers had taken Thalidomide, an over-the-counter sedative, while pregnant. Three years later, spurred by the Thalidomide scandal, Congress directed the FDA to tighten its drug safety standards.

The agency declared that pharmaceutical companies had to demonstrate drugs' safety and effectiveness in elaborate studies. The tests required by the agency were very expensive—millions of dollars per drug in the 1960s and, by some estimates, hundreds of millions today. Oddly, the original FDA ruling made no distinction between new drugs and drugs already on the market.

The makers of over-the-counter (OTC) pharmaceuticals screamed that the FDA had no right to require costly testing of drugs that had been used safely for decades. As a compromise, the agency appointed panels of physicians, pharmacists, and pharmacologists to review the safety and effectiveness of OTC ingredients. These panels wrote reports, called monographs, that served as the basis for grandfathering approval of drugs determined to be safe and effective. The FDA began appointing OTC Review Panels in 1972. The final monographs were completed by 1985.

When the OTC review process began, more than 100 herbal medicines were listed as safe and effective in the *U.S. Pharmacopoeia*, a standard drug reference. They deserved to be approved as OTC medicines. Unfortunately, the OTC Review Panels did not undertake a comprehensive review of the medical literature. The only information examined by the panels was what OTC manufacturers submitted in support of products that they wanted to keep on pharmacy shelves.

By the end of the review process, hundreds of medicines had been incorporated into the OTC monographs, including about two dozen herbs. Among these were the active ingredients in most OTC laxatives (senna, psyllium seed, and cascara sagrada) and a few decongestants (peppermint oil, eucalyptus oil, and two ingredients derived from Chinese ephedra).

The approved herbs represented only a tiny fraction of the hundreds of botanical medicines that had extensive historical and clinical evidence of safety and efficacy. For example, before World War II, U.S. pharmacies carried several valerian-based sleep aids. By the time of the OTC review process, the drug companies had dropped valerian in favor of sedative antihistamines such as diphenhydramine (Benadryl). As a result, no valerian products were presented to the OTC Review Panel, and none were approved. Dozens of other herbs were also ignored by the panels.

Why didn't medicinal herb companies present their products to the OTC Review Panels? There were several reasons.

❧ During the 1970s and early 1980s, botanical medicine was just beginning to come back from its lowest ebb in U.S. history. The few herb companies in existence were, by and large, mom-and-pop enterprises run by herbalists whose marketing efforts consisted mainly of brewing medicinal teas for friends and selling them at local health food stores. Many of these entrepreneurs had no idea that the OTC review process was even taking place, let alone how to participate. When they found out, it was too late.

❧ At the time, many herbalists felt uncomfortable with the word *drug*. During the 1970s, most herbalists saw their products as foods, not drugs, despite the fact that their teas and tinctures were used for pharmacological, not nutritive, purposes. A few herbalists tried to organize participation in the OTC review process, but their efforts largely fell on deaf ears.

❦ Finally, to herbalists, the OTC Review Panels did not look sympathetic. They were composed of mainstream health professionals who were largely unfamiliar with herbs. Except for the few herbs that were approved, the OTC Review Panels basically ignored medicinal plants.

Once the OTC review process was completed in 1985, it was closed. Any drug or herb that was not already approved had to undergo the expensive and time-consuming tests that the FDA required of new drugs.

When a new drug wins approval, the company that owns it gets a patent, the exclusive right to market that medication for many years and recoup its investment. But who's going to spend millions to prove, for example, that garlic lowers cholesterol or that valerian is an effective sleep aid? These claims are true, demonstrated in many well-designed studies, but since no herb company can patent garlic or valerian, there's no way to recoup the huge investment in the approval process.

FDA regulations have left healing herbs in limbo. Many herbs have been used for thousands of years, but to be approved as drugs, they must be tested as though they were brand-new compounds. This makes no sense economically because they can't be patented. Thus, the vast majority of medicinal herbs are sold as dietary supplements, a designation several rungs down the regulatory ladder.

The catch is that dietary supplements cannot make medicinal claims. That's why product labels are vague about the herbs' effects.

In 1994, Congress passed the Dietary Supplement Health and Education Act (DSHEA), which directed the FDA to consider petitions that would allow herbs (and vitamin and mineral supplements) to make medicinal claims. To date, a few claims have been approved, notably that soy protein helps lower cholesterol. But the FDA has declined many requests by people in the herb industry to reopen the OTC review process to accommodate healing herbs.

That's what Germany has done. Herbal medicine is considerably more mainstream there than in the United States. Like our own FDA, the German government requires pre-approval safety and efficacy testing for all newly synthesized pharmaceuticals. However, it does not hold herbs, which the Germans call traditional medicines, to quite so high a standard.

In 1978, the counterpart of the FDA in the former West Germany convened an expert panel, Commission E, to study the extensive scientific literature for about 650 herbs. In a process quite similar to the FDA's earlier OTC review, the commission published monographs declaring several hundred herbs safe and effective for dozens of ailments. The commission also recommended dosages and warned of possible side effects.

German herb companies are allowed to make medicinal claims in line with the Commission E monographs as long as they market unadulterated, properly labeled herbs and adhere to the commission's dose recommendations. Currently, Commission E monographs stand as the world's most authoritative government-sponsored, expert-developed information on medicinal herbs' benefits, dosages, and side effects.

In this country, the National Institutes of Health's Office of Complementary and

Alternative Medicine (OCAM) has sponsored meetings between officials of the FDA and advocates of herbal medicine. The dialogue has focused on the possibility of the FDA reopening the OTC review process with an American panel similar to Commission E. Some FDA officials support the idea, but at this time, the agency has taken no action.

Without clear labeling to specify benefits, side effects, and recommended dosage—labeling that the FDA currently prohibits for all but a few medicinal herbs—many Americans remain confused about how best to use herbal remedies. This consumer information is essential as herbs become increasingly popular in the 21st century.

Chapter 2

TEMPEST IN A TEAPOT

Are Healing Herbs Safe?

Before you take anyone's advice about using medicinal herbs, ask the person, "Are healing herbs safe?" If the answer is a blanket "yes," you'd best consult someone else.

The fact is that some of the most potent poisons known to humanity are herbal. One example is poison hemlock, also known as wild parsley. This is why you should *never* pick parsley in the wild. Another example is the *Amanita* mushroom (aptly called the death cap), which is why you should *never* forage for mushrooms in the wild unless you're *certain* you can identify them correctly.

So are herbal medicines safe? Here's the correct answer: Most popular medicinal herbs, including all the herbs discussed in this book, are reasonably safe for most people most of the time when taken in recommended amounts. But medicinal herbs contain pharmacologically active compounds that have drug effects on the body, and while drugs can heal, all drugs have the potential to cause harm—allergic reactions, side effects, possible fetal injury, and interactions with other herbs and drugs.

Overall, herbs are safer than pharmaceuticals, but they can still cause harm, and anyone who uses them should do so cautiously and responsibly.

Herbs in the Headlines

In recent years, headlines have proclaimed the hazards of healing herbs.

- Potentially serious surgery-related bleeding complications have developed in people taking herbs with anticoagulant action, including garlic and ginseng. (Ginkgo was also blamed, but it appears that was a false accusation. See page 248.)

- Kava has been blamed for serious liver failure, including some deaths.

- St. John's wort can interfere with the action of several prescription drugs.

- Chinese ephedra (ma huang) has been abused by some people seeking amphetamine-like intoxication. At very high doses, it can cause death.

- Herbal laxatives (buckthorn, cascara sagrada, rhubarb, and senna) have also caused problems: abdominal cramps, bloody stool, and even potentially serious electrolyte imbalances from regular use of unusually high doses.

There's no question about it: Herbal medicines can cause problems. That's why this book contains extensive information on safety and side effects for every herb discussed.

However, by any reasonable measure of drug safety, pharmaceuticals cause much more harm.

Around the same time that the above reports of problems with medicinal herbs were published, the following reports about pharmaceuticals also appeared.

🍀 According to the most recent report from the American Association of Poison Control Centers, pain relievers, cough and cold preparations, antibiotics, sedatives, and antidepressants accounted for more than 400,000 poisonings (both accidental overdoses and intentional suicide attempts) in 2006. Among the hazardous substances listed in each category, almost none were medicinal herbs. In fact, the most hazardous plants turned out to be *houseplants*, because infants and toddlers sometimes munched on them and became ill.

🍀 For a report published in the April 15, 1998, edition of the *Journal of the American Medical Association*, researchers at the University of Toronto combed through 30 years of medical literature for reports of drug side effects among hospital patients. Extrapolating from the most scientifically rigorous 39 studies, the researchers estimated that drug side effects kill an astonishing 106,000

U.S. hospital patients a year and cause 2.2 million serious but nonfatal medical problems. In other words, adverse reactions to pharmaceuticals rank as this country's fourth leading cause of death, accounting for more fatalities than AIDS, suicide, and homicide combined. These side effects did not result from medical errors. They occurred when drugs were administered in accordance with FDA dosage guidelines.

Clearly, pharmaceuticals have safety issues of their own. But which are more hazardous, pharmaceuticals or herbal medicines? Conventional medications win that contest hands down. Even the regrettable death tolls from all potentially hazardous herbs combined are dwarfed by the problems caused by the pharmaceuticals mentioned above.

Of course, many more Americans take drugs than use herbs. From a cost-benefit perspective, it's reasonable to prescribe potentially hazardous drugs to treat serious conditions. The point here is not to condemn pharmaceuticals but rather to point out that despite some problems, herbal medicines do not pose a major public health hazard.

A Double Standard

Herbal medicines are the unfortunate victims of a double standard. Doctors and the public generally believe that pharmaceuticals are more trustworthy than herbs because, as discussed in Chapter 1, the former are more tightly regulated by the FDA. In many cases, though, the FDA's supposedly tight pharmaceutical regulations deliver little more than the illusion of safety—as evidenced by the fact that use of prescription pharmaceuticals within FDA prescribing guidelines is responsible for more than 100,000 U.S. deaths a year and more than 2 million serious adverse reactions.

The FDA requires pharmaceutical companies to conduct clinical trials to demonstrate the safety and effectiveness of new drugs, but most of these trials involve at most only a few thousand people. What about side effects that affect only 1 person in 10,000 or 50,000 or 1 million? They don't show up until the drug has become widely used. Within 5 years of approval, an estimated 50 percent of pharmaceuticals have their labels revised to include side effects—some potentially serious—that were discovered after the drugs were released.

Herbal medicines may not be as tightly regulated as pharmaceuticals, but they usually have much longer histories of use: decades, centuries, even millennia. They have withstood the test of time. Every now and then, an age-old herb turns out to pose a new hazard: The potentially liver-damaging pyrrolizidine alkaloids in comfrey are one example. But such findings are rare compared with the unanticipated side effects that come to light in recently approved pharmaceuticals.

Another aspect of the double standard concerning herb safety has to do with the mass media. Because herbal medicines are less familiar than pharmaceuticals to the vast majority of experts to whom the media turn for health information, these authorities tend to be anxious about herb safety and overstate herb hazards. Because these same authorities are much more familiar with pharmaceuticals, however, they tend to understate drug hazards.

That's why reports of relatively minor herb hazards tend to generate big headlines and persist in the media. By comparison, reports of drug hazards—for example, the fact that pharmaceuticals are the nation's fourth leading cause of death—make headlines for a day and then are largely forgotten.

Of course, as more people with a greater variety of medical conditions begin using healing herbs, especially in combination with pharmaceuticals, some new problems are bound to turn up. The interactions between St. John's wort and several drugs are good examples. Herbs should always be used cautiously, especially by people who are taking other medications for chronic conditions. By and large, however, herbal medicines are gentler and safer than pharmaceuticals.

The Issue of Dose Control

Some critics of herbal medicine contend that herbs are hazardous because typical preparation directions—1 to 2 teaspoons of dried herb per cup of boiling water, steeped for 10 to 20 minutes—yield infusions with highly variable doses of the medicinally active compounds. In contrast, when people take pharmaceuticals, they know precisely how much of the active ingredients they're getting.

The critics have a point. Herb potency depends on plant genetics, growing conditions, maturity at harvest, time in storage, the possibility of adulteration, and preparation method. A cup of instant coffee contains about 65 milligrams of caffeine. Cappuccino drinks may contain more than 300.

On the other hand, you need look no further than the statistics on suicide to know that precise dose control is no guarantee that pharmaceuticals will be used safely. In addition, drug effects depend on body weight. A standard dose of a pharmaceutical taken by a person who weighs 120 pounds has a greater effect than the same dose ingested by someone who weighs 200 pounds. Finally, individuals vary. Different people often have very different reactions to the same drugs.

How do you react to drugs? For headache, the standard adult aspirin dose is two tablets every 4 hours. Through experience, some people learn that one tablet provides sufficient relief, while others must take three.

In general, healing herbs cause fewer side effects than pharmaceuticals. Pharmaceuticals tend to be highly concentrated, and pills and capsules have little taste, factors that make taking an overdose easier. The active constituents in herbs are typically less concentrated, and most herbs taste bitter, both of which help discourage overdose. Nonetheless, anyone who uses healing herbs must strive for good dose control.

The doses recommended in this book represent a consensus of the opinions found in both traditional herbals and scientific references. In the few cases where sources disagreed significantly, this book recommends the smaller amount, in the belief that it's best to err on the side of caution.

These days, an increasing number of herbal medicines are available in pills and capsules as standardized extracts. This means that the plants were grown from seeds or clones known to produce a certain concentration of the pharmacologically active compounds. Then the plants were harvested, stored, and prepared under controlled conditions to produce dose uniformity.

Standardized extracts are not quite as dose-controlled as laboratory-synthesized pharmaceuticals, but they're considerably more dose-controlled than bulk herbs. When you buy commercial preparations, look for standardized extracts.

How to Use Herbs Safely

Fortunately, you don't need to be a master herbalist or an M.D. or Ph.D. to use herbal medicines safely. All you need is a little information.

BEFORE YOU TAKE ANY HERB, READ UP ON IT. Don't just listen to friends and neighbors. Each herb profile in this book contains extensive information on safety and side effects. Take any warnings seriously. When in doubt about the appropriateness of any herb for your particular medical condition or medical history, don't use it, or consult a health professional.

DON'T TAKE HERB IDENTITY FOR GRANTED. Look for products that identify herbs by their Latin binomial names—that is, genus and species. For example, garlic's binomial name is *Allium sativum*. Latin binomial identification is no guarantee that the herb is labeled properly. But it suggests that the marketer understands the importance of proper identification, and has taken steps to do that.

STICK WITH THE RECOMMENDED DOSAGE. Do not exceed it. Some people assume that if a little herb is good, more must be better. Wrong. Herbal dosage recommendations are based on scientific research and, often, centuries of clinical experience. Don't put yourself at risk by taking more than is suggested. As a general rule, whenever you use a commercial preparation (such as tea, a tincture, pills, or capsules), follow the label directions carefully.

RESPECT YOUR INDIVIDUALITY. Individuals vary. You may be allergic to one or more herbs or develop other unusual reactions. When you take herbal medicines, stay alert for adverse reactions such as abdominal upset, diarrhea, headache, itching, rash—anything out of the ordinary. If you notice any unusual symptoms that appear to be linked to the medicinal herb, stop taking it and discuss your reaction(s) with your doctor.

Who is most sensitive to healing herbs? Generally, people who have hay fever, those with illnesses often linked to allergies (such as asthma and eczema), and those who have had hives or experienced a serious allergic reaction called anaphylaxis.

It's extremely unlikely that medicinal herbs will cause anaphylaxis, but it's still remotely possible. The main symptom is difficulty breathing. If you develop any trouble breathing, call your emergency medical number immediately and tell the operator that you're having suspected anaphylaxis. Then give your address and phone number and do what the operator says. Paramedics should respond immediately, as anaphylaxis can be fatal.

BE AWARE OF YOUR REACTIONS. Even if you're not allergic, you may still be unusually sensitive to one or more medicinal herbs. Doctors refer to this as an idiopathic reaction. In medical lingo, idiopathic means "for unknown reasons"—in other words, just one of those things. Out of the blue, you may react badly to an herb that's generally considered safe. It happens.

Pay attention to your body. If things go awry and you suspect that an herb is to blame, stop taking it and consult your physician.

IF YOU'RE OVER AGE 65, START WITH A LOW DOSE. As people grow older, they often become more sensitive to drug effects, so a low dose might suffice. In addition, older people often take other medications. Starting with a low dose of medicinal herbs reduces the risk of adverse herb-drug interactions. You can always increase the dose later.

IF YOU'RE PREGNANT OR NURSING, USE HERBS WITH EXTREME CAUTION. With a few exceptions, such as raspberry or ginger, women who are pregnant or nursing should not take medicinal amounts of healing herbs. Herbs that cause no problems for adults may harm the unborn and newborns. Moms-to-be and nursing moms who wish to try any herbal medicine should do so only with the consent and supervision of their professional health care providers.

WITH FEW EXCEPTIONS, DON'T GIVE HEALING HERBS TO CHILDREN UNDER AGE 2. While some herbalists contend that herbal medicines are okay for children 6 months and older, this book takes a more conservative position. As gentle as most herbs are, they're usually not appropriate for the very young. The few exceptions include cinnamon, chamomile, cranberry, dill water, and ginger—and even these should be given cautiously.

When administering an herb to a child, dilute the remedy in accordance with the child's weight. Standard herb doses are appropriate for a 150-pound person. A child who weighs 50 pounds should get one-third of the adult dose.

BE WARY OF INTERACTIONS. Exercise caution when using herbs if you already take pharmaceuticals or other herbs for a chronic condition. Do not duplicate a drug's effects with herbs. If you're already taking an antidepressant drug, for example, don't use the herbal antidepressant St. John's wort without your doctor's approval. If you're taking a pharmaceutical blood thinner (anticoagulant) such as aspirin, don't add garlic or white willow to your treatment plan. If you're already taking a tranquilizer or an anti-anxiety medication, steer clear of kava, an herbal tranquilizer.

THINK TWICE BEFORE JUMPING ON ANY NEW HERB'S BANDWAGON. Be extra careful when taking a newly popular herb or an old herb with a new use. In the mid-1990s, when the age-old herb St. John's wort was shown to have an important new benefit as an antidepressant, it flew off the shelves of health food stores. As the number of users jumped into the millions, rare side effects that strike only one person in a million suddenly began showing up.

That's how St. John's wort's interactions with several pharmaceuticals were identified. Until St. John's wort became popular, too few people took it for these problems to be noticed.

BE PRUDENT WHEN USING HERB OILS. Aromatic herbs' essential or volatile oils are highly concentrated, and amounts that seem small may cause serious harm. For example, as little as a teaspoon of pennyroyal oil can cause death.

Many herbal oils are available commercially. They are best used topically. If you ingest any, take only a drop or two at a time. Keep herbal oils well out of the reach of children.

PAY ATTENTION TO ANY SYMPTOMS OF TOXICITY. If you develop stomach upset, nausea, diarrhea, or headache within an hour or two of using any healing herb, stop taking it and see if your symptoms subside. When in doubt, call your local Poison Control Center or your physician or pharmacist. If you experience a severe reaction, call your doctor or 911 immediately.

KEEP YOUR PHYSICIAN INFORMED. In any medical consultation, tell the doctor which herbs you take and why. Forthrightness helps prevent potentially harmful herb-drug interactions.

DISCONTINUE HERBS BEFORE SURGERY. If you're scheduled for surgery, stop taking anticoagulant herbs at least 2 weeks beforehand. Anticoagulant herbs include evening primrose oil, garlic, ginger, turmeric, and white willow.

Potentially Problematic Herbs

Some popular herbs are more likely than others to cause problems. Consumers should become familiar with these herbs and exercise extra caution when taking them.

Stimulants. Stimulants are the herbs most likely to cause trouble. As mentioned earlier, large doses of Chinese ephedra can cause amphetamine-like effects and potentially fatal heart problems. Unusually large doses of other herbal stimulants can also cause problems.

Herbs with stimulant action include ginseng and all those that contain caffeine: coffee, tea, cocoa (chocolate), maté, and kola. Don't exceed the recommended doses; in the case of the herbs that contain caffeine, don't take more than what you're used to. In addition, don't take two or more stimulant herbs at the same time. The effects are additive.

Laxatives. Aloe, buckthorn, cascara sagrada, and senna all contain potent laxative compounds called anthraquinones. Even in recommended doses, these herbs may cause violent purging and abdominal distress. In larger doses, they cause bloody diarrhea and a host of other problems.

Chemical laxatives—both herbal and pharmaceutical—should be last-resort treatments for constipation. First, increase your intake of dietary fiber by eating more plant foods, drink more fluids, and get more exercise. If that doesn't work, try a fiber supplement. Switch to a bran cereal for breakfast, or try the fiber-rich herb psyllium, conveniently available in products such as Metamucil. If that doesn't provide sufficient relief, try a chemical laxative such as senna—but if you need to use it more than once a week, consult your doctor.

Tranquilizers and sedatives. Just as overstimulation can be hazardous, so can oversedation. The herbal tranquilizers and sedatives include valerian, catnip, chamomile, hop, kava, lavender, lemon balm, and passionflower.

Beware of using more than one of these herbs at a time medicinally—that is, in infusions steeped for longer than a minute or two. Don't take any of these herbs with alcohol, which is a very potent tranquilizer-sedative, and don't combine them with pharmaceutical tranquilizers or sedatives.

Undoubtedly, more herbs-can-be-hazardous headlines will appear in the future, as more people use herbal medicines more frequently, for more ailments, and in combination with more drugs. And unfortunately, some people are likely to suffer harm. But by following the advice in this chapter and in the individual herb entries, you should be able to avoid most problems.

Chapter 3

STORING AND PREPARING HEALING HERBS

Getting the Most from Nature's Medicines

These days, most medicinal herbs are available in pills and/or capsules. It's as easy to take them as it is to take Tylenol.

Some herbs come in tinctures, which are alcohol extracts. Typically, the bottle includes an eyedropper cap, so it's easy to add the recommended number of drops to a glass of water, juice, or beverage herb tea.

Still, you may enjoy growing and preparing your own herbs. Or you may choose to use some herbs that are available only as dried bulk plant material. That can feel daunting. Don't let it intimidate you.

Directions for Drying

Culinary herbs that also have medicinal applications, such as peppermint, rosemary, and ginger, can be used fresh. But the convention among herbalists is to start with dried plant material, which is more convenient to store and doesn't rot or spoil as easily.

Traditionally, most herbs were simply tied in bunches and hung in a warm, dry, shady place until they crumbled easily. Roots were washed,

split, and spread in a single layer on a clean tray. These drying methods are still used today. In fact, some herb shops sell herbs in dried bunches.

Traditional drying has two disadvantages, however: It often requires more room than foragers or gardeners have, and it takes time—a few days to a few weeks for many leaves, stems, and flowers, and sometimes many months for barks or roots. To preserve the volatile aromatic oils in many herbs, the faster the drying time, the better. That's why most commercial herb producers use special equipment for drying herbs.

An easy way to dry herbs at home is to place them on a baking sheet or a piece of clean window screen in a 95°F oven. Oven drying is convenient and inexpensive, but it has two drawbacks. First, if you harvest herbs in the heat of summer, the last thing you may want to do is turn on your oven. Second, many ovens don't heat evenly, so some plant material may char while some remains too moist.

Another approach is to purchase a small produce dryer, a tabletop appliance with built-in removable trays that uses a hot-air fan to dry not only herbs but also other garden produce. To purchase one, ask a local nursery, check garden catalogs or Web sites, or search the Internet for "herb dryers."

Power for Powdering

Once herbs are dry, herbalists usually reduce them to powder, the form that's most convenient to use. Traditional herbalists made their powders with mortars and pestles, a method that still works well for those who process only small amounts.

A more modern approach is to use a small electric coffee grinder (carefully cleaned to remove all traces of coffee). For gardeners who produce large amounts of herbs, larger grinders are available.

Setup for Storing

This may come as a shock to those who store their kitchen spices in clear glass jars, but light is one of the two biggest destroyers of herb flavor and medicinal potency. The other is oxygen.

To best preserve herbs' medicinal constituents, store them in opaque glass or ceramic containers. Fill containers to the top to limit the amount of oxygen in them. As you use your herbs, add cotton wadding to prevent oxygen from seeping inside.

When stored carefully, aromatic herbs such as sage, rosemary, and thyme can remain potent for more than a year. Nonaromatic herbs such as alfalfa and uva-ursi last considerably longer.

Moisture is another herb killer. If your herbs get wet, redry them quickly to prevent the growth of mold.

Insects also take their toll. Drying kills many pests, but watch for signs of infestation. When not using your herbs, keep the containers closed tight.

Procedures for Preparation

Healing herbs are typically used as infusions, decoctions, tinctures, capsules, ointments, and compresses. They may also be added to baths.

How to Make an Infusion

Infusions are hot-water extracts made from herbs with medicinal constituents in their flowers, leaves, and stems. Some herbalists use the terms *infusion* and *tea* interchangeably, but the two are quite different. Infusions are prepared like teas, but they are steeped longer so they become considerably stronger.

The standard traditional infusion recipe calls for $1/2$ to 1 ounce of dried herb steeped in a pint of boiling water for 10 to 20 minutes, then strained. But infusions do not have long shelf lives and should be made as needed. So modern herbalists generally recommend 1 to 2 rounded teaspoons of dried herb per cup of boiling water and steeped for the same amount of time.

Of course, after 20 minutes, infusions are no longer hot. They may be drunk at room temperature or reheated on the stove or in a microwave.

You can use fresh herbs instead of dried to make an infusion. Simply double the amount of herb. (Fresh herbs contain more moisture, which makes them bulkier, so you need more of them.)

Making infusions can be as therapeutic as drinking them. While your infusion is steeping, inhale the warm, steamy vapors. They can act as a nasal decongestant and may help relieve the discomfort of colds, flu, cough, bronchitis, and allergies. As you inhale the vapors, close your eyes and visualize your immune system attacking your illness and making you well. Studies show that such meditative visualizations stimulate the immune system to more effectively fight many diseases.

Some herbal infusions, such as chamomile, ginger, and peppermint, are quite tasty. But others are unpalatably bitter. This is nature's way of discouraging overdose, but if you can't get your medicine down, it can't do any good. To make bitter infusions more palatable, add sugar, honey, or lemon, or mix them with herbal beverage blends or fruit juice. If you still can't stomach an infusion, try a different preparation.

How to Make a Decoction

Similar to infusions, decoctions are extracts made from roots and barks. Compared with flowers, leaves, and stems, roots and barks give up their active compounds less readily. So instead of steeping, you must bring the water to a boil, reduce the heat, and gently simmer the dried herb material for 10 to 20 minutes, then strain.

How to Make a Tincture

Tinctures are extracts made with alcohol instead of water. They are highly concentrated, so they're more portable than infusions or decoctions or even the herbs themselves. They also remain potent longer—up to several years.

To make tinctures, commercial manufacturers typically use pure grain alcohol, which is 198 proof. But home tincture makers can use 100 proof vodka or brandy. Vodka is less expensive.

The standard tincture recipe calls for 1 ounce of powdered dried herb steeped in 5 ounces of distilled spirits for 6 weeks. Here are some tips for tincture making.

- Seal tincture containers tightly.
- Despite sealing, some containers may ooze. Don't store developing tinctures on valuable furniture.
- Label each tincture with the herb used and the date you put it up to steep. That way, you'll know when 6 weeks have passed.
- Shake each mixture every few days to encourage alcohol uptake of the herb's medicinal constituents.
- Keep tinctures out of direct sunlight.
- If possible, use brown glass containers to minimize light damage.
- Don't be surprised if a tincture changes color as it develops. It happens.
- As the liquid level in a developing tincture goes down, top it off with more distilled spirits.
- After 6 weeks, strain out the plant material, if you wish. Many herbalists recommend doing this, but it's not necessary.
- Store tinctures in a cool place.
- Keep tinctures out of the reach of children. They are quite potent, and a small amount might trigger a harmful reaction.

People who do not drink alcohol can make tinctures using warm (but not boiled) vinegar. Herbalists recommend wine or apple cider vinegar, not white vinegar. The directions are the same as for alcohol tinctures.

Using Capsules

Powdered herbs can also be packed inside standard pharmaceutical gelatin capsules. Capsules are a convenient way to carry healing herbs while you travel or to take herbs that taste unpleasant. Many herb supply catalogs offer empty capsules and capsule-packing devices.

Capsules come in different sizes. The "00" size is standard. If you make capsules, measure how much powdered herb fits into the capsules you're using so you won't exceed the dosage recommended in this book.

Store capsules away from light and out of the reach of children.

External Preparations: Ointments, Compresses, and Baths

You can make your own herbal ointment by adding 1 to 2 teaspoons of tincture per ounce of commercial skin lotion.

For compresses to treat cuts, burns, and other skin problems, dip a clean cloth in a cool infusion or decoction and drape it over the affected area for 20 minutes. Repeat as needed.

To make baths more relaxing, fill a cloth bag with a few handfuls of aromatic herbs, then allow water to run over it. For additional aroma, leave the herb bag in the water as you bathe.

Chapter 4

HOW TO OBTAIN HEALING HERBS

The Best Sources Are Close at Hand

There are three ways to obtain healing herbs: Gather them, grow them, or buy them.

Gathering Your Own

If you enjoy long walks in meadows and forests, gathering herbs can be great fun. Of course, not all healing herbs grow in the United States, but many do.

To go "herbing," you need a good field guide. The best ones are *A Field Guide to Medicinal Plants: Eastern and Central North America* by noted herbalists Steven Foster and James A. Duke, Ph.D., and *A Field Guide to Western Medicinal Plants and Herbs* by Steven Foster and another distinguished herbalist, Christopher Hobbs. Both books are part of the Peterson Field Guides series. Each book discusses more than 500 healing herbs. The Eastern book includes 500 pen-and-ink drawings and 200 color photos. The Western book features more than 600 color photos. Both are excellent.

Some herbs, such as dandelion, are easy to recognize and safe to pick. In fact, with dande-

lion, your neighbors will probably thank you for pulling it out of their lawns. (If you're going to be harvesting dandelion anywhere other than your own lawn, though, it's wise to first make sure the area hasn't been treated with pesticides or other chemicals. Your best bets are vacant lots and open land that's not being cared for.) Unfortunately, other herbs, particularly ginseng, are more difficult to find.

Some healing herbs—including blackberry, raspberry, nettle, and rose—have thorns. Wear gloves, long pants, and long sleeves to gather these favorites.

Other herbs, such as angelica root and cascara sagrada bark, are safe to ingest when dried but hazardous to consume when fresh.

In a few herbs, the medicinal parts are safe but other parts cause problems. Blue cohosh is a good example. Its medicinal root is safe when used properly, but its berries are poisonous. Likewise, rhubarb's medicinal root can be used safely, but its leaf blades are poisonous.

Finally, a few poisonous plants resemble healing herbs. Three poisonous species of hemlock look like parsley. Some herb gatherers have died because they mistook poison hemlock—also known as fool's parsley—for the familiar garnish. Never ingest any wild parsley.

If you stalk the wild healers, dress appropriately, read up on the herbs in Chapter 5 to see if they're safe or problematic, and use a good field guide. Most important, when in doubt about any plant's identity, don't ingest it.

Growing Your Own

The herb entries in Chapter 5 contain directions for cultivating the healing herbs that grow in the United States. To get started, you'll still need cuttings, seeds, or root divisions.

Cuttings can be difficult to obtain. You have to know an herb gardener. But cuttings are rarely necessary. Most nurseries carry quite a few culinary herb seeds. Standard seed catalogs usually contain dozens of herbs as well. Most nurseries also carry herb seedlings. If you don't see the herbs you want, ask if your nursery can obtain them for you.

For the committed herb gardener, nothing compares with the specialty catalogs published by many of the nation's hundreds of commercial herb growers. Most charge a small fee for the catalog. Here are some of the best mail-order companies.

- Companion Plants features more than 300 varieties of plants and 100 varieties of seeds. Write to 7247 North Coolville Ridge Road, Athens, OH 45701, or visit the Web site at www.companionplants.com.

- The Rosemary House offers more than 100 varieties of plants and 200 varieties of seeds. Its address is 120 South Market Street, Mechanicsburg, PA 17055.

- Mountain Rose Herbs sells more than 100 varieties of herbs, seeds, herbalist supplies, and other herbal products. Write to P.O. Box 50220, Eugene, OR 97405, or try the Web site at www.mountainroseherbs.com.

- Sandy Mush Herb Nursery features more than 1,000 herbs and other plants. Contact the nursery at 316 Surrett Cove Road, Leicester, NC 28748. Or at the Website, www.sandymushherbs.com

- The International Herb Association (IHA) provides an enormous number of services to herb growers. It publishes a member directory and newsletter and sponsors conferences. Membership cost varies from $25 to $200 per year. The mailing address is P.O. Box 5667, Jacksonville, FL 32247-5667; the Web address is www.iherb.org.

You Can Always Buy

Supermarkets now carry many herbal beverage teas, some of which can be brewed into medicinal infusions. For a better selection, try a health food store. Most carry dozens of bulk herbs, medicinal herb blends, tinctures, oils, and tablets.

Bulk herbs, tinctures, oils, and tablets can also be purchased by mail. Many of the gardeners' resources listed above sell dried herbs and herb preparations. In addition, the following catalog companies offer large selections.

- Jean's Greens features more than 200 varieties of organic and wildcrafted herbs, along with other herbal products. Write to 1545 Columbia Turnpike, Castleton, NY 12033; call 888-845-TEAS; or log on to www.jeansgreens.com.

- Wild Weeds offers more than 100 herbs and herbal products. You can contact them at P.O.

Box 1016, Blue Lake, CA 95525. Or call 800-553-9453 or log on to www.wildweeds.com.

❧ Monterey Bay Spice Company sells more than 500 herbs and spices. Write to 719 Swift Street, Suite 62, Santa Cruz, CA 95060. You can also contact them at 800-500-6148 or www.herbco.com.

❧ HerbPharm features more than 250 herb products. Write to P.O. Box 116, Williams, OR 97544; call 800-348-4372; or log on to www.herb-pharm.com.

Noteworthy Herb Publications

Another way to find herbs—and to learn more about them—is to read the herb press. Recommended publications include:

❧ *HerbalGram*, the quarterly magazine of the American Botanical Council and the Herb Research Foundation. It's an excellent, authoritative source of the latest herb research, with an emphasis on herbal healing. To order it, write to the American Botanical Council at 6200 Manor Rd, Austin, TX 78723; call 512-926-4900; or log on to www.herbalgram.org.

❧ *The Herb Quarterly* is a wonderful magazine with a broad scope, including herb gardening, cookery, crafts, history, and herbal medicine. Their mailing address is 4075 Papazian Way, Fremont, CA 94538; their Web address is www.herbquarterly.com.

❧ Consumer Lab. This independent laboratory tests supplements and herbal products to see if they stand up to their label claims for purity and dosage. Results are available online to members. Membership costs $29.95 per year and is well worth it. To subscribe, log on to www.consumerlab.com.

PART II

He causeth the grass to grow for the cattle

and herbs for the service of humanity.

—Psalm 104:14

Chapter 5

130 HEALING HERBS
The Cream of the Herbal Crop

This chapter features profiles of 130 of the world's widely used medicinal plants. Why these 130? There are several reasons.

THEY'RE AVAILABLE. The selected herbs are generally Western in origin, from the Egyptian, European, and Native American healing traditions. Some of the more familiar Asian herbs have also been included, such as cinnamon, ginger, ginseng, rhubarb, and tea. Plants unique to Chinese herbalism have been omitted, however, despite their medical effectiveness, because they're not widely available in the United States.

THEY'RE USEFUL. All of the selected herbs have practical applications for everyday health concerns.

THEY'RE REASONABLY SAFE. The selected herbs should not cause serious side effects or other problems when used as recommended. Each profile provides detailed information on dosage limits, precautions, and potential hazards. (See Chapter 2 for a general discussion of herb safety.)

THEY'RE OFTEN IN KITCHEN SPICE RACKS. Centuries ago, all of the herbs and spices used in cooking today were prized mainly for their food preservation and healing powers. Few people realize that they have fully stocked pharmacies right in their own kitchens.

THEY'RE FASCINATING. The Pied Piper was as much an herbalist as a musician (see page 469). The makers of Bayer were originally skeptical of aspirin (see page 478). A 19th-century battle over abortion popularized a modern remedy for menstrual cramps (see page 107). And cowboys who drank sarsaparilla were less interested in refreshment than in preventing venereal diseases (see page 419).

THEY'RE POPULAR. Every year, *Whole Foods Magazine*, the health food industry trade journal, ranks medicinal herbs by popularity based on sales. All of the top-rated herbs are represented here.

ALFALFA

Hope for the Heart

Family: Leguminosae; other members include beans and peas

Genus and species: *Medicago sativa*

Also known as: Chilean clover, buffalo grass, and lucerne (in Britain)

Parts used: Seeds and leaves

Alfalfa is the world's oldest forage crop. Farmers have prized it since before the dawn of history. Since the 1970s, people who graze on salads have come to appreciate the herb's sprouts as well. But it's the seeds and leaves that contain the real healing power. They reduce cholesterol, which helps prevent heart disease and most strokes.

Healing History

What's good for cattle is good for people, too, or so the ancient Chinese thought. Their animals ate alfalfa so enthusiastically that the Chinese began preparing the herb's tender young leaves as a vegetable. Soon, traditional Chinese physicians were using the plant to stimulate appetite and to treat digestive problems, particularly ulcers.

Ancient India's traditional Ayurvedic physicians also used alfalfa to treat ulcers, and they prescribed it for arthritis pain and fluid retention as well.

Ancient Arabs fed their horses alfalfa, believing that it made the animals swift and strong. They called it *al-fac-facah*, or "father of all foods." The Spanish changed the name to alfalfa.

Spain introduced alfalfa into the Americas, where it became a popular forage crop, particularly in the Great Plains. Like the ancient Chinese, the pioneers believed that what was good for their cattle was good for themselves, so they used alfalfa to treat arthritis, boils, cancer, scurvy, and urinary and bowel problems. Pioneer women used it to bring on menstruation.

After the Civil War, alfalfa fell out of favor as a healing herb. It wasn't until the 1970s that it returned to popularity via the salad bowl.

Therapeutic Uses

Most of alfalfa's traditional therapeutic uses have long been disproved. Modern scientists may have discovered a potential healing benefit that our ancestors never dreamed of, however: alfalfa as an agent in the war against heart disease, stroke, and cancer, the nation's top three killers.

HEART DISEASE AND STROKE. Animal studies show that alfalfa leaves and seeds reduce blood cholesterol levels. High cholesterol levels raise the risk considerably for heart attack and most strokes. (Alfalfa sprouts produce a similar, but less pronounced, effect.) Scandinavian researchers gave alfalfa seeds (1.5 ounces three times a day) to 15 people with high cholesterol. After 8 weeks, their cholesterol was significantly lower.

CANCER. One study suggests that alfalfa helps neutralize cancer-causing substances in the intestine. Another, published in the *Journal of the National Cancer Institute*, shows that the herb binds carcinogens in the colon and helps speed their elimination.

WOMEN'S HEALTH CONCERNS. Alfalfa seeds contain two chemicals, stachydrine and homostachydrine, that promote menstruation. They can also cause miscarriage, which is why pregnant women should not eat alfalfa seeds. Nor should women consider the herb a reliable contraceptive.

BAD BREATH. Alfalfa is a source of chlorophyll, the active ingredient in most commercial breath fresheners. Sip an alfalfa infusion if you're concerned about bad breath.

Intriguing Possibility

In laboratory studies, alfalfa helps fight disease-causing fungi. One day, it may be used to treat fungal infections.

Medicinal Myths

While some herbalists still espouse the age-old view that alfalfa treats ulcers, they may have to eat their words. Scientific research has found no support for this traditional use of the herb.

Herbalists also recommend alfalfa for bowel problems and as a diuretic to treat fluid retention. Unfortunately, these traditional uses have not held up under scientific scrutiny either.

Although some supplement manufacturers promote alfalfa tablets as a treatment for asthma and hay fever, a study published in the *Journal of the American Medical Association* shows that these claims have no merit. Alfalfa contains neither bronchodilators, which arrest an asthma attack, nor antihistamines, which relieve hay fever.

Rx Recommendations

Save alfalfa sprouts to dress up your salads; it's the leaves and seeds that are used in herbal healing. Alfalfa leaf and seed tablets and capsules are available in most health food stores and supplements shops. Take them according to package directions.

When using the bulk herb, prepare medicinal infusions with 1 to 2 teaspoons of dried leaves and/or bruised seeds per cup of boiling water and steep for 10 to 20 minutes. Enjoy up to 3 cups a day to take advantage of alfalfa's cholesterol-reducing potential. The infusion has a hay-like aroma and tastes like chamomile, with a slightly bitter aftertaste.

The Safety Factor

Do not consume more than the recommended amounts of alfalfa seeds. They contain the potentially toxic amino acid canavanine. Over time, eating large quantities of seeds may introduce enough canavanine into the body to cause the reversible blood disorder pancytopenia, according to a report in *Lancet*. This condition impairs blood platelets, which are necessary for clotting, and white blood cells, which fight infection.

The canavanine in alfalfa seeds has also been linked to systemic lupus erythematosus, a serious inflammatory disease that can attack many organs, particularly the kidneys. Alfalfa seeds have reactivated the disease in some people who were in remission, according to a report published in the *New England Journal of Medicine.* Another study shows that the seeds actually induce lupus in monkeys. If you have lupus or have ever had pancytopenia, do not use alfalfa.

Pregnant and nursing women should not use alfalfa, except the sprouts.

Do not give alfalfa to children under 2. In older children, adjust the recommended dose based on the child's weight. Give a 50-pound child one-third of the dose a 150-pound adult would take.

If you're over 65, start with a low dose, and increase only if necessary.

Inform health care professionals of the herbs you use. Problematic herb-drug interactions are possible.

Alfalfa may cause allergic reactions or other unexpected side effects. If any develop, reduce your dose or stop taking it.

For more on herb safety, see Chapter 2.

If symptoms get worse or persist longer than 2 weeks, consult a health care professional promptly.

Growing Information

Alfalfa grows throughout most of the United States. The plant is a deep-rooting, bushy perennial that grows to 3 feet and resembles tall clover. The leaves are divided into three leaflets. The herb's lavender, pale blue, or yellow flowers bloom from May through October, depending on location.

Alfalfa grows best in loamy soil. It tolerates clay but not sand, which lacks sufficient nutrients. Seeds are usually sown in autumn in rows 18 inches apart. Prepare the soil with manure and rock phosphate. Young plants require regular watering, but once established, they become fairly drought tolerant. Harvest plants when they bloom by cutting them back to within 3 inches of the ground, then hang them to dry. When dry, pick off the leaves.

ALOE

Soothe Those Wounds

Family: Liliaceae; other members include lily, tulip, garlic, and onion

Genus and species: *Aloe vera* and an estimated 500 other species

Also known as: Cape, Barbados, Curaiao, Socotrine, and Zanzibar aloe

Parts used: Leaves (gel and juice, or latex)

Every kitchen should have a potted aloe on the windowsill. That way, when minor burns, scalds, or cuts occur, it's easy to cut off one of the plant's thick, fleshy leaves and scoop the clear gel onto the injury. Aloe gel dries into a natural bandage. It also promotes wound healing and helps prevent infection.

Another part of aloe, the latex (extracted from special cells on the leaf's inner skin), is a powerful laxative. It's so potent, in fact, that many authorities say it should not be taken internally.

Healing History

Our word *aloe* comes from the Arabic *alloeh*, meaning "bitter and shiny"—an apt description of the plant's wound-healing inner leaf gel. Drawings of aloe have been found in Egyptian temples dating to 3000 B.C. The Bible mentions aloe several times, in passages such as "I have perfumed my bed with myrrh, aloes, and cinnamon" (Proverbs 7:17), but it's unlikely that biblical aloe was *Aloe vera*. In the ancient world, many bitter, resinous plants were called aloe.

Aloe has played a role in healing since the dawn of history. Egyptian medical writings from 1500 B.C. recommend it for infections and skin problems and as a laxative, uses that are supported by modern science.

Aloe is one of the few nonnarcotic plants to cause a war. When Alexander the Great conquered Egypt in 332 B.C., he heard of a plant with amazing wound-healing powers on an island off Somalia. Intent on healing his soldiers' wounds—and on denying this healer to his enemies—Alexander sent an army to seize the island and the plant, which turned out to be aloe.

The Greek physician Dioscorides recommended aloe externally for wounds, hemorrhoids, ulcers, and hair loss. The Roman naturalist Pliny prescribed it for internal use as a laxative.

Arab traders carried aloe from Spain to Asia around the 6th century. They introduced the herb to India's traditional Ayurvedic physicians, who used it to treat skin problems, intestinal worms, and menstrual discomforts. Chinese healers used it similarly.

More recently, American pioneers relied on aloe gel to treat wounds, burns, and hemorrhoids. These uses continue today.

Therapeutic Uses

Contemporary herbalists use aloe in at least one of the ways that Dioscorides suggested almost 2,000 years ago—externally, to treat wounds.

WOUNDS (INCLUDING BURNS, SCALDS, SCRAPES, AND SUNBURN). Aloe contains various compounds—bradykinase, salicylic acid, and magnesium lactate—that reduce the inflammation, swelling, and redness of wounds. They also help relieve pain and itching. Scientific evidence of aloe's wound-healing power was first documented in 1935, when an American medical journal reported the case of a woman whose x-ray burns were successfully treated with aloe gel scooped straight from leaves cut from the plant. Since then, many studies have supported the herb's ability to stimulate healing of first- and second-degree burns. Asian researchers analyzed many studies of aloe for wound healing. Compared with standard care, the wounds of those using aloe healed significantly faster—up to 8 days faster.

Aloe works best for superficial wounds. In a study published in the *Journal of Dermatology and Surgical Oncology*, the herb sped the healing of pimples by 3 days compared with standard medical treatment. For deep wounds, however, it actually slows healing. That was what researchers found when they studied the effect of aloe on cesarean section incisions. In the study, published in *Obstetrics and Gyne-*

cology, the incisions not treated with aloe gel healed in 53 days, but for those treated with aloe, healing took 83 days. As a rule of thumb, use aloe gel on wounds that don't require stitches, but don't use it to treat deep wounds that require stitches.

INFECTIONS. Aloe gel not only spurs wound healing, it also helps keep injured skin from getting infected. Several studies have found aloe to be effective against many different bacteria and fungi that can invade a wound, including *Escherichia coli* and strains of staphylococcus, streptococcus, salmonella, shigella, and candida. It also boosts the immune system, which helps the body fight infection.

ACNE AND RASHES FROM POISONOUS PLANTS. Beyond wounds, aloe also helps heal other minor skin conditions, including acne and rashes caused by poison ivy, oak, and sumac.

PSORIASIS. This skin condition, which affects some 5 million Americans, causes eruptions of red, raised skin patches that are usually topped with gray, white, or silvery scaly tissue. At Malmo University Hospital in Sweden, researchers gave 60 people with psoriasis either a medically inactive placebo cream or a cream containing 0.5 percent aloe gel. The participants were instructed to use the creams three times a day, 5 days a week for 16 weeks. Among those using the placebo cream, 7 percent experienced substantial clearing of their psoriasis skin patches. Among those using the aloe cream, that figure rose to 83 percent.

GENERAL SKIN CARE. Cleopatra massaged aloe gel into her skin to make it shine, and the herb remains a popular ingredient in skin-care products. But if you're after beautiful skin, do what the legendary beauty did: Use the fresh leaf gel. The "stabilized" (preserved) gel found in commercial skin-care products and shampoos may not provide the fresh herb's skin-enhancing benefits. If you enjoy the fragrance of aloe shampoos and skin lotions, that's fine. Just don't expect them to turn you into Cleopatra.

DIABETES. Several studies show that aloe juice reduces blood sugar (glucose) levels in animals. Further, Thai researchers gave 72 people with diabetes either a placebo or aloe juice (1 tablespoon twice a day). After 6 weeks, the aloe group's blood sugar fell significantly.

Intriguing Possibilities

Aloe juice and aloe-based beverages are widely available in health food stores. Their labels claim that these products are good for the digestive tract. Anecdotal reports suggest possible benefits for inflammatory bowel disease (colitis and Crohn's disease), but there is no rigorous research to support this.

Studies show that aloe may kill the fungus (*Candida albicans*) that causes vaginal yeast infections. Its possible effectiveness against the yeast fungus has led some herbalists to recommend using it to treat the infection itself. But just because it kills the fungus in laboratory tests doesn't mean that it can wipe out the infection in the human body. No scientific studies support this use, and an FDA advisory panel found insufficient evidence to recommend aloe as a yeast treatment.

In laboratory tests, a chemical in aloe called aloe-emodin has shown promise against leukemia. But National Cancer Institute scientists say that experimental preparations are still too toxic to give to people with leukemia.

Although aloe has been used in folk medicine as an external treatment for skin cancer, its effectiveness has never been studied scientifically.

Rx Recommendations

To help soothe wounds, including burns, scalds, scrapes, and sunburn, and to help prevent infection, select a lower (older) aloe leaf and cut off several inches. Then slice it lengthwise, scoop the gel onto the wound, and let it dry. Be sure to clean the wound properly with soap and water first. As for the injured leaf, it quickly closes its own wound. You can use the rest of it in the future.

To enjoy the cosmetic benefits of aloe, apply the leaf gel to freshly washed skin. Discontinue use if it seems to irritate your skin.

The Safety Factor

Aloe gel is safe for external use by anyone who does not develop an allergic reaction. If a wound treated with aloe does not heal significantly within 2 weeks or if it appears worse, consult a doctor.

Commercial aloe juice may have a mild laxative effect, but stay away from laxatives containing aloe latex. The latex contains laxative compounds (anthraquinones) with such powerful purgative action that they are called cathartics. Other laxative herbs, such as senna, rhubarb, buckthorn, and cascara sagrada, also contain anthraquinones, but aloe's action is considered the most drastic—and least recommended—because it often causes severe intestinal cramps and diarrhea.

Although many herbalists discourage the use of aloe as a laxative, some supplement companies sell aloe laxative tablets on the strength of approval by Commission E, the expert panel that evaluates herbal medicines for the German counterpart of the FDA. If you take aloe as a laxative, never exceed the dosage recommendations on the package, and reduce the dosage or stop using the product if you develop intestinal cramps. If you're looking for a natural laxative, your best bet is to seek other herbs with proven, but milder, effects, such as psyllium (see page 375).

Women who are pregnant or trying to conceive should not take aloe latex, as its cathartic nature may stimulate uterine contractions and trigger miscarriage. Nor should aloe latex be used by nursing mothers. The latex enters the mother's milk and may cause stomach cramps and violent catharsis in infants.

Aloe latex's cathartic power may also aggravate ulcers, hemorrhoids, diverticulosis, diverticulitis, colitis, Crohn's disease, or irritable bowel syndrome. Anyone with a gastrointestinal illness should not use aloe latex as a laxative.

In general, aloe latex is not recommended for internal use in children or adults.

Inform health care professionals of the herbs you use. Problematic herb-drug interactions are possible.

Aloe may cause allergic reactions or other unexpected side effects. If any develop, reduce your dose or stop taking it.

For more on herb safety, see Chapter 2.

If symptoms get worse or persist longer than 2 weeks, consult a health care professional promptly.

Growing Information

Aloe is the perfect houseplant for people with brown thumbs because it requires little water and no other care. Aloe prefers sun, but it tolerates shade and doesn't mind poor soil. The only conditions this hardy succulent cannot tolerate are poor drainage and cold temperatures. Bring potted aloe indoors before the temperature falls below about 40°F.

Aloe periodically produces offshoots, which you may remove and replant when they are a few inches tall. Simply uproot or unpot the plant, work the soil gently to separate the offshoot, and return the mother plant to its bed or pot.

ANDROGRAPHIS

The "King of Bitters" Fights Colds— And More

Family: Acanthaceae; other members include acanthus

Genus and species: *Andrographis paniculata*

Also known as: Kalmegh

Parts used: Mostly leaves, sometimes root

Many healing herbs taste bitter. But andrographis, an annual herb native to India, is so bitter that centuries ago, Indians named it *kalmegh*, meaning "king of the bitters" in Bengali. It's a garden herb in India and parts of China and Thailand, where it has long been incorporated into herbal medicine.

Healing History

India's traditional Ayurvedic physicians used andrographis—like so many other bitter herbs—to promote digestion, increase appetite, and treat stomach distress and snakebite. In addition, the herb was used to treat fever and jaundice (liver disease). Traditional Chinese physicians considered andrographis a "cold" herb and used it to treat conditions involving too much heat, such as fever.

Therapeutic Uses

IMMUNE STIMULATION. Andrographis boosts the ability of white blood cells to gobble up invading germs, including *E. coli*, the digestive-tract bacteria that cause urinary tract infections, and shigella, which causes infectious diarrhea (dysentery).

COLDS, FLU, AND SINUS INFECTIONS. Andrographis also improves the body's ability to fight viruses, including the viruses that cause colds and flu. Swedish researchers gave either a placebo or the herb to 179 adults with cold symptoms—sore throat, nasal congestion, runny nose, watery eyes, and cough. After 3 days, the andrographis group showed highly significant benefit, especially in relief of sore throat. Other studies by Armenian, Russian, and Chilean researchers agree that treatment with andrographis results in shorter, milder colds in both adults and children, without significant side effects. The Armenian study also dealt with sinus infection and found the herb to be beneficial.

Russian researchers gave a placebo or andrographis to 540 people with symptoms of flu (cold symptoms plus fever and muscle aches). The herb, they concluded, "contributes to quicker recovery and reduces risk of post-influenza complications," such as bronchitis. Andrographis caused no significant side effects.

Finally, Thai researchers analyzed all

studies of andrographis as a treatment for colds and flu. They concluded that the research "supports the usefulness of andrographis in reducing the severity of upper respiratory tract infections."

RELIEF OF FEVER, PAIN, AND INFLAMMATION. At a dose of 6 grams, the herb reduces fever, thus validating this use by traditional Chinese physicians. In one Chinese study, the herb reduced fevers in 70 of 84 subjects within 48 hours. In another, Thai researchers gave either a placebo or andrographis (6 grams per day) to 152 people with fever and sore throat caused by tonsillitis. After 1 week, the herb group reported significantly greater relief, results on a par with what one would expect from acetaminophen (Tylenol).

URINARY TRACT INFECTIONS. Thai researchers gave either andrographis (1,000 milligrams per day) or standard antibiotics to people with UTIs. The herb was as effective as the antibiotics for eliminating blood and pus from their urine.

LIVER PROTECTION. When liver-damaging toxic chemicals are ingested, or when the liver is infected (hepatitis), the organ produces more of specific enzymes. In animal studies, andrographis helps return these enzyme levels to normal, especially for liver damage caused by alcohol, certain carcinogens, and parasites. Liver protection from andrographis is similar to that achieved by the milk thistle extract, silymarin (see page 328).

Intriguing Possibilities

One animal study shows that pretreatment with andrographis reduced deaths from cobra venom, possibly validating the traditional Indian practice of using the herb to treat snakebite.

Some animal studies suggest that andrographis lowers blood sugar, which might help control diabetes. Further, pilot studies suggest that andrographis might treat malaria.

The herb also appears to reduce blood clotting, including the internal blood clots that cause heart attack and most strokes. This finding, if confirmed, might lead to its use in preventing these conditions.

Rx Recommendations

For immune stimulation, the traditional adult dose is 1 to 2 teaspoons (2 to 3 grams) of liquid extract per day. To treat colds and other infections, the dose is 4 teaspoons (6 grams) per day. But liquid extracts are too bitter to be palatable. Most andrographis products are sold as capsules. Follow package directions.

The Safety Factor

Andrographis is considered nontoxic. If taken at doses several times higher than recommended, however, stomach distress, loss of appetite, nausea, and vomiting are possible.

Andrographis reduces blood clotting. If you have a clotting disorder or are taking anticoagulant medication (including aspirin), talk to your doctor before using andrographis.

At high doses, andrographis suppresses the fertility of both male and female laboratory animals. The one human trial showed sperm suppression. Couples hoping to conceive should not use it.

Pregnant and nursing women should not use andrographis.

Do not give andrographis to children under 2. In older children, adjust the recommended dose based on the child's weight. For example, give a 50-pound child one-third of the dose a 150-pound adult would take.

If you're over 65, start with a low dose, and increase only if necessary.

If you use this herb, inform your health care professionals. Problematic herb-drug interactions are possible.

Andrographis may cause allergic reactions or other unexpected side effects. If unusual symptoms develop, reduce your dose or stop taking it.

For more on herb safety, see Chapter 2.

If symptoms get worse or persist longer than 2 weeks, consult a health care professional promptly.

Growing Information

Andrographis is not grown in the United States.

ANGELICA
An Angel of an Herb

Family: Umbelliferae; other members include carrot, parsley, celery, fennel, and dill

Genus and species: *Angelica archangelica* (European), *A. atropurpurea* (American), *A. sinensis* (Chinese), and other species

Also known as: Wild celery and masterwort; in China, dang gui and dong quai

Parts used: Roots, leaves, and seeds

Tall, striking, and attractive, angelica has played a role in magic and medicine for several thousand years. But the species used in Western and Chinese herbal medicine have always differed. So, too, have opinions of the herb's medicinal value.

In the West, European angelica has been a minor player. But in Asia, Chinese angelica, usually called dang gui, has long been considered a major herb for treating gynecological complaints. This claim is controversial, but still, Western researchers may have been too quick to dismiss Chinese angelica as medically worthless.

Healing History

In Asia, where Chinese angelica has been used since the dawn of history, the herb has always been considered the premier tonic for menstrual problems, menopausal complaints, and other women's health concerns. Traditional Chinese practitioners and Indian Ayurvedic physicians continue to prescribe it for gynecological conditions, arthritis, abdominal pain, colds, and flu.

European angelica has been viewed as a magical herb for more than 1,000 years. European peasants made angelica leaf necklaces to protect their children from illness and witchcraft. Angelica was reputed to be the only herb that witches never used, and its presence in a woman's garden or cupboard was once considered a defense against charges of witchcraft.

During the 16th and 17th centuries, the juice from crushed angelica roots was combined with other herbs to make "Carmelite water." This medieval drink was said to cure headache, promote relaxation and long life, and protect against poisons and witches' spells.

In 1665, Europe was decimated by bubonic plague. Legend has it that a monk dreamed that he met an angel, who showed him an herb that could cure the scourge. The herb was angelica, and the monk named it in honor of the angel in his dream. The name stuck, and angelica water was incorporated into the official English plague remedy, developed by the Royal College of Physicians in London and called the King's Excellent Plague Recipe.

History provides no clear verdict on the effectiveness of the "excellent recipe," but perhaps the old monk's dream was prophetic. Bubonic plague is a bacterial disease, and modern science has discovered that certain substances isolated from angelica have some antibacterial action.

During the 17th century, European angelica also became a popular treatment for colds and other respiratory ailments. Its stems are hollow, allowing air to pass through them. Under the Doctrine of Signatures—the medieval belief that an herb's physical appearance reveals its healing benefits—hollow-stemmed plants were considered beneficial for respiratory problems.

When European colonists arrived in North America, they found many Native American tribes using American angelica the same way their own healers used the European species—to treat respiratory ailments, particularly tuberculosis. Eventually, the colonists began using large doses to induce abortion. The 19th-century American Eclectic physicians, forerunners of today's naturopaths, recommended angelica for heartburn, indigestion, bronchitis, malaria, and typhoid.

Therapeutic Uses

Contrary to legend, angelica does not deliver humanity from epidemic disease, but the Chinese species of the herb has delivered a good deal of controversy. Two studies show benefit for menopausal discomforts, while one does not. Meanwhile, most of the traditional uses for European angelica have not stood up to scientific scrutiny all that well.

Contemporary herbalists generally recommend angelica mostly for digestive problems and to help clear mucus. These uses may have some validity.

MENOPAUSAL COMPLAINTS. Israeli researchers gave 55 women complaining of hot flashes either a placebo or a combination of dang gui and chamomile (75 milligrams of dang gui and 30 milligrams of chamomile, five times a day). After 12 weeks, the herb group reported significantly greater relief.

In the second study, researchers at the National College of Naturopathic Medicine in Portland, Oregon, and Bastyr University, the naturopathic medical school in Kenmore, Washington, gave 13 menopausal women either medically inactive placebos or a Chinese herbal formula containing dang gui, licorice root, hawthorn leaf, burdock root, and wild yam root. After 3 months, the women who took the herbal formula reported significantly greater relief.

In the one negative study, researchers at Kaiser Permanente Medical Center in Oakland, California, treated 71 menopausal women with dang gui for 3 months. This time, however, the women showed no improvement. Experts in Chinese herbal medicine have criticized the Kaiser Permanente study because it used only dang gui. In Chinese herbal medicine, the herb is never used alone; it's combined with other herbs in formulas, as was done in the other studies.

HEART DISEASE AND STROKE. Angelica species contain compounds, called coumarins, that have anticoagulant (blood-thinning) action. Blood thinners are used to prevent the internal blood clots that trigger heart attacks and most strokes. Chinese studies show that dang gui extract administered by injection helps dissolve the clots that cause stroke.

RESPIRATORY AILMENTS. Score one for the Doctrine of Signatures. German researchers have determined that angelica relaxes the windpipe, suggesting that it may have some value in treating colds, flu, bronchitis, and asthma.

DIGESTIVE PROBLEMS. The same German investigators found that angelica relaxes the intestines. This lends some credence to the herb's traditional use in treating digestive complaints.

ARTHRITIS. Japanese researchers have reported that angelica has anti-inflammatory effects, so there may be something to angelica's traditional Asian use as an arthritis treatment.

Intriguing Possibilities

Preliminary research from China suggests that dang gui increases red blood cell counts, indicating that the herb may someday prove beneficial in treating anemia.

The Chinese have also found that dang gui improves liver function in people with cirrhosis or chronic hepatitis. Their research is preliminary, however, and no specific recommendations can be made at this time about using angelica for liver problems.

A pilot study in China suggests that dang gui may help treat ulcerative colitis.

Rx Recommendations

If you'd like to use Chinese angelica to treat gynecological problems, consult a practitioner of Chinese herbal medicine for a multi-herb formula.

Commission E, the expert panel that evaluates herbal medicines for the German counterpart of the FDA, endorses European angelica as a treatment for appetite loss, abdominal distress, and flatulence.

There are many ways to prepare this herb,

depending on your personal preference. To make an infusion, use 1 teaspoon of powdered seeds or leaves per cup of boiling water. Steep for 10 to 20 minutes and strain if you wish.

For a decoction, use 1 teaspoon of powdered root per cup of water. Bring to a boil and simmer for 2 minutes. Remove from the heat, let stand for 15 minutes, and strain if you wish. Drink up to 2 cups a day. Angelica decoctions have a bitter taste.

As a homemade tincture, use $1/2$ to 1 teaspoon up to twice a day.

When using commercial preparations, follow the package directions.

The Safety Factor

Angelica has never been shown to stimulate uterine contractions, but given its traditional use to induce menstruation and abortions, women who are pregnant or trying to conceive should not use medicinal amounts.

Angelica contains chemicals known as psoralens. Exposure to sunlight may cause a rash in people who have ingested psoralens, a reaction known as photosensitivity. Psoralens may also promote tumor growth, leading the authors of a report in the journal *Science* to advise against taking angelica internally.

On the other hand, an animal study showed that the angelica constituent alpha-angelica lactone has an anticancer effect. Angelica's role in human cancer, if any, remains unclear. People with a history of cancer probably should not take the herb until questions about it have been answered.

Fresh angelica roots are poisonous, but drying eliminates the hazard. Herb gardeners should be sure to dry the roots thoroughly before using them.

Unless you are a confident field botanist, do not collect angelica in the wild. It's easy to confuse angelica with water hemlock (*Cicuta maculata*), an extremely poisonous plant.

For adults who are not pregnant or nursing, do not have a history of cancer or photosensitivity, and are not taking other anticoagulant medications, angelica is considered relatively safe in the amounts typically recommended.

Do not give angelica to children under 2. In older children, adjust the recommended dose based on the child's weight. For example, give a 50-pound child one-third of the dose a 150-pound adult would take.

If you're over 65, start with a low dose, and increase only if necessary.

Inform health care professionals of the herbs you use. Problematic herb-drug interactions are possible.

Angelica may cause allergic reactions or other unexpected side effects. If any develop, reduce your dose or stop taking it.

For more on herb safety, see Chapter 2.

If symptoms get worse or persist longer than 2 weeks, consult a health care professional promptly.

Growing Information

Angelica often blooms around May 8, the feast day of St. Michael the Archangel, which is the source of European angelica's species name, *archangelica*. The plant grows to 8 feet and resembles celery—hence its common name, wild celery—and is a biennial that dies after producing seeds. It grows from seeds or root divisions. Seed viability is relatively brief, only about 6 months, but refrigeration extends it up to a year. Germination may take a month. Sow angelica in the fall or spring $1/2$ inch deep in well-prepared beds. Space plants 2 feet apart in all directions.

Angelica thrives in rich, moist, well-drained, slightly acidic soil. It prefers partial shade. Leaves may be harvested in the fall of the first year and roots during the spring or fall of the second year.

Angelica is not usually considered a culinary herb, but fresh leaves provide a zesty accent to soups and salads. It has a fragrant aroma and a warm, vaguely sweet taste reminiscent of juniper, followed by a bitter aftertaste. You can eat steamed stems with butter, and chopped stems add flavor to roast pork.

APPLE
A Daily Dose of Protection

Family: Rosaceae; other members include rose, peach, almond, and strawberry

Genus and species: *Malus sylvestris* or *Pyrus malus*

Also known as: No other common names

Parts used: Fruits

"An apple a day keeps the doctor away." The old rhyme is truer than ever, particularly if the doctor is a gastroenterologist, oncologist, or cardiologist. Apples help treat both diarrhea and constipation, and they may help prevent cancer, heart disease, and some types of stroke—America's top three killers.

Although few contemporary herbalists consider the apple to be an herb, it has a venerable tradition as a healing agent. So much of what the ancient herbalists believed about the therapeutic powers of this delectable fruit has been scientifically supported that it's time to let the apple resume its respected place on the herbal roster.

Healing History

The Bible never identifies the Garden of Eden's "forbidden fruit," but since ancient times, people have believed that it was an apple. Legend has it that a piece got stuck in Adam's throat; hence the term *Adam's apple*.

The "apple of discord" started the Trojan War. Snow White's coma was induced by a poisoned apple. And William Tell shot an apple off his young son's head.

Then there was early America's own apple eccentric, John "Johnny Appleseed" Chapman. This pioneer spent most of his life wandering around Pennsylvania, Ohio, and Indiana sowing apple seeds—and becoming a legend.

The ancient Egyptians, Greeks, and Romans loved apples and developed dozens of varieties, but it was ancient India's traditional Ayurvedic physicians who first prescribed them to relieve diarrhea. Applesauce is still a popular home remedy for diarrhea.

Traditional Chinese physicians have used apple bark for centuries to treat diabetes, another use that's supported by modern science.

The medieval German abbess/herbalist Hildegard of Bingen prescribed raw apples as a tonic for healthy people and cooked apples as the first treatment for any sickness.

Around the same time in England, people said, "To eat an apple before going to bed/ Will make the doctor beg his bread." This evolved into our saying about an apple a day.

Not everything the English had to say about apples was so apt, however. Seventeenth-century English herbalist Nicholas Culpeper recommended apples "for hot and bilious stomachs . . . inflammations of the breast and lungs . . . [and] asthma." He also suggested boiled apples mixed with milk as a treatment for gunpowder burns.

The Americas had no native apples, but the Pilgrims brought apple seeds with them, and the fruit quickly became, well, as American as apple pie. Apples, apple bark, and apple cider soon became mainstays of American folk medicine.

Speaking of apple pie, when the poor baked pies, they used only a bottom crust. Richer bakers could afford to add a top crust—hence our description of the wealthy as "upper crust."

A century ago, American Eclectic physicians, forerunners of today's naturopaths, recommended apples in many forms: raw apples for constipation, baked or stewed apples for minor fevers, apple bark decoction for intermittent fever (malaria), and apple cider "as a refreshing drink for patients with fever."

Therapeutic Uses

Modern medical science has found that Johnny Appleseed's favorite fruit has tremendous value in healing thanks to its pulp, which is high in pectin, a soluble form of fiber.

DIARRHEA. Studies show that pectin helps relieve diarrhea because intestinal bacteria transform it into a soothing, protective coating for the irritated intestinal lining. In addition, pectin adds bulk to the stool, which helps resolve diarrhea.

Some diarrhea results from bacterial infection. One study found that apple pectin is effective against several types of bacteria that are known to cause diarrhea, among them salmonella, staphylococcus, and *Escherichia coli*. In fact, pectin is the "pectate" in the over-the-counter diarrhea preparation Kaopectate.

CONSTIPATION. Physicians recommend diets high in fiber to add bulk to stool. Since pectin is a type of fiber, it can help with constipation by adding bulk and stimulating bowel contractions.

HEART DISEASE AND STROKE. A diet high in fiber helps reduce blood cholesterol, a key risk factor for heart disease and some types of stroke. In the presence of fiber, the cholesterol we eat remains in the intestinal tract until it is eliminated. So if you eat a pectin-rich, high-fiber apple for dessert when you have meat and dairy products, you will enjoy some protection from their cholesterol.

In a long-term study involving 805 Dutch men, researchers discovered that those who ate the most apples experienced the fewest heart attacks. The scientists concluded that in addition to pectin, compounds in apples called flavonoids played an important protective role. Flavonoids are antioxidants that help prevent the cell damage that's at the root of the arterial narrowing that leads to heart disease.

CANCER. The American Cancer Society recommends a high-fiber diet to help prevent several forms of cancer, particularly colon cancer. Pectin binds certain cancer-causing compounds in the colon, speeding their elimination from the body, according to a study published in the *Journal of the National Cancer Institute*.

The antioxidant flavonoids in apples also help prevent the cell damage that causes many cancers.

DIABETES. Physicians also recommend a high-fiber diet to control diabetes. A study published in the *Annals of Internal Medicine* showed that apple pectin helps reduce blood sugar (glucose) levels in people with the disease.

TOXIN EXPOSURE. European studies suggest that apple pectin helps eliminate lead, mercury, and other toxic heavy metals from the body. Cleansing the body of these poisons is yet another reason for people who live in polluted cities to enjoy the proverbial apple a day.

WOUNDS. Although pectin is the apple's major medicinal component, the fruit's leaves contain an antibiotic called phloretin. If you cut yourself out in the orchard, you can use apple leaves as immediate first aid.

Intriguing Possibility

A few studies, including one published in the *Journal of the National Cancer Institute*, hint that pectin may help keep cancer from spreading around the body (metastasizing).

Rx Recommendations

For handy first aid for minor wounds, crush some apple leaves and apply them to the cut or scrape until you can wash and bandage it.

Eat the whole fresh fruit to enjoy a wide range of healthful benefits. Green apples tend to be tart, but they usually have more "snap." Red apples are usually sweeter but may have a mealy texture. Wash apples with soap and water before eating to eliminate any pesticide residue.

The Safety Factor

James A. Duke, Ph.D., retired USDA herbal medicine authority (and poet), sums up apple safety this way:

> *An apple a day keeps the doctor away,*
> *Or at least that's what some people say.*
> *But one man, we read,*
> *Ate a cupful of seed,*
> *And this man died.*
> *Overdosed. Cyanide.*

It's strange but true: Apple seeds contain high levels of cyanide, the powerful poison. About $1/2$ cup of seeds can be deadly for the average adult, but considerably less is fatal for children and the elderly. Many parents are familiar with the stomachaches that young children develop when they eat apple cores. The few seeds in the typical core pose little risk of serious poisoning. But to be prudent, teach children not to eat apple seeds, and stay away from them yourself.

If apples or applesauce cause minor discomfort, such as diarrhea or constipation, reduce your consumption. If diarrhea or constipation does not improve within a week, consult a physician.

Growing Information

Archeologists have found evidence that humans have been enjoying apples since at least 6500 B.C. Prehistoric apples resembled today's crab apples—small, dry, and mealy. But as agriculture developed, apples became one of the world's first hybridized orchard fruits.

Today, about 300 apple varieties grow in the 50 states. Special varieties have been developed for just about every set of growing conditions in North America. Consult a nursery for the varieties best suited to your locale.

Full-size apple trees grow to about 40 feet and spread over 1,600 square feet (40 by 40). Genetic dwarf apple varieties produce delicious, full-size fruits but grow to only 6 to 12 feet and spread over less than 150 square feet (12 by 12).

Plant the rootstock in a sunny location and water regularly. Prune at planting, then annually. Different apple varieties have different fertilizer requirements and different pest problems. Consult a nursery for advice.

ARNICA

Controversial Homeopathic Wound Treatment

Family: Asteraceae; other members include daisy

Genus and species: *Arnica montana*

Also known as: Mountain daisy, wolfsbane, leopard's bane

Parts used: Dried flower heads

Arnica is homeopathic first aid for wounds, injuries, and muscle soreness. But mainstream physicians scoff at homeopathy in general and homeopathic arnica in particular. The studies go both ways, some showing benefit, others showing none. But the weight of the evidence tilts in favor of arnica.

Healing History

For centuries, European herbalists used arnica in salves and ointments as a topical treatment for injuries, bruising, and pain. They also prescribed teas and tinctures made from arnica for a variety of conditions, including menstrual problems, paralysis, and typhoid fever.

The German philosopher Johann Wolfgang von Goethe drank arnica tea to ease his angina, chest pain caused by heart disease. But he used a very low dose because arnica was also well known for its toxicity. Even modest amounts cause nausea, vomiting, and diarrhea. Larger amounts suppress respiration and cause coma and death. As a result, America's 19th-century Eclectic physicians used this herb externally only to treat wounds, bruising, pain, and inflammation.

Arnica is most widely prescribed by homeopaths. Homeopathy, developed in the 1830s by the German physician Samuel Hahnemann (1755–1843), is very controversial because it uses microdose medicines, treatments so dilute that standard pharmacology insists they could not possibly have any effect. Nonetheless, for reasons science cannot currently explain, many treatments using homeopathic doses of herbal medicines, including arnica, have shown benefits in rigorous scientific studies.

Therapeutic Uses

Recent studies of arnica are confusing. Some show benefit. Others do not. Results showing benefit are often barely statistically significant. But results that show no benefit often miss statistical significance by very little. So the scientific cases for and against arnica are not very compelling. Nonetheless, the majority of studies show benefit, and in homeopathic doses, this herb is safe and inexpensive.

SURGICAL PAIN AND BRUISING. Homeopaths prescribe arnica most often for pain caused by injuries. As a result, most of the arnica research has dealt with pain.

German researchers gave 88 people having bunion surgery either a standard drug for pain and inflammation (diclofenac, brand name Voltaren) or homeopathic arnica (10 tiny pills three times a day). Both groups took their medication for 4 days after surgery. The drug and homeopathic arnica were equally effective for bruising, swelling, and wound tenderness. Diclofenac was more effective for pain. But those taking arnica got back on their feet more quickly and comfortably. The researchers concluded: "After foot operations, arnica can be used instead of diclofenac."

Welsh scientists gave 190 adults having tonsillectomies either a placebo or homeopathic arnica (two tiny pills six times the day after surgery, then two tiny pills a day for the next week). The arnica group reported significantly less pain.

German researchers gave 60 people having surgery to remove varicose veins either a placebo or arnica (five tiny pills three times a day for 2 weeks). The arnica group reported significantly less bruising and pain.

Plastic surgeons in Farmington, Connecticut, gave 29 people having face-lifts either a placebo or arnica for 10 days after surgery. The people taking arnica had less bruising.

But not all the research involves homeopathic doses taken by mouth. Swiss researchers gave 204 people with osteoarthritis of the hands either a standard topical ointment containing ibuprofen (Motrin, Advil) or an arnica ointment. After 21 days, both groups reported the same relief.

MUSCLE SORENESS. Norwegian researchers tested arnica in runners in two Oslo mara-

thons (1990 and 1995). A total of 82 runners were given either a placebo or arnica (five tiny pills starting the evening before the races, then morning and evening of race day and for 3 days after). The arnica group reported less muscle soreness.

Commission E, the expert panel that evaluates herbal medicines for the German counterpart of the FDA, approves arnica ointments for muscle aches, inflammation, and insect bites and stings.

Intriguing Possibility

Animal studies suggest that arnica may stimulate the immune system.

Rx Recommendations

When using arnica ointments or homeopathic pills, follow package directions. Or consult a homeopath for advice.

The Safety Factor

Do not ingest arnica plant material. It's poisonous. It causes nausea, vomiting, gastrointestinal distress, and in high doses, coma, cardiac arrest, and death. If you grow arnica, keep the plant away from young children, and warn older children not to ingest it.

Ingest this herb *only* in homeopathic doses, which are too low to cause problems. Consult a homeopath for appropriate dosages for children and those over the age of 65.

Pregnant and nursing women should not ingest arnica. Use of topical ointments is fine.

If you use this herb, inform your health care

professionals. Problematic herb-drug interactions are possible.

Arnica may cause allergic reactions or other unexpected side effects. If unusual symptoms develop, reduce your dose or stop taking it.

For more on herb safety, see Chapter 2.

If symptoms get worse or persist longer than 2 weeks, consult a health care professional promptly.

Growing Information

Arnica is native to cool, mountainous regions of Europe and Russia. It also grows at higher elevations in the northwestern United States. Arnica is a perennial that grows to 12 inches and produces bright yellow, daisylike flowers, hence the name mountain daisy. Sow seed in the spring in a mix of loam, peat moss, and sand. Arnica likes acid pH, full sun, moisture, and a high altitude. The flowers smell unpleasant, but the odor subsides as they dry. Pulverize dried flowers and make a tincture. Mix some tincture with hand lotion or skin cream for a topical ointment.

ARTICHOKE

The Delicious Vegetable with Surprising Medical Benefits

Family: Compositae or Asteraceae; other members include thistle

Genus and species: *Cynara scolymus*

Also known as: Garden artichoke, globe artichoke

Parts used: The flower and lower portions of the barbed scales that enclose it

Quick: What's the best herb for preventing and treating liver problems? If you're familiar with herbal medicine, you know the answer: milk thistle (see page 327). But artichoke, though less well known, is almost as beneficial. It's a close botanical relative of milk thistle; its species name, *scolymus*, derives from the Greek word for thistle. In traditional European herbal medicine, the two were used almost interchangeably.

But artichoke is more than just a tasty vegetable that helps maintain liver health. It also soothes the stomach, lowers cholesterol, and treats irritable bowel syndrome.

Healing History

Twenty-five hundred years ago, the ancient Greek naturalist Theophrastus wrote about a plant native to the Mediterranean, particularly to Sicily: "The head [flower bud] is most pleasant, being boiled." He called the plant scolymus, which is now artichoke's species name. Theophrastus's scolymus was wild artichoke, or cardoon (*Cynara cardunculus*). Ancient farmers cultivated it as well as bred it, selecting for larger flower buds. By the Middle Ages, they had produced today's globe artichokes, which continued to be called cardoons (or cardone, cardoni, carduni, or cardi) until the 19th century.

The ancient Greeks, Romans, and Egyptians used cardoon/artichoke as both a food and a medicine. As a food, it was considered a delicacy. As a medicine, the flower and the plant's juice were used to promote digestion and treat upset stomach and liver problems (jaundice).

One type of artichoke, blessed thistle, was so popular in 17th-century England that in his famous *Complete Herbal* (1652), the noted English herbalist Nicholas Culpeper wrote: "I shall spare the labour of writing a description as almost everyone may describe them from their own knowledge." Culpeper called blessed thistle "an excellent remedy" for jaundice and gallbladder problems, and recommended it for plague, boils, and "the bites of mad dogs and venomous beasts." He also said it "cures the French pox," that is, syphilis.

In France, for centuries artichoke juice has been a traditional liver tonic.

America's 19th-century Eclectic physicians recommended artichoke for liver disease, gout, and muscle aches (rheumatism). They also considered artichoke juice an aphrodisiac.

Therapeutic Uses

LIVER PROBLEMS. Like milk thistle, artichoke has considerable antioxidant action that spurs regeneration of liver cells. Several studies indicate that in animals treated with liver-damaging chemicals, artichoke minimizes liver damage and increases survival.

INDIGESTION. German researchers gave 244 adults with chronic indigestion either a placebo or artichoke extract (640 milligrams twice a day). After 6 weeks, the artichoke group reported significantly greater relief and improved quality of life. In a similar study, British scientists reported the same findings.

Commission E, the expert panel that evaluates herbal medicines for the German counterpart of the FDA, approves fresh artichoke and its leaf extract and juice for indigestion.

IRRITABLE BOWEL SYNDROME (IBS). This common condition causes chronic digestive problems including abdominal pain, bloating, diarrhea or constipation, and a general feeling that one's digestion is out of control. Because artichoke helps treat indigestion, British researchers thought it might also alleviate IBS. They gave 208 adult IBS sufferers either a placebo or artichoke extract (320 or 640 milligrams per day). Two months later, compared with the placebo group, the artichoke group reported 41 percent greater relief than did the placebo group.

HIGH CHOLESTEROL. A few studies show

that artichoke lowers cholesterol. In one trial, German researchers gave people with high cholesterol either a placebo or 450 milligrams of artichoke extract daily. After 6 weeks, the placebo group's total cholesterol fell 9 percent, but in the artichoke group, it dropped 19 percent, a 10 percent difference. For every 1 percent decrease in total cholesterol, heart attack risk drops 2 percent. So thanks to artichoke, participants' risk of heart attack decreased 20 percent. The researchers called their findings "clear evidence for recommending artichoke" as a treatment for high cholesterol. And an Italian study shows that in addition to lowering cholesterol, artichoke juice (about 1 cup a day) also improves arterial health by reducing the deposits that narrow them.

ANTIMICROBIAL. Artichoke inhibits the activity of several bacteria and fungi.

Intriguing Possibilities

Pilot studies suggest that artichoke may have some pain-relieving and anti-inflammatory action.

Artichoke may also reduce blood sugar and help manage diabetes.

Finally, one study shows that when male laboratory animals are exposed to chemicals that damage testicular tissue, artichoke treatment minimizes the damage.

Medicinal Myths

In some folk medicine traditions, artichokes were recommended to treat hangover. British researchers gave 15 adults either artichoke extract (three standard capsules) or a placebo immediately after the participants drank enough alcohol to cause intoxication and hangover. One week later, the treatments were switched so that the artichoke group took the placebo and vice versa. There were no differences in hangover duration or discomfort between the artichoke and placebo groups. Artichoke does not reduce hangover.

Rx Recommendations

Artichoke extract is available at some health food stores or on the Internet. But why buy extract when artichokes themselves are available cheaper as a vegetable? Steam them for 30 to 45 minutes. Pull off and discard the outer scales. Dip the inner scales in melted butter, yogurt, or mustard and eat the fleshy base. When you get down to the flower, remove the immature scales and central hairs, and eat the heart.

The Safety Factor

Frequent contact with artichoke may cause allergic reactions, notably skin irritation or hives.

Commission E warns that people with gallstones or obstructed bile ducts should consult a physician before using artichoke medicinally.

Growing Information

Don't confuse this plant with Jerusalem artichoke (*Helianthis tuberosus*), which is a species of sunflower.

Artichoke is a perennial that can grow to 6 feet tall and 4 feet wide. Flower buds (heads) appear in July in the southern United States, or in August in the northern United States and Canada.

Growing requires 100 frost-free days a year. Soil should be rich with compost and manure, and well drained. Artichokes like slightly acid soil (pH 6.0). Seeds can be started indoors in early spring and transplanted after the last frost. Watering well encourages large artichokes.

Replace some older plants each year. Take suckers or side roots from your healthiest plants to propagate.

ASHWAGANDHA
India's Potent Adaptogen

Family: Solanaceae; other members include tomato, potato, and bell pepper

Genus and species: *Withania somnifera*

Also known as: Withania, Indian ginseng, winter cherry, dunal

Parts used: Roots

Ashwagandha is known as Indian ginseng because its effects are similar to the revered Chinese herb. Known as an adaptogen, it strengthens the whole body and treats fatigue, weakness, debility, and many age-related conditions.

Healing History

Ashwagandha is a small evergreen shrub native to India, though it also grows in the Middle East and in East Africa. It produces a small, smooth, round, fleshy fruit that contains many seeds and turns reddish orange when ripe, hence the name winter cherry.

Ashwagandha has been used in India's traditional Ayurvedic medicine for at least 3,000 years. It was discussed in several ancient Ayurvedic medical texts, including the *Charak,* which recommends it as a whole-body tonic, particularly for those suffering from emaciation, and as an aid for enhancing reproductive function and longevity. It has also been used to treat arthritis, muscle aches, inflammation, and conditions associated with aging.

Therapeutic Uses

Like ginseng, rhodiola, and a few other herbs, ashwagandha is considered a "tonic" or "adaptogen" in Chinese and Ayurvedic medicine. The term was coined in 1947 by Russian scientist N. V. Lazarev, Ph.D, of the Academy of Sciences of the former Soviet Union, who was interested in drugs that help the body adapt to physical and emotional stress. His student, Israel I. Brekhman, Ph.D., popularized the term and showed that the most powerful adaptogens are not drugs, but herbs. Dr. Lazarev and Dr. Brekhman believed that adaptogens should:

- Counteract the adverse effects of stress
- Increase energy
- Increase the body's resistance to a broad range of adverse influences
- Have a normalizing effect, improving many conditions while aggravating none
- Cause minimal side effects

Since Dr. Brekhman's death in 1994, the term *adaptogen* has been generalized to include herbs that don't necessarily boost energy or counteract stress, but still have a number of benefits including enhanced immune function, antioxidant action, and physiological normalization.

Unfortunately, in American medical history, the term *tonic* has negative connotations. Many 19th-century patent medicines sold as "rejuvenating tonics" contained mostly alcohol and/or opium. In addition, drug advertising has socialized Americans to expect that individual drugs treat just one problem. We're not used to the idea that one drug—or herb—can have a broad range of physical and mental health benefits. But ashwagandha has quite a few.

ENHANCED IMMUNITY. Several Indian animal studies show that ashwagandha stimulates the immune system, boosts antibody and red blood cell levels, and spurs white blood cells to devour germs.

STAMINA. Animal studies show that the herb improves physical stamina and endurance.

STRESS RESISTANCE. In one Indian study, laboratory animals were subjected to mild electrical shocks that produced chronic stress, resulting in learning problems, immune suppression, high blood sugar, increased levels of stress hormones, stomach ulcers, and male sexual dysfunction. But when the animals were given ashwagandha before the shocks, their stress symptoms were significantly reduced. Other studies agree and "support the use of ashwagandha as an anti-stress adaptogen."

PREVENTION OF DEGENERATIVE DISEASES. Ashwagandha is also a powerful antioxidant that neutralizes dangerous free radical molecules in the bloodstream, thus preventing and reversing the cellular damage at the root of heart disease and most cancers. In addition, animal studies show that the herb's antioxidant action also helps protect the liver and kidneys.

HEART DISEASE. Indian researchers gave laboratory animals drugs that damage the heart. Before this, some of the animals were treated with ashwagandha. The drugs damaged their hearts significantly less, prompting the researchers to conclude that ashwagandha "exerts a strong cardio-protective effect."

HIGH CHOLESTEROL. Adding to the herb's heart benefits, ashwagandha also lowers cholesterol. In a study published in the *Indian Journal of Experimental Biology*, researchers gave ashwagandha daily to people with both diabetes and high cholesterol. After a month, their cholesterol levels had declined significantly.

DIABETES. In the same Indian cholesterol study, the participants' blood sugar levels also declined. The decrease "was comparable to that produced by oral diabetes medication."

CANCER. Indian animal studies show that this herb reduces the risk of skin cancer and other tumors, and boosts the effectiveness of radiation treatments.

Intriguing Possibilities

Ashwagandha appears to have some antidepressant and anti-anxiety action. It may also protect against seizures and loss of cognitive function due to toxic chemicals.

Rx Recommendations

The recommended dose is 1 to 6 grams per day (2 to 12 teaspoons) in capsules or tea. In tincture or liquid extract, use 2 to 4 milliliters three times a day.

The Safety Factor

Very high doses of ashwagandha may cause stomach upset, diarrhea, nausea, vomiting, drowsiness, dulling of reflexes, and loss of motor abilities.

Large doses may trigger abortion. Pregnant and nursing women should not use ashwagandha.

Do not give ashwagandha to children under 2. In older children, adjust the recommended dose based on the child's weight. For example, give a 50-pound child one-third of the dose a 150-pound adult would take.

If you're over 65, start with a low dose, and increase only if necessary.

If you use this herb, inform your health care professionals. Problematic herb-drug interactions are possible.

Ashwagandha may cause allergic reactions or other unexpected side effects. If unusual symptoms develop, reduce your dose or stop taking it.

For more on herb safety, see Chapter 2.

If symptoms get worse or persist longer than 2 weeks, consult a health care professional promptly.

Growing Information

Ashwagandha is hardly grown in the United States, but it can be grown in the South and Southwest. The plant is an erect shrub that grows to 3 feet in the wild, but cultivated plants grow larger. This herb grows primarily in dry, subtropical areas of India to an elevation of about 5,000 feet. It also grows from Pakistan to Egypt, and in Spain, Morocco, the Canary Islands, and South Africa.

Keep seeds moist but not too wet. Seeds germinate within 2 weeks at 70°F. This herb prefers full sun and sandy soil. The fruit is harvested in the late fall, and the bright yellow seeds are dried for planting the following spring. Harvest the medicinal root in the fall after the first frost. Roots are either dried whole or cut into pieces and dried.

ASTRAGALUS
An Asian Immunity Booster

Family: Leguminosae; other members include beans and peas

Genus and species: *Astragalus membranaceus*

Also known as: Huang qi, yellow leader, and milk vetch

Parts used: Roots

The Chinese refer to astragalus as huang qi, which, loosely translated, means "strengthener of qi." *Qi* (or *chi*) is the Chinese term for life force, vitality, stamina, disease resistance, and the ability to cope with physical and emotional stress. As a strengthener of qi, astragalus is powerful medicine.

Healing History

The medicinal use of astragalus was first recorded in China some 2,000 years ago.

Modern-day practitioners of Chinese medicine believe that the herb strengthens all body systems and that it's particularly effective for treating illnesses that cause fatigue. They consider it similar to ginseng, and they prescribe it for diabetes, heart disease, and high blood pressure.

Therapeutic Uses

Western scientists began to study astragalus only in the past few decades, so there are still more questions than answers about the herb's effects. But research to date confirms the Chinese claims.

ENHANCED IMMUNITY. The first Western study of astragalus took place in 1983 at the University of Texas M. D. Anderson Cancer Center in Houston. The herb improved immune function in 19 cancer patients who were being treated with immune-suppressing chemotherapy drugs.

Since then, several studies—both animal and human—have shown that astragalus, administered either orally or by injection, improves various measures of immune function. In one study, infection-fighting human T cells became significantly more vigorous after being treated with astragalus. In another, astragalus injected into mice improved the ability of their infection-fighting macrophages (a type of white blood cell) to devour bacteria, viruses, and fungi.

In a Chinese study, 10 people with viral heart infections and depressed immune systems were given daily injections of 8 grams of astragalus extract. The patients' immune system functions improved significantly.

In another Chinese study, 235 women with various chronic viral infections, among them herpes, were treated with immune-boosting interferon and/or astragalus. The herb by itself did not provide much benefit. But astragalus plus interferon produced the best antiviral effect.

Currently, Americans are most likely to use astragalus while taking immune-suppressing cancer chemotherapy drugs.

HEART DISEASE. Chinese researchers gave astragalus to 92 people with angina, a form of heart disease that causes chest pain on minor exertion. The herb reduced chest pain in 83 percent of them. In another Chinese study, compared with heart attack sufferers who did not take the herb, those treated with it showed significantly improved heart function.

LIVER DAMAGE. Chinese researchers exposed mice to stilbenemide, a cancer chemotherapy drug that causes liver damage as a side effect. Animals that received only the drug developed serious liver damage, while those given the drug plus an oral astragalus extract did not.

Intriguing Possibilities

Other Chinese studies suggest that astragalus improves sperm motility, reduces blood pressure, improves heart function, and enhances immune function in people infected with HIV, the virus that causes AIDS.

Rx Recommendations

When using the dried root sticks, finely chop four or five sticks and simmer them in 4 cups of boiling water for 1 hour. Drink 1 cup in the morning and 1 cup in the evening. Astragalus tastes mildly sweet, but you may prefer it blended with other herbal beverages.

Astragalus is also available in a variety of commercial preparations, including tinctures, capsules, and tablets. Follow the package directions.

The Safety Factor

Astragalus is generally considered safe when used as recommended. One laboratory test, however, found that a strong decoction caused chromosome mutations, a hint that the herb might be carcinogenic. Traditional Chinese herbalists recommend using astragalus for only a few weeks during an illness, and not routinely. This would be prudent advice if the herb's mutagenic action is confirmed.

Chinese practitioners advise against taking astragalus for acute infections; instead, they recommend reserving it to strengthen the body after it has begun to heal.

Pregnant and nursing women should not use astragalus.

Do not give astragalus to children under 2. In older children, adjust the recommended dose based on the child's weight. For example, give a 50-pound child one-third of the dose a 150-pound adult would take.

If you're over 65, start with a low dose, and increase only if necessary.

Inform health care professionals of the herbs you use. Problematic herb-drug interactions are possible.

Astragalus may cause allergic reactions or other unexpected side effects. If any develop, reduce your dose or stop taking it.

For more on herb safety, see Chapter 2.

If symptoms get worse or persist longer than 2 weeks, consult a health care professional promptly.

Growing Information

Astragalus is not grown in the United States. It is a perennial plant native to northern China and Mongolia that produces small yellow flowers. Its thick, carrotlike root has a tough fibrous skin with a yellowish interior, which is the medicinal part. The root has a sweetish, licorice-like taste.

In China, the root is peeled and dried, sometimes after being soaked in honey. Then it's cut into long slices that resemble ice-pop sticks. Chinese herb shops sell the sticks, but for U.S. consumers, the herb is typically powdered and sold in capsules.

BACOPA

This Herb Can Make You Smarter

Family: Scrophulariaceae; other members include snapdragon

Genus and species: *Bacopa monnieri*

Also known as: Brahmi, water hyssop

Parts used: Whole plant

Bacopa is an age-old Ayurvedic remedy for the nervous system. Another Ayurvedic herb, gotu kola (*Centella asiatica,* see page 264), was used similarly. As a result, both of these herbs share the Sanskrit name *brahmi*. This has caused confusion. To avoid mix-ups, most herbalists have stopped using the term *brahmi*, and refer to these herbs as bacopa and gotu kola.

Healing History

In India's traditional Ayurvedic medicine, bacopa was used to improve learning, memory, and concentration. It was also recommended to treat anxiety, seizures, and mental illness. In addition to nervous complaints, bacopa is also a traditional Ayurvedic treatment for respiratory conditions, urinary incontinence, and heart problems. Modern research has shown that bacopa offers so many health benefits that Indian researchers consider it an adaptogen—an herb that enhances total well-being—like ginseng, ashwagandha, or rhodiola.

Therapeutic Uses

LEARNING, MEMORY, AND CONCENTRATION. Many of bacopa's traditional uses have been confirmed by modern research, particularly its brain-boosting power. The herb contains compounds, bacosides, that enhance nerve impulse transmission. As early as 1966, a study showed that bacopa increases neurotransmitter levels in the brain involved in learning and reasoning. Since then, many animal studies and a few clinical trials have shown that this herb is a brain-booster.

In several studies, Australian and Indian researchers gave middle-aged adults either a placebo or bacopa (300 milligrams a day), and then administered a series of standard cognitive function tests. In one study, after 5 weeks, the herb improved speed of learning and other measures of mental function. In another, after 12 weeks, the bacopa group showed significant improvement in speed of processing new information, learning, and memory consolidation.

But bacopa is not a quick fix for students who want to cram for exams. No improvement in cognitive function is seen shortly after it's taken. Instead, it takes several weeks for cognitive benefits to become measurable.

Indian studies also show that 3 to 9 months of daily bacopa improve children's IQ scores.

ATTENTION DEFICIT/HYPERACTIVITY DISORDER (ADHD). Indian psychiatrists gave 36 children with ADHD either a placebo or bacopa (50 milligrams twice a day). After 12 weeks, the bacopa group showed improvement in memory and learning.

PREVENTION OF DEGENERATIVE DISEASES. How do the bacosides in bacopa boost brain power? They have antioxidant action. Antioxidants prevent or reverse the cellular damage caused by highly reactive oxygen ions, known as free radicals. Antioxidants reduce risk of heart disease and cancer. But for reasons that still puzzle scientists, bacosides appear to focus their antioxidant action on the parts of the brain involved in reasoning and memory, the frontal cortex and hippocampus.

LIVER PROTECTION. The antioxidants in bacopa also protect the liver from drug-induced damage.

ANXIETY. Animal studies show that bacopa has anti-anxiety action comparable to drugs in the Valium family. In one Indian study, 35 people suffering severe anxiety took large doses of the herb (12 grams per day). After 2 weeks, they were significantly less anxious.

THYROID DISEASE. Bacopa stimulates production of thyroid hormone, suggesting value in treating hypothyroidism.

INFLAMMATION. Bacopa also has anti-inflammatory action. One study suggests that it's as effective as the standard nonsteroidal anti-inflammatory drug (NSAID) indomethacin (Indocin), but without the stomach upset common with NSAIDs.

Intriguing Possibilities

Traditional Ayurvedic physicians used bacopa to treat epileptic seizures. Animal studies show it does have anticonvulsant action—but only at very high doses.

In other animal studies, bacopa has been shown to open the airway into the lungs, serving as a bronchodilator. As a result, it may help treat bronchitis and asthma.

Bacopa may also act as a stomach soother. Pilot studies suggest that bacopa has a relaxing effect on the digestive tract and may be beneficial for indigestion and irritable bowel syndrome. Bacopa suppresses *Helicobacter pylori*, the bacteria that causes ulcers.

Finally, the herb has been shown to inhibit growth of certain cancer cells.

Rx Recommendations

The traditional adult dose is 5 to 10 grams of powdered herb (or 5 to 12 milliliters of fluid extract) per day in divided doses. Or you can take 200 to 400 milligrams per day of bacopa extracts standardized to 20 percent bacosides. When using commercial preparations, follow package directions.

The Safety Factor

At recommended doses, bacopa causes no known side effects. But at unusually high doses, it becomes a sedative.

Pregnant and nursing women should not use bacopa.

Do not give bacopa to children under 2. In older children, adjust the recommended dose based on the child's weight. For example, give a 50-pound child one-third of the dose a 150-pound adult would take.

If you're over 65, start with a low dose, and increase only if necessary.

Inform health care professionals of the herbs

you use. Problematic herb-drug interactions are possible.

Bacopa may cause allergic reactions or other unexpected side effects. If any develop, reduce your dose or stop taking it.

For more on herb safety, see Chapter 2.

If symptoms get worse or persist longer than 2 weeks, consult a health care professional promptly.

Growing Information

Bacopa is a hardy, creeping ground cover with small oblong leaves and white or purple flowers. It likes marshy soil and can be grown in temperate or warmer areas at elevations to 4,500 feet with adequate water. Water frequently.

BARBERRY
A Powerful Infection Fighter

Family: Berbericlaceae; other members include May apple and mandrake

Genus and species: *Berberis vulgaris*; Oregon grape: *B. aquifolium* or *Mahonia aquifolium*

Also known as: Berberry, berberis, and jaundice berry

Part used: Root bark

Who says herbs can't compete with pharmaceutical drugs? In one study, berberine, the active constituent in barberry, proved more potent against bacteria than chloramphenicol, a powerful pharmaceutical antibiotic.

But there's a lot more to this herb than mere infection treatment. Barberry, and its close relative Oregon grape, may also stimulate the immune system, reduce blood pressure, and even shrink some tumors.

Healing History

Barberry has played a prominent role in herbal healing for more than 2,500 years. The ancient Egyptians relied on it to prevent plague, a use that was probably beneficial considering the herb's antibiotic action. India's traditional Ayurvedic healers prescribed barberry for dysentery, another use that's been confirmed by modern science.

During the early Middle Ages, European herbalists were guided by the Doctrine of Signatures, the belief that a plant's physical appearance revealed its therapeutic benefits. Barberry has yellow flowers, and its roots produce a yellow dye. These features were linked to the yellowing of the skin and eyes associated with jaundice, a symptom of liver disease. As a result, barberry was widely used to treat liver and gallbladder ailments, earning it the name jaundice berry.

In addition to treating liver and gallbladder ailments, traditional Russian healers recommended it for skin inflammations, high blood pressure, and abnormal uterine bleeding.

When colonists introduced barberry into North America, the Native Americans recognized it as a relative of the native Oregon grape, a hollylike plant that they considered a powerful healer. Many tribes adopted barberry enthusiastically and used it to treat dysentery, mouth ulcers, sore throat, wound infections, and intestinal complaints.

The 19th-century American Eclectic physicians, forerunners of today's naturopaths, prescribed barberry as a purgative and treatment for jaundice, dysentery, eye infections, cholera, fevers, and "impurities of the blood," which was a euphemism for syphilis.

Barberry was also an ingredient in the popular but highly controversial Hoxsey Cancer Formula, an alternative cancer therapy marketed from the 1930s to the 1950s by ex–coal miner Harry Hoxsey (see page 33).

Therapeutic Uses

Most present-day herbalists limit their recommendations to gargling barberry decoction for sore throat and drinking it for diarrhea and constipation. But if they were reading the medical journals, they'd be recommending it for a great deal more.

INFECTIONS. The berberine in barberry has remarkable infection-fighting properties. Studies around the world show that it kills microorganisms that cause wound infections (staphylococcus and streptococcus), diarrhea (salmonella and shigella), dysentery (*Entamoeba histolytica*), cholera (*Vibrio cholerae*), giardiasis (*Giardia lamblia*), urinary tract infections (*Escherichia coli*), and vaginal yeast infections (*Candida albicans*).

ENHANCED IMMUNITY. Berberine may also fight infection by stimulating the immune system. Studies show that it activates macrophages (literally, "big eaters"), the white blood cells that devour harmful microorganisms.

LIVER DAMAGE. Score one for the Doctrine of Signatures and "jaundice berry." Pakistani researchers gave laboratory animals large doses of acetaminophen to produce liver damage, as measured by significant increases in blood levels of liver enzymes. Then some of the animals were treated with a barberry preparation. Levels of liver enzymes remained abnormally high in the animals that didn't receive barberry, but in those that did, the enzymes declined, showing significant normalization of liver function. The researchers concluded, "This study provides a scientific basis for the traditional use of barberry in liver disorders."

PSORIASIS. Barberry's traditional use as a treatment for skin problems was confirmed by German researchers in a 4-week study involving 82 people with psoriasis, a condition that produces red, raised, scaly skin eruptions. Each study participant was given two tubes of ointment—one with barberry extract, the other without. The tubes were marked "left" and "right," and people were instructed to apply each ointment to the respective sides of their bodies. The barberry ointment produced significantly greater shrinkage of skin eruptions.

PINKEYE. Barberry's traditional use for treating eye problems is alive and well in Germany, where a berberine preparation called Ophthiole is prescribed to treat sensitive eyes, inflamed lids, and pinkeye (conjunctivitis). Unfortunately, the product is not available in the United States. A compress made from an herbal infusion may prove helpful, however.

HIGH BLOOD PRESSURE. Barberry contains chemicals that may help reduce elevated blood pressure by enlarging blood vessels. This lends support to the herb's traditional Russian use as a treatment for high blood pressure.

Intriguing Possibilities

Perhaps old Harry Hoxsey was right. Animal studies suggest that barberry helps shrink some tumors. Pilot studies found that the herb also may have anti-inflammatory activity, suggesting possible value in treating arthritis. More research needs to be done in both areas before any specific recommendations can be made.

Rx Recommendations

To prepare a decoction, boil $1/2$ teaspoon of powdered root bark in 1 cup of water for 15 to 30 minutes, then strain if you wish. Let it cool, and drink up to 1 cup a day. The taste is quite bitter, but you can mask it with honey or an herbal beverage blend.

When using commercial preparations, follow the package directions.

To make a compress to treat pinkeye, soak a clean cloth in a barberry infusion.

The Safety Factor

In large doses, barberry can cause nausea, vomiting, convulsions, hazardous drops in blood pressure, and depression of heart rate and breathing. People with heart disease or chronic respiratory problems should be careful not to take large doses and should take this herb only with the knowledge and approval of their physicians.

Berberine may stimulate uterine contractions. For this reason, women who are pregnant or trying to conceive should not use it. Nursing women should also avoid it.

If barberry causes minor discomfort, such as stomach upset or diarrhea, decrease the dosage or stop using it. Likewise, stop using it if it causes dizziness or faintness. Let your doctor know if you experience any unpleasant effects or if the symptoms for which you are using the herb do not improve significantly within 2 weeks.

Do not give barberry to children under 2. In older children, adjust the recommended dose based on the child's weight. For example, give a 50-pound child one-third of the dose a 150-pound adult would take.

If you're over 65, start with a low dose, and increase only if necessary.

Inform health care professionals of the herbs you use. Problematic herb-drug interactions are possible.

Barberry may cause allergic reactions or other unexpected side effects. If any develop, reduce your dose or stop taking it.

For more on herb safety, see Chapter 2.

If symptoms get worse or persist longer than 2 weeks, consult a health care professional promptly.

Growing Information

Barberry is a perennial shrub that reaches 10 feet. It has smooth gray bark, long spines, and hanging clusters of bright yellow flowers that bloom in spring.

Barberry grows easily in the Northeast and Midwest. Plant seeds in the fall in fertile, moist, well-drained soil. Germination occurs the following spring. The shrub can also be propagated from cuttings.

Barberry prefers sun but tolerates shade. Prune and thin the branches in the spring after the shrub flowers. Neglected shrubs become overgrown and unhealthy, but they can be rejuvenated by fertilizing and cutting back to within a foot of the ground in late winter. In areas with cold winters, shelter the plant from the wind. Harvest the root bark in spring or fall, and dry it.

The herb's edible berries are used to make jams and jellies. The berry juice may be substituted for lemon juice.

BAYBERRY
An All-American Fever Treatment

Family: Myricaceae; other members include myrtle

Genus and species: *Myrica cerifera*

Also known as: Wax myrtle, candleberry, and tallow shrub

Part used: Root bark

Before electric lights were commonplace, bayberry was highly prized as the source of a fragrant candlewax that produced considerably less smoke than tallow. Today, bayberry candles are still with us, but only as Christmas curiosities.

Healing History

In early America, bayberry trees grew throughout the East. But bayberry was used medicinally mainly in the South, where Choctaw tribes boiled the leaves and drank the decoction as a treatment for fever. Later, white settlers adopted the plant and drank bayberry wax in hot water "as a certain cure for the most violent cases of dysentery," according to a medical account from 1722.

During the early 19th century, bayberry was popularized by Samuel A. Thomson, a New England herbalist and creator of some of the first patent medicines. He touted the herb as second only to red pepper for producing "heat" within the body. Thomson recommended bayberry for colds, flu, and other infectious diseases as well as for diarrhea and fever.

Thomson's herbalism lost popularity after the Civil War, when it was replaced by the teachings of the more scientific Eclectic physicians, forerunners of today's naturopaths. They prescribed bayberry topically for bleeding gums and internally for diarrhea, dysentery, sore throat, scarlet fever, menstrual difficulties, and even typhoid.

Although bayberry has since waned in popularity, some contemporary herbalists recommend using it externally for varicose veins and internally for diarrhea, dysentery, colds, flu, bleeding gums, and sore throat. One modern herbal calls it one of the most useful herbs in botanical medicine and goes so far as to advocate treating uterine bleeding by packing the vagina with cotton soaked in bayberry tea. (Do not try this remedy; see a physician for unusual uterine bleeding.)

Therapeutic Uses

Two hundred years ago, bayberry was widely used medicinally. It's a shame that this native American herb has been all but forgotten, because science has shown that bayberry may have some real benefits in treating diarrhea and fever.

DIARRHEA. Bayberry root bark contains myricitrin, an antibiotic chemical that fights a broad range of bacteria and protozoa. Myricitrin's antibiotic action supports bayberry's traditional use against diarrhea and dysentery.

Bayberry also contains astringent tannins, which add to its value in treating diarrhea.

FEVER. The antibiotic myricitrin also helps reduce fever, thus lending credence to bayberry's traditional use among the Choctaws.

Intriguing Possibilities

Myricitrin promotes the flow of bile, so bayberry may potentially be of value in treating liver and gallbladder ailments. As yet, however, no research demonstrates this use.

Indian researchers have discovered that a closely related Asian species of bayberry, *Myrica sapida*, opens the bronchial tubes, acting as a bronchodilator. This action suggests that this plant—and American bayberry—might treat asthma.

Rx Recommendations

To prepare a decoction, boil 1 teaspoon of powdered root bark in 1 pint of water for 10 to 15 minutes, then strain if you wish. Add a bit of milk and drink up to 2 cups a day of the cooled beverage. You'll find the taste bitter and astringent. A tincture might go down more easily. If you use a homemade tincture, take $1/_2$ teaspoon up to twice a day.

When using commercial preparations, follow the package directions.

The Safety Factor

Bayberry's high tannin content makes the herb of questionable value for anyone with a history of cancer. In various studies, tannins show both pro-cancer and anticancer actions. Their cancer-promoting action has received more publicity, notably from a study published in the *Journal of the National Cancer Institute*, which showed that tannins produce malignant tumors in laboratory animals. But tannins have also been found to have an anticancer effect on some animal tumors.

Tannins' effects on human cancer remain unclear. Small quantities have never been implicated in human tumors, but Asians who drink large quantities of tea, which contains tannins, show unusually high rates of stomach cancer. The British also love tea, but their rates of stomach cancer remain low. One reason may be that they drink their tea with milk, which neutralizes the tannins.

People with a history of cancer, particularly stomach or colon cancer, should exercise caution and not use bayberry. Others should consume no more than the recommended amounts.

In large doses, bayberry root bark may cause stomach distress, nausea, and vomiting. People with chronic gastrointestinal conditions, such as colitis, should use it cautiously.

Bayberry changes the way the body uses sodium and potassium, so people who must watch their sodium/potassium balance, such as those with kidney disease, high blood pressure, or congestive heart failure, should consult their physicians before using it.

Pregnant and nursing women should not use bayberry.

Do not give bayberry to children under 2. In older children, adjust the recommended dose based on the child's weight. For example, give a 50-pound child one-third of the dose a 150-pound adult would take.

If you're over 65, start with a low dose, and increase only if necessary.

Inform health care professionals of the herbs you use. Problematic herb-drug interactions are possible.

Bayberry may cause allergic reactions or other unexpected side effects. If any develop, reduce your dose or stop taking it.

For more on herb safety, see Chapter 2.

If symptoms get worse or persist longer than 2 weeks, consult a health care professional promptly.

Growing Information

Bayberry is native to the area from New Jersey to the Great Lakes and south to Florida and Texas. In the Southeast, it matures into an evergreen tree that reaches about 35 feet. Farther north, the plant does not grow that tall. Around the Great Lakes, mature plants rarely grow taller than 3 feet.

Bayberry has grayish bark; waxy branches; and dense, narrow, delicately toothed leaves dotted with resin glands, which produce a fragrant aroma when crushed. Yellow flowers appear in spring and produce nutlike fruits thickly covered with the wax once so highly valued in candle making.

Bayberry grows from seeds planted in spring or early fall. It prefers peaty soil under full sun but tolerates poorer, sandy soil along streams and in swampy areas. Plants require little care other than pruning. Harvest the root bark after a few years.

BILBERRY

An Herb for the Eyes

Family: Ericaceae; other members include azalea, blueberry, cranberry, and uva-ursi

Genus and species: *Vaccinium myrtillus*

Also known as: European blueberry, bogberry, and whortleberry

Parts used: Fruits

Bilberries, sometimes called European blueberries, are small blue berries that have been used in herbal medicine for at least 800 years. But it wasn't until World War II that the herb's real value was discovered—not by scientists, but by aviators.

Healing History

No one knows exactly when bilberries began to be used for healing. The first written recommendations date from the 12th century, when Hildegard of Bingen, an abbess, herbalist, and composer, recommended the berries to treat a variety of complaints, including respiratory problems.

Bilberries are astringent, meaning that they draw tissue together. Bilberry and other astringent herbs, such as tea, have been used for thousands of years to treat wounds, mouth sores, and diarrhea.

In Elizabethan England, a combination of bilberries and honey, called rob, was a popular remedy for diarrhea. Later, bilberries were typically prepared as jam, but their use for treating diarrhea continued. Over time, people who ate bilberries or the jam reported clearer vision, and folk herbalists began touting the berries for eyesight. Herbalists also recommended them to treat diabetes.

During World War II, British fliers ate bilberry jam before nighttime bombing missions. They swore that the berries prevented night blindness and sharpened their vision. After the war, researchers began studying the herb and discovered that it did indeed improve night vision and accelerate adjustment to glare.

Therapeutic Uses

Bilberries owe their color to high levels of potent antioxidant compounds called anthocyanosides. Antioxidants help prevent and reverse the cell damage inflicted by highly reactive oxygen molecules called free radicals. Scientists now agree that the oxidative damage produced by free radicals is an underlying cause of heart disease, many cancers, and other degenerative illnesses.

GENERAL DISEASE PREVENTION. Antioxidants—including vitamins C and E, the mineral selenium, carotenoids (including beta-carotene), and anthocyanosides—are found in plant foods. At the Jean Mayer USDA Human Nutrition Research Center on Aging at Tufts University, researchers analyzed the antioxidant content of dozens of common plant foods. Those richest in antioxidants turned out to be the dark-colored fruits and berries that contain generous amounts of anthocyanosides: blueberries, blackberries, raspberries, cherries, cranberries, red grapes, plums, raisins, and prunes.

The study did not include bilberries because they are not common in the United States, but they are about as rich in anthocyanosides as blueberries, which ranked near the top in terms of antioxidant content.

CATARACTS. In the United States, cataracts are a major cause of vision impairment and blindness among older adults. The condition results from oxidative damage to the normally clear lens of the eye, which leads to the development of cloudy spots.

For reasons that remain unclear, the anthocyanosides in bilberry have unusually powerful effects on the eyes. In one Italian study, 50 people with early-stage cataracts were given bilberry extracts three times a day in combination with another antioxidant, vitamin E. The treatment stopped the progression of cataracts in 97 percent of the study participants.

GLAUCOMA. Italian researchers gave 120 milligrams per day of a standardized extract of bilberry to 20 adults with elevated intra-ocular fluid pressure (IOP), the key risk factor for glaucoma. Nineteen other study participants were not treated. Baseline IOP was comparable in both groups. After 6 months, 1 of the 19 people in the control group had significantly lower IOP. But in the bilberry group, 19 of 20 did.

MACULAR DEGENERATION. The nerve-rich retina in the back of the eye plays a key role in vision. Macular degeneration involves deterioration of the macula, the most sensitive part of the retina. It's the part that's responsible for seeing what's directly in front of you (central vision) as well as fine detail.

In a European study, 31 people with various types of retinal problems, including macular degeneration, were given bilberry extract. Those with macular degeneration experienced significant vision improvement.

For another study, a South Dakota researcher recruited 10 men and women, ages 61 to 77, all with macular degeneration. He gave his volunteers a list of antioxidant-rich fruits and vegetables and asked them to eat two servings of fruit and three servings of vegetables from the list every day. He also instructed the participants to take supplements containing antioxidant vitamins and minerals plus extracts of bilberry and ginkgo (like bilberry, ginkgo is an antioxidant). One year later, all 10 people showed significant vision improvement in at least one eye.

DIABETIC RETINOPATHY. Diabetes damages all the blood vessels in the body, including the tiny capillaries in the eye that nourish the retina. When these capillaries develop diabetes-related damage, they leak blood into the eye, causing the blurred vision of retinopathy.

Bilberry's powerful antioxidants help strengthen retinal blood vessels, reducing blood leakage from the capillaries. In the European study mentioned above, people with diabetic retinopathy showed significant improvement when treated with bilberry.

VARICOSE VEINS. Varicose veins result from weakness of the biological "glue" that holds together the veins' cell structure. Once weakened, the veins stretch abnormally, allowing blood to pool in them. Varicose veins usually occur in the legs; when they affect the anal area, they're known as hemorrhoids.

Because bilberry strengthens the structure of veins, it can help treat varicose veins. When Italian researchers gave bilberry extract to 47 people with this condition, their symptoms improved significantly.

DIARRHEA AND MOUTH SORES. Commission E, the expert panel that evaluates herbal medicines for the German counterpart of the FDA, endorses bilberry as a treatment for diarrhea and mouth sores—the herb's primary traditional uses.

Intriguing Possibilities

Some studies suggest that bilberry lowers blood sugar levels in people with diabetes, a finding that supports another of the herb's traditional uses. In addition, animal studies suggest that it helps prevent and treat ulcers.

Rx Recommendations

European herbalists have bred a variety of bilberry that is processed into a standardized extract containing 25 percent anthocyanosides. Check the labels of commercial preparations. In most studies that showed the herb's benefit, participants took one or two 80- to 160-milligram capsules of standardized bilberry extract three times a day. Follow the package directions.

The Safety Factor

Bilberry is a food. Pregnant and nursing women may use it in consultation with their health care providers.

Inform health care professionals of the herbs you use. Problematic herb-drug interactions are possible.

Bilberry may cause allergic reactions or other unexpected side effects. If any develop, reduce your dose or stop taking it.

For more on herb safety, see Chapter 2.

If symptoms get worse or persist longer than 2 weeks, consult a health care professional promptly.

Growing Information

Bilberry is a shrubby perennial that grows to about 18 inches in forested areas of Northern and Central Europe. The leaves are oval, bright green, and about 1 inch long. Red or pink bell-shaped flowers appear in spring, with blue-black or blue-purple berries forming in late summer and fall. Bilberry does not grow well in the United States and is rarely cultivated here.

BITTER MELON

Diabetes? Obesity? Try This Herb

Family: Cucurbitaceae; other members include melons, gourds, cucumber, pumpkin, squash

Genus and species: *Momordica charantia*

Also known as: Bitter cucumber, bitter gourd, balsam pear

Parts used: Fruit, leaves, seed, and seed oil

Bitter melon is an annual vine that grows to 6 feet in Asia, Africa, South America, and the southeastern United States. It produces a bitter orange-yellow fruit shaped like a cucumber, gourd, or small melon—hence its common names. The fruit is eaten as a vegetable.

Healing History

Bitter melon has a long history of use in folk medicine on several continents. Externally applied to the skin, it has been used to treat wounds and abscesses. Internally, it was recommended for asthma, constipation, diabetes, intestinal parasites, kidney stones, psoriasis, stomach upset, and some tumors.

Therapeutic Uses

DIABETES. All parts of bitter melon, but especially the fruit, contain compounds chemically similar to the hormone insulin. Several animal studies show that the insulin-like compounds in bitter melon reduce blood sugar and help treat diabetes. For example, researchers at India's University of Mumbai (Bombay) gave an extract of bitter melon fruit to diabetic rats. It reduced their blood sugar by 48 percent, an effect comparable to that of the widely prescribed diabetes drug glibenclamide (Glyburide, Micronase).

Several small studies have shown that bitter melon reduces blood sugar levels in people with type 2 diabetes. If you have diabetes, talk to your doctor about supplementing your diet and medication with the herb. In addition, one report shows that bitter melon reduces blood sugar in children.

OBESITY. Being overweight raises the risk for diabetes. Several animal studies show that diets supplemented with bitter melon reduce weight gain and fat accumulation. University of Hong Kong researchers placed rats on a high-fat diet with or without supplemental bitter melon extract. The animals in the herb group gained less weight and accumulated less body fat. The researchers concluded that the herb "strongly counteracts the [harmful] effects of a high-fat diet."

IMMUNE STIMULATION. Bitter melon boosts production of interferon, a component of the immune system that prevents infection.

Intriguing Possibilities

A protein in bitter melon fruit and seed inhibits the replication of several viruses, including polio, herpes, and HIV, the virus that causes AIDS.

Bitter melon also seems to reduce cholesterol. Japanese researchers at Miyazaki University fed rats a bitter melon extract and documented a "marked reduction in cholesterol."

The herb also increases levels of key antioxidants, notably glutathione and superoxide dismutase. Antioxidants help prevent cancer. Japanese researchers added bitter melon extract to rats' drinking water. A known percentage of rats spontaneously develop breast cancer. But among those ingesting the herb, the rate of breast cancer was significantly less than expected. Indian researchers have found that bitter melon also reduces risk of animal stomach cancer.

It's too early to call the herb a treatment for herpes, HIV, high cholesterol, and cancer, but in the future, that's a possibility.

Rx Recommendations

Some herbalists recommend bitter melon juice for diabetes; they suggest a dose of $1/2$ to 1 cup a day. When using the fruit, the typical dose is 900 milligrams three times a day with meals.

Several supplements are available. Most are capsules containing 250 to 500 milligrams of fruit extract. Follow package directions.

The Safety Factor

There are no published reports of serious side effects in adults taking recommended doses of bitter melon. However, large amounts of juice have sickened children, causing vomiting. In some animal studies, bitter melon has suppressed fertility and raised liver enzyme levels, an indication of liver damage. Couples trying to conceive and people with liver disease should not use bitter melon.

People with diabetes who try bitter melon should inform their physicians, monitor their blood sugar closely, and be prepared to reduce their dose of insulin and other medications.

Pregnant and nursing women should not use bitter melon.

Do not give this herb to children under 2. In older children, adjust the recommended dose based on the child's weight. For example, give a 50-pound child one-third of the dose a 150-pound adult would take.

If you're over 65, start with a low dose, and increase only if necessary.

Inform health care professionals of the herbs you use. Problematic herb-drug interactions are possible.

Bitter melon may cause allergic reactions or other unexpected side effects. If any develop, reduce your dose or stop taking it.

For more on herb safety, see Chapter 2.

If symptoms get worse or persist longer

than 2 weeks, consult a health care professional promptly.

Growing Information

Bitter melon grows in the Caribbean, so it can be cultivated in Florida and near the Gulf Coast. It's a climbing annual vine with long-stalked leaves and yellow flowers. The fruits look like small warty cucumbers.

BLACKBERRY

More Than Jam and Jelly

Family: Rosaceae; other members include rose, peach, almond, apple, and strawberry

Genus and species: *Rubus fruticosus* (European); *R. villosus* (American); and other species

Also known as: Bramble, dewberry, goutberry

Parts used: Leaves, bark, roots, and fruits

If your acquaintance with the blackberry is confined to jam and jelly, it's time to branch out. The blackberry bush was once as highly prized for its medicinal leaves, bark, and roots as for its sweet fruit.

Until recently, however, blackberry had fallen from healing fashion. Now that's changing, based on research showing that the pigment that gives blackberries their color is a potent antioxidant with remarkable health benefits.

Healing History

The ancient Greeks relied on blackberry to treat gout. They were the only people to use the herb for this condition, but Greek medicine was so influential in Europe that well into the 18th century, the herb was called goutberry.

The ancient Chinese used the unripe berries to treat kidney problems, urinary incontinence, and impotence. The Romans chewed the leaves and bark for bleeding gums and drank a decoction for diarrhea.

Tenth-century Arab physicians considered the fruit to be an aphrodisiac (it isn't). During the Middle Ages, blackberry leaves were applied to the skin to soothe burns and scalds.

In his influential *Herbal*, 17th-century English herbalist Nicholas Culpeper described blackberry as "very binding" and good for "fevers, ulcers, putrid sores of the mouth and secret parts [genitals], spitting blood [tuberculosis], piles [hemorrhoids], stones of the kidney, too much flowing of women's courses [menstruation], and hot distempers of the head, eyes, and body."

Nineteenth-century American Eclectic physicians, forerunners of today's naturopaths, recommended a preparation made from blackberry fruit as "an excellent syrup which is of much service in dysentery, being pleasant to the taste, mitigating the sufferings of the patient, and ultimately effecting a cure." They also recommended blackberry leaves for gonorrhea, vaginal discharges, recovery from childbirth, and "cholera infantum," an old term for infant infectious diarrhea, which, in the days before antibiotics, was often fatal (and still is in many parts of the world).

Few contemporary herbalists recommended blackberry for anything beyond treating diarrhea until the mid-1990s, when scientists discovered the value of the pigment that gives the berries their dark color.

Therapeutic Uses

Contrary to the claims of Nicholas Culpeper, blackberry doesn't do much for the genitals. But the fruit and leaves of this herb help prevent and treat quite a few common ills.

Blackberries owe their healing power to high levels of anthocyanosides, compounds in the pigment that give the fruits their dark color. Anthocyanosides are potent antioxidants, helping to prevent and reverse the cell damage produced by highly reactive oxygen molecules called free radicals. Scientists now agree that the damage resulting from free radicals (oxidative damage) is the underlying cause of heart disease, many cancers, and other degenerative illnesses.

GENERAL DISEASE PREVENTION. Antioxidants such as vitamins C and E, the mineral selenium, carotenoids (including beta-carotene), and anthocyanosides are found only in plant foods. In a study conducted at the Jean Mayer USDA Human Nutrition Research Center on Aging at Tufts University, researchers assessed the antioxidant content of dozens of common plant foods. The scientists determined that the best sources of antioxidants are the dark-colored fruits that contain generous amounts of anthocyanosides, including blackberries, blueberries, cherries, red grapes, plums, raisins, and prunes.

CATARACTS. Cataracts are a major cause of vision impairment and blindness among older Americans. The condition occurs when oxidative damage to the normally clear lens of the eye leads to the development of cloudy spots.

For reasons that scientists can't yet explain, anthocyanosides have unusually powerful effects on the eyes. Most of the research into their benefits has been performed in Europe using bilberry, a distinctly European fruit that's similar to the American blueberry and rich in the same pigment. But medicinal herb experts, including James A. Duke, Ph.D., retired USDA herbal medicine authority and author of several highly regarded herbal medicine references, agree that all fruits rich in anthocyanosides should produce similar benefits.

In one Italian study, 50 people with early-stage cataracts were given bilberry extracts containing anthocyanosides three times a day, along with vitamin E, which is also an antioxidant. In 97 percent of the study participants, cataract progression stopped.

MACULAR DEGENERATION. At the back of the eye is a nerve-rich structure called the retina, which plays an important role in vision. The most sensitive part of the retina, called the macula, is responsible for discerning what's directly in front of you (central vision) as well as fine detail. Macular degeneration involves deterioration of the macula, which can lead to the loss of central vision.

In a European study, 31 people with macular degeneration and various other types of retinal problems were treated with anthocyanosides in the form of bilberry extract. Those with macular degeneration showed significant vision improvement.

On this side of the Atlantic, a South Dakota researcher conducted a study involving 10 men and women between the ages of 61 and 77, all with macular degeneration. The researcher presented his volunteers with a list of antioxidant-rich fruits and vegetables, along with instructions to eat two servings of fruit and three servings of vegetables from the list every day. He also asked each person to take supplements containing antioxidant vitamins and minerals, plus bilberry (with its antioxidant anthocyanosides) and ginkgo (also an antioxidant). One year later, all 10 people showed significant vision improvement in at least one eye.

DIABETIC RETINOPATHY. Diabetes damages all of the blood vessels in the body, including the tiny capillaries in the eye that nourish the retina. The injured capillaries leak blood into the eye, setting the stage for the blurred vision of diabetic retinopathy.

With their powerful antioxidant action, anthocyanosides help strengthen retinal blood vessels, thus reducing leakage into the eye. In the European study mentioned above, the participants with diabetic retinopathy showed significant improvement when treated with anthocyanosides from bilberry.

VARICOSE VEINS. Varicose veins occur when the biological "glue" that holds together the veins' cell structure begins to weaken. This allows the veins to stretch abnormally, causing blood to pool in them. The condition can affect veins in the legs or in the anal area, where they're known as hemorrhoids.

Anthocyanosides can help treat varicose veins by strengthening their structure. In an Italian study, when 47 people received anthocyanosides (in the form of bilberry extract) for their varicose veins, they experienced significant improvement in their symptoms.

DIARRHEA. Blackberry leaves contain large amounts of astringent tannins. In the digestive tract, the action of tannins helps control diarrhea and dysentery, confirming a traditional use for the herb. Commission E, the expert panel that evaluates herbal medicines for the German counterpart of the FDA, endorses blackberry leaf as a treatment for diarrhea.

WOUNDS. The astringent action of tannins also helps to constrict blood vessels and stop minor bleeding. This would tend to explain blackberry's traditional use as an external treatment for wounds. Blackberry thorns often cause minor cuts, so it's nice to know that first aid is close at hand.

MOUTH SORES AND SORE THROAT. The astringent properties of blackberry leaf tea may help soothe mouth sores and sore throat.

HEMORRHOIDS. The herb's astringent nature may also help explain its traditional use as a hemorrhoid remedy.

Intriguing Possibilities

One study found that a strong infusion of blackberry leaves reduces blood sugar levels in rabbits with diabetes, hinting at the herb's possible value in diabetes management.

Research has shown that blackberry's close relative, raspberry, relaxes the uterus. Women might try blackberry for painful menstrual cramps.

Rx Recommendations

To help protect yourself against degenerative conditions such as heart disease, cancer, cataracts, and macular degeneration, eat blackberry fruit. It doesn't matter how you eat the berries—fresh, frozen, canned, or in preserves, jams, or jellies. In any form, blackberries contain generous amounts of anthocyanosides.

To treat diarrhea or soothe a sore throat, try an infusion, decoction, or tincture. To prepare an infusion, use 2 to 3 teaspoons of dried leaves per cup of boiling water. (If you prefer, you can use a handful of dried or fresh crushed berries or 1 to 2 teaspoons of dried powdered bark instead of dried leaves.) Steep for 10 to 20 minutes, strain, and add a bit of milk. Drink up to 3 cups a day.

For a decoction, use 1 teaspoon of powdered root per cup of water. Boil for 30 minutes and strain if you wish. Drink up to 1 cup a day with a bit of milk.

If you're using a homemade tincture, take up to 1 teaspoon up to twice a day.

To treat wounds or hemorrhoids, soak a clean cloth in a tincture or strong infusion and apply it externally.

When using commercial preparations, follow the package directions.

The Safety Factor

Blackberries are considered safe for anyone who is not allergic to them, but questions have been raised about the tannins in medicinal preparations of blackberry leaf. In various studies, tannins show both pro-cancer and anticancer actions. Their cancer-promoting action has attracted a lot more attention, primarily because of a study published in the *Journal of the National Cancer Institute*, which showed that tannins produce malignant tumors in laboratory animals. But tannins appear to also have an anticancer effect on some animal tumors.

The relationship between tannins and human cancer remains unclear. In small quantities, such as the amount found in blackberry fruits, the compounds have never been shown to cause human tumors. It has been noted that Asians who drink large quantities of tea, which is high in tannins, show unusually high rates of stomach cancer. The British also love tea, but their rates of stomach cancer remain low. One reason may be that they drink their tea with milk, which neutralizes the tannins.

People with a history of cancer, particularly stomach or colon cancer, should exercise caution and not ingest blackberry leaf tea. Others should take no more than the recommended amount of infusion or decoction and, for extra safety, add a bit of milk.

In large amounts, tannins may cause stomach distress, nausea, and vomiting. Blackberry root bark contains the most tannins, followed by the leaves and, in distant third, the fruits. People with chronic gastrointestinal conditions, such as colitis, probably should not use the roots.

Pregnant and nursing women should not use blackberry leaf tea. However, blackberries are a food and may be eaten by anyone.

Do not give blackberry leaf tea to children under 2. In older children, adjust the recommended dose based on the child's weight. For example, give a 50-pound child one-third of the dose a 150-pound adult would take.

If you're over 65, start with a low dose, and increase only if necessary.

Inform health care professionals of the herbs you use. Problematic herb-drug interactions are possible.

Blackberry leaf may cause allergic reactions or other unexpected side effects. If any develop, reduce your dose or stop taking it.

For more on herb safety, see Chapter 2.

If symptoms get worse or persist longer than 2 weeks, consult a health care professional promptly.

Growing Information

Blackberry bushes grow wild around most of North America. They have long, tangled, thorny stems; lush foliage; and a profusion of berries that turn red as they ripen and become a juicy, purplish blue-black by midsummer.

Blackberry bushes are so vigorous and invasive that they quickly become a thick, thorny, impenetrable mass. Rooting them out is almost impossible, as any gardener who has tried can attest. Even when the bushes are removed, stray root fragments continue to send up new shoots. To minimize problems, plant this shrub in containers or surround its roots with sheet metal.

Blackberries grow easily from $\frac{1}{2}$-inch root cuttings taken in autumn and stored through the winter in cool sand (around 50°F). Plant cuttings vertically 1 to 3 feet apart in 3 to 4 inches of soil.

Blackberries adapt to many conditions but grow best in loose, moist, rich soil amended with manure or finished compost. The plants flower in spring and bear fruit throughout the summer.

Harvest the leaves and roots anytime. For ease of harvesting the berries, train the branches along supports and prune them mercilessly.

BLACK COHOSH

The Classic Women's Herb

Family: Ranunculaceae; other members include buttercup, larkspur, and peony

Genus and species: *Actea racemosa* (formerly *Cimicifuga racemosa*) or *Macrotys actaeoides*

Also known as: Squawroot, snakeroot, cimicifuga

Parts used: Rhizomes and roots

One of the 19th century's most popular patent medicines was Lydia E. Pinkham's Vegetable Compound, introduced in 1876 to treat "female weakness," that is, premenstrual syndrome, menstrual cramps, and menopausal complaints. Pinkham's compound—developed by its namesake, a Lynn, Massachusetts, homemaker and practitioner of folk herbalism—contained several medicinal herbs. Chief among them was black cohosh, an age-old Algonquin treatment for gynecological complaints.

Pinkham's product also contained an enormous amount of alcohol. During the 19th century, respectable ladies did not drink liquor. Critics charged that the main weakness treated by the Vegetable Compound was a thirst for alcohol. Based on modern research findings, however, it seems clear that the black cohosh in Pinkham's product helped treat menstrual and menopausal symptoms.

After World War II, Pinkham's Vegetable Compound was reformulated to contain very little alcohol. Ironically, the revamped version also contained no black cohosh, the ingredient that supported the product's advertising as a remedy for female complaints.

Healing History

The *black* in black cohosh refers to the plant's dark medicinal roots. The word *cohosh* is Algonquin for "rough," another reference to the roots.

Native Americans boiled black cohosh's gnarled roots in water and drank the decoction for fatigue, sore throat, arthritis, and rattlesnake bite—hence another of the plant's popular names, snakeroot. But black cohosh was used primarily by Native American women for gynecological problems and for recovery after childbirth.

Wild black cohosh grew most profusely in the Ohio River valley, which seems fitting. After all, the herb was championed by 19th-century American Eclectic physicians, forerunners of today's naturopaths, whose medical school was located in Cincinnati on the banks of the Ohio. The Eclectics called the herb by a different name, macrotys, and recommended it for fever, rashes, insomnia, malaria, yellow fever, and all "hysterical" (gynecological) ailments. The Eclectic medical text *King's American Dispensatory* (1898) stated, "In dysmenorrhea [menstrual cramps], it is of greatest utility, being surpassed by no other drug."

Non-Eclectic ("regular") physicians remained unimpressed by black cohosh. But Lydia Pinkham sided with the Eclectics and included the herb in her compound.

Black cohosh does not grow in China, but Chinese physicians use several related plants to treat headache, measles, diarrhea, bleeding gums, and some gynecological problems. Homeopaths recommend microdoses of black cohosh for menstrual problems and childbirth.

Contemporary herbalists recommend the herb primarily for premenstrual syndrome (PMS), menstrual cramps, and menopausal symptoms. Since the mid-1990s, its popularity for women's health concerns has been growing, with many herb companies now marketing black cohosh products.

Therapeutic Uses

Black cohosh owes its medicinal properties to several compounds in its root: acetein, formononetin, and triterpenes. In the 1940s, German scientists discovered that these compounds are estrogenic, meaning that they mimic the effects of the female sex hormone estrogen. By the 1950s, a commercial standardized extract, Remifemin, was in wide use in Germany as a treatment for PMS, menstrual cramps, and menopausal hot flashes. (Herbal medicine is much more mainstream in Germany than in the United States.) Remifemin is now also widely available in the United States.

Most contemporary herbalists consider black cohosh estrogenic. It is, but indirectly. The herb suppresses the secretion of luteinizing hormone (LH), which is produced by the pituitary gland. But this produces an estrogenic effect.

PREMENSTRUAL SYNDROME (PMS). Germany's Commission E, the expert panel that evaluates herbal medicines for the German counterpart of the FDA, endorses black cohosh as a treatment for PMS. The panel's position is based on more than 40 years of testimonials and clinical experience in Germany.

MENSTRUAL CRAMPS. For the same reasons, Commission E also endorses black cohosh as a treatment for menstrual cramps.

MENOPAUSAL COMPLAINTS. Most studies of black cohosh have examined the herb as a treatment for hot flashes and other menopausal discomforts. Occasionally a study shows no benefit. But the great weight of the evidence supports the herb as a treatment for hot flashes.

From 1982 through 1991, eight clinical trials involving a total of 1,170 women were conducted by German researchers. The studies differed somewhat in design, but all of them investigated the effectiveness of the black cohosh extract Remifemin (40 drops twice a day or two 40-milligram tablets daily for 6 to 12 weeks). All of these trials produced the same results: fewer, briefer hot flashes; less vaginal dryness; improved mood; and relief from fatigue. In the largest of the studies, involving 629 women, 80 percent of the participants reported significant improvement in their discomfort within a month. Many experienced complete relief within 6 to 8 weeks. The herb caused no significant side effects. Commission E endorses black cohosh as a treatment for menopausal discomforts.

Since 1991, a dozen other studies have been

published showing that black cohosh relieves menopausal complaints. For example, German researchers asked 6,141 women to rate their menopausal symptoms using a standard rating index and then gave them black cohosh (Remifemin, label dosage). A year later, physical symptoms had declined significantly. (For emotional upsets, a combination of Remifemin and St. John's wort was effective.)

HORMONE REPLACEMENT ALTERNATIVE. The ovaries manufacture most of the estrogen in women's bodies. During menopause, production of the hormone slowly declines. Among women of any age who have their ovaries removed, estrogen production also declines, but more suddenly.

To make up for the loss of estrogen, mainstream physicians prescribe hormone replacement therapy. German researchers compared pharmaceutical hormone replacement with black cohosh (two tablets of Remifemin twice a day) in 60 women who had their ovaries removed before age 40. After 6 months, both groups reported similar satisfaction with their treatment, but the black cohosh caused no significant side effects.

BREAST CANCER. Estrogen spurs the growth of breast tumors, and anything with estrogenic effects can be presumed to do the same. For a while, scientists speculated that breast cancer survivors and women at high risk for the disease should not use black cohosh because of its estrogenic effect. However, as mentioned, the herb is only indirectly estrogenic. University of Missouri researchers gave the herb to menopausal women and measured both its effect on hot flashes and biomarkers for estrogenic effects. After 12 weeks, the women reported significant relief from hot flashes—but they showed no increase in markers of estrogen effects. In other words, black cohosh does not have typical estrogenic action, and should not stimulate the growth of breast cancer.

In fact, it appears that black cohosh may reduce the risk of breast cancer. In laboratory studies, German scientists have shown that the herb inhibits the growth of breast cancer cells. University of Pennsylvania researchers surveyed 2,473 older women about their use of black cohosh. Some were breast cancer survivors. Others had never had the disease. The researchers concluded that the "use of black cohosh had a significant breast-cancer-protective effect."

HIGH BLOOD PRESSURE. A study published in *Nature* revealed that black cohosh reduces blood pressure by opening blood vessels in the limbs (peripheral vasodilation). The herb may help manage high blood pressure, but consult your physician before using it for this purpose.

Intriguing Possibilities

One study found that black cohosh relieves pain and has anti-inflammatory activity, possibly explaining its traditional use as a treatment for arthritis. Another report suggests that it helps preserve bone, promoting its potential use in osteoporosis prevention. Other research involving the herb showed cholesterol and blood pressure reduction, anti-ulcer effects, and blood sugar regulation, pointing toward the herb's possible value in controlling diabetes. Finally, black cohosh appears to inhibit the growth of prostate cancer cells.

More research needs to be done to determine

whether black cohosh will prove useful in treating any of those conditions. Other preliminary findings of animal studies hint that the herb may have antibiotic, sedative, and stomach-soothing properties.

Rx Recommendations

For a decoction, use $1/2$ teaspoon of powdered root per cup of water and boil for 30 minutes, then strain if you wish. Let cool before drinking. Black cohosh has an unpleasant aroma and a sharp, bitter taste; you can add lemon and honey and/or mix the herb with an herbal beverage. Take 2 tablespoons every few hours, up to 1 cup a day.

As a homemade tincture, take 2 to 4 teaspoons twice a day.

When using commercial preparations, follow the package directions.

The Safety Factor

If you want to use black cohosh, double-check the label to be sure that you have black cohosh, not *blue* cohosh. The latter should not be used by most women. Or simply buy Remifemin, which is black cohosh.

Nineteenth-century researchers gave laboratory animals doses of black cohosh 90 times the recommended human equivalent. They reported that the herb may cause dizziness, diarrhea, vomiting, tremors, depressed heart rate, miscarriage, and other worrisome side effects. These studies continue to be cited today. On the other hand, in the eight studies that examined black cohosh as a treatment for menopausal discomforts, no significant side effects turned up. In fact, the only side effect was stomach upset,

which was reported by just 7 percent of the participants in the largest study. The consensus of the modern scientific research is that black cohosh is safe when used in recommended doses.

Since 2000, a few case reports have documented liver damage in women taking black cohosh, raising the possibility that the herb might be toxic to the liver. On closer examination, however, all of the women involved in these case reports were taking other herbs and/or drugs known to increase risk of liver damage. There is currently no compelling evidence that recommended doses of black cohosh cause liver damage.

Women who are pregnant or nursing or whose physicians have advised them not to take birth control pills should not use black cohosh.

There is no reason to give black cohosh to children.

If you're over 65, start with a low dose, and increase only if necessary.

Inform health care professionals of the herbs you use. Problematic herb-drug interactions are possible.

For more on herb safety, see Chapter 2.

If you are taking postmenopausal hormone replacement therapy, consult your physician before taking black cohosh.

Let your doctor know if you experience any unpleasant effects or if the symptoms for which you are using the herb do not improve significantly within 4 weeks.

Growing Information

Black cohosh is native to the area from Ontario south to Tennessee and west to Missouri. A leafy perennial, it reaches 9 feet. It has knotty black roots and a smooth stem with large, toothed, compound leaves and small, multiple white flowers that develop in midsummer on long projections called racemes.

Black cohosh grows from seeds sown in spring or root divisions taken in spring or fall. Harvest the roots in fall after the fruits have ripened and cut them lengthwise to dry.

BLACK HAW

An Herb with Southern Roots

Family: Caprifoliaceae; other members include honeysuckle and elder

Genus and species: *Viburnum prunifolium*

Also known as: Viburnum

Part used: Bark

Indiana poet James Whitcomb Riley wrote, "What is sweeter, after all / Than black haws in early fall?" He was referring to the shrub's blue-black fruits, which are the size of small olives.

It's the reddish brown bark of this native American shrub, however, that has a long folk history as a remedy for gynecological complaints— a history that has been confirmed by modern science.

Native American women drank a decoction of black haw bark for menstrual cramps, childbirth recovery, and menopausal discomforts, but especially to prevent miscarriage.

Healing History

Before the Civil War, black haw's miscarriage-preventing action played a small but telling role in relations between slave women and their owners. Slaves were valuable assets, and slaveholders wanted the women to bear as many children as possible. Slave women were often raped by plantation owners or foremen, and many slaves attempted to terminate the resulting pregnancies as a quiet protest against this abuse. In reaction, many slave owners forced slave women to take black haw to prevent them from ending their pregnancies with abortion-inducing herbs.

A popular abortion-inducing herb was cotton root, which was readily available to slaves on Southern plantations. As explained in *King's American Dispensatory* (1898), the textbook of the 19th-century American Eclectic physicians who were forerunners of today's naturopaths, "It was customary for planters to compel female slaves to drink an infusion of black haw daily whilst pregnant to prevent abortion from taking the cotton root."

An Eclectic physician from Mississippi introduced black haw to the North, where it quickly became an herbal mainstay for gynecological complaints. The Eclectics valued it highly: "As a uterine tonic, it is unquestionably of great utility . . . for menstrual pains . . . and a good remedy for menopause. . . . But the condition for which black haw is most valued is threatened abortion. By its quieting effect upon the irritable womb, women who have been previously unable to go to term have been aided to pass through pregnancy without mishaps."

Today, black haw is a minor medicinal herb. But it's still recommended for menstrual cramps and threatened abortion. Some herbals encourage women to drink black haw tea throughout pregnancy, but this turns out not to be a good idea.

Therapeutic Uses

Here is another case where modern science supports folk wisdom, or at least some of it. Scientists have confirmed that black haw may be a good treatment for certain gynecological complaints.

MENSTRUAL CRAMPS. A study published in the British journal *Nature* found that black haw contains a uterine relaxant called scopoletin, thus supporting the herb's value in treating menstrual cramps. In Germany, where herbal medicine is more mainstream than in the United States, black haw preparations are widely recommended for menstrual cramps. These products are not available in the United States, but the herb itself is fairly easy to obtain.

MISCARRIAGE. Black haw has been used for centuries to prevent miscarriage. As a uterine relaxant, it may indeed do the job. Unfortunately, it also contains salicin, a close chemical relative of aspirin. Because aspirin has been linked to birth defects, pregnant women should not take black haw, except possibly under a physician's supervision to prevent premature delivery.

FEVER AND PAIN (INCLUDING HEADACHE AND ARTHRITIS). The aspirin-like chemical in black haw may reduce fever and relieve pain.

Rx Recommendations

For relief of menstrual cramps, fever, headache, and general aches and pains, prepare a decoction using 2 teaspoons of dried black haw bark per cup of water. Boil for 10 minutes, then strain and cool. Drink up to 3 cups a day. The herb has an extremely bitter taste, so you may want to add lemon and honey or mix it with a beverage tea.

As a homemade tincture, take up to 2 teaspoons three times a day.

When using commercial preparations, follow the package directions.

The Safety Factor

Like aspirin, the salicin in black haw is a pain reliever (analgesic), which may contribute to the herb's ability to relieve menstrual cramping. But aspirin has been implicated as a cause of birth defects in the children of women who take it while pregnant. Aspirin is most hazardous to the unborn early in pregnancy. Recognizing this, the classic British herbal *Potter's New Cyclopaedia of Botanical Drugs and Preparations* says that black haw should be used only during the final 5 weeks of pregnancy as a means of preventing potential premature delivery.

Any woman facing a possible premature birth should discuss her situation with her obstetrician. Drugs (including herbs) are a last resort and should be used only with the consent of a doctor.

There is no reason to give black haw to children. There is no reason for postmenopausal women to use it.

Inform health care professionals of the herbs you use. Problematic herb-drug interactions are possible.

Black haw may cause allergic reactions or other unexpected side effects. If any develop, reduce your dose or stop taking it.

For more on herb safety, see Chapter 2.

If symptoms get worse or persist longer than 2 weeks, consult a health care professional promptly.

Growing Information

In the North, black haw is a deciduous spreading shrub with reddish brown bark. In the South, it becomes a small tree. The leaves are pointed, serrated ovals resembling plum leaves. They turn red in the fall.

Depending on location, black haw blooms from early spring to summer. The flowers are large, clustered, white, and showy.

Black haw grows best in rich, moist, well-drained soil under full sun. It tolerates poorer soil and partial shade as long as it gets adequate moisture.

The branch bark may be collected in summer; the trunk bark should be collected in fall. Dry it in the shade.

BONESET

A Traditional Remedy for Colds and Flu

Family: Compositae; other members include daisy, dandelion, and marigold

Genus and species: *Eupatorium perfoliaturn*

Also known as: Feverwort, agueweed, and sweat plant

Parts used: Leaves and flowers

Let's clear up one matter right away: Boneset has nothing to do with mending broken bones. The name comes from its traditional use as a treatment for breakbone fever, an old term for dengue (pronounced *DENG-ee*) fever. Dengue is a mosquito-borne viral disease that causes muscle pain so intense that people imagine that their bones are breaking, hence the condition's traditional name. Today, dengue is rare in the United States, except in southern Florida and Texas and among overseas travelers, who sometimes return from the tropics with it.

Ironically, boneset has never been shown to provide significant relief from dengue fever. But it may help treat minor viral and bacterial illnesses by revving up the immune system's response to infection.

Healing History

Native Americans introduced boneset to early colonists as a sweat inducer, an old treatment for fever. They used the herb for all fever-producing illnesses, including influenza, cholera, dengue, malaria, and typhoid. This is how boneset earned its other popular names: feverwort, sweat plant, and agueweed (*ague* is an archaic term for fever).

Native Americans also used boneset to relieve arthritis and to treat colds, indigestion, constipation, and loss of appetite.

White settlers adopted boneset so enthusiastically that it became one of early America's most popular healing herbs. During the Civil War, soldiers used it not only to treat fever but also as a tonic to keep them healthy. (Modern science shows this is not a good idea; see "The Safety Factor" on page 110.)

In his classic book *American Medicinal Plants*, Dr. C. F. Millspaugh had this to say about boneset: "There is probably no plant more extensively or frequently used than this. The attic or woodshed of almost every farm house has bunches hanging from the rafters, ready for immediate use should some family member or neighbor be taken with a cold."

Dr. Millspaugh also considered boneset excellent against malaria, a major health problem in 19th-century America. He wrote that he'd seen the herb cure cases of malaria that didn't respond to Peruvian cinchona bark, the source of the antimalarial drug quinine.

Boneset was listed as a treatment for fever in the *U.S. Pharmacopoeia*, a standard drug reference, from 1820 through 1916 and in the *National Formulary*, the pharmacists' reference, from 1926 through 1950. But the herb fell from favor over time, replaced by another fever fighter, aspirin.

Some contemporary herbalists continue to recommend boneset for fever.

Therapeutic Uses

Modern critics of herbs tend to ridicule boneset as passionately as physicians a century ago praised it. One expert says, "It simply doesn't work." Another claims, "Boneset lacks therapeutic merit." A third writes, "In view of [boneset's] singular lack of effectiveness, it seems incredible that the plant held official status from 1820 to 1950."

The critics have a point: Boneset has never been shown to suppress fever as well as aspirin. But several studies seem to suggest that the herb has some therapeutic value after all.

COLDS AND FLU. European studies show that boneset helps treat minor viral and bacterial infections by stimulating white blood cells to more effectively destroy disease-causing microorganisms. In Germany, where herbal medicine is more mainstream than in the United States, physicians currently use boneset to treat viral infections such as colds and flu.

ARTHRITIS. One study suggests that boneset is mildly anti-inflammatory, lending some support to its traditional use in treating arthritis.

Intriguing Possibility

Studies conducted worldwide suggest that possible immune-stimulating compounds in boneset have anticancer effects. More research is needed, however, before the herb can be used to treat tumors.

Medicinal Myth

Despite its traditional use, boneset has never been shown to be effective against dengue fever or malaria.

Rx Recommendations

To treat colds, flu, and arthritis and relieve minor inflammation, use an infusion or tincture of boneset. To prepare an infusion, use 1 to 2 teaspoons of dried leaves per cup of boiling water and steep for 10 to 20 minutes. Drink up to 3 cups a day. You'll find the taste very bitter and astringent, so you might want to add sugar or honey and lemon or mix it with an herbal beverage tea.

As a homemade tincture, take $1/2$ to 1 teaspoon up to three times a day.

When using commercial preparations, follow the package directions.

The Safety Factor

In large amounts, boneset may cause nausea, vomiting, and violent diarrhea. In addition, the herb contains pyrrolizidine alkaloids (PAs), chemicals that cause liver damage when administered in large amounts. Boneset's effect on human cancer, if any, is unclear, because the plant also contains anticancer substances.

The PAs in some healing herbs, such as comfrey (see page 173), have caused liver damage in a few cases in which people have taken more than the recommended dose for long periods of time. It's not a good idea to take boneset frequently as a tonic.

Also, do not eat fresh boneset. It contains tremerol, a toxic chemical that causes nausea, vomiting, weakness, muscle tremors, increased respiration, and possibly—at high doses—even coma and death. Drying the herb eliminates the tremerol and the possibility of poisoning.

Pregnant and nursing women should not use boneset.

Do not give boneset to children under 2. In older children, adjust the recommended dose based on the child's weight. For example, give a 50-pound child one-third of the dose a 150-pound adult would take.

If you're over 65, start with a low dose, and increase only if necessary.

Inform health care professionals of the herbs you use. Problematic herb-drug interactions are possible.

Boneset may cause allergic reactions or other unexpected side effects. If any develop, reduce your dose or stop taking it.

For more on herb safety, see Chapter 2.

If symptoms get worse or persist longer than 2 weeks, consult a health care professional promptly.

Growing Information

Boneset is easy to identify because its long, narrow, pointed leaf pairs are not distinct; rather, they are connected and pierced by the stem. The herb has round, erect, hairy, hollow stems that grow to 5 feet, then split into three branches, each of which produces tiny, densely clustered white to bluish florets from midsummer through fall.

A hardy perennial, boneset grows easily from seeds planted in spring or root divisions planted in spring or fall. It prefers rich, moist, well-drained soil under full sun but tolerates poorer soil and partial shade.

Harvest it as it flowers by cutting the entire plant a few inches above the ground.

BORAGE

"Essential" to Healing

Family: Boraginaceae; other members include comfrey and forget-me-not

Genus and species: *Borago officinalis*

Also known as: Star flower, bee bread, bee fodder, cool tankard

Part used: Seed oil

Borage is an annual native to Syria that grows to 2 feet. The stem and leaves are covered with prickly hairs. It produces large star-shaped flowers, hence the common name star flower. The flowers are magnets for bees, hence the names bee bread and bee fodder. When steeped in water or wine, fresh borage imparts a cool, vaguely cucumber flavor. For centuries, it was mixed in wine, producing a beverage known as cool tankard, which became one of the plant's common names.

Healing History

The ancient Greek naturalist Dioscorides documented the earliest known medicinal use of borage—as an additive to wine that made drinkers more forgetful than wine by itself.

The early English herbalist John Parkinson recommended borage to revive hypochondriacs and "expell melancholie."

From ancient times until the early 19th century, borage infusion was also used as a diuretic and as a treatment for colds and bronchitis, and to increase milk production in lactating women.

Therapeutic Uses

Borage seeds yield an oil that is the richest plant source of the essential fatty acid (EFA) gamma-linolenic acid (GLA). In fact, borage seed oil contains about twice the GLA of a more popular medicinal herb, evening primrose oil (see page 211). Essential fatty acids play many important roles in the body. The brain is about 20 percent EFAs, and they are crucial in proper brain and nervous system functioning. EFAs also play important roles in hormone production, the formation of healthy cell membranes, the regulation of blood pressure and blood clotting, and liver function. Though some EFAs have inflammatory effects that can harm the body, others—notably GLA—have potent anti-inflammatory action. Essential fatty acids cannot be synthesized by the body; instead, they must be obtained from the diet. Cold-water fish such as salmon contain EFAs, notably omega-3s, but many Americans who eat a meat-centered diet are deficient in EFAs, especially GLA.

In studies, when animals are placed on diets lacking GLA, they develop a number of health problems, including eczema-like skin conditions, immune suppression, cardiovascular disease, poor wound healing, liver abnormalities, and infertility. This led researchers to try GLA supplementation in people with these conditions. The results have been remarkably positive.

Borage seed oil has not been studied as extensively as evening primrose oil. But a considerable amount of research has been conducted. The studies discussed below are specific to borage seed oil. But presumably, borage seed oil also offers all the benefits of evening primrose oil—or greater benefits—because it contains more GLA.

DRY SKIN. GLA helps maintain moisture in the skin. Older people often develop dry skin, and German researchers wondered if borage oil might help. They gave borage oil (in doses of 360 or 720 milligrams per day) to 20 people, average age 69, who complained of dry skin. After 2 months, their skin was significantly less dry. A common symptom of dry skin is itching. Before borage oil treatment, 34 percent of the participants reported frequent itching. After treatment, that number was reduced to zero.

ECZEMA. Study results have been mixed on the effectiveness of borage oil for treating eczema, known medically as atopic dermatitis. While a few studies showed no benefit, several others showed that its anti-inflammatory action provides significant benefit. German researchers treated a dozen people with eczema using either a placebo or borage seed oil, applied topically. In the placebo group, 20 percent of the participants showed benefit using standard scales for measuring eczema severity. But in the borage oil group, the figure was 71 percent.

Japanese researchers gave new undershirts to 32 children with eczema. Half of the shirts had been coated with borage oil. After 2 weeks, the children wearing the borage oil–coated shirts showed significant relief from skin welts.

ASTHMA. Asthma involves inflammation of the bronchial tubes. Canadian researchers gave 35 asthma sufferers either a placebo or a combination of GLA and another essential fatty acid with anti-inflammatory action. After 4 weeks, the GLA group reported fewer asthma symptoms and less use of inhalers.

ACUTE RESPIRATORY DISTRESS SYNDROME (ARDS). ARDS, often caused by serious infection, involves airway inflammation and potentially fatal breathing impairment. Ohio State University researchers fed 146 people with ARDS either a standard hospital diet or that diet with added GLA from borage oil and another essential fatty acid possessing anti-inflammatory action. After a week, the borage oil group showed significantly less airway inflammation and better oxygenation of their blood.

PRETERM INFANTS. Preemies can have many health problems that retard normal growth and development. British researchers gave 238 preemies either standard formula or formula supplemented with borage oil and fish oil, another source of GLA. Compared with the group given standard formula, the preemies given the GLA showed greater growth and weight gain.

RHEUMATOID ARTHRITIS. Because of GLA's anti-inflammatory action, researchers speculated that it might be helpful for people with rheumatoid arthritis, which involves painful joint inflammation. University of Pennsylvania researchers gave either cottonseed oil, which contains no GLA, or borage oil (1.4 grams per day of GLA) to 37 people with rheumatoid arthritis. After 6 months, "treatment with GLA resulted in clinically important reduction in signs and symptoms of the disease." GLA reduced the number of tender joints by 36 percent and the number of swollen joints by 28 percent. GLA reduced joint pain, tenderness, and swelling by 40 percent.

University of Maryland researchers analyzed 13 studies of GLA treatment of rheumatoid arthritis. They found that, overall, it was beneficial.

BREAST CANCER. British researchers gave 38 women with breast cancer either a standard regimen of the drug tamoxifen, or tamoxifen plus GLA (8 capsules per day totaling 2.8 grams). Biopsies before and after the regimen assessed changes in estrogen receptors. Those receiving the drug and herb oil showed a significant decrease in estrogen receptors, which is associated with less risk of recurrences.

Intriguing Possibility

Pilot studies suggest that borage oil improves bone mineral density, which could be helpful in the prevention and treatment of osteoporosis.

Rx Recommendations

In studies, researchers have used 1 to 3 grams per day.

The Safety Factor

Borage seed oil is considered safe in recommended doses for those who do not have liver disease. However, borage leaves, flowers, and seeds contain compounds (pyrrolizidine alkaloids) that are toxic to the liver. Concentrations of these chemicals are low, and there are no reports of liver damage. But because of the theoretical possibility of liver damage, people with liver disease should not ingest borage.

Pregnant women who would like to use borage oil should discuss it with their physicians.

Breast milk is rich in GLA, so nursing women may use borage oil in consultation with their physicians.

Do not give borage oil to children under 2. In older children, adjust the recommended dose based on the child's weight. For example, give a 50-pound child one-third of the dose a 150-pound adult would take.

If you're over 65, start with a low dose, and increase only if necessary.

Inform health care professionals of the herbs you use. Problematic herb-drug interactions are possible.

Borage oil may cause allergic reactions or other unexpected side effects. If any develop, reduce your dose or stop taking it.

For more on herb safety, see Chapter 2.

If symptoms get worse or persist longer than 2 weeks, consult a health care professional promptly.

Growing Information

Borage grows in most warm and temperate climes. It prefers sandy, well-drained soil. Plant seeds, cuttings, or root divisions in spring. Thin seedlings to space plants about every 15 inches. Borage self-seeds and will grow year after year.

BOSWELLIA

Hello Boswellia, Good-Bye
Inflammation

Family: Burseraceae; other members include
myrrh and frankincense

Genus and species: Boswellia serrata

Also known as: Indian frankincense, Indian
olibanium

Part used: Gum resin

Christians believe that the three wise men who
visited the baby Jesus presented him with frankincense. In Leviticus (24:5–7), frankincense was
offered in sacrifices to God. And in Isaiah (60:6),
the prophet imagined pilgrims arriving in Jerusalem bearing gifts of gold and frankincense.

Frankincense, like its botanical relative
myrrh, is an aromatic resin exuded from the
bark of tropical boswellia trees that grow from
North Africa, across the Middle East, and into
India as well as in tropical regions of the
Western Hemisphere. In the Bible, frankincense
was burned on sacrificial altars, imparting a
distinctive fragrance to the proceedings.
Scholars believe that biblical frankincense was
Boswellia carterii, found in Arabia. Indian
frankincense is very similar. In herbal medicine,
the terms *boswellia* and *Indian frankincense* are
used interchangeably.

Healing History

India's traditional Ayurvedic healers have used
boswellia resin for thousands of years. They
applied it topically for acne, boils, wounds, and
scars, and to smooth wrinkles. Internally, they
used it to treat dysentery, ulcers, respiratory
problems, menstrual problems, and muscle aches
(rheumatism). The herb was also widely used as
a perfume on hair and clothing, and as an indoor
air freshener. It was also used in Indian weddings and religious ceremonies.

Therapeutic Uses

Boswellia resin contains anti-inflammatory
compounds called boswellic acids that inhibit
leukotrienes, chemicals in the body that maintain inflammation.

OSTEOARTHRITIS. Several studies show
that boswellia reduces the pain of osteoarthritis.
Indian researchers gave 66 people with arthritis
of the knee either a standard pharmaceutical or
boswellia (333 milligrams three times a day).
After 6 months, both treatments produced similar benefit. The herb had no effect for the first
month. The drug began working faster. But after
treatments were terminated, boswellia produced
longer residual benefit.

Another group of Indian scientists gave 30 people with osteoarthritis either a placebo or boswellia. After 8 weeks, the groups were switched. While taking the herb, every participant reported less pain. Other Indian studies using multi-herb formulas containing boswellia (with turmeric, myrrh, and ashwagandha) have produced similar benefits.

RHEUMATOID ARTHRITIS. In India, boswellia gum resin has been marketed to treat rheumatoid arthritis since 1982—and with good reason. A German review of the research called it effective. And a British review of seven studies showed that it's "clinically effective."

PAIN. An animal study conducted in China shows that boswellia has pain-relieving action. This would also help in the treatment of arthritis.

ULCERATIVE COLITIS. The intestinal inflammation that causes colitis results, in part, from leukotrienes. Boswellia suppresses leukotrienes. Indian scientists gave patients with colitis either boswellia resin (350 milligrams three times a day) or a standard pharmaceutical (sulfasalazine). After 6 weeks 75 percent of participants in the drug group went into remission. In the herb group, the figure was 82 percent. The researchers repeated this study in 30 subjects, and the results were even better for boswellia—40 percent remission in the drug group, but 90 percent among those taking boswellia.

ASTHMA. Inflammation plays a key role in asthmatic airway constriction. German researchers gave 40 people with asthma either a placebo or boswellia (300 milligrams three times a day). Six weeks later, 27 percent of the placebo group showed improvement. But in the herb group, the figure was 70 percent.

Intriguing Possibilities

Pilot studies in India suggest that boswellia reduces cholesterol and triglyceride (blood fat) levels, and that an herbal formula containing boswellia may reduce the inflammation linked to the arterial damage that causes heart disease.

In laboratory studies, the herb also suppresses replication of DNA in leukemia, hinting that it might have potential as a cancer treatment.

Rx Recommendations

For asthma, osteoarthritis, and colitis, take 300 milligrams of powdered resin three times a day. For rheumatoid arthritis, take 400 milligrams three times a day. Or follow package directions.

The Safety Factor

At recommended doses, boswellia is considered safe. In studies, mild stomach distress, nausea, diarrhea, and heartburn have been reported. If you have chronic heartburn, avoid boswellia.

Boswellia may stimulate menstruation. Pregnant and nursing women should not use it.

Do not give boswellia to children under 2. In older children, adjust the recommended dose based on the child's weight. For example, give a 50-pound child one-third of the dose a 150-pound adult would take.

If you're over 65, start with a low dose, and increase only if necessary.

Inform health care professionals of the herbs you use. Problematic herb-drug interactions are possible.

Boswellia may cause allergic reactions or

other unexpected side effects. If any develop, reduce your dose or stop taking it.

For more on herb safety, see Chapter 2.

If symptoms get worse or persist longer than 2 weeks, consult a health care professional promptly.

Growing Information

Boswellia serrata is a moderate-size deciduous tree that grows in hot, mountainous, arid areas of central India. It requires limestone-rich soil. It is not grown commercially in the United States, but might grow in places like the hill country of Texas or mountain areas of the Southwest, possibly with lime added. Resin harvesters cut a thin strip of bark near the base of the tree and tap the tree in a manner similar to harvesting maple sap for syrup. Tapping takes place from November to May.

BUCHU

A South African Diuretic

Family: Rutaceae; other members include orange, lemon, and rue

Genus and species: *Barosma betulina* or *Agathosma betulina, B. crenulata,* and *B. serratifolia*

Also known as: Bookoo, buku, bucku, and bucco

Parts used: Leaves

The leaves of this 5-foot shrub from southern Africa contain an oil that increases urine production.

Healing History

The native people of what is now Namibia and South Africa used buchu for urinary problems long before they had any contact with Europeans.

In the 17th century, when Dutch (Afrikaner) colonists settled the region, they adopted buchu as a treatment for urinary tract infections, kidney stones, arthritis, cholera, and muscle aches.

Later, English settlers adopted buchu and relied on it to treat so many illnesses that medical botanists now claim that it has been used for "almost every disease that afflicts mankind."

In 1847, New York patent medicine entrepreneur Henry T. Helmbold introduced Helmbold's Compound Extract of Buchu as a remedy for urinary problems, kidney stones, and "diseases arising from imprudence [venereal diseases]." The American public responded as enthusiastically as the African colonists had. Helmbold grew rich and called himself Helmbold, the Buchu King.

Therapeutic Uses

The Buchu King has long been forgotten, but herbalists have considered buchu an effective diuretic ever since.

PREMENSTRUAL SYNDROME (PMS). Many women complain of bloating from water retention before their periods. Buchu is an ingredient in several teas marketed in health food stores to relieve the bloating of PMS.

URINARY TRACT INFECTIONS. Most modern herbals continue to recommend buchu as a treatment for urinary tract infections. One study of the herb's effects on the bacteria that cause the infections showed no benefit. Still, herbal experts stand behind buchu as an infection fighter.

HIGH BLOOD PRESSURE AND CONGESTIVE HEART FAILURE. Physicians prescribe diuretics to treat high blood pressure and congestive heart failure. These are serious conditions requiring professional care, so consult your physician about including buchu in your treatment plan.

Medicinal Myth

For years, buchu was an ingredient in herbal weight-loss products. Diuretics can cause temporary loss of excess water weight, but no science-based weight-loss program endorses the use of diuretics for permanent weight control.

Rx Recommendations

For relief of premenstrual bloating, try an infusion or tincture of buchu. You might also try these preparations for relief of chronic urinary tract infections.

To prepare an infusion, use 1 to 2 teaspoons of dried, crumbled leaves per cup of boiling water and steep for 10 to 20 minutes. Drink up to 3 cups a day. Buchu has a minty aroma and a pleasant, minty taste.

As a homemade tincture, take $1/2$ to 1 teaspoon up to three times a day.

When using commercial preparations, follow the package directions.

The Safety Factor

There are no reports of significant hazards from using recommended amounts of buchu.

Diuretics deplete the body's stores of potassium, an important nutrient. If you take buchu, you should increase your consumption of foods rich in potassium, such as bananas and fresh vegetables.

Pregnant and nursing women should not use buchu.

Do not give buchu to children under 2. In older children, adjust the recommended dose based on the child's weight. For example, give a 50-pound child one-third of the dose a 150-pound adult would take.

If you're over 65, start with a low dose, and increase only if necessary.

Inform health care professionals of the herbs you use. Problematic herb-drug interactions are possible.

Buchu may cause allergic reactions or other unexpected side effects. If any develop, reduce your dose or stop taking it.

For more on herb safety, see Chapter 2.

If symptoms get worse or persist longer than 2 weeks, consult a health care professional promptly.

Growing Information

This 5-foot shrub with finely toothed opposite or alternate leaves is not grown in the United States.

BUCKTHORN
An Old-Time Constipation Cure

Family: Rhamnaceae; other members include cascara sagrada

Genus and species: *Rhamnus cathartica* and *R. frangula*

Also known as: Purging buckthorn, frangula, and alder buckthorn

Parts used: Berries and bark

The species name for buckthorn, *cathartica*, is no joke. This herb is a potent laxative—so powerful, in fact, that authorities recommend using it only as a last resort, after other, gentler laxatives have failed.

Healing History

Buckthorn became popular in herbal healing in Europe around the 13th century. At the time, physicians believed that the key to curing disease lay in purging "foul humors." With such a focus on purging, powerful laxatives were widely prescribed. Buckthorn was a favorite because it produced quick, reliable results—while often leaving people with intestinal cramps.

Down through the ages, herbalists have also recommended buckthorn for treating jaundice, hemorrhoids, gout, arthritis, and promoting menstruation. In addition, this herb has a long history as a cancer treatment. In America, it was an ingredient in the popular but highly controversial Hoxsey Cancer Formula (see page 33).

Therapeutic Uses

Buckthorn doesn't treat jaundice or arthritis, and it's more likely to aggravate hemorrhoids than to relieve them. But its laxative action is so powerful that it's considered a purgative.

CONSTIPATION. No one disputes buckthorn's laxative action. It has been an ingredient in many pharmaceutical and herbal laxatives. Commission E, the expert panel that evaluates herbal medicines for the German counterpart of the FDA, approves the herb as a laxative.

Buckthorn contains chemicals called anthraquinones. They're dramatic purgatives—too powerful for most people. That's why buckthorn should be considered a last-resort treatment for constipation.

Intriguing Possibility

Harry Hoxsey may have been on the right track. Buckthorn has an anti-tumor effect, according to research published in the *Journal of the National Cancer Institute*. But one study does not establish efficacy as a cancer treatment. Research continues on buckthorn as a possible cancer therapy, but to date, no clinical trials have been conducted, which means this herb is many years away from use as a cancer treatment—if it's ever used that way.

Rx Recommendations

In Germany, physicians prescribe an infusion containing 1/2 teaspoon each of dried buckthorn bark, fennel seeds, and chamomile flowers (which soothe the stomach). Steep the blend in 1 cup of boiling water for 10 minutes, then strain. Drink it before going to bed. You'll find the taste initially sweet, then bitter.

If you prefer a decoction, boil 1 teaspoon of dried buckthorn in 3 cups of water. Steep for 30 minutes, then strain. Drink it cool, 1 tablespoon at a time, before going to bed.

As a homemade tincture, take 1/2 teaspoon before going to bed.

When using commercial preparations, follow the package directions.

The Safety Factor

Because of buckthorn's powerful laxative action, people who have chronic gastrointestinal problems, including ulcers, colitis, Crohn's disease, diverticulitis, and hemorrhoids, should not use it.

Don't take buckthorn for more than 2 weeks at a time. If you use it for too long, it causes lazy bowel syndrome, an inability to have bowel movements without chemical stimulation.

If you use bulk buckthorn, be sure that it has

been dried thoroughly. Otherwise, it causes vomiting, severe abdominal pain, and violent diarrhea. Most herbalists recommend drying the berries or bark for at least a year (some say 2 years) before using them. Commercial preparations use aged bark.

You can artificially dry fresh buckthorn by baking it at 250°F for several hours. If you experience nausea and abdominal distress after taking the herb, seek professional medical attention immediately.

Pregnant and nursing women should not use buckthorn.

Do not give buckthorn to children.

If you're over 65, start with a low dose, and increase only if necessary.

Inform health care professionals of the herbs you use. Problematic herb-drug interactions are possible.

Buckthorn may cause allergic reactions or other unexpected side effects. If any develop, reduce your dose or stop taking it.

For more on herb safety, see Chapter 2.

If symptoms get worse or persist longer than 2 weeks, consult a health care professional promptly.

Growing Information

Buckthorn is a shrub or small tree that reaches about 20 feet. It has shiny, dark green leaves and produces black, pea-size berries. It is not a garden plant.

BURDOCK
Likely to Stick Around

Family: Compositae; other members include daisy, dandelion, and marigold

Genus and species: *Arctium lappa*

Also known as: Great burdock and burr

Parts used: Primarily roots; also leaves and seeds

The term *burdock* is a combination of *bur-*, for its tenacious burrs, and *-dock*, an Old English term for "plant." The name is apt. Burdock seems to reach out and grab anything that comes near it. The same could be said for its place in modern herbal healing. While many scientists have dismissed burdock as useless, it seems destined to hang on as a healing herb, particularly as a potential treatment for cancer.

Healing History

Burdock has had its ups and downs in the past. When it wasn't being reviled as a weed, it was being recommended as a healing treatment for a surprising variety of conditions.

Early Chinese physicians considered burdock a remedy for colds, flu, throat infections, and pneumonia. India's traditional Ayurvedic healers used it in similar ways.

The medieval German abbess/herbalist Hildegard of Bingen prescribed burdock to treat cancerous tumors. And during the 14th century in Europe, the herb's leaves were used to make wine and treat leprosy.

England's overly imaginative 17th-century herbalist Nicholas Culpeper recommended burdock for uterine prolapse, a condition in which the ligaments supporting the uterus weaken and cause it to fall into the vagina. Culpeper's bizarre prescription: Place burdock on the crown of the head to draw the womb back up.

Later European herbalists prescribed burdock root for fever, cancer, eczema, psoriasis, acne, dandruff, gout, ringworm, skin infections, syphilis, gonorrhea, and problems associated with childbirth. And America's 19th-century Eclectic physicians, forerunners of today's naturopaths, considered the herb an excellent diuretic. They prescribed it for urinary tract infections, kidney problems, and painful urination in addition to skin infections and arthritis.

Centuries after Hildegard recommended burdock for cancer, the herb's reputation as a tumor treatment spread to Russia, China, India, and the Americas. From the 1930s to the 1950s, burdock was an ingredient in the alternative cancer treatment marketed by ex–coal miner Harry Hoxsey (see page 33).

Contemporary herbalists have abandoned burdock as a cancer treatment (perhaps prematurely). But they continue to recommend it for skin problems, wound healing, urinary tract infections, arthritis, sciatica, ulcers, and even anorexia nervosa.

Therapeutic Uses

Many modern herb experts give a thumbs-down to burdock as a healing herb. In *Natural Product Medicine*, Ara Der Marderosian, Ph.D., and Lawrence Liberti write, "There is little evidence to suggest burdock is useful in treatment of any human disease." And in *Tyler's Honest Herbal*, the late Varro E. Tyler, Ph.D., writes, "However, despite its long folkloric use, no solid evidence exists that burdock exhibits any useful therapeutic activity."

Most traditional claims for burdock have not withstood scientific scrutiny. The herb does not treat leprosy, arthritis, uterine prolapse, or congestive heart failure. Still, several studies suggest that it may prove to be therapeutic after all.

INFECTIONS. Burdock's traditional use against fungal and bacterial infections has been experimentally confirmed. German researchers have discovered that fresh burdock root contains chemicals called polyacetylenes, which kill disease-causing bacteria and fungi. Brazilian researchers have shown that the herb inhibits the growth of *Candida albicans*, the fungus that causes yeast infections, and several types of bacteria, including staphylococcus, pseudomonas, and enterococcus.

Intriguing Possibilities

Burdock has been used extensively around the world as a cancer treatment. Several studies have shown that certain substances in the herb do, in fact, have anti-tumor activity. An article published in *Chemotherapy* identified arctigenin, a chemical in burdock, as an "inhibitor of experimental tumor growth." And a study reported in *Mutation Research* determined that burdock decreases mutations in cells exposed to mutation-causing chemicals. (Most substances that cause genetic mutations also cause cancer.)

Burdock may also have potential as a cough suppressant. Researchers in Slovakia induced coughs in laboratory animals, and then gave them a variety of herbs. Marshmallow, an herbal cough suppressant with a long history of effectiveness, worked best. But burdock also worked quite well.

In addition, burdock could help fight allergic reactions. In an animal study, German researchers have discovered that burdock, applied topically, interferes to some extent with the type of allergic swelling that causes hives.

Finally, burdock has an as-yet-unexplained anti-poisoning effect. Experimental animals that were fed the herb were somehow protected against several chemicals known to be toxic.

In view of these tantalizing findings, let's hope that scientists cling to burdock research as tenaciously as the plant's burrs cling to just about anything.

Rx Recommendations

Use burdock as a decoction or tincture. To prepare a decoction, boil 1 teaspoon of root in 3 cups of water for 30 minutes, then let cool. Drink up to 3 cups a day. Burdock has a sweet taste similar to celery root. When using a tincture, take $1/2$ to 1 teaspoon up to three times a day.

When using commercial preparations, follow the package directions.

The Safety Factor

No one questioned the safety of burdock until the *Journal of the American Medical Association* linked the herb to one case of poisoning that could have proved fatal. A woman who drank a strong decoction experienced blurred vision, dry mouth, and hallucinations, all classic symptoms of atropine poisoning. Burdock does not contain atropine, but belladonna, a plant that looks similar, does. Presumably, some belladonna accidentally adulterated the woman's burdock.

One case of adulteration is not cause for alarm. Still, if you use burdock and develop any of the symptoms of atropine poisoning mentioned above, seek emergency medical treatment immediately.

Pregnant and nursing women should not use burdock.

Do not give burdock to children under 2. In older children, adjust the recommended dose based on the child's weight. For example, give a 50-pound child one-third of the dose a 150-pound adult would take.

If you're over 65, start with a low dose, and increase only if necessary.

Inform health care professionals of the herbs you use. Problematic herb-drug interactions are possible.

Burdock may cause allergic reactions or other

unexpected side effects. If any develop, reduce your dose or stop taking it.

For more on herb safety, see Chapter 2.

If symptoms get worse or persist longer than 2 weeks, consult a health care professional promptly.

Growing Instructions

Burdock's medicinal root has brown bark and a white, spongy, fibrous interior that becomes hard when dried. Its stem is multibranched, with long, egg-shaped leaves. Each branch is topped by a bristled "flower"—actually a clump of many purplish flowers—that produces its infamous burrs.

Burdock grows easily from seeds planted in spring. Thin seedlings to 6-inch spacing. Burdock prefers moist, rich, deeply cultivated soil and full sun, but it tolerates poorer soils. Many herbalists mix wood chips and sawdust into burdock beds to keep the soil loose so the roots are easier to harvest.

Burdock roots deeply, so it's not advisable to transplant established plants. Harvest the roots during the fall of the first year or the spring of the second.

BUTCHER'S BROOM

Sweep Away Varicose Veins and Hemorrhoids

Family: Liliaceae; other members include lilies, tulips, and onions

Genus and species: *Ruscus aculeatus*

Also known as: Ruscus, box holly, knee holly, sweet broom

Parts used: Rhizomes and roots

For centuries, European butchers bound the stiff twigs of this plant into bundles and used the small brooms to keep their cutting boards clean. However, many plants were used to make brooms and acquired the name "broom." If you want butcher's broom, confirm that the herb you're buying is *Ruscus aculeatus.*

Butcher's broom is native to the Mediterranean and Middle East, but grows throughout much of Europe. Its leaves resemble holly leaves, hence some of its common names and its generic name, *ruscus*, which is derived from the Anglo-Saxon word for holly.

Healing History

In ancient times, butcher's broom was used as a laxative and diuretic. A root decoction in wine was used to treat kidney stones.

Seventeenth-century English herbalist Nicholas Culpeper recommended a decoction of the root and a poultice of the berries for broken bones.

Then the plant fell into disuse. In the 1950s, scientists discovered that butcher's broom's underground stems, called rhizomes, made veins less likely to leak fluid (a condition known as venous permeability, or venous insufficiency) and might be useful in treating circulatory problems, such as edema and varicose veins.

Therapeutic Uses

Most of the studies have used a French proprietary formula, Cyclo 3 Fort. It contains butcher's broom (150 milligrams per capsule) extract plus vitamin C (100 milligrams) and hesperidin methyl chalcone (150 milligrams), a compound from citrus fruits that also helps reduce venous permeability.

VARICOSE VEINS/CHRONIC VENOUS INSUFFICIENCY. Chronic venous insufficiency means that the veins, particularly the leg veins, don't properly return blood to the heart. Blood pools in the legs, eventually causing varicose veins. An estimated 80 million Americans, about 40 percent of the adult population, have varicose veins in their legs. While not life-threatening, they can be painful, unsightly, and costly to treat. Italian researchers analyzed 20 studies of Cyclo 3 Fort for treating chronic venous insufficiency. Compared with placebo treatment, the herb product "significantly reduces" swelling, the severity of pain, heaviness, cramping, and tingling. The researchers called their analysis "a strong demonstration of the efficacy of Cyclo 3 Fort in treating chronic venous insufficiency."

Several studies also show that Cyclo 3 Fort relieves pregnancy-related varicose veins. The research to date has not established the absolute safety of butcher's broom during pregnancy, but an article in *Alternative and Complementary Therapies* says, "Both animal and human studies indicate a high degree of safety during pregnancy."

Commission E, the expert panel that evaluates herbal medicines for the German counterpart of the FDA, approves butcher's broom for varicose veins.

LYMPHEDEMA. Lymph is a fluid that circulates throughout the body and contains white blood cells that fight infection. When lymph vessels become damaged, lymph drainage becomes blocked, and excess fluid accumulates, causing swelling and discomfort. When lymph nodes are removed from the underarm as part of breast cancer surgery, lymphedema is a common side effect. French researchers gave fluid-draining arm massage, a standard therapy, to 57 women who had developed lymphedema after breast cancer surgery. The women also took either a placebo or Cyclo 3 Fort daily. After 3 months, the herb group had significantly less residual arm swelling.

HEMORRHOIDS. Hemorrhoids are varicose veins around or near the anus. French researchers gave Cyclo 3 Fort to 124 people with hemorrhoids. They took six capsules a day for 3 days, followed by four capsules a day for 4 days. Using standard measures of hemorrhoid symptoms, the herb produced significant pain relief. Commission E approves butcher's broom for hemorrhoids.

Intriguing Possibility

Pilot studies suggest that Cyclo 3 Fort helps relieve the bloating some women experience before their periods.

Rx Recommendations

Take two to four capsules of Cyclo 3 Fort a day. Or follow package directions.

The Safety Factor

Butcher's broom is considered safe in recommended doses, but stomach upset and diarrhea have been reported.

Pregnant women interested in trying Cyclo 3 Fort for varicose veins should discuss this with their physicians.

Do not give butcher's broom to children under

2. In older children, adjust the recommended dose based on the child's weight. For example, give a 50-pound child one-third of the dose a 150-pound adult would take.

If you're over 65, start with a low dose, and increase only if necessary.

Inform health care professionals of the herbs you use. Problematic herb-drug interactions are possible.

Butcher's broom may cause allergic reactions or other unexpected side effects. If any develop, reduce your dose or stop taking it.

For more on herb safety, see Chapter 2.

If symptoms get worse or persist longer than 2 weeks, consult a health care professional promptly.

Growing Information

Butcher's broom is a prickly, low-growing evergreen shrub that thrives throughout much of the southern United States. Its shoots look like asparagus and are edible, but the berries are toxic. This plant grows best in moist, chalky soil. Though it can grow in many parts of the United States, most of the herb used medicinally is imported.

BUTTERBUR

For Hay Fever and Migraine Relief

Family: Asteraceae; other members include daisy

Genus and species: *Petasites hybridus*

Also known as: Pestilence wort, bog rhubarb, butter dock, butterfly dock

Parts used: Leaf and root extract

Butterbur is a perennial shrub native to Europe. Its leaves are downy and very large, hence its generic name, *Petasites*, from the Greek word, *petasos*, for the broad-brimmed felt hats worn by shepherds. During the Middle Ages, the leaves were used to wrap butter in warm weather, hence the name butterbur. This herb has a long history of use as a healer. But for the last century it was largely forgotten. Then studies in the 1990s showed that it deserves a place in herbal medicine.

Healing History

The ancient Greeks used butterbur to treat asthma. This use continued through the Middle Ages, when butterbur was also used to treat fevers, cough, headache, ulcers, and plague, hence one of its names, pestilence wort.

Therapeutic Uses

The medicinally active constituent in butterbur is petasin.

MIGRAINE PREVENTION. Mention herbs for migraines, and people knowledgeable about herbal medicine immediately think of feverfew (see page 222). It works, but so does butterbur, validating one of the herb's folk uses. German researchers gave 60 people with migraines either butterbur (pyrrolizidine-free, 50 milligrams twice a day) or a placebo. After 12 weeks, the herb group experienced significantly fewer migraines than the placebo group—and 60 percent fewer migraines than their baseline rate.

In a 4-month study at Albert Einstein College of Medicine in the Bronx, New York, butterbur extract (pyrrolizidine-free, 75 milligrams twice a day) reduced migraine frequency by 48 percent. Another German group found that among 33 people with migraines, the herb butterbur (pyrrolizidine-free, 50 milligrams twice a day) reduced migraine frequency by at least half in 45 percent of participants. A third German team treated 108 children, ages 6 to 17, with the herb (pyrrolizidine-free, 50 to 150 milligrams per day, depending on age). After 4 months, 77 percent reported attack frequency reduced by at least 50 percent.

HAY FEVER. Swiss scientists gave 125 allergy sufferers either a popular antihistamine (Zyrtec) or butterbur (pyrrolizidine-free, 50 milligrams four times a day). The herb worked as well as the drug. But while the drug caused drowsiness in 75 percent of users, the herb did not.

Other studies—but not all of them—support butterbur's anti-allergy action. To settle the matter, British researchers conducted a meta-analysis, a statistically sophisticated review. They included all published studies that met standard criteria for scientific rigor—subjects were randomly assigned to either herb or placebo groups (or a popular antihistamine), and neither the subjects nor the researchers knew who was in which group. The researchers found six rigorous butterbur trials. Five showed that the herb was effective. It worked better than the placebo and as well as standard antihistamines.

Intriguing Possibility

One study suggests that butterbur (pyrrolizidine-free, 50 milligrams three times a day) reduces the number, duration, and severity of asthma attacks.

Rx Recommendations

Look for tablets containing 50 milligrams of a standardized carbon dioxide extract containing 8 milligrams of petasin per tablet. Take one tablet two or three times a day. Or follow package directions.

The Safety Factor

Butterbur contains pyrrolizidine alkaloids, which are toxic to the liver. The root contains more than the leaves. Commission E, the expert panel that evaluates herbal medicines for the German counterpart of the FDA, says intake of pyrrolizidine alkaloids should be limited to no more than 1 microgram per day. Butterbur roots contain as much as 100 micrograms per gram. However, commercial preparations use carbon dioxide to remove the pyrrolizidine alkaloids. Look for butterbur products that specify no pyrrolizidines, or a CO_2 extract.

Headache, itchy eyes, stomach upset, constipation, and diarrhea have been reported after butterbur use.

Pregnant and nursing women should not use butterbur.

Do not give butterbur to children under 2. In older children, adjust the recommended dose based on the child's weight. For example, give a 50-pound child one-third of the dose a 150-pound adult would take.

If you're over 65, start with a low dose, and increase only if necessary.

Inform health care professionals of the herbs you use. Problematic herb-drug interactions are possible.

Butterbur may cause allergic reactions especially in those with ragweed allergies, or other unexpected side effects. If any develop, reduce your dose or stop taking it.

For more on herb safety, see Chapter 2.

If symptoms get worse or persist longer than 2 weeks, consult a health care professional promptly.

Growing Information

Butterbur grows in temperate climates, including North America. It prefers wet, marshy soil adjacent to streams. Once established, it spreads aggressively. Snip flowers before they open to stop spreading. Traditionally, stems were cooked as a vegetable, hence the name bog rhubarb. Because scientists have found that they contain pyrrolizidine alkaloids, however, eating the stems is not recommended.

CARAWAY
A Digestive Aid from Ancient Egypt

Family: Umbelliferae; other members include carrot, celery, parsley, fennel, dill, and angelica

Genus and species: *Carum carvi*

Also known as: Carum

Parts used: Fruits (seeds)

Caraway is best known as the seed that flavors rye bread. The reason it came to be used in rye bread, as well as many other foods, is that its seeds have been used since ancient times to calm the digestive tract and expel gas.

Caraway seeds have been found in prehistoric food remains from 3500 B.C. The ancient Egyptians loved the aromatic seeds. They were recommended for digestive upsets in the *Ebers Papyrus*, one of the world's oldest surviving medical documents, dating to about 1500 B.C.

Healing History

Caraway is one of only a handful of herbs whose major medicinal uses have remained unchanged throughout history. The Greek physician Dioscorides mentioned the seeds as a digestive aid, and herbals down through the ages have recommended them for indigestion, gas, and infant colic.

In Shakespeare's day, baked apples with caraway seeds were considered a stomach-soothing dessert. In *Henry IV*, a meal ends with "a pippin and a dish of caraway."

Seventeenth-century English herbalist Nicholas Culpeper said that caraway "helpeth digestion . . . and easeth the pains of the wind colic." America's 19th-century Eclectic physicians, forerunners of today's naturopaths, believed that the seeds "gently excite the digestive powers . . . [and can be] used in flatulent colic, especially of children."

Throughout history, in Europe, the Middle East, and early America, caraway was a favorite addition to laxative herbs because it tempered their frequently violent effects.

Caraway's only other traditional uses relate to women's health—for relieving menstrual cramps, promoting menstruation, and aiding milk production in nursing mothers.

Therapeutic Uses

The Egyptians were right about caraway. It's amazing that a treatment used 3,500 years ago can still be effective today.

DIGESTIVE PROBLEMS. Modern researchers have discovered that two chemicals in caraway seeds, carvol and carvene, soothe the smooth muscle tissue of the digestive tract and help expel gas.

In Germany, where herbal medicine is more mainstream than in the United States, a popular over-the-counter digestive product called Enteroplant has two active ingredients: peppermint oil (90 milligrams) and caraway oil (50 milligrams). German researchers gave 45 people with chronic indigestion either a placebo or Enteroplant (one capsule three times a day with meals). After 4 weeks, those taking the placebo reported no change in abdominal distress. Of those taking Enteroplant, 94.5 percent reported significant improvement in their symptoms, with 63 percent declaring that they were free from pain.

In a separate German study, another herbal digestive aid—this one containing peppermint, caraway, fennel, and wormwood—produced similar relief from indigestion symptoms in only 2 weeks. No wonder Commission E, the expert panel that evaluates herbal medicines for the German counterpart of the FDA, endorses caraway as a treatment for indigestion and abdominal distress.

WOMEN'S HEALTH CONCERNS. Antispasmodics, which appear to be present in caraway, soothe not only the digestive tract but also other smooth muscles, such as those of the uterus. Thus, caraway may relax the uterus, not stimulate it. Women might try the herb for relief of menstrual cramps.

Rx Recommendations

You can chew fresh caraway seeds a teaspoon at a time or mix them into food. Add them to any recipe that would benefit from their unique flavor. They're often used in breads, soups, salads, stews, cheeses, sauerkraut, pickling brines, and meat dishes.

Caraway oil is also used to flavor two digestive-aid liqueurs: Scandinavian Aquavit and German Kummel.

For a pleasant-tasting infusion that may aid digestion or relieve gas or menstrual cramping, use 2 to 3 teaspoons of crushed seeds per cup of boiling water. Steep for 10 to 20 minutes, then strain. Drink up to 3 cups a day.

If you prefer a homemade tincture, take $1/2$ to 1 teaspoon up to three times a day.

When using commercial preparations, follow the package directions.

You may give low-strength caraway infusions to infants for colic and gas.

The Safety Factor

There have been no reports of harm from caraway.

Although the herb has antispasmodic properties, which means that it may relax the uterus, it has been used throughout history to promote menstruation. Pregnant women should exercise caution and not take the herb medicinally.

Inform health care professionals of the herbs you use. Problematic herb-drug interactions are possible.

Caraway may cause allergic reactions or other unexpected side effects. If any develop, reduce your dose or stop taking it.

For more on herb safety, see Chapter 2.

If symptoms get worse or persist longer than 2 weeks, consult a health care professional promptly.

Growing Information

Caraway is an attractive biennial that reaches 2 feet. It has feathery leaves and umbrella-like clusters of tiny white flowers, which bloom in early summer.

Caraway grows easily from seeds planted in spring $1/2$ inch deep and 8 inches apart. The plants like rich, well-drained soil and full sun. Keep them moist but not wet.

The first year, caraway produces a small rosette of leaves and a long taproot. Don't transplant it once it has become established. During the second year, caraway sends up its stem, reveals its feathery leaves, and produces its seeds.

Seeds appear in midsummer. Harvest them as soon as they ripen. Leave some seeds behind, and the plants will self-sow.

CASCARA SAGRADA

An Effective Laxative

Family: Rhamnaceae; other members include buckthorn

Genus and species: *Rhamnus purshiana* or *Frangula purshiana*

Also known as: Cascara, sacred bark, and chittem bark

Part used: Bark

The 16th-century Spanish explorers who first visited northern California had a problem—constipation. The Native Americans in the area had the solution, a tea made from a healing herb they held sacred. The herb worked, and the Spanish named it *cascara sagrada*, or "sacred bark." It has been the answer to millions of prayers ever since. But the FDA thinks it's too hazardous to use.

Healing History

The Spanish recognized cascara sagrada as a relative of buckthorn, the powerful laxative herb used in Europe since ancient times. But cascara was much gentler. The explorers sent some back to Spain, where its comparatively mild action was hailed as a wonder of the New World.

But the Spanish explorers were more interested in finding gold than in spreading laxatives around the newly discovered continent. For a long time, cascara remained a West Coast folk remedy, known as chittem bark, a polite variant of the Gold Rush '49ers' name, sh—tin' bark.

In 1877, an Eclectic physician in Detroit extolled cascara's mildness in a home medical guide, prompting Parke, Davis, the pharmaceutical firm, to market a commercial preparation. Cascara sagrada has been popular ever since. It entered the *U.S. Pharmacopoeia*, a standard drug reference, in 1890 and remains there today.

In Appalachian folk medicine, cascara sagrada has also been used to treat cancer. It was an ingredient in the popular but highly controversial Hoxsey Cancer Formula, an alternative therapy marketed from the 1930s to the 1950s by ex–coal miner Harry Hoxsey (see page 33).

Therapeutic Uses

Modern herbals recommend cascara sagrada for constipation and endorse the assertion of Eclectic physicians, who were forerunners of today's naturopaths, that it "restores bowel tone."

CONSTIPATION. Commission E, the expert panel that evaluates herbal medicines for the German counterpart of the FDA, endorses cascara sagrada as a safe, effective laxative. Many European laxative products contain the herb.

At one time in the United States, cascara was an ingredient in dozens of over-the-counter laxatives. But senna (see page 429) has largely taken its place. In 2002, the FDA banned cascara sagrada from over-the-counter laxatives, saying that the herb is too powerful and cathartic. However, it continues to be the active ingredient in a few prescription laxatives, among them Cascara Aromatic and Aromatic Cascara Fluid Extract.

Intriguing Possibility

Harry Hoxsey may have been on the right track. Cascara sagrada contains aloe-emodin, which has demonstrated anti-leukemia action in laboratory animals, supporting the herb's use as a cancer treatment. Unfortunately, aloe-emodin is also quite toxic, and scientists say more research is needed before it can be used to treat leukemia.

Rx Recommendations

Over-the-counter laxatives in the United States can no longer contain cascara sagrada. If you'd like to use it, buy dried, year-old bark and prepare a decoction or ask your doctor for a prescription.

To prepare a decoction, boil 1 teaspoon of well-dried bark in 3 cups of water for 30 minutes, then strain and let cool to room temperature. Drink 1 to 2 cups a day. The taste is quite bitter. You may find that a tincture is more palatable; take $1/2$ teaspoon at bedtime.

When using a prescription product, follow the pharmacist's directions.

The Safety Factor

Cascara sagrada contains chemicals called anthraquinones that stimulate the intestinal contractions known as "the urge." However, laxatives that contain anthraquinones are considered last resorts for constipation. First, increase your fiber intake, drink more fluids, and exercise more. If that doesn't work, try a bulk-forming laxative, such as psyllium (see page 375). And if that doesn't provide relief, try cascara sagrada.

Do not use cascara for more than 2 weeks. Over time, it causes lazy bowel syndrome, an inability to have bowel movements without chemical stimulation. If constipation persists, consult a physician.

Cascara bark must be stored and dried for at least a year before use. The fresh herb contains chemicals that can cause violent diarrhea and severe intestinal cramps. Drying changes these chemicals and gives the herb milder action. Fresh bark may also be artificially dried by baking it at 250°F for several hours.

Cascara sagrada should not be used by anyone with ulcers, ulcerative colitis, Crohn's disease, irritable bowel syndrome, hemorrhoids, or other gastrointestinal conditions.

Pregnant and nursing women should not use cascara sagrada.

Do not give this herb to children.

If you're over 65, start with a low dose, and increase only if necessary.

Inform health care professionals of the herbs you use. Problematic herb-drug interactions are possible.

Cascara sagrada may cause allergic reactions or other unexpected side effects. If any develop, reduce your dose or stop taking it.

For more on herb safety, see Chapter 2.

If symptoms get worse or persist longer than 2 weeks, consult a health care professional promptly.

Growing Information

Cascara sagrada is an unassuming, 20-foot tree with reddish brown bark and thin, finely serrated leaves. It grows in the northwestern United States and is not a garden herb.

CATNIP

Enjoy It with Kitty

Family: Labiatae; other members include mints

Genus and species: *Nepeta cataria*

Also known as: Catmint, catnep, catswort, and field balm

Parts used: Flowers and leaves

You don't have to be an herbalist to appreciate catnip's effect on cats. But here's a case where one species' intoxicant is another's calmer. In people, catnip helps soothe the nerves and digestive tract. It may also help relieve menstrual cramps and can provide handy first aid for gardeners.

Healing History

From Europe to China, catnip has been used medicinally for at least 2,000 years. In teas, its pleasant, lemon-minty vapors were considered a cold and cough remedy, relieving chest congestion and loosening phlegm. Old herbals praised catnip's ability to promote sweating, a traditional treatment for fever.

Catnip has a long history of use as a tranquilizer, sedative, digestive aid, menstruation promoter, and treatment for menstrual cramps, flatulence, and infant colic. Parents used to give weak catnip tea to colicky infants and even hang a small bag of the herb around their babies' necks so they could inhale its soothing vapors.

A blend of equal parts of catnip and saffron was once recommended as a remedy for smallpox and scarlet fever. Catnip leaves were chewed to relieve toothache and, as crazy as this sounds today, smoked to treat bronchitis and asthma.

Catnip was a popular beverage tea in pre-Elizabethan England. During the Age of Exploration, it was replaced by the more stimulating Chinese herb that we call tea (*Camellia sinensis*). But not all English catnip lovers switched to Chinese tea without regrets. In her book *The Herb Garden*, a certain Miss Bardswell clucked, "Catmint Tea was . . . a good deal more wholesome."

Colonists introduced catnip into North America. The plant quickly went wild and now grows across the continent. Native Americans adopted it and used it as the settlers did, for indigestion and infant colic and as a beverage.

Early Americans believed that catnip roots made even the kindest person mean. Hangmen used to consume the roots before executions to get in the mood for their work.

Catnip was listed as a stomach soother in the *U.S. Pharmacopoeia*, a standard drug reference, from 1842 to 1882 and in the *National Formulary*, the pharmacists' reference, from 1916 to 1950.

A report published in the *Journal of the American Medical Association* in 1969 claimed that catnip produces marijuana-like intoxication. The wire services picked up the story, newspapers ran screaming headlines, and bewildered pet shop owners reported a sudden run on cat toys.

The report was quickly discredited by correspondents who flooded the medical journal with letters pointing out that the catnip photos that were printed with the article actually showed marijuana. Catnip has no history as a human intoxicant, and authorities quickly dismissed the notion that smoking catnip causes anything— except a sore throat.

Unfortunately, the same cannot be said for the popular press. As the late Varro E. Tyler, Ph.D., wrote in *Tyler's Honest Herbal*, "It is unfortunate that once an erroneous statement has appeared in print, it is almost impossible to eradicate. Catnip now is listed in practically all books devoted to drugs of abuse as a mild intoxicant." For the record: It isn't.

Cat intoxication is another matter. All cats are attracted to catnip, but only about two-thirds exhibit strong "feline catnip euphoria," according to a report published in *Economic Botany*. Kitty euphoria is an inherited trait, and not all cats have the necessary gene.

Contemporary herbalists continue to have great faith in catnip. One writes, "Surely a plant with such a powerful impact on our feline friends . . . could not be destitute of medicinal value in humans." Modern herbals recommend catnip as a tranquilizer, sedative, digestive aid, and treatment for colds, colic, diarrhea, flatulence, and fever.

Therapeutic Uses

Studies confirm that catnip is definitely not just for cats. While modern herbalists tend to overstate the herb's value, scientists have confirmed several of its traditional uses.

DIGESTIVE PROBLEMS. Like other mints, catnip is an antispasmodic. It soothes the smooth muscles of the digestive tract. Have a cup of catnip tea after meals if you're prone to indigestion or heartburn.

INSOMNIA AND ANXIETY. German researchers report that the chemicals in catnip responsible for cat intoxication (nepetalactone isomers) are similar to the natural sedatives in valerian (valepotriates). This finding supports catnip's traditional use as a mild tranquilizer and sedative. Try a cup of tea when you feel tense or before bed and see if it works for you.

INFECTIONS. Catnip has some, but rather weak, antibiotic action, which lends credence to the herb's traditional use in some cases of diarrhea and fever. But since it's not a particularly powerful antibiotic, you cannot rely on it to prevent infection.

WOMEN'S HEALTH CONCERNS. Antispasmodics calm not only the digestive tract but also other smooth muscles, such as the uterus. Catnip's antispasmodic effect supports its traditional role in relieving menstrual cramps.

Intriguing Possibility

Research at Iowa State University shows that compounds in catnip oil are "highly effective" mosquito repellants—more effective than DEET. If you grow it, you can see for yourself. In late afternoon when mosquitoes come out, crush a few leaves, rub them on your skin, and see if you get bitten.

Rx Recommendations

Enjoy a pleasant, minty infusion of catnip as a digestive aid, as a mild tranquilizer, or to soothe menstrual cramps.

For an infusion, use 2 teaspoons of dried herb per cup of boiling water. Steep for 10 to 20 minutes, then strain. (Do not boil catnip; boiling dissipates its healing oil.) Drink up to 3 cups a day.

If you prefer a homemade tincture, take $1/2$ to 1 teaspoon up to three times a day.

When using commercial preparations, follow the package directions.

For infant colic, you may give weak, cool catnip infusions cautiously in consultation with the child's doctor.

If you grow catnip, to prevent infection from minor garden mishaps, press some crushed leaves on cuts and scrapes until you can wash and bandage them.

The Safety Factor

Catnip was also used traditionally as a menstruation promoter. Current research suggests that it should not stimulate the uterus, but pregnant women should still exercise caution and not take medicinal amounts.

Catnip is considered nontoxic, but some people may experience upset stomach or allergic reactions.

In children over 2, adjust the recommended dose based on the child's weight. For example, give a 50-pound child one-third of the dose a 150-pound adult would take.

If you're over 65, start with a low dose, and increase only if necessary.

Inform health care professionals of the herbs

you use. Problematic herb-drug interactions are possible.

Catnip may cause allergic reactions or other unexpected side effects. If any develop, reduce your dose or stop taking it.

For more on herb safety, see Chapter 2.

If symptoms get worse or persist longer than 2 weeks, consult a health care professional promptly.

Growing Information

Catnip is a gray-green aromatic perennial that grows to 3 feet and bears all the hallmarks of the mint family: a square stem, fuzzy leaves, and twin-lipped flowers.

The herb grows easily from seeds or root divisions planted in spring or fall. It thrives in almost any well-drained soil with full sun or partial shade. Some growers say that keeping the soil on the dry side produces more aromatic plants. Thin seedlings to 18-inch spacing.

Harvest the leaves and flowers in late summer when the plants are in bloom. Dry and store them in opaque, tightly sealed containers to preserve the volatile oil.

Gardeners' mythology holds that cats are not attracted to catnip in the ground. An old rhyme says, "If you set it / The cats will get it. / But if you sow it / The cats won't know it." Don't believe it. Euphoric cats often destroy sown plants.

The current consensus is that sowing, per se, does not keep cats away. The key is to prevent bruising of the leaves. Carefully cultivated, completely unbruised plants reportedly hold little attraction for cats. Any bruising, however, releases the plant's aromatic oil, and the cats come running.

CAT'S CLAW

The Peruvian "Life-Giver"

Family: Rubiaceae; other members include coffee and gardenia

Genus and species: *Uncaria tomentosa, U. guianensis*

Also known as: Una de gato and life-giving vine of Peru

Part used: Inner bark

Cat's claw—in Spanish, *una de gato*—is a climbing, woody, South American vine whose strands can grow longer than 1,000 feet. It climbs trees with the help of curved spines that resemble—guess what? It first attracted North American herbalists' attention in the early 1990s. It's still a minor medicinal herb, but that may change as its benefits become more widely known.

Healing History

Indigenous South Americans have used cat's claw's inner root bark for centuries to spur wound healing and treat intestinal distress. In Peru, where cat's claw is a popular medicinal herb, it is also used to treat dysentery, gonorrhea, and cancers. Some Amazon Indian tribes believe that cat's claw has "life-giving" powers. They drink a cup of decoction weekly to prevent all manner of disease.

Therapeutic Uses

OSTEOARTHRITIS. Several studies confirm that cat's claw has anti-inflammatory and pain-relieving action. At the National University Medical School in Lima, Peru, researchers gave either a placebo or cat's claw to 45 people with osteoarthritis (OA) of the knee. After 4 weeks of treatment, the herb group reported significantly less pain. The researchers concluded: "Cat's claw is an effective treatment for osteoarthritis."

RHEUMATOID ARTHRITIS. Rheumatoid arthritis (RA) is not as common as osteoarthritis—2.5 million Americans have RA—but it's the more severe condition and may cause joint deformity and impairment. At Innsbruck University Hospital in Austria, scientists gave 40 people with RA a placebo or cat's claw in addition to standard drugs. After 6 months, the herb group reported significantly fewer painful, swollen joints.

ENHANCED IMMUNITY. Life-giving may not be too far off the mark. Cat's claw is an immune booster in three ways. It increases the number of germ-fighting white blood cells.

It stimulates them to gobble up more germs. And it increases levels of the key immune proteins interleukin-1 and -6. Writing in the *Journal of Ethnopharmacology*, Canadian researchers say it is a "strong immunostimulant," just as the Amazon Indians believed. The herb's immune-boosting action should make it useful in preventing and treating all manner of infections.

PREVENTION OF DEGENERATIVE DISEASES. Cat's claw also has antioxidant action. Antioxidants help prevent the DNA damage at the root of heart disease, cancer, and many other conditions. The herb has been shown to prevent cell mutations that can lead to cancer. Swedish researchers studied a dozen people being treated with a drug, one of whose side effects is the possibility of DNA damage. Subsequently, four of them took a placebo while the eight others took cat's claw (four took 250 milligrams per day; four took 350 milligrams per day). After 8 weeks, the herb groups showed significantly greater DNA repair and less DNA damage.

It's still too early to call cat's claw a cancer treatment, but in a laboratory study, Italian researchers exposed rapidly dividing human breast cancer cells to an extract of the herb. It reduced cancer-spreading cell division by 90 percent.

Intriguing Possibilities

Animal studies suggest that cat's claw lowers cholesterol and relaxes the arteries, lowering blood pressure. If it has the same effects in humans, it might be used to prevent and treat heart disease and stroke.

Rx Recommendations

To make a decoction, boil 1 teaspoon of powdered bark per cup of water for 10 minutes, then strain. Drink 1 to 3 cups a day.

If using tincture, the recommended dose is 1 to 2 teaspoons two to three times a day.

When using a standardized extract, the recommended dose ranges from 350 to 700 milligrams per day. Follow label directions.

The Safety Factor

Cat's claw is nontoxic and rarely causes side effects, but headache, dizziness, and stomach upset have been reported.

Because it stimulates the immune system, cat's claw should not be used by those with autoimmune conditions, such as lupus or multiple sclerosis. Those taking immune-suppressing medication, such as organ transplant or skin graft recipients, should also avoid it.

Pregnant and nursing women should not use cat's claw.

Do not give cat's claw to children under 2. In older children, adjust the recommended dose based on the child's weight. For example, give a 50-pound child one-third of the dose a 150-pound adult would take.

If you're over 65, start with a low dose, and increase only if necessary.

Inform health care professionals of the herbs you use. Problematic herb-drug interactions are possible.

Cat's claw may cause allergic reactions or other unexpected side effects. If any develop, reduce your dose or stop taking it.

For more on herb safety, see Chapter 2.

If symptoms get worse or persist longer than 2 weeks, consult a health care professional promptly.

Growing Information

Cat's claw is not grown in the United States.

CELERY

Good for Gout and High Blood Pressure

Family: Umbelliferae; other members include carrot and parsley

Genus and species: *Apium graveolens*

Also known as: Marsh parsley and wild celery

Parts used: Stalks and fruits (seeds)

Dieters often eat celery stalks, believing that chewing the stringy vegetable burns more calories than it contains. Most experts dismiss this as a myth.

Celery does more than add crunch to salads, however. Scientists have discovered a surprising number of healing benefits in its stalks and seeds. This herb may help relieve gout, insomnia, high blood pressure, and high cholesterol.

Healing History

The ancient Greeks gave celery wine to winning athletes, and celery elixirs have been used in healing throughout history. A contemporary echo of this, minus any medicinal claims, is the soft drink Dr. Brown's Cel-Ray Soda, which contains extract of celery seed.

India's traditional Ayurvedic physicians have prescribed celery seed since ancient times as a diuretic to treat water retention. They also recommend it as a treatment for colds, flu, indigestion, arthritis, and diseases of the liver and spleen.

The medieval German abbess/herbalist Hildegard of Bingen wrote, "Whoever is plagued by [the arthritis of] gout . . . should powder celery seeds . . . because this is the best remedy." English herbalist John Gerard claimed celery "provoketh urine" as an aid to weight loss and expelled "phlegm out of the head." And in 17th-century England, Nicholas Culpeper recommended celery seed as a diuretic for dropsy (congestive heart failure).

Later herbalists suggested celery to treat insomnia, obesity, nervousness, and several cancers, to promote menstruation, and to induce abortion. It has even been recommended as an aphrodisiac.

Oddly, America's 19th-century botanical physicians, the Eclectics, forerunners of today's naturopaths, were not impressed with celery. They considered the herb a mere footnote to its close relative, parsley. If parsley was unavailable, the Eclectics grudgingly recommended celery as "a nerve tonic" and a remedy for arthritis and chest congestion.

Contemporary herbalists recommend celery

as a diuretic, tranquilizer, sedative, and menstruation promoter and as a treatment for gout, arthritis, obesity, anxiety, and lack of appetite (gustatory, not sexual).

Therapeutic Uses

There hasn't been that much research on the medicinal benefits of celery, but the studies to date validate several of the herb's age-old uses in healing.

GOUT. Some 800 years after Hildegard of Bingen endorsed celery as "best" for gout, science has validated her claim. Gout is caused by a buildup of uric acid that forms crystals in the joints, notably the big toe.

In the mid-1990s, James A. Duke, Ph.D., retired USDA herbal medicine authority and author of several highly regarded herbal medicine references, developed gout. As he recalls, "My doctor had urged me to take the gout-preventive drug allopurinol—one pill a day for the rest of my life. I did, for a while. Then I read a study showing that celery extract can eliminate uric acid. It seemed as though four daily 800-milligram tablets of celery seed extract would provide protection equivalent to the allopurinol I'd been taking. Now, I'm a believer. My uric acid level has stayed below the level that triggers gout. I haven't had any gout attacks since I began taking celery seed extract."

Of course, one testimonial does not prove that celery seed extract works. If you'd like to try it, talk with your doctor.

HIGH BLOOD PRESSURE. In Chinese medicine, celery is recommended as a treatment for high blood pressure. Until the 1990s, this seemed ludicrous to mainstream physicians. As a vegetable, celery contains an unusually large amount of salt (sodium), which raises blood pressure in many people.

In 1992, Minh Le, the father of a University of Chicago medical student, was diagnosed with high blood pressure. His doctor prescribed standard antihypertensive medication. Le ignored his doctor's advice and began eating $1/4$ pound of celery a day (about four stalks). Before long, his blood pressure dropped from 158/96 to 118/82.

Le's son, Quang Le, and University of Chicago pharmacologist William Elliot, Ph.D., isolated a compound from celery (3-n-butyl phthalide) and injected rats with an amount equal to four stalks of celery. The animals' blood pressure dropped 13 percent, and their cholesterol declined 7 percent.

If you want to add celery to a treatment plan for high blood pressure, consult your doctor. It might help. But if you're especially sensitive to salt, it may do more harm than good.

HIGH CHOLESTEROL. A high-fiber diet helps reduce cholesterol, and celery supplies an abundance of fiber. In addition, the 3-n-butyl phthalide it contains helped cut cholesterol in the animal study mentioned above.

CONGESTIVE HEART FAILURE. Diuretics are often prescribed to treat both high blood pressure and congestive heart failure, which involves serious fluid buildup in the body. Celery seed has been shown to have diuretic action, which supports its traditional role as a treatment for congestive heart failure. If you'd like to use celery seed for this purpose, discuss it with your doctor.

DIABETES. Several studies have indicated that celery seed reduces blood sugar (glucose) levels, an important part of managing diabetes.

Diabetes requires professional treatment. If you'd like to use celery seed as part of your treatment plan, discuss it with your physician.

ANXIETY AND INSOMNIA. Celery seed oil contains phthalides, chemicals that have sedative effects in animals. Of course, findings in animals don't always apply to humans, but if you're anxious, nervous, or wakeful, try the herb and see if it works for you.

WOMEN'S HEALTH CONCERNS. Celery seed stimulates uterine contractions in animals, lending support to its traditional uses in promoting menstruation and inducing abortion. For this reason, pregnant women should exercise caution and not consume the seeds. The stalks, however, are not harmful.

Other women may want to try celery seed to bring on their periods. But don't use the herb to try to induce abortion.

Diuretics help relieve the bloated feeling caused by premenstrual fluid retention. Women who are bothered by premenstrual syndrome might try some celery seed during the uncomfortable days right before their periods.

Intriguing Possibilities

Celery contains psoralens, chemicals that have been used to treat psoriasis and, more recently, a form of cancer called cutaneous T-cell lymphoma. Further research is needed to determine whether celery is indeed effective for these diseases.

Medicinal Myth

Celery seed's diuretic action lends some credence to its traditional use in treating obesity, because it would tend to eliminate water weight. Keep in mind, however, that lost water weight usually returns.

Celery may aid weight loss in the short term, but the key to permanent weight control is a low-fat, high-complex-carbohydrate diet and regular aerobic exercise.

Rx Recommendations

To treat gout, try adding four 800-milligram tablets of celery seed extract a day to your treatment program, in consultation with your physician.

To treat high blood pressure, high cholesterol, or congestive heart failure, add four stalks of celery a day to your treatment program, in consultation with your doctor.

For a pleasant-tasting, relaxing infusion that might help treat diabetes, use 1 to 2 teaspoons of freshly crushed seeds per cup of boiling water. Steep for 10 to 20 minutes, then strain. Drink up to 3 cups a day.

As a tincture, take $1/2$ to 1 teaspoon up to three times a day.

The Safety Factor

All diuretics should be used in consultation with a physician. They can deplete the body's stores of potassium, an essential nutrient, so people who use them should also eat foods high in potassium, such as bananas and fresh vegetables, to replace lost electrolytes.

High blood pressure, elevated cholesterol, congestive heart failure, and diabetes are serious conditions. Celery seed may help manage them, but it should be used in consultation with your physician as part of an overall treatment plan.

If symptoms get worse or persist longer than 2 weeks, consult a health care professional promptly.

Growing Information

Celery grows best in well-watered, richly organic soil. Less ideal conditions produce tougher, stringier, more bitter stalks.

In mild areas, celery grows virtually year-round. Elsewhere, start seeds indoors in January and plant seedlings in early spring after the danger of frost has passed. Soak the seeds before planting.

Germination typically takes about 10 days. Transplant at approximately 3 months, when the seedlings are about 3 inches high. Space the plants about 6 inches apart, and water copiously. The juiciness of the stalks depends on how much water the plants receive. Harvest seeds when they mature.

The psoralens in celery sometimes cause rashes in agricultural workers. Gardeners take note: Wearing sunscreen prevents this reaction.

CHAMOMILE

Pretty Flowers, Potent Medicine

Family: Compositae; other members include daisy, dandelion, and marigold

Genus and species: *Matricaria chamomilla* (German or Hungarian) and *Anthemis nobilis* (Roman or English)

Also known as: Camomile, matricaria, anthemis, and ground apple

Parts used: Flowers

In *The Tale of Peter Rabbit*, the young bunny eats himself sick in Mr. McGregor's garden, then gets chased out at the wrong end of the angry man's hoe. When Peter gets home, his mother gives him chamomile tea.

Peter's mother was a wise herbalist. Chamomile helps treat indigestion and soothes jangled nerves. Perhaps Peter's mother feared that his ordeal might give him an ulcer. Chamomile helps prevent them. Or perhaps Mr. McGregor's hoe grazed Peter's tender skin. A chamomile compress can help heal superficial wounds.

Unfortunately, few people who sip tasty, apple-flavored chamomile tea realize what a healer they hold in their paws . . . sorry, hands.

Healing History

Chamomile is not one herb but two: German (or Hungarian) chamomile and Roman (or English) chamomile. The two plants are botanically unrelated, but oddly, both produce the same light blue oil that's been healing people since ancient times.

Chamomile's daisylike flowers reminded the ancient Egyptians of the sun. They used the herb to treat fever, particularly the recurring fevers of malaria.

The Greek physician Dioscorides and the Roman naturalist Pliny recommended chamomile to treat headaches and kidney, liver, and bladder problems. India's ancient Ayurvedic physicians used the herb in similar ways.

Germans have used chamomile since the dawn of history to ease digestive upsets, promote menstruation, and relieve menstrual cramps.

The 17th-century English herbalist Nicholas Culpeper recommended chamomile for fevers, digestive problems, aches, pains, jaundice, kidney stones, dropsy (congestive heart failure), and "to bring down women's courses" (promote menstruation).

British and German immigrants introduced both chamomiles into North America. Most of the chamomile grown here today is the German variety.

America's 19th-century Eclectic physicians, forerunners of today's naturopaths, recommended chamomile poultices to speed wound healing and prevent gangrene. They prescribed infusions for digestive problems, malaria, typhus, menstrual cramps, and menstruation promotion as well as for all birth-related difficulties: to quiet fetal kicking, stop premature labor, relieve sore breasts and nipples, suppress milk production, and relieve infant colic.

Today, chamomile is one of the nation's best-selling herbs, not as a medicine, but as a beverage tea, by itself or in blends. Its apple aroma gives many herbal skin care products their fragrance, and it has been used in shampoos since the days of the Vikings because it adds luster to blond hair.

Medicinally, contemporary herbalists recommend chamomile as an external treatment for wounds and inflammation and as an internal treatment for fever, digestive upsets, anxiety, and insomnia.

Therapeutic Uses

In Germany, where herbal healing is more mainstream than in the United States, one pharmaceutical company markets a popular chamomile product called Kamillosan. The Germans use it externally for wounds and inflammations and internally for indigestion and ulcers. (The product is not available in the United States.)

Chamomile is so popular in Germany that many there call the herb *alles zutraut*, or "capable of anything." An exaggeration, to be sure, but chamomile has a lot going for it.

DIGESTIVE PROBLEMS. Dozens of studies support chamomile's traditional use as a digestive aid. Several chemicals in chamomile oil—primarily bisabolol—have a relaxing effect on the smooth muscle lining the digestive tract, making the herb an antispasmodic. In fact, one study found that chamomile relaxes the digestive tract as well as the opium-based drug papaverine.

Commission E, the expert panel that evaluates herbal medicines for the German counterpart of the FDA, endorses chamomile for gastrointestinal conditions.

ULCERS. Chamomile may help prevent stomach ulcers and speed their healing. In one experiment, two groups of animals were fed a chemical known to cause ulcers. The animals that also received chamomile developed significantly fewer sores. When the animals that got ulcers were divided into two groups, those that were fed chamomile recovered more quickly.

ANXIETY. Chamomile's long history as a tranquilizer has a scientific basis. Argentinean researchers discovered that a compound in chamomile oil, apigenin, binds to the same cell receptors as the family of tranquilizers and anti-anxiety drugs that includes diazepam (Valium). This suggests that chamomile would have similar effects.

A British study has shown that chamomile has a mild sedative effect, which confirms its tranquilizing action. In another British report, researchers massaged people who complained of chronic anxiety. Some were massaged with a placebo lotion, the rest with a lotion infused with chamomile oil. Both treatments reduced anxiety levels, but, according to researchers, "the addition of chamomile oil seems to enhance the effect and to improve physical and psychological symptoms, as well as quality of life."

STRESS. Japanese researchers worked with chamomile oil vapors in a study of animals under stress. Among the animals exposed to the chamomile vapor, stress hormone levels fell significantly.

DIARRHEA. German researchers gave either a placebo or chamomile tea to 79 children with diarrhea. The kids ranged from 6 months to 6 years. After 3 days, those taking chamomile were significantly more likely to be cured.

DEPRESSION. British researchers used standard psychological tests to assess the mood of 20 people, and then gave them chamomile. Their mood shifted from negative toward positive. Chamomile's mood-elevating effects are mild. It's unlikely to have any effect on those with serious depression. But for minor everyday blues, a cup of chamomile tea might help.

INFECTIONS. The Eclectic physicians were onto something when they suggested using chamomile compresses to keep wounds from becoming infected. Some studies show that chamomile oil applied to the skin reduces the time required for burns to heal. The herb also has anti-inflammatory action, thanks to the azulene compounds it contains. Commission E endorses chamomile topically as a wound treatment.

Other studies show that the herb kills *Candida albicans*, the yeast fungi that cause vaginal infections, as well as staphylococcus bacteria. Chamomile also impairs replication of the polio virus.

ENHANCED IMMUNITY. No one knew why chamomile prevented infections until British researchers discovered that it stimulates the immune system's infection-fighting white blood cells (macrophages and B-lymphocytes). Drink some chamomile tea when you have a cold or the flu. It does no harm, and it just might help.

WOMEN'S HEALTH CONCERNS. Antispasmodics relax not only the digestive tract but also other smooth muscles, such as the uterus.

Chamomile's antispasmodic properties support its age-old use to soothe menstrual cramps and reduce the risk of premature labor.

Oddly, however, chamomile was also used to stimulate menstruation. The apparent contradiction remains unresolved, but European researchers have isolated a substance in chamomile that stimulates uterine contractions.

Women should feel free to try chamomile both to soothe menstrual cramps and to promote the onset of menstruation, but women who are pregnant or trying to conceive should steer clear of medicinal amounts.

ARTHRITIS. In animal studies, chamomile successfully relieves arthritis-related joint inflammation. Findings in animals don't necessarily apply to people, but chamomile has been used traditionally to treat arthritis. Try it and see if it works for you.

Intriguing Possibility

A Japanese pilot animal study suggests that chamomile tea helps control blood sugar levels, which could mean it would be helpful in diabetes management.

Rx Recommendations

Use an infusion or tincture to take advantage of chamomile's many proven healing benefits.

For a pleasant, refreshing, apple-flavored infusion, use 2 to 3 heaping teaspoons of flowers per cup of boiling water. Steep for 10 to 20 minutes, then strain. Drink up to 3 cups a day.

As a homemade tincture, take $1/2$ to 1 teaspoon up to three times a day.

When using commercial preparations, follow the package directions.

You can give weak infusions of chamomile cautiously to children under age 2 for colic. For older children and adults over age 65, start with low-strength preparations and increase the strength if necessary.

Try a chamomile infusion when you feel anxious, or add chamomile flowers to a hot bath. Just tie a handful of chamomile flowers inside a cloth and run the bathwater over it. Don't forget to inhale the vapors.

For cuts, scrapes, and burns, brew a strong infusion, then soak a clean cloth in the liquid and apply it as a compress.

The Safety Factor

Controversy about chamomile erupted in 1973, when a report in the *Journal of Allergy and Clinical Immunology* claimed that chamomile tea might cause a potentially fatal allergic reaction, called anaphylaxis, in people who were allergic to its botanical relative, ragweed. Herb conservatives immediately urged the millions of people with ragweed allergy to shun chamomile. Outraged herb advocates insisted that chamomile had been vilified unfairly.

To settle the issue, researchers compiled all of the reports of chamomile-induced allergic reactions from all of the world medical literature for the 95-year period from 1887 to 1982. The grand total: no deaths and 50 allergic reactions—45 involving Roman chamomile and just 5 involving German chamomile, the type typically grown in the United States.

Chamomile poses no significant health hazard. The only people who should think twice about using the herb (and its close relative, yarrow) are those who have previously experienced anaphylaxis from ragweed.

This doesn't mean that adverse reactions are impossible. Large amounts of highly concentrated chamomile preparations—much more concentrated than the typical tea—have caused nausea and vomiting. If you experience an allergic reaction or other unexpected side effect, reduce your dose or stop taking it.

Inform health care professionals of the herbs you use. Problematic herb-drug interactions are possible.

For more on herb safety, see Chapter 2.

If symptoms get worse or persist longer than 2 weeks, consult a health care professional promptly.

Growing Information

German chamomile is an annual that reaches 3 feet. The Roman herb is a perennial ground cover that rarely exceeds 9 inches. Both have downy stems, feathery leaves, and daisylike flowers with yellow centers and white rays.

Most chamomile seed available in the United States is the annual German variety. It grows easily when sown in spring after the danger of frost has passed. Scatter the tiny seeds on well-prepared beds, then gently tamp them down.

Seedlings up to 2 inches tall transplant well; taller plants do not.

German chamomile prefers sandy, well-drained soil in partially shaded gardens and tends to shrivel under full sun. It flowers at about 6 weeks, producing lush flowers even in the short summers of northern climes. The flowering lasts for several weeks, and if some flowers are left unharvested, the plant will sow itself. Don't leave too many, though, as this herb may become a pest.

Perennial Roman chamomile comes in two subtypes: single-flower and double-flower. Herbalists prefer the double-flower variety, which adapts to almost any soil but favors moist, well-manured loam. The tiny seeds may be sown, but most gardeners prefer to propagate the plant from offshoots. Plant them about 18 inches apart in early spring. Roman chamomile is quite hardy, but if your winters are particularly severe, protect the plants with mulch.

Oddly enough, Roman chamomile does best when it's stepped on. In Britain, it is often used as a ground cover on garden paths. Walking on it releases the herb's lovely apple fragrance and does not hurt the plant. After harvesting, dry the flowers and store them in sealed containers to preserve their volatile oil.

CHAPARRAL

A Cavity-Preventive Mouthwash

Family: Zygophyllaceae; other members include caltrop, star thistle, and bean caper

Genus and species: *Larrea divaricata* and *L. tridentata*

Also known as: Stinkweed, greasewood, and creosote bush

Parts used: Twigs and leaflets

Chaparral stinks. Literally. And it tastes down-right unpleasant. Because of these characteristics, one of the herb's major benefits may come as something of a surprise: It's used as a mouthwash.

We're not talking minty fresh here. You wouldn't want to reach for it before puckering up for your morning kiss. But don't let that stop you. The unassuming chaparral shrub, native to the American Southwest, contains a chemical that may spell death to some of the germs that cause tooth decay. The same chemical, called NDGA (nordihydroguaiaretic acid), also kills other microorganisms that turn fats and oils rancid.

Healing History

If, as some people believe, effective medicine smells foul and tastes terrible, chaparral should be a wonderful healer. Its leaves exude a waxy resin that smells like creosote and is the source of its popular names: stinkweed, greasewood, and creosote bush (although the plant contains no actual creosote).

Native Americans in the Southwest rubbed chaparral resin on burns. They used chaparral tea to treat colds, bronchitis, chickenpox, snakebite, and arthritis. And they heated the tips of chaparral twigs and applied the hot resin to painful teeth.

White settlers adopted the plant, using it externally for bruises, rashes, dandruff, and wounds and internally for diarrhea, upset stomach, menstrual problems, venereal diseases, and cancers of the liver, kidney, and stomach.

Chaparral was listed as an expectorant (to clear mucus from the respiratory system) and bronchial antiseptic in the *U.S. Pharmacopoeia*, a standard drug reference, from 1842 to 1942. Today, few herbalists mention it. Those who do suggest using it externally to prevent wound infections and internally to treat intestinal parasites and bacterial and viral illnesses.

Therapeutic Uses

Chaparral is a very intriguing herb, as well as a controversial one.

WOUNDS. The NDGA in chaparral is a potent antiseptic with antibacterial and antifungal action, lending credence to the herb's traditional use as a wound treatment. It was approved by the USDA as a preservative in lard and animal shortenings, although since the 1960s, it has been supplanted by other commercial preservatives.

TOOTH DECAY AND GUM DISEASE. Because of chaparral's traditional use as a treatment for toothache, scientists tested the herb against the bacteria that cause tooth decay and gum disease. A study published in the *Journal of Dental Research* showed that chaparral mouthwash reduces cavity formation by 75 percent.

Oral microorganisms also cause gum disease, the leading cause of tooth loss in adults. Chaparral mouthwash is no substitute for regular brushing and flossing, but it may provide added protection.

GENERAL DEGENERATIVE ILLNESS PREVENTION. NDGA is a powerful antioxidant. It helps prevent the cell damage that's at the root of many degenerative diseases, including heart disease, cataracts, and, especially, many cancers.

CANCER. Investigations of chaparral's effects on cancer have been mixed. Laboratory studies by the National Cancer Institute (NCI) show that the herb has definite anti-tumor effects, but NCI animal studies have shown no cancer-treating benefit.

Meanwhile, the medical literature contains several case studies of tumor shrinkage in people who have used chaparral. One such study, published in *Cancer Chemotherapy Reports*, tells of a man diagnosed with malignant melanoma, the most serious skin cancer. His doctors urged surgery, but the man refused, saying that he would treat himself with chaparral tea. Eight months later, the man showed "marked regression" of his cancer. Of course, a case study cannot be considered scientific proof, but it suggests that something might be going on.

Melanoma is a life-threatening disease that requires professional medical care. Do not rely solely on chaparral as a treatment. Cancer patients might decide—in consultation with their physicians—to use the herb in conjunction with other therapies.

ARTHRITIS. Some animal studies confirm that chaparral has anti-inflammatory action, lending support to its traditional use in treating arthritis.

Intriguing Possibility

Life-extension advocates say that antioxidants such as NDGA help slow the aging process and may even extend the human life span. One French study found that NDGA significantly lengthens the average life span of laboratory animals. Other scientists claim that the chemical almost doubles the average life span of laboratory insects. While science has not yet found a way to extend the human life span, these results are certainly intriguing.

Rx Recommendations

To prepare a mouthwash or an infusion, use 1 tablespoon of dried leaves and stems per quart of boiling water. Steep for 1 hour, then strain. Gargle or drink up to 3 cups a day. Because of its unpleasant taste, you may want to add honey and lemon to the infusion or mix it with a beverage tea.

The Safety Factor

Chaparral is safe for use as a mouthwash, assuming that you spit it out.

Since 1990, there have been 18 reports of liver damage in people taking chaparral. All but a few were using tablets or capsules, not the tea traditionally preferred in herbal medicine. One person developed liver damage after only 3 weeks, but most took chaparral for at least 3 months. Several were using other substances that damage the liver, such as alcohol and a variety of over-the-counter and prescription drugs, at the same time. In all cases, the liver abnormalities cleared up after treatment with chaparral was discontinued.

In 1992, after six cases of liver damage had been reported, the American Herbal Products Association (AHPA) asked member herb marketers to voluntarily suspend chaparral sales pending the outcome of an investigation. Scientists at the University of Texas Health Sciences Center reviewed case reports supplied by the FDA. They found no pattern clear enough to warrant action against chaparral. So, in 1995, the AHPA rescinded its voluntary suspension of chaparral sales. The FDA has taken no action against sale of the herb.

Still, in light of the possibility of liver damage, no one with liver disease or a history of it should ingest chaparral. Nor should it be used by anyone who is an alcoholic or taking any medication—including over-the-counter drugs—regularly.

Others who wish to try chaparral should use an infusion, not tablets or capsules, and should not take it for longer than a few months. Stop using chaparral if you develop any signs of liver trouble, such as nausea, fatigue, fever, or jaundice (dark-colored urine or yellowing of the eyes).

Pregnant or nursing women should not take chaparral.

Do not give chaparral to children under age 2. Older children and adults over age 65 may use a full-strength gargle, but for internal use, they should start with low-strength preparations and increase the strength if necessary.

Inform health care professionals of the herbs you use. Problematic herb-drug interactions are possible.

Chaparral may cause allergic reactions or other unexpected side effects. If any develop, reduce your dose or stop taking it.

For more on herb safety, see Chapter 2.

If symptoms get worse or persist longer than 2 weeks, consult a health care professional promptly.

Growing Information

Chaparral is not a garden herb. It's a woody, olive green or yellow shrub that dominates the Southwest's arid landscape. It grows to about 10 feet and resembles a dwarf oak. Its roots radiate far beyond its aboveground parts and contain chemicals that kill other plants.

CHASTE TREE

Balancing Hormones Naturally

Family: Verbenaceae; other members include verbenas and many tropical trees and shrubs

Genus and species: *Vitex agnus-castus*

Also known as: Vitex, monk's pepper, and wild pepper

Parts used: Fruits (berries)

Since ancient times, Europeans believed that the small, dark, peppercorn-like fruits of the chaste tree suppressed a woman's libido. Those who took religious vows of chastity used the fruits to suppress their sexual urges, hence the name chaste tree.

This herb has no documented effect on libido, but it does change the balance of female sex hormones in ways that make it helpful in treating several women's health conditions.

Healing History

As a native Mediterranean plant, chaste tree was well known to ancient Greek physicians. Hippocrates, the father of mainstream Western medicine, recommended it as a treatment for injuries and inflammations.

Dioscorides, author of the West's first guide to herbal medicine, *De Materia Medica* (*On Medicines*), recognized chaste tree's effect on the female reproductive system, especially its ability to increase milk production in nursing mothers. He recommended the leaves and berries to treat lactation problems and to expel the placenta and control bleeding after delivery. "If blood flows from the womb," Dioscorides wrote, "let the woman drink dark red wine in which the leaves of the chaste tree have been steeped."

During the 1st century A.D., the Roman naturalist Pliny cited chaste tree as an aphrodisiac, but most ancient writers believed that it put a damper on sexuality. In Homer's *Iliad*, the herb is mentioned as a symbol of virginity. In ancient Rome, the vestal virgins carried chaste tree twigs as symbols of their chastity. (The plant's species name, *agnus-castus*, means "chaste lamb.")

During the Middle Ages, chaste tree flowers were strewn on the ground before the feet of novitiates as they entered convents and monasteries, symbolically preparing them for their vows of chastity. Monks ate the fruits to suppress sexual urges, hence one of the plant's common names, monk's pepper.

During times of war or social upheaval, when Asian black pepper was difficult to obtain, Europeans used peppery chaste tree fruits as a substitute. This gave rise to another of the plant's common names, wild pepper.

Nineteenth-century American Eclectic physicians, forerunners of today's naturopaths, prescribed chaste tree berries to increase milk production in nursing women.

Therapeutic Uses

Modern research has shown that chaste tree affects the pituitary gland, increasing production of luteinizing hormone and decreasing secretion of follicle-stimulating hormone. These changes influence the balance of female sex hormones, reducing levels of estrogen and increasing levels of progesterone.

PREMENSTRUAL SYNDROME (PMS). Shifting the estrogen-progesterone balance can help relieve the irritability, breast tenderness, fluid retention, and other symptoms of PMS. In Germany, where herbal medicine is more mainstream than in the United States, an over-the-counter tincture of chaste tree (called Agnolyt) has been marketed since the 1950s as a treatment for PMS discomforts. German women consider the herb particularly effective for relieving PMS-related bloating and breast tenderness.

Several studies support the use of chaste tree for PMS symptoms. In one German trial, 1,542 women took 50 drops of tincture of chaste tree every day for 6 months. Ninety percent reported significant or complete relief of PMS symptoms.

In another German trial, this one lasting 3 months, 175 women with PMS took either chaste tree or 200 milligrams of vitamin B_6, a treatment with demonstrated effectiveness for premenstrual complaints. Among the women taking B_6, 61 percent found the treatment helpful. But chaste tree helped 77 percent.

British researchers gave a placebo or chaste tree to 600 women. After 3 months, the herb showed significant benefit for relieving premenstrual discomfort.

Commission E, the expert panel that evaluates herbal medicines for the German counterpart of the FDA, approves chaste tree for the prevention and treatment of premenstrual discomforts.

MENSTRUAL PROBLEMS. Chaste tree's hormonal effects also help regulate the menstrual cycle. In one German study, 126 women with a variety of menstrual problems—scant flow, heavy flow, and midcycle spotting—took 40 drops of chaste tree tincture every day for several months. The women experienced statistically significant normalization of their menstrual cycles.

Women with erratic cycles, scant or unusually heavy menstrual flow, midcycle spotting, nonovulatory periods, or menstrual cramps might try chaste tree in consultation with a physician.

Commission E approves chaste tree for menstrual irregularity.

MENSTRUAL-RELATED BREAST PAIN. Studies by Czech researchers show that chaste tree relieves cyclic breast pain, called mastalgia. In one study, 97 women with breast pain were given either a placebo or the herb (30 drops of tincture twice a day). After three cycles, those using chaste tree reported significantly greater relief.

Commission E approves chaste tree for cyclic mastalgia.

LACTATION PROBLEMS. The ancients were right: Chaste tree fruits help increase milk production in nursing women. A German study demonstrated this benefit when the participants took the herb for at least several weeks. The researcher who led the study described chaste tree as safe for breastfed infants.

LIBIDO REDUCTION. In men, chaste tree reduces levels of androgens, the male sex hormones. Most men produce much more testosterone and other androgens than is necessary to fuel normal libido, so suppressing androgens probably has little effect. But in men with low levels of androgens, the herb might reduce libido, suggesting that some of the monks who took it to inhibit sexual urges may have indeed gotten what they hoped for.

Intriguing Possibilities

German researchers gave a placebo or chaste tree to 96 women suffering infertility. After 3 months, 36 percent of the women in the placebo group became pregnant. In the herb group, the figure was 57 percent. However, these results did not quite reach statistical significance, so they might have occurred by chance. Nonetheless, chaste tree may well help treat infertility.

In laboratory studies, chaste tree has suppressed the growth of cervical, uterine, ovarian, and breast cancer cells. It's too early to call the herb a treatment for these diseases, but in the future, that's possible.

Rx Recommendations

Most studies with chaste tree have used tinctures in which 100 milliliters of the solution has been standardized to contain the equivalent of 9 grams of berries. The standard dose is 40 drops daily for at least 12 weeks.

Chaste tree is a slow-acting herb. It usually takes several months to show benefit, except in the case of lactation, which often improves within a few weeks.

Capsules of chaste tree are also now available. Recommended doses vary from 30 to 175 milligrams per day. Follow the package directions.

The Safety Factor

Chaste tree has never been linked to any significant side effects, but minor problems are possible. In the 6-month German study of PMS, 17 women dropped out because of stomach upset. A few cases of itching, rash, fatigue, and hair loss have also been reported.

Pregnant women should not use this herb.

Do not give chaste tree to girls who have not reached puberty.

Inform health care professionals of the herbs you use. Problematic herb-drug interactions are possible.

Chaste tree may cause allergic reactions or other unexpected side effects. If any develop, reduce your dose or stop taking it.

For more on herb safety, see Chapter 2.

If symptoms get worse or persist longer than 2 weeks, consult a health care professional promptly.

Growing Information

Chaste *tree* is something of a misnomer. The plant is more of a shrub, generally growing to about 10 feet, although in favorable conditions, it may reach 20. It's most commonly found along moist riverbanks in southern Europe and around the Mediterranean.

Chaste tree has finger-shaped leaves, slender violet flowers that bloom in summer, and dark brown or black berrylike fruits the size of peppercorns that appear in fall. The berries are edible and have a peppery fragrance and flavor.

European colonists introduced chaste tree to the United States. Today, it grows along the Eastern Seaboard from Maryland to Florida and throughout the South as far west as Arkansas, Oklahoma, and Texas.

CINNAMON
Spice with a Punch

Family: Lauraceae; other members include bay, avocado, nutmeg, and sassafras

Genus and species: *Cinnamomum zeylanicum*, *C. cassia*, and *C. saigonicum*

Also known as: Cassia, Ceylon cinnamon, and Saigon cinnamon

Part used: Inner bark

We sprinkle it on toast, add it to cookie dough, stir it into hot apple cider, and find it in candies. But cinnamon is more than a sweet treat. It's one of the world's oldest healers. Modern science has confirmed its value for preventing infection and indigestion—and recent research shows that it helps manage diabetes.

Healing History

Cinnamon originally grew in southern Asia. Ancient Chinese herbals from as early as 2700 B.C. mention the aromatic herb as a treatment for fever, diarrhea, and menstrual problems. India's ancient Ayurvedic healers used it in similar ways.

When ancient travelers introduced the herb to the Egyptians, they added it enthusiastically to their embalming mixtures. The Egyptian demand for cinnamon (and other Asian spices) played a major role in ancient trade.

The biblical Hebrews, Greeks, and Romans adopted cinnamon as a spice, perfume, and treatment for indigestion. After the fall of Rome, trade with Asia came to a virtual halt, but somehow, cinnamon still found its way to Europe. The 12th-century German abbess/herbalist Hildegard of Bingen recommended it as "the universal spice for sinuses" and as a treatment for colds, flu, cancer, and "inner decay and slime."

By the 17th century, Europeans considered cinnamon primarily a kitchen spice. In healing, they used it only to mask the bitterness of other herbs.

As time passed, however, cinnamon slowly regained its former reputation as a healer. America's 19th-century Eclectic physicians, forerunners of today's naturopaths, prescribed it for stomach cramps, flatulence, nausea, vomiting, diarrhea, and infant colic. The Eclectic medical text *King's American Dispensatory* (1898) also endorsed it for uterine problems: "[Cinnamon's] most direct action is on the uterine muscle fibers, causing contraction and arresting bleeding. For postpartum and other uterine hemorrhages, it is one of the most prompt and efficient remedies."

Modern herbalists recommend cinnamon to relieve nausea, vomiting, diarrhea, and indigestion and as a flavoring agent for bitter-tasting healing herb preparations. They can't quite agree about how it affects the uterus. Some say it stimulates uterine contractions, while others say it calms the uterus.

Therapeutic Uses

Of course, cinnamon delights the tastebuds, but it benefits other parts of the body as well.

INFECTIONS. Cinnamon oil is included in toothpaste and dental floss for more than just flavor. Like all of the other culinary spices, it's a powerful antiseptic. It kills many decay- and disease-causing bacteria, fungi, and viruses. Try sprinkling some on minor cuts and scrapes after they've been thoroughly washed.

Perhaps toilet paper should be permeated with cinnamon. One German study showed that it "suppresses completely" the bacteria that cause most urinary tract infections (*Escherichia coli*) and the fungus responsible for vaginal yeast infections (*Candida albicans*). Cinnamon also suppresses salmonella bacteria, a cause of food poisoning.

PAIN. Beyond its antimicrobial action, there's another reason to dust a bit of cinnamon on cuts and scrapes. It contains eugenol, a natural anesthetic oil that may help relieve the pain of household mishaps.

DIGESTIVE PROBLEMS. Along with lending flavor to foods, cinnamon assists the body in digesting cakes, cookies, ice cream, and other high-fat treats. According to a study published in the British journal *Nature*, cinnamon helps break down fats in the digestive system, possibly by boosting the activity of a particular digestive enzyme (trypsin).

Commission E, the expert panel that evaluates herbal medicines for the German counterpart of the FDA, endorses cinnamon for indigestion, abdominal distress, bloating, and flatulence.

CHOLESTEROL. In 2003, Pakistani researchers gave cinnamon (1 gram a day, about a heaping teaspoon) to 60 people with high cholesterol and type 2 diabetes. After 40 days, their total cholesterol dropped 12 to 26 percent, significantly reducing their risk of heart disease. If you have high cholesterol, it can't hurt to sprinkle a teaspoon a day on your food.

DIABETES. Animal studies have shown that cinnamon reduces blood sugar. The Pakistani study just mentioned showed that cinnamon reduced blood sugar by about 20 percent.

Intriguing Possibilities

Japanese researchers report that cinnamon helps reduce blood pressure. If yours is high, it can't hurt to use more of this tasty spice.

Cinnamon may also help retard food spoilage. Spanish researchers impregnated food-wrapping paper with cinnamon oil. The herb wrapping extended the mold-free shelf life of fruits, vegetables, breads, and meats.

Rx Recommendations

For a warm, sweet, spicy infusion, use $1/2$ to $3/4$ teaspoon of powdered herb per cup of boiling water, steep for 10 to 20 minutes, and strain if you wish. Drink up to 3 cups a day.

To treat minor cuts and scrapes, wash the affected area thoroughly, then sprinkle on a little powdered cinnamon.

The Safety Factor

Culinary amounts of powdered cinnamon are nontoxic. Cinnamon oil is a different story. On the skin, it may cause redness and burning. Used internally, it can cause nausea, vomiting, and possibly even kidney damage. Do not ingest the oil.

Despite some modern herbalists' contention that cinnamon helps calm the uterus, the weight of historical evidence suggests the opposite. For this reason, pregnant women should limit their use of cinnamon to culinary amounts.

Inform health care professionals of the herbs you use. Problematic herb-drug interactions are possible.

Cinnamon may cause allergic reactions or other unexpected side effects. If any develop, reduce your dose or stop taking it.

For more on herb safety, see Chapter 2.

If symptoms get worse or persist longer than 2 weeks, consult a health care professional promptly.

Growing Information

Cinnamon is not grown in the United States. Most of our supply comes from Asia and the West Indies. The trees reach a height of 30 feet. Collectors strip the aromatic bark from young branches no more than 3 years old.

CLOVE
Your Dentist Loves It

Family: Myrtaceae; other members include myrtle, tea tree, and eucalyptus

Genus and species: *Eugenia caryophyllata* or *Syzygium aromaticum*

Also known as: Clavos and caryophyllus

Parts used: Flower buds

Step into any spice shop, take a deep breath, and enjoy the rich, warm aroma that fills the air. Chances are the dominant fragrance is clove, one of the world's most aromatic healing herbs.

Step into your dentist's supply room and, although things smell quite different, chances are that clove oil is one of the items on the shelf. It's a dental anesthetic—and more.

Healing History

Clove is the bud of a highly aromatic Asian tropical evergreen tree. During the Han dynasty (207 B.C. to A.D. 220), those who addressed the Chinese emperor were required to hold cloves in their mouths to mask bad breath.

Traditional Chinese physicians have long used clove to treat indigestion, diarrhea, hernia, and ringworm, along with athlete's foot and other fungal infections. Likewise, India's traditional Ayurvedic healers have prescribed clove since ancient times to treat respiratory and digestive ailments.

Clove first arrived in Europe around the 4th century A.D. as a highly coveted luxury. The medieval German abbess/herbalist Hildegard of Bingen recommended the rare herb in her anti-gout formula.

Demand for clove and other Asian herbs helped launch the Age of Exploration. The remnants of Magellan's flotilla carried some back to Spain in 1512, when the explorers completed their first voyage around the world.

Once the herb became readily available in Europe, it was prized as a treatment for indigestion, flatulence, nausea, vomiting, and diarrhea. It was also used to treat cough, infertility, warts, worms, wounds, and toothache.

America's 19th-century Eclectic physicians, forerunners of today's naturopaths, recommended clove to treat digestive complaints and added it to bitter herbal medicine preparations to make them more palatable. The Eclectics were also the first to extract clove oil from the herbal buds. They used it on the gums to relieve toothache, a practice adopted by modern dentists.

Contemporary herbalists recommend clove for digestive complaints and its oil for toothache.

Therapeutic Uses

Clove oil is 60 to 90 percent eugenol, which is the source of its anesthetic and antiseptic properties.

TOOTHACHE AND ORAL HYGIENE. Dentists use clove oil as an oral anesthetic and to disinfect root canals. It is an ingredient in some over-the-counter toothache remedies, such as Dentapaine. These days the topical anesthetic benzocaine is more popular than clove oil, but that might change if a Kuwaiti study gets publicized. The Kuwaiti researchers gave 73 adults with dental pain one of four treatments: clove oil, a placebo resembling clove oil, benzocaine, or a placebo resembling the drug. Both clove oil and benzocaine provided significantly greater pain relief than the placebos—and there was "no significant difference" between the effectiveness of clove oil and benzocaine.

Commission E, the expert panel that evaluates herbal medicines for the German counterpart of the FDA, endorses clove oil as an oral anesthetic. Keep in mind, though, that toothaches require professional care. Clove oil and products that contain either it or eugenol may provide temporary relief, but you need to see a dentist promptly.

DIGESTIVE PROBLEMS. Like all culinary spices, clove helps relax the smooth muscle lining the digestive tract, supporting the herb's age-old use as a digestive aid.

PARASITES AND INFECTIONS. Clove kills intestinal parasites and "exhibits broad antimicrobial properties against fungi and bacteria," according to one of many reports supporting the herb's traditional use as a treatment for diarrhea, intestinal worms, other digestive ailments, and ringworm.

HAY FEVER. Research shows that clove has some antihistamine action. If you have hay fever, clove probably won't replace pharmaceutical antihistamines, but it may provide additional relief.

Rx Recommendations

For temporary relief of toothache prior to professional care, dip a cotton swab in clove oil and apply it to the affected tooth and surrounding gum. When using commercial clove oil or eugenol preparations, follow the package directions.

To make a warm, pleasant-tasting infusion, use 1 teaspoon of powdered herb per cup of boiling water and steep for 10 to 20 minutes, then strain if you wish.

The Safety Factor

Small amounts of clove oil are used in some foods, beverages, and toothpastes. However, clove oil should never be ingested in amounts greater than one or two drops. As little as 1 teaspoon can cause serious toxicity. Externally, clove oil may cause skin irritation.

Some smokers switch to clove cigarettes, thinking that they're safer than tobacco. They aren't. Most clove cigarettes are 50 to 60 percent tobacco, and when clove burns, it releases many carcinogens. The *Journal of the American Medical Association* has reported many toxic reactions to clove cigarettes.

Use clove oil only temporarily for dental pain. See a dentist promptly.

Clove oil may cause allergic reactions or

other unexpected side effects. If any develop, reduce your dose or stop taking it.

For more on herb safety, see Chapter 2.

Growing Information

Clove does not grow in the United States. The aromatic clove evergreen, which has leathery leaves and reaches 60 feet in height, is native to the Philippines.

Today, Tanzania produces about 80 percent of the world's clove supply. The plant also grows in Indonesia, Sri Lanka, Brazil, and the West Indies.

COCOA (CHOCOLATE)

Great News! It's Good for You!
(Dark Chocolate, That Is)

Family: Sterculiaceae; other members include kola

Genus and species: *Theobroma cacao*

Also known as: Chocolate and cacao

Parts used: Seeds (beans)

Chocoholics of the world, rejoice! Your favorite vice may be just what the doctor ordered for a long, sweet life with reduced risk of heart attack and stroke. The only catch is that you must eat *dark* chocolate. Milk and white chocolate offer minor health benefits, but nowhere near as many as dark chocolate.

Healing History

Imagine a world without chocolate. It would be desolate indeed. But that's how the Old World was until 1519, when Spanish conquistador Hernando Cortez saw Mexico's Aztec ruler, Montezuma, sip a bitter drink called *xocoatl* from a golden goblet. Cortez was more interested in the goblet's gold than in its contents—until the Aztecs informed him that the drink was made from beans so valuable that 100 could buy a healthy human slave. The Aztecs also claimed that *xocoatl* was an aphrodisiac. Montezuma insisted on having some before visiting his harem. After conquering Mexico, Cortez shipped some *xocoatl*, which he called *chocolatl*, back to Spain as a gift for the king.

Before the arrival of the Spanish, the Aztecs and Mayans drank enormous amounts of *xocoatl* (the name means "bitter water"). The common folk could afford it only for special occasions, such as the sealing of marriage vows. Priests used it in prayer offerings. But royalty couldn't get enough. Surviving records suggest that a century before the arrival of Cortez, the Aztec royal court consumed an astonishing 32,000 cocoa beans a day.

Cortez's gift to his king became an instant sensation with the Spanish court. Chocolate proved so popular that the Spanish tried to keep it secret from the rest of Europe—and they succeeded for more than 100 years. During the late 16th century, Mexico was exporting some 200 tons of cocoa beans to Spain each year. Some ships carrying the beans were captured by pirates or other European powers, and eventually, the secret got out.

By the mid-17th century, chocolate had spread throughout Western Europe. It became especially popular in Switzerland, England, Belgium, and Holland. In 1875, Daniel Peter, a Swiss candy maker, figured out how to combine milk and cocoa powder. Voilà, milk chocolate.

Peter and his neighbor, Henri Nestlé, started a company that quickly became the world's leading makers of chocolate candies.

Oddly, until the 19th century, chocolate was consumed only as a beverage—sometimes dark and bitter, sometimes sweetened with sugar or made creamier with milk, but always a liquid. It was only about 150 years ago that chocolate was first fashioned into the blocks and candies that we so love today.

For centuries, Central Americans have used cocoa to treat fever, coughs, and problems associated with pregnancy and childbirth. They have also applied cocoa butter to soothe burns, chapped lips, balding heads, and the sore nipples of nursing mothers.

America's 19th-century Eclectic physicians, forerunners of today's naturopaths, recommended cocoa butter externally as a wound dressing and salve. They prescribed hot cocoa internally as a treatment for asthma, as a substitute for coffee, and as "a very useful nutritive for invalids and persons convalescing from acute illness."

Therapeutic Uses

Cocoa's generic name, *Theobroma*, means "food of the gods," a high tribute to a humble bean. But its derivative, chocolate, is much more than a revered sweet treat. It possesses remarkable healing powers, thanks largely to the antioxidants, caffeine, and theobromine that it contains.

APHRODISIAC POWER? Cocoa and chocolate contain 10 to 20 percent of the amount of caffeine found in coffee. (A cup of cocoa contains about 13 milligrams of caffeine, compared to 65 milligrams of caffeine in a cup of instant coffee and 100 to 150 milligrams in a cup of drip coffee.) But that's sufficient to have stimulant action if you consume enough. In traditional herbal medicine worldwide, stimulant herbs have always been considered sex stimulants.

In addition, chocolate contains a compound called phenylethylamine, or PEA, that plays a key role in the biochemistry of feeling in love. PEA is an antidepressant chemically similar to amphetamine. It's what makes lovers feel as if they're walking on clouds. When a love affair ends, PEA levels drop precipitously.

Some scientists argue that chocolate contains too little PEA to produce amorous emotions. But the skeptics can't explain why chocolate is among the world's favorite Valentine's Day gifts. Perhaps it's a coincidence, or maybe this custom developed because chocolate boosts lovers' PEA levels and heightens their feelings of emotional attachment and erotic interest. It may also explain why those with broken hearts sometimes binge on chocolate—perhaps it's an unconscious desire to replace their lost PEA and recoup some of its mood-elevating effects.

PREVENTION OF DEGENERATIVE DISEASES. Although chocolate is high in fat (more on this later), oddly, it doesn't spoil when left unrefrigerated. This observation led researchers around the world to speculate that cocoa might contain antioxidant compounds, because antioxidants prevent fat spoilage. They discovered that cocoa and dark chocolate contain large amounts of flavonoids and phenolics, both important categories of antioxidant nutrients. Antioxidants—among them vitamins A, C, and E, and the mineral selenium—help prevent the cell damage at the root of heart disease, stroke, and many cancers.

Korean researchers compared the antioxidant content of cocoa with other foods renowned for their antioxidants, including red wine and tea. Cocoa was the clear winner.

- Cocoa powder (2 tablespoons dissolved in 200 milliliters of water): phenolics, 611 milligrams; flavonoids, 564 milligrams
- Red wine (merlot, 140 milliliters): phenolics, 340 milligrams; flavonoids, 163 milligrams
- Green tea (2-gram bag steeped in 200 milliliters of water for 2 minutes): phenolics, 165 milligrams; flavonoids, 47 milligrams
- Black tea (2-g bag steeped in 200 milliliters of water for 2 minutes): phenolics, 124 milligrams; flavonoids, 34 milligrams

Dark chocolate's antioxidant content is similar to cocoa's. But milk chocolate contains considerably less because it is diluted with milk and sugar.

HEART DISEASE, HIGH BLOOD PRESSURE, AND HIGH CHOLESTEROL. Many studies have shown that consumption of tea and red wine (limited to one to two glasses a day) reduces risk of heart attack. When researchers learned that cocoa is richer in antioxidants than tea and red wine, they began investigating dark chocolate to see if it could help prevent heart disease—often with funding from Nestlé (maker of Kit Kat) or Mars (M&M's).

Swiss researchers used sophisticated tests to measure bloodflow through 25 men's arteries, then gave them 1 1/2 ounces of dark chocolate (74 percent cocoa) or white. Tests taken 24 hours later showed no improvement in bloodflow in the white chocolate group, but significantly improved bloodflow in those who'd eaten the dark chocolate. Compared with the white chocolate group, the dark chocolate group also showed blood platelets less likely to form clots. Increased arterial bloodflow and reduced clotting both help prevent heart attack and stroke.

A study by German researchers shows that in people with high blood pressure, daily consumption of 3$\frac{1}{2}$ ounces of dark chocolate lowers blood pressure as much as some pharmaceutical blood pressure medications—atenolol (Tenormin) and propranolol (Inderal). An analysis of five studies by other German researchers agrees: Dark chocolate reduces blood pressure significantly.

Harvard researchers analyzed 136 studies of cocoa and dark chocolate's effects on cardiovascular health. They found consistent evidence that cocoa and dark chocolate reduce blood pressure, raise HDL (good) cholesterol, reduce LDL (bad) cholesterol, reduce inflammation, and prevent internal blood clots—all of which reduce risk of heart disease and stroke.

CANCER. Cocoa also reduces cancer risk. Panamanian researchers compared cancer deaths among mainland Panamanians and the Kuna tribe that lives in relative isolation and drinks a great deal of cocoa. The Kunas' risk of cancer death (and death from heart disease and diabetes) was much lower.

A lower risk of cancer can also be inferred from a Harvard study that tracked the diet and health of 7,814 male Harvard graduates for many years. Compared with men who ate no chocolate bars, those who ate one to three bars a month had a 36 percent lower death rate from all causes.

PHYSICAL AND PSYCHOLOGICAL WELL-BEING. Finnish scientists tracked the physical and emotional health of 1,367 men from their thirties into their seventies. Those who ate the most chocolate were the healthiest. They were also the most optimistic.

FATIGUE AND LETHARGY. The caffeine and theobromine in cocoa and chocolate can help relieve drowsiness and provide mild stimulation without causing as much jitteriness, insomnia, and irritability as coffee. Try some when you feel lethargic (purely as herbal medicine, of course).

DIGESTIVE PROBLEMS. The theobromine in cocoa relaxes the smooth muscle lining of the digestive tract, which may be why many people have room for chocolate after a heavy meal. Try some to soothe your stomach after eating.

BRONCHIAL CONGESTION. Theobromine and caffeine are close chemical relatives of theophylline, which, until recently, was a standard asthma medication. Theophylline opens the bronchial passages; theobromine and caffeine have similar effects.

If you're really congested, or if you have asthma, the large dose of decongestant caffeine found in coffee may be more beneficial. But even the low dose in cocoa or chocolate may provide some relief from the chest congestion of colds and flu.

Rx Recommendations

Kiss guilt good-bye. Now you have some genuine, good-for-you reasons to make yourself a heavenly cup of cocoa. Try the herb as a gentle pick-me-up or digestive aid. And if you have respiratory congestion from a cold, flu, or asthma, there's no harm in sipping steamy hot cocoa, as long as you combine it with appropriate professional medical care.

To make cocoa, use 1 to 2 heaping teaspoons of herb per cup of hot water or low-fat or fat-free milk.

Milk chocolate shows some health benefits, but nowhere near as many as dark chocolate.

For those who grew up eating just milk chocolate, the dark variety does not taste as sweet and creamy, and may even taste bitter. If you'd like to wean yourself from milk chocolate, many chocolate makers now label their products based on how much cocoa they contain. Start with dark chocolate that's around 50 percent cocoa, and slowly work up to around 70 percent.

The Safety Factor

Chocolate cake is sometimes called devil's food, and it's no wonder. Chocolate has long been vilified as a cause of obesity, heart disease, tooth decay, acne, kidney stones, infant colic, headaches, and heartburn. Much of this reputation is undeserved. Chocolate's fat content may contribute to obesity, but a good deal of that saturated fat is in the form of stearic acid, which does not raise cholesterol. Cocoa and dark chocolate contain no cholesterol. (Milk chocolate does.) So, the chocolate in confections is rarely as much of a problem as the high-fat, high-cholesterol butter and cream used in them.

As for chocolate's contribution to tooth decay, it has been blown out of proportion. Some research even suggests that the antioxidants in cocoa help inhibit the growth of bacteria that cause tooth decay. Again, the problem with chocolate candy is not its cocoa content but rather its sugars.

There is no evidence that chocolate causes acne, kidney stones, or infant colic. It does contain chemicals called tyramines that can trigger headaches in some people, particularly those prone to migraines.

Some children and adults are extra-sensitive to the stimulant compounds in cocoa and chocolate. If insomnia, irritability, or hyperactivity becomes a problem, reduce consumption.

Many people find that a cup of hot chocolate soothes their stomachs after meals. The only glitch here is that cocoa and chocolate may cause heartburn. The herb relaxes the valve at the end of the esophagus, the tube that carries food into the stomach. When this valve (the lower esophageal sphincter) does not shut tightly, it allows stomach acid to splash up into the esophagus, causing heartburn. If cocoa or chocolate gives you heartburn, reduce your consumption or give it up.

The real safety issue with cocoa and chocolate has to do with their caffeine content. Caffeine is a powerfully stimulating, classically addictive drug. It has been linked to insomnia, irritability, and anxiety attacks; elevated blood pressure, cholesterol, and blood sugar (glucose) levels; and increased risk of birth defects. (For a complete discussion of caffeine's many effects, see Coffee on page 164.)

Although cocoa and chocolate contain only 10 to 20 percent as much caffeine as coffee, consuming large amounts of them may trigger caffeine's classic effects. People with insomnia, anxiety problems, high cholesterol, high blood pressure, diabetes, or heart disease should limit their caffeine intake.

Cocoa and chocolate may cause allergic reactions or other unexpected side effects. If any develop, reduce your dose or stop taking it.

For more on herb safety, see Chapter 2.

If symptoms get worse or persist longer than 2 weeks, consult a health care professional promptly.

Growing Information

Cocoa (or cacao) should not be confused with coconut or with coca, the source of cocaine. Cocoa trees are small, oval-leafed evergreens that grow in tropical lowlands. They do not grow in the United States.

Wild cocoa trees grow to 30 feet, but cultivated trees are pruned to about 15 feet to allow easier harvesting of the seeds (beans). Central and South America still grow and export cocoa beans, but an estimated 80 percent of the world crop now comes from Africa.

Once harvested, cocoa beans are roasted and ground into a liquid known as cocoa liquor. The liquor then undergoes Dutching, the addition of a minute amount of lye to enhance its flavor (the amount is so small that it poses no health hazard). Then the liquor is further processed to remove its fat, known as cocoa butter. The final product, chocolate, is a combination of the defatted cocoa powder with some cocoa butter added back.

The powder that we know as cocoa is simply dried cocoa liquor, perhaps with a little sugar added. Baker's chocolate is processed cocoa liquor with no sugar added. Bittersweet chocolate has some sugar added, semisweet contains more sugar, and milk chocolate has the most, plus milk to make it creamy.

COFFEE
Plenty of Uses beyond the Boost

Family: Rubiaceae; other members include gardenia, cat's claw, and cinchona

Genus and species: *Coffea arabica, C. liberica,* and *C. robusta*

Also known as: Arabica, mocha, java, espresso, cappuccino, and latté

Parts used: Seeds (beans)

The next time one of your skeptical friends starts giving you a hard time about using medicinal herbs, here's the perfect comeback: "Do you drink coffee?"

Coffee is America's most widely used herbal medicine. The average American drinks 28 gallons a year, using 10 pounds of coffee beans—and for clearly medicinal reasons, to gain the stimulant effects of this herb's caffeine.

But coffee does more than wake us up in the

morning. It also helps treat colds, flu, allergies, and asthma. It improves athletic performance. It helps prevent kidney stones and jet lag. It relieves pain and combats depression, possibly even reducing the risk of suicide. It may also promote weight loss in some people who are seriously obese.

On the other hand, coffee impairs women's fertility and can produce significant side effects. Its active constituent, caffeine, is an addictive drug. Over time, regular users develop a tolerance, and if they suddenly give up caffeine, they experience symptoms of withdrawal.

Caffeine has also been accused, often mistakenly, of causing or contributing to many other health problems. Ironically, its main downside—its effect on women's fertility—has not been well publicized.

Caffeine is definitely not risk-free. No drug is. Authorities generally agree, however, that for most people, it's safe to drink 1 or 2 cups of coffee a day.

Healing History

Our word *coffee* comes from Caffa, the name of the region in Ethiopia where the fabled beans were first discovered. Archeological evidence suggests that prehistoric East Africans loved coffee's remarkable stimulant properties. They ate the red, unroasted beans ("cherries") before tribal wars, extended hunts, and other activities that required alertness, strength, and stamina.

The beverage that we know as coffee emerged around A.D. 1000, when Arabs began roasting and grinding coffee beans and drinking the hot beverage as we do today. Around the same time, the noted Arab physician Avicenna penned the first medical description of coffee's stimulant effects.

Although coffee is enormously popular today, it took centuries to become a worldwide favorite. From 100 to 1500, coffee was consumed only in the Middle East. Then, in 1517, Sultan Selim I introduced the beverage into Constantinople (now Istanbul). At around the same time, spice traders introduced it into Italy. Over the next 100 years, it spread throughout Europe.

The first coffeehouse opened at Oxford University in England in 1650. It was remarkably similar to Starbucks and other contemporary coffeehouses—a place to enjoy coffee, conversation, reading, and writing. Coffeehouses quickly spread to London, where they became hotbeds of political discussion and dissent. In 1675, King Charles II ordered all of London's coffeehouses closed, claiming that they contributed to sedition.

Coffee arrived in New York City in 1696, 30 years before it reached Brazil, which is now one of the world's major coffee-exporting nations.

Until the 17th century, Arabia supplied all of the world's coffee through the port of Mocha (hence one popular name for coffee). Then the Dutch introduced the plant into Java, and the island quickly became synonymous with coffee.

In 1732, Bach composed the "Coffee Cantata" in celebration of his favorite beverage, despite some feeling that it threatened Germany's traditional brew, beer. As coffee became more popular in Germany, the backlash in favor of beer intensified. In 1777, Frederick the Great of Prussia issued a manifesto denouncing coffee in favor of beer.

Fernando Illy of Italy invented the espresso machine in 1904. Merck, the pharmaceutical manufacturer, introduced decaffeinated coffee in 1910. And in 1938, Nestlé introduced Nescafé instant coffee. It is still the leading brand.

Coffee has always been more popular as a beverage than as a healing herb, but European herbalists believed that its stimulant effect could help treat opium and alcohol sedation.

In their medical text *King's American Dispensatory* (1898), America's 19th-century Eclectic physicians, forerunners of today's naturopaths, prescribed coffee as "an agreeable stimulant . . . that frequently overcomes the soporific [sedative] effects of opium, morphine, and alcohol." They also recommended it to treat asthma, constipation, menstrual cramps, and dropsy (congestive heart failure).

The Eclectics also recognized coffee's downside, however. As noted in *King's*: "If taken too freely, [coffee causes] irritability, trembling, confusion, ringing in the ears, and disorders of the bowel. On the other hand, if one is accustomed to moderate amounts, headache will result if the coffee be withdrawn."

Folk healers have used coffee for centuries to treat asthma, fever, headache, colds, and flu. But few modern herbalists include it among the healing herbs. This is odd, considering that coffee is America's most popular medicinal herb.

Therapeutic Uses

Caffeine, the stimulant in coffee (as well as in tea, cocoa, chocolate, cola, maté, and guarana), is also an ingredient in many cold, flu, antidrowsiness, and menstrual remedies. These uses are direct outgrowths of coffee's role in traditional herbal healing.

The caffeine content of coffee depends on how it's prepared. A cup of instant contains about 65 milligrams, a cup of drip or percolated has 100 to 150 milligrams, and a cup of espresso delivers about 350 milligrams.

Caffeine is such an integral part of our culture that we seldom realize how much of a drug it is. The fact is, caffeine is classically addictive. Regular users develop a tolerance and require increasing amounts to obtain the expected stimulant effect. Deprived of caffeine, these people usually develop withdrawal symptoms, primarily headache and constipation that can last for up to 2 weeks.

The media regularly report health problems linked to caffeine and coffee, many of which have been debunked, but they never discuss coffee's many potential therapeutic benefits. Herbal medicine users deserve a more balanced perspective.

FATIGUE AND LETHARGY. No doubt about it: Coffee is a powerful central nervous system stimulant. For those who drive long distances, it helps prevent dozing at the wheel. It also counteracts the sedative effects of antihistamines, one reason it's included in many cold remedies. It does not, however, help people sober up after overindulging in alcohol.

ENHANCED ATHLETIC PERFORMANCE. Attention, athletes: Coffee improves physical stamina and athletic performance. British researchers had 18 runners race about a mile on nine different days after giving them 1 to 2 cups of either regular or decaffeinated coffee. With the help of caffeine, the runners ran 4.2 seconds faster.

In a similar study, researchers had runners run and cyclists ride until they were clinically exhausted. A few days later, the athletes were retested an hour after drinking 5 cups of coffee. With caffeine in their systems, their stamina improved by 44 percent in the running test and by 51 percent in the cycling test.

The International Olympic Committee regulates caffeine use by Olympic athletes, allowing no more than 12 micrograms of caffeine per milligram of urine. To reach that level, an athlete would have to drink at least 5 cups of coffee within 3 hours before Olympic events.

To experience caffeine's performance-enhancing benefit, you must consume more than you already tolerate. A person who uses no caffeine might improve performance by drinking just a cup or two of coffee, but a 1-cup-a-day athlete might have to drink 2 to 3 cups before noticing any benefit.

COLDS, FLU, AND ALLERGIES. Caffeine is a decongestant. As such, it can be used to treat ailments that cause chest congestion, such as colds, flu, and allergies. That's another reason it's included in many cold formulas.

ASTHMA. Some years ago, North Carolina pharmacists Joe and Terry Graedon, authors of *The People's Pharmacy* books and syndicated column, received a letter from a woman who had just returned from her honeymoon. While in Hawaii, the woman, who had asthma, began wheezing. She reached for the inhaler she always carried with her, but it was nowhere to be found. Wheezing more and feeling panicky, she ransacked her luggage. Nothing. In all of the wedding and honeymoon commotion, she'd forgotten to pack it.

She imagined her honeymoon ruined by a trip to the emergency room. Then she recalled something that she'd read in *The People's Pharmacy*. Caffeine is chemically similar to some asthma medications. In a pinch, the Graedons had written, it can be used to stop an asthma attack. It's a bronchodilator, which means that it opens narrowed bronchial tubes and eases breathing.

The wheezing newlywed rushed to the hotel snack bar and quickly downed 3 cups of coffee. Within minutes, she was breathing easier. She wrote the Graedons: "You saved my honeymoon."

This woman's experience is not unique. A survey of 70,000 Italian households shows that as coffee consumption increases, incidence of asthma decreases.

PAIN RELIEF. Compared with plain aspirin or ibuprofen (Motrin, Advil), a combination of aspirin and a small amount of caffeine (60 milligrams, about the amount in 1 cup of instant coffee, or half a cup of brewed coffee, or a strong cup of tea, or a 12-ounce cola) relieves pain faster and more effectively. Caffeine has no intrinsic pain-relieving effect, but it is a mild antidepressant. Pain and mood are connected. Pain hurts less when you feel happier, and more when you feel depressed. Researchers believe that coffee's mood-elevating effect is the reason it boosts the action of pain-relieving drugs. Next time you have a headache or any injury that makes you reach for aspirin or ibuprofen, wash it down with a caffeinated beverage or take Excedrin, a combination of aspirin and caffeine.

PREVENTION OF DEGENERATIVE DISEASES. Like other plants, coffee beans contain antioxidant nutrients. Compared with tea and cocoa (chocolate), coffee has considerably lower levels of antioxidants. However, according to researchers at the University of Scranton in Pennsylvania, because Americans drink so much coffee, many get more antioxidants from coffee than from sources richer in these nutrients (tea, cocoa, and fruits and vegetables). Antioxidants help prevent and reverse the cell damage at the root of heart disease, cancer, and many other conditions.

DIABETES. Several studies show that coffee reduces risk of type 2 diabetes. A Harvard study published in *Diabetes Care* shows that 1 cup a day reduces diabetes risk by 13 percent and 2 to 3 cups a day reduces risk by 42 percent. Other studies have come up with somewhat different findings, but they all agree that moderate coffee consumption reduces risk of type 2 diabetes. Why would coffee lower risk? That remains unclear, but coffee's antioxidant content may play a role. In addition, coffee is a modest aid to weight loss (see below), and type 2 diabetes is strongly associated with obesity.

SUICIDE PREVENTION. Caffeine's mood-elevating effect also appears to explain why regular coffee consumers have a lower-than-expected risk of suicide. For more than 20 years, Harvard researchers have been following the diet, lifestyle, and health of a group of about 85,000 female nurses in the ongoing Nurses' Health Study. Participants who drink no coffee have a somewhat higher suicide rate than those who drink 2 to 3 cups a day.

KIDNEY STONES. Kidney stones cause excruciating pain in the lower back and groin. The traditional preventive measure involves drinking plenty of water to keep the urine dilute, which minimizes risk of stone formation. But the Nurses' Health Study, mentioned above, shows that compared with no preventive efforts, a daily glass of water cuts kidney stone risk by 2 percent, while a daily cup or two of coffee reduces risk by 10 percent. (Tea cuts risk by 8 percent.)

GALLSTONES. Gallstones affect 20 million Americans and send 800,000 to hospitals each year. Harvard researchers followed 46,008 male health professionals who were initially free of gallstones. More than 8 years later, 1,081 had developed the condition. Compared with study participants who drank no coffee, those who consumed 2 to 3 cups a day had a 40 percent lower risk of developing gallstones. Those who drank 1 cup a day also enjoyed some, though less, protection.

MENSTRUAL FLOW. Coffee appears to protect against heavy menstrual flow, which not only is inconvenient but also might contribute to iron-deficiency anemia. Researchers surveyed 403 healthy premenopausal women enrolled in California's Kaiser Permanente health maintenance organization about their health, diet, and lifestyle. Compared with those who drank no coffee, the women who drank more than 2 cups a day (supplying them with 300 milligrams of caffeine) had a significantly lower risk of menstrual periods lasting at least 8 days. Caffeine is a vasoconstrictor, the researchers explain. It constricts blood vessels, including those in the uterus, which might explain reduced menstrual flow.

JET LAG. Jet lag is the disorientation, insomnia, and fatigue that develop after flying across time zones. Coffee may help shift the body's natural time cycle (known as its circadian rhythm) after abrupt time-zone changes. Some jet-lag authorities recommend drinking coffee in the morning when traveling west and in the late afternoon when traveling east.

WEIGHT LOSS. The caffeine in coffee raises basal metabolic rate (BMR), the speed at which the body burns calories while at rest. As BMR increases, fat accumulation decreases, and the body may shed unwanted pounds. In medically supervised weight-loss programs, severely obese individuals who supplement a low-calorie diet and regular exercise with caffeine and other stimulants lose a little more weight—not much, but enough to keep caffeine a part of some weight-loss programs. However, the side effects can be a problem (see below). And caffeine helps only those who are severely obese, weighing well over 20 percent more than their recommended weight. It does not help those with more modest weight-loss goals, such as losing 5 to 10 pounds.

GOUT. Canadian and Harvard researchers correlated gout attacks and coffee drinking in 45,000 men over the course of 12 years. Drinking up to 3 cups a day had no effect on gout risk. But 4 cups a day reduced risk by 40 percent, and 6 cups a day reduced it by 59 percent. Decaf coffee produced similar results.

Rx Recommendations

Coffee has a wonderful, rich, pleasantly bitter taste. The growing sales of decaffeinated coffee demonstrate that taste alone is sufficient incentive for millions of people to drink it regularly. You might also enjoy regular coffee as a stimulating pick-me-up, stamina-booster, decongestant, antidepressant, preventive measure for kidney stones, gallstones, and jet lag, or as part of a medically supervised weight-loss program.

To make an infusion (otherwise known as a cup of java), use 1 heaping tablespoon of ground beans per cup of water. Brew it using your favorite method, or buy instant and follow the directions on the label. Drink up to 3 cups a day.

Coffee-flavored food items such as yogurt and ice cream also contain some caffeine. If you use them, be aware that they add to your caffeine consumption and may increase your tolerance and side effects.

The Safety Factor

Coffee is classically addictive and causes so many side effects that one report noted: "If caffeine were a newly synthesized drug, its manufacturer would almost certainly have great difficulty getting it licensed under current [Food and Drug Administration] regulations. If it were licensed, it would almost certainly be available only by prescription."

More Than Just Jitters

If you're a coffee drinker, you know that when you drink more than you're used to, you get jittery, irritable, and impatient and have trouble falling asleep. If you're concerned about having a short temper, consider reducing your coffee consumption or switching to decaf. If you don't sleep as soundly as you'd like, drink less coffee, switch to decaf, or drink caffeinated coffee only in the morning, so the caffeine's stimulant effect wears off by bedtime.

Individual reactions to caffeine vary, but over time, large amounts—on the order of 8 or more cups per day—may cause caffeinism, a condition with the same symptoms as anxiety neurosis: nervousness and irritability, chronic muscle tension, insomnia, heart palpitations, diarrhea, heartburn, and stomach upset. In fact, many people are misdiagnosed with anxiety neurosis when the problem is actually caffeinism, according to a report in the *American Journal of Psychiatry*.

Java Junkies—For Real

Regular use of caffeine produces a tolerance, meaning that over time, you need more coffee than you used to drink to produce the desired stimulation. Once you're addicted to caffeine, suddenly eliminating coffee produces a withdrawal syndrome: a headache that may last several days, and often sluggishness and constipation. If you want to cut down on coffee, or stop drinking it, or switch to decaf, do it gradually. This minimizes or prevents the discomforts of withdrawal. To switch to decaf, over the course of several weeks, mix increasing amounts of decaf with decreasing amounts of regular coffee until you're drinking 100 percent decaf.

Be aware that coffee increases the secretion of stomach acid. Those with ulcers or other chronic digestive disorders should use it sparingly, if at all.

Links to Serious Illnesses?

Coffee has been accused of increasing the risk of several serious conditions, including high blood pressure, high cholesterol, heart attack, cancer, birth defects, and hyperactivity in children. The news here is largely reassuring.

HIGH BLOOD PRESSURE? As mentioned earlier, caffeine is a vasoconstrictor. As blood vessels narrow, blood pressure rises. Caffeine produces a sharp spike in blood pressure in those using it for the first time, but several studies show that in people with normal blood pressure, the rise is temporary, and blood pressure soon returns to normal. If your blood pressure is normal, modest caffeine consumption—1 to 2 cups a day—does not cause hypertension. But if you take blood pressure medication, discuss your caffeine intake with your doctor.

HIGH CHOLESTEROL? Some years ago, a Scandinavian study that followed 38,500 men and women for 3 years showed that as coffee consumption increased, so did cholesterol levels and heart attack risk. Rising coffee consumption

was associated with higher cholesterol levels, and compared with those who abstained from coffee, those who consumed 9 cups a day had about three times the risk of heart attack. Of course, very few people drink 9 cups a day. Nonetheless, risk increased with every daily cup, so the association was troubling.

It's considerably less troubling today. The same researchers continued their study for 12 years, during which time the association between coffee drinking and elevated cholesterol and heart attack risk plummeted. After 12 years, the 9-cup-a-day coffee drinkers have only 1.3 times the risk of heart attack of their no-coffee counterparts, which is barely statistically significant, and those who drink a cup or two show hardly any elevated risk at all.

What changed? The Scandinavians' preferred coffee-brewing method. They used to boil their coffee, which extracts compounds from the beans that raise cholesterol and increase risk of heart attack. But as this study was taking place, Scandinavians switched to drip coffee, which filters out these harmful compounds. Instant coffee does not contain these compounds either.

The vast majority of Americans drink instant or drip coffee. A recent analysis of long-term data from the Nurses' Health Study shows no increase in heart disease risk based on coffee consumption.

Most recently, Swedish researchers discovered that coffee raises blood levels of homocysteine, an amino acid that has been identified as another risk factor for heart disease. But the increase was small, and the researchers concluded that a cup or two a day does not pose a heart disease risk. Public health authorities are no longer concerned that typical coffee consumption increases heart attack risk.

HEART DISEASE? Despite accusations over the years that coffee increases the risk of heart disease, it contains antioxidants that help prevent heart disease, and it raises neither blood pressure nor cholesterol. As a result, we would not expect it to increase heart disease risk, and indeed—as mentioned earlier—that's what Harvard researchers found when they analyzed the data of more than 85,000 women nurses who took part in the Nurses' Health Study. In another huge study, they tracked 44,005 men and 84,488 women for 14 years, and again found no evidence that drinking up to 6 cups a day increases risk of heart disease.

CANCERS? In various studies over the years, coffee has been linked to cancers of the breast, bladder, ovaries, pancreas, and prostate gland. All of these reports have been disputed. Most have been thoroughly debunked. In fact, the researchers who accused caffeine of increasing the risk of bladder cancer later repudiated their own findings.

At this point, there is no evidence that a daily cup or two increases cancer risk significantly. In fact, a few studies have shown that coffee reduces the risk of liver cancer; some studies have also shown a reduced risk of breast cancer in high-risk women. It's true that roasting coffee introduces carcinogens into the beans, but apparently, the antioxidant content of coffee more than compensates for this.

OSTEOPOROSIS? Caffeine pulls calcium out of bone. As a result, coffee drinking has been accused of increasing the risk of osteoporosis. Since 1975, 23 studies have investigated caffeine as a risk factor for osteoporotic fractures. Ten studies (43 percent) show that caffeine increases fracture risk. Four (17 percent) are inconclusive. Nine (39 percent) show that caffeine has no effect on fracture risk. The evidence tilts slightly toward caffeine as a risk factor for fractures, but it's far from compelling.

There may be a simple explanation for the studies' disagreement. It looks as though there's a caffeine threshold for fracture risk. Up to 2 cups of coffee a day (or 4 cups a day of tea or cola) does not increase risk. But any more does. Most coffee drinkers consume only 1 to 2 cups a day, below the threshold for caffeine-related bone damage. If you limit coffee to 2 cups a day or less (or 4 cups of tea), you probably don't have to worry about the caffeine you're consuming contributing to fractures. But if you drink more, you might consider cutting down to protect your bones.

BIRTH DEFECTS? Studies from the early 1980s showed that animals that were fed extraordinarily high doses of caffeine bore young with an increased risk of birth defects. But no human study has ever shown that a daily cup or two of coffee increases birth defect risk. Still, the Food and Drug Administration warns pregnant women to limit their caffeine intake or eliminate it altogether. Nature seems to have the same opinion, since many women lose their taste for coffee while pregnant.

HYPERACTIVITY IN CHILDREN? Caffeine is clearly a stimulant, but there is no evidence that it contributes to hyperactivity. In fact, stimulant drugs such as methylphenidate (Ritalin) are often used to treat this condition. It's not clear why stimulants calm hyperactive children, but they often do. Researchers at the University of Chicago analyzed 12 studies of caffeine and behavior in children. None showed any increase in hyperactivity. A few showed calming benefits.

STUNTING CHILDREN'S GROWTH?

Many parents tell their kids: "Don't drink coffee. It will stunt your growth." Wrong. Studies have found no effect from coffee drinking on children's growth.

Problems for Women

For all the publicity given to reports of coffee's side effects, the media have generally underreported the problems caffeine can cause women.

IMPAIRED FERTILITY. In a 10-year study, researchers at Johns Hopkins University School of Medicine tracked 1,430 mothers, analyzing their diet and lifestyle habits, including their coffee consumption. The women experienced 2,501 pregnancies during the study. The more coffee they drank, the longer it took them to get pregnant. A 3-cup-a-day coffee habit reduced fertility by about 26 percent.

If you're trying to get pregnant, limit your caffeine consumption or go caffeine free. On the other hand, be aware that, even in large amounts, coffee should not be considered a contraceptive because its fertility-reducing effect is highly unreliable.

FIBROCYSTIC BREASTS. A few studies have linked caffeine to painful, noncancerous breast lumps called fibrocysts, a normal but annoying condition. Women bothered by fibrocystic breasts might try cutting out all sources of caffeine—including coffee, tea, cocoa, chocolate, soft drinks, and over-the-counter drugs—and seeing if it helps.

PREMENSTRUAL SYNDROME. In one study, researchers found that compared with those who drank none, women who drank 2 to 4 cups of brewed coffee a day suffered five times the rate of premenstrual syndrome (PMS) symptoms. If PMS is a problem for you, consider cutting back on coffee or switching to decaf.

STRESS INCONTINENCE. Coffee contributes to stress incontinence, the urine leakage that can occur with coughing, laughing, or sneezing. For reasons that remain unclear, coffee consumption is associated with a weakening of the muscles that hold the urine tube (the urethra) closed, a condition known as detrusor instability. Brown University researchers surveyed 259 women with various types of urinary incontinence. Compared with those who drank little or no coffee, the women who consumed 5 cups a day were 2.4 times more likely to suffer stress incontinence.

A Cup or Two a Day

Because coffee is America's most popular herbal medicine, the debate over its safety is sure to continue, with headlines trumpeting any research findings of adverse effects. But public health experts generally agree that for people with no medical reason to abstain, it's safe to drink 1 to 2 cups of coffee a day. Beyond that, the risk of side effects increases.

Inform health care professionals of the amount of coffee you drink. Problematic herb-drug interactions are possible.

Coffee may cause allergic reactions or other unexpected side effects. If any develop, reduce your dose or stop taking it.

For more on herb safety, see Chapter 2.

Growing Information

Coffee grows in tropical areas around the world. The plant is an evergreen shrub or small tree with two-seeded, bright crimson fruits. The green seeds (beans) are extracted and roasted to produce the dark brown, oily beans recognized the world over. (Most of the world's supply consists of the Arabian *arabica* species. But *liberica*, from Liberia, and *robusta*, from the Congo, are also cultivated worldwide.)

You can, however, grow a coffee plant purely as an ornamental if you live in a sunny, humid area where the temperature does not dip below 60°F. The plant requires full sun, moist air, moist soil, good drainage, and regular feeding.

Coffee plants are also available as houseplants. Again, they require full sun and high humidity. They grow well in greenhouses but not in homes with forced-air heat, which tend to be too dry. Consult your local nursery or plant store.

COMFREY

A Controversial Wound Treatment

Family: Boraginaceae; other members include borage and forget-me-not

Genus and species: *Symphytum officinale*

Also known as: Bruisewort, knitbone, boneset, and healing herb

Parts used: Roots

Well into the 1980s, many herbalists touted comfrey as "an absolute must," "ideal for the amateur herbalist," and "perfectly safe and harmless." Then the herb was found to contain chemicals capable of causing severe liver damage. Today, responsible herbalists recommend comfrey for external use only.

Healing History

The early Greeks used juicy comfrey root externally to treat wounds, believing that it encouraged torn flesh to grow back together. The Roman naturalist Pliny "verified" this practice with the observation that boiling comfrey in water produces a sticky paste capable of binding chunks of meat together. Comfrey paste hardens like plaster, and on ancient battlefields, cloths soaked in it were often wrapped around broken bones. When the paste dried, the result was a primitive but effective cast. This treatment earned comfrey the popular names knitbone and boneset (although comfrey shouldn't be confused with the herb boneset).

During the 1st century A.D., the Greek physician Dioscorides began prescribing comfrey tea internally for respiratory and gastrointestinal problems.

By the 1500s, herbalists were recommending comfrey tea, not paste, to mend broken bones. One early English herbal suggested that it "helpeth [people who have] broken the bone of the legge."

The 17th-century English herbalist Nicholas Culpeper recommended comfrey roots, "full of glutinous and clammy juice," for "all inward hurts, and for outward wounds and sores in [all] fleshy or sinewy parts of the body. . . . [It] is especially good for ruptures and broken bones." Culpeper also prescribed the herb for fever, gout, hemorrhoids, gangrene, and respiratory and menstrual problems.

As plaster replaced comfrey paste for casting broken bones, names like knitbone were discarded. Comfrey came to be used internally to soothe inflamed mucous membranes. America's 19th-century Eclectic physicians, forerunners of today's naturopaths, prescribed it for diarrhea, dysentery, cough, bronchitis, and "female debility" (menstrual discomfort).

Mexican midwives still apply comfrey to torn vaginal tissue. In the Philippines, the herb is used to treat arthritis, diabetes, anemia, lung infections, and even leukemia.

By the mid-1990s, responsible herbalists had stopped recommending comfrey for internal use because of its potential to cause liver damage. Today, it's primarily used to heal wounds and provide pain relief for musculoskeletal injuries.

Therapeutic Uses

The ancient Greeks and Romans were right about comfrey aiding wound healing. But the herb's stickiness has nothing to do with it.

WOUNDS. Comfrey contains allantoin, a chemical that helps protect the skin and promotes the growth of new skin cells. These properties validate the herb's more than 2,500 years of external use on everything from minor cuts and burns to major battle wounds. Studies show that comfrey also helps relieve inflammation, adding to its wound-treating effects. Be sure to wash wounds thoroughly with soap and water before applying the herb.

The FDA considers allantoin safe in concentrations of up to 2 percent. It is an ingredient in many over-the-counter products for dry skin, diaper rash, and herpes.

Such widespread commercial use of allantoin suggests that whole comfrey root preparations may provide similar benefits. Commission E, the expert panel that evaluates herbal medicines for the German counterpart of the FDA, approves comfrey root powder for the treatment of minor wounds.

Small amounts of comfrey can be absorbed through the skin, but because transdermal comfrey is not digested, it poses no hazard to the liver.

ARTHRITIS. German researchers gave 220 people with painful arthritis of the knee either a placebo ointment or a comfrey cream (2 grams three times a day). After 3 weeks, the comfrey cream provided significantly greater pain relief. A different group of German scientists gave a placebo or comfrey ointment to 142 men with sprained ankles. Again, the herb group reported significantly greater pain relief.

Rx Recommendations

To use comfrey on minor wounds, wash them with soap and water, and then sprinkle some dried, powdered root on the wound. Another option is to make a paste from some powdered root and a few drops of water. Apply the paste to the wound and cover with a clean bandage. Change the bandage and reapply the comfrey daily.

For pain relief, buy a comfrey lotion or add powdered root to any skin cream.

The Safety Factor

Comfrey contains chemicals called pyrrolizidine alkaloids (PAs), which, in large amounts, cause serious liver damage. Animals fed plants containing PAs showed symptoms of poisoning, and some died. In humans, several cases of poisoning have also been reported after long-term ingestion of comfrey.

Tests by FDA researchers have shown that the PA content of comfrey varies greatly, with the root—the part most widely used in herbal medicine—containing the highest levels. Some herbalists have claimed that PAs are not water-soluble and that, as a result, comfrey tea should be free of PAs. But the FDA scientists have found PAs in comfrey tea as well.

The American Herbal Products Association, the herb industry trade organization, recommends that all comfrey products be labeled for external use only.

Do not ingest comfrey. Use it topically only.

Growing Information

Comfrey is a hardy 5-foot perennial with large, hairy, lance-shaped leaves; thick, spreading roots; a hollow, bristly stem; and bell-like flowers, which may be white, blue, or purple.

Comfrey can be started from seeds, but it grows best from root cuttings taken in spring or fall. An inch-long piece of root planted in 3 inches of soil almost always produces a plant. Set cuttings 3 feet apart. The herb grows in any well-drained soil and tolerates full sun or partial shade. It spreads vigorously, so contain it in a pot or border it with sheet metal to a depth of 12 inches.

Gather the roots in autumn, after the first frost, or in spring before the first leaves appear. Wash harvested roots thoroughly and cut them into slices to dry. Grind them to a powder in a blender or coffee grinder and store in a sealed container.

CORDYCEPS

The Parasitic "Worm" That Heals

Family: Clavicipitaceae; other members include other mushrooms

Genus and species: *Cordyceps sinensis*

Also known as: Caterpillar fungus and dong chong xia cao, which means "summer plant/winter worm"

Parts used: Whole fungus

Cordyceps is native to high-altitude locales—above 10,000 feet—in Asia. It's a parasite that infests and kills insect larvae and caterpillars, hence the name caterpillar fungus. The fungus emerges from its dying host looking like a worm. The ancient Chinese considered cordyceps a plant during the summer and an animal in winter, hence the name summer plant/winter worm.

Healing History

Cordyceps was widely used in traditional medical systems of the Himalayas. An ethnomedical survey published in 2006 shows that it continues to be among the most common treatments in parts of Nepal.

Not much cordyceps found its way from the Himalayas into lowland China. The fungus was so rare in China that it was used only by the emperor and his family. It was first mentioned in a Chinese medical text in 1757. In 1843, an American physician reported in the *New York Journal of Medicine* that cordyceps had actions similar to ginseng: improved stamina, greater energy, less fatigue, greater sexual vitality, and enhanced longevity.

Therapeutic Uses

IMMUNE STIMULATION. Canadian scientists have shown that cordyceps activates infection-fighting white blood cells. In a Chinese study, it was found to improve immune function in people with cancer, who also reported improved quality of life.

PREVENTION OF DEGENERATIVE DISEASES. A Japanese study shows that cordyceps possesses "potent antioxidant activity." Antioxidants help prevent the cell damage at the root of heart disease, cancer, and many other conditions. Hong Kong researchers agree, calling the fungus a "strong antioxidant."

HEART ATTACK AND STROKE. A Chinese report shows that cordyceps reduces levels of both cholesterol and blood fats (triglycerides), meaning reduced risk of heart attack and stroke. A Japanese study shows that it slows the growth of the cholesterol-rich deposits that narrow the arteries and increase risk of heart attack and stroke. Other Chinese studies show that cordyceps (3 grams a day) normalizes heart rhythm; it also was shown to improve congestive heart failure by reducing shortness of breath.

KIDNEY DISEASE. Chinese scientists have found that cordyceps reduces risk of kidney failure and organ rejection after kidney transplantation. They called the fungus an "ideal" treatment for people receiving kidney transplants.

Other Chinese researchers have discovered that cordyceps prevents lupus-related kidney inflammation, known as lupus nephritis. They studied 61 people with lupus who had already had at least one episode of this condition. Half were treated with a Chinese herb formula, and half received cordyceps (3 grams a day before meals) plus another Chinese herb, artemisinin (0.6 gram a day after meals). After 3 years, 77 percent of people in the herb-formula group experienced reduced lupus nephritis recurrence, while the figure for the cordyceps/ artemisinin group was significantly greater, 97 percent.

LIVER DISEASE. Chinese studies show that cordyceps improves liver function in people with chronic hepatitis and cirrhosis.

ASTHMA AND BRONCHITIS. Several Chinese studies show that cordyceps improves lung function in people with asthma and bronchitis. In a review of five studies, 4 weeks of cordyceps treatment (3 to $4^{1}/_{2}$ grams a day) was found to improve lung function in 78 to 92 percent of participants.

FATIGUE-FIGHTER AND STAMINA-BUILDER? In the elderly, cordyceps appears to live up to its traditional use as a fatigue-fighter and stamina-builder. Chinese researchers tested the endurance of 30 elderly people, and then gave them either a placebo or 3 grams of the fungus a day. Six weeks later, both groups were retested. The placebo users showed no improvement in exercise capacity, but those taking cordyceps showed significantly improved stamina.

In another Chinese study, compared with those who took a placebo, elderly people who used 3 grams of cordyceps per day reported significantly less fatigue, dizziness, ringing in the ears (tinnitus), and intolerance to cold.

However, four studies show that cordyceps does not improve athletic performance in younger people. Two of these trials involved competitive cyclists who were tested before and after taking 3 grams of the fungus daily for 2 weeks or 5 weeks. In none of the four trials did cordyceps improve athletic performance. It's possible that cordyceps helps the elderly, but not younger people.

Intriguing Possibilities

Korean scientists have shown that cordyceps treatment kills liver cancer cells. This is presumably because the herb has two cancer-fighting actions: It's an antioxidant and it stimulates the immune system. It's too early to call cordyceps a cancer treatment, but one day it might be.

Cordyceps may also be helpful in the treatment of sexual problems. In one Chinese study of 155 people with unspecified sexual problems, almost two-thirds reported improvement after taking cordyceps.

Rx Recommendations

Most studies have used 3 grams per day (approximately 1 tablespoon). For weakness, debility, and recovery from illness, Chinese medical practitioners recommend 3 to 9 grams per day (1 to 3 tablespoons) of powdered fungus. It can also be mixed into soup and eaten.

The Safety Factor

Animal studies show low toxicity, if any.

Pregnant and nursing women should not use cordyceps.

Do not give cordyceps to children under 2. In older children, adjust the recommended dose based on the child's weight. For example, give a 50-pound child one-third of the dose a 150-pound adult would take.

If you're over 65, start with a low dose, and increase only if necessary.

Inform health care professionals of the herbs you use. Problematic herb-drug interactions are possible.

Cordyceps may cause allergic reactions or other unexpected side effects. If any develop, reduce your dose or stop taking it.

For more on herb safety, see Chapter 2.

If symptoms get worse or persist longer than 2 weeks, consult a health care professional promptly.

Growing Information

Medicinal *Cordyceps sinensis* is not found outside of the Himalayas. A related species, *C. militaris*, parasitizes some caterpillars in North America.

Aloha Medicinals of Carson City, Nevada (alohamedicinals.com), grows *Cordyceps sinensis* in the United States under simulated high-altitude conditions—low temperature and low oxygen equivalent to an elevation of 18,000 feet. The company claims to be the world's largest producer of this fungus.

CRANBERRY

Not Just for UTIs

Family: Ericaceae; other members include azalea, blueberry, and uva-ursi

Genus and species: *Vaccinium macrocarpon* or *Oxycoccus quadripetalus*

Also known as: No other common names

Parts used: Berries

Cranberry, or, more specifically, cranberry juice, is *the* herbal choice for preventing urinary tract infections (UTIs). The berries are also rich in antioxidant nutrients, which help prevent degenerative diseases, particularly those that affect the eyes.

Healing History

Cranberries were eaten for their tangy, refreshing taste long before anyone thought of them as healing herbs. The Pilgrims reportedly dined on cranberry dishes at the first Thanksgiving in 1621, but cranberry sauce did not become a national tradition until after the Civil War. General Ulysses S. Grant considered cranberry sauce an essential part of Thanksgiving, and he ordered it served to Union troops during the siege of Petersburg in 1864. Soldiers who were unfamiliar with the tart berries liked them, and the custom stuck.

Although the colonists were unaware of their high vitamin C content, the bright red berries became a favorite among New England sailors because those who ate them did not develop scurvy.

America's 19th-century Eclectic physicians, forerunners of today's naturopaths, did not consider the cranberry particularly beneficial. Their medical reference *King's American Dispensatory* (1898) contained this curious prescription, however: "A split cranberry, held in position by a daub of starch paste, will quickly relieve the pain and inflammation attending boils on the tip of the nose."

Today, we Americans eat cranberries not only at Thanksgiving but year-round. Our annual consumption is somewhere around 400 million pounds, an amount that's valued at more than $1 billion.

Therapeutic Uses

Cranberry's claim to fame as a UTI preventive comes not from herbal tradition but rather from 19th-century German chemists.

URINARY TRACT INFECTIONS. During the 1840s, German researchers discovered that people who eat cranberries pass a bacteria-fighting chemical called hippuric acid in their urine. Sixty years later, American researchers speculated that urine acidified by a steady diet of cranberries might prevent UTIs, a common, recurrent, and often chronic health problem among women.

Women began drinking cranberry juice with gusto, and several studies endorsed the practice. But by the late 1960s, naysayers claimed that the tart berries did not significantly acidify urine and therefore could not prevent UTIs.

More recent research shows that cranberry juice is indeed an effective UTI preventive. A 1984 study, reported in the *Journal of Urology*, showed that 73 percent of women with recurrent UTIs experienced significant protection from infection after drinking a pint of commercial cranberry juice cocktail every day for 3 weeks. The researchers theorized that urinary acidity has nothing to do with the herb's effectiveness. Instead, they explained, the juice prevents the germs that cause UTIs from adhering to the lining of the urinary tract, reducing the likelihood of infection.

Many subsequent studies in the *New England Journal of Medicine* (1991), the *Journal of the American Medical Association* (1994 and 1998), the *Journal of Family Practice* (1997), and the *Journal of Urology* (2008) reached the same conclusion. In addition, a British review of 10 studies concluded that cranberry juice reduces risk of recurrent UTIs. The reason: Cranberries contain antioxidant compounds called proanthocyanidins that inhibit bacterial adherence in the bladder.

PREVENTION OF DEGENERATIVE DISEASES. Proanthocyanidins are members of the chemical family of antioxidants known as anthocyanosides. These compounds help prevent and reverse the cell damage that's at the root of heart disease, most strokes, many cancers, and other degenerative diseases. Researchers at the Jean Mayer USDA Human Nutrition Research Center on Aging at Tufts University in Boston analyzed and ranked dozens of common plant foods according to their total antioxidant contents. The best antioxidant sources turned out to be the dark-colored fruits and berries, such as cranberries, that contain generous amounts of anthocyanosides.

CATARACTS. Cataracts are a major cause of vision impairment and blindness among older adults in the United States. The condition occurs when the normally clear lens of the eye develops cloudy spots as a result of oxidative damage.

Though scientists aren't sure why, anthocyanosides have unusually powerful effects on the eyes. In one Italian study, 50 people with early-stage cataracts were given an extract of bilberry (another berry rich in anthocyanosides) three times a day, along with antioxidant vitamin E. The treatment stopped cataract progression in 97 percent of the study participants. Because cranberries contain generous amounts of anthocyanosides, they may also help prevent cataracts.

MACULAR DEGENERATION. The nerve-rich retina in the back of the eye plays a key role in vision. One area of the retina, called the macula, is responsible for central vision (seeing what's directly in front of you) and fine detail. Macular degeneration is characterized by deterioration of the macula.

In a European study, 31 people with various types of retinal eye problems, including macular degeneration, were given an extract of bilberry. Those with macular degeneration experienced significant improvement in their vision. Since cranberries have many of the same eye-friendly nutrients as bilberries, they may also help this condition.

DIABETIC RETINOPATHY. Diabetes damages all of the blood vessels in the body, including the tiny capillaries that nourish the retina. When injured, these capillaries can leak blood into the eye, causing the blurred vision of diabetic retinopathy.

Anthocyanosides strengthen retinal blood vessels, thus reducing leakage. In the European study of retinal eye problems mentioned above, people with diabetic retinopathy showed significant improvement when taking the bilberry extract. Cranberries may also help.

INCONTINENCE. Cranberry juice helps deodorize urine. A report in the *Journal of Psychiatric Nursing* suggests that people with urinary incontinence incorporate cranberry juice into their diets to reduce embarrassing odor.

Rx Recommendations

Most of the studies showing that cranberry helps prevent UTIs have used cranberry juice cocktail, which is available in most supermarkets. Pure cranberry juice is highly acidic and too sour to drink, which is why water and sugar are added to the commercial juice, turning it into "cocktail." If you're prone to UTIs, try drinking a couple of glasses of cranberry juice cocktail daily to see if it helps prevent recurrence.

In the study of UTIs reported in the *Journal of Family Practice*, participants did not drink juice. Instead, they took one capsule of concentrated cranberry extract, containing 400 milligrams of cranberry solids, twice a day for at least a month. The solids were as effective as the juice. If you'd like to try an extract, they are available in many health food stores.

Another option is to munch on dried cranberries. Many health food stores and supermarkets sell them as a snack food similar to raisins.

The Safety Factor

Cranberries are unlikely to cause allergic reactions or other unexpected side effects. But if any develop, reduce your dose or stop taking them.

Inform health care professionals of the herbs you use. Problematic herb-drug interactions are possible.

For more on herb safety, see Chapter 2.

If symptoms get worse or persist longer than 2 weeks, consult a health care professional promptly.

Growing Information

Cranberry is a small evergreen shrub that grows in mountain forests and damp bogs from Alaska to Tennessee. Its pink or purple flowers bloom from late spring to late summer and produce bright red fruits in fall.

Few gardeners have the conditions necessary to grow this herb. It requires wet, boggy, acidic soil amended with peat moss or leaf mold. Check with your local nursery to see if cranberry is viable in your area.

DANDELION

Much More Than a Weed

Family: Compositae; other members include daisy and marigold

Genus and species: *Taraxacum officinale*

Also known as: Lion's tooth, wild endive, and piss-abed

Parts used: Primarily roots; also leaves

Dandelion is so widely despised as a weed that many people have a hard time seeing it for what it really is: a nutritious healing herb with a medicinal reputation dating back more than 1,000 years.

Dandelion stimulates the flow of bile, and as a diuretic, it may help treat premenstrual syndrome, high blood pressure, and congestive heart failure. It may also help prevent gallstones and have other medically intriguing benefits as well.

Healing History

Chinese physicians have prescribed dandelion since ancient times to treat colds, bronchitis, pneumonia, hepatitis, boils, ulcers, obesity, dental problems, itching, and internal injuries. They also made poultices of chopped dandelion to treat breast cancer.

India's traditional Ayurvedic physicians used the herb for similar therapeutic purposes. Tenth-century Arab physicians were the first to recognize that dandelion increases urine production.

During the Middle Ages, Europeans believed in the Doctrine of Signatures, the idea that plants' physical characteristics reveal their healing virtues. Under this doctrine, anything yellow was linked to the liver's yellow bile and was considered a liver remedy. That's why dandelion gained a reputation as a treatment for jaundice and gallstones.

The Doctrine of Signatures also supported the observation that dandelion is diuretic. The plant has a juicy root, stem, and leaves. Anything juicy was linked to urine production.

By the 17th century, dandelion was so well known as a diuretic that the English referred to it as piss-abed, from the French *pissenlit*. Meanwhile, the French thought the herb's leaves were shaped like lion's teeth and so dubbed it *dent de lion*, which became anglicized as dandelion.

Thanks to such herbal exaggerators as 17th-century English herbalist Nicholas Culpeper, dandelion's medicinal reputation spread as widely as the plant itself across an untended lawn. Culpeper recommended the herb for every "evil disposition of the body."

In fact, dandelion was used for so many ailments that it became known as "the official remedy for disorders." This designation lives on today in dandelion's genus name, *Taraxacum*, from the Greek *taraxos*, meaning "disorder," and *akos*, for "remedy."

Early American colonists introduced dandelion to North America, and Native Americans quickly adopted the herb as a tonic. Dandelion root was an ingredient in Lydia E. Pinkham's Vegetable Compound, a popular 19th-century patent medicine for menstrual discomforts. Because it's a diuretic, dandelion no doubt helped relieve the bloating that many women experience before they menstruate.

Even though dandelion was included in the *U.S. Pharmacopoeia*, a standard drug reference, from 1831 to 1926, many 19th-century herbalists despised it for the weed it had become. According to *King's American Dispensatory* (1898), the text used by the American Eclectic physicians, who were forerunners of today's naturopaths, dandelion was "overrated. . . . Dandelion root possesses little medicinal virtue [except] slightly diuretic action."

Contemporary herbalists recommend dandelion almost exclusively as a diuretic for premenstrual syndrome, menstrual discomforts, swollen feet, high blood pressure, congestive heart failure, and weight loss.

Therapeutic Uses

Most people treat dandelion as a weed. They might want to read Ralph Waldo Emerson. "What is a weed?" the distinguished author wrote. "A plant whose virtues have not yet been discovered." As far as dandelion is concerned, truer words were never penned, although this plant's virtues have been well documented.

GALLSTONES. The Doctrine of Signatures was right on at least one count. Two German studies suggest that dandelion stimulates the flow of bile, which helps digest fats.

In Germany, where herbal medicine is more mainstream than in the United States, physicians routinely recommend dandelion to help improve the flow of bile and prevent gallstones. A German preparation called Chol-Grandelat— a combination of dandelion, milk thistle, and rhubarb—is prescribed for gallbladder disease. (This product is not available in the United States.)

Commission E, the expert panel that evaluates herbal medicines for the German counterpart of the FDA, endorses dandelion root and leaves as bile flow stimulants.

PREMENSTRUAL SYNDROME (PMS). Animal studies suggest that dandelion does indeed have diuretic action. Findings in animals don't always apply to people, but this one seems to.

Commission E recognizes dandelion as an effective diuretic. Because diuretics may help relieve the bloated feeling of PMS, women may want to try some before their periods to see if it works for them.

HIGH BLOOD PRESSURE. As the fluid volume of blood decreases, so does blood pressure. That's why physicians often prescribe diuretics to treat high blood pressure. Dandelion may help.

Of course, high blood pressure is a serious condition that requires professional treatment. Use dandelion only in consultation with your physician.

CONGESTIVE HEART FAILURE. Congestive heart failure is characterized by chronic fatigue of the heart muscle. The condition is often treated with diuretics because they reduce blood volume, so the weakened heart has less fluid to pump around the body. As a natural diuretic, dandelion may be appropriate when taken in conjunction with other medications and therapies prescribed by a physician.

Like high blood pressure, congestive heart failure is a serious condition that cannot be self-treated. If you'd like to try dandelion, discuss it with your physician and use it in addition to standard medication.

CANCER. Dandelion leaves contain noteworthy amounts of beta-carotene and vitamin C. Both nutrients are antioxidants that help prevent the cell damage that sets the stage for cancer, not to mention other degenerative diseases.

OVERWEIGHT. In one study, animals fed dandelion lost a significant amount of weight. As a diuretic, the herb could help eliminate water weight.

Experts do not recommend diuretics for permanent weight control. Most advocate a low-fat diet, moderate portion size, and regular exercise. Lost water weight eventually returns as the body, which is mostly water, adjusts to ongoing treatment with diuretics and decreases its urine output.

Intriguing Possibilities

Dandelion may help reduce the amount of sugar in the blood, which means that it may help manage diabetes. If you have diabetes, use dandelion only in consultation with your physician.

Some studies have also shown that dandelion root has anti-inflammatory properties, suggesting the herb's possible value in treating arthritis.

What's more, a Japanese study hinted at dandelion's anti-tumor activity, although it's much too early to consider the herb a cancer treatment.

Finally, one study found that dandelion inhibits the growth of *Candida albicans*, the fungus responsible for vaginal yeast infections.

Rx Recommendations

Eat fresh leaves in a salad or steam them as a vegetable.

If you're using dandelion as a diuretic (for premenstrual syndrome, high blood pressure, or congestive heart failure) or as a digestive aid, take it as a leaf infusion, root decoction, or tincture. The taste is reasonably pleasant, with a slightly bitter sharpness.

To make a leaf infusion, use $1/2$ ounce of dried leaves per cup of boiling water. Steep for 10 minutes, then strain. Drink up to 3 cups a day.

For a root decoction, gently boil 2 to 3 teaspoons of powdered root per cup of water for 15 minutes, let cool, and strain if you wish. Drink up to 3 cups a day.

As a homemade tincture, take 1 to 2 teaspoons up to three times a day.

When using commercial preparations, follow the package directions.

The Safety Factor

Long-term use of diuretics such as dandelion can be hazardous. Diuretics deplete the body of potassium, an essential nutrient, so people who are using them should be sure to eat foods rich in potassium, such as bananas and fresh vegetables.

Fortunately, dandelion causes less potassium

loss than other diuretics because the herb itself is high in potassium. Nevertheless, if you use dandelion for long periods, be sure to eat potassium-rich foods.

Women who are pregnant or nursing should not take diuretics in any form without a doctor's approval.

Do not give medicinal preparations of dandelion to children under 2. In older children, adjust the recommended dose based on the child's weight. For example, give a 50-pound child one-third of the dose a 150-pound adult would take.

If you're over 65, start with a low dose, and increase only if necessary.

Inform health care professionals of the herbs you use. Problematic herb-drug interactions are possible.

Dandelion may cause skin rash, allergic reactions, or other unexpected side effects. If any develop, reduce your dose or stop taking it.

For more on herb safety, see Chapter 2.

If symptoms get worse or persist longer than 2 weeks, consult a health care professional promptly.

Growing Information

If you cultivate dandelions, be careful whom you tell. You may end up with some unhappy neighbors.

As every gardener knows, dandelions grow like weeds. This low-growing perennial has a deep taproot, a rosette of jaggedly toothed leaves that radiate from its base, and a smooth, hollow, 6- to 12-inch stem capped by a single yellow flower that gives rise to hundreds of tufted single-seed fruits. The root, leaves, and stem contain a milky fluid.

Harvest young leaves as they develop; as they mature, they become unpleasantly bitter. Herbalists generally recommend harvesting the root at the end of the second growing season. To prevent spreading, clip the flowers before seed tufts form.

Dandelion seeds may not be readily available, but check seed catalogs. Better yet, check nearby lawns or vacant lots. It's unlikely that anyone will mind if you take a few. Plant the seeds in early spring. They grow in almost any soil but prefer moist, well-drained loam.

DEVIL'S CLAW

An Angel of a Pain Reliever

Family: Pedaliaceae; other members include sesame

Genus and species: *Harpagophytum procumbens*

Also known as: Grapple plant and harpago

Parts used: Tubers

Are you bothered by stiff, achy, arthritic joints or lower-back pain? Then devil's claw can be an angel of a healer to you.

Devil's claw is a perennial ground cover that grows only in the dry highlands of Angola, Zimbabwe, Namibia, Botswana, and South Africa. Its fierce-looking, hook-shaped fruits are the source of its satanic name as well as its other common name, grapple plant. The herb's Latin generic, *Harpago*, means hook. The plant's taproot produces secondary tubers, the part used medicinally.

Healing History

The indigenous people of southern Africa have used devil's claw for centuries to treat upset stomach, fever, inflammation, and pain. German researchers first became interested in the plant more than 40 years ago. Since then, European researchers have amassed considerable scientific evidence that the herb is a safe, effective treatment for lower-back pain and osteoarthritis, the form of joint pain most people simply call arthritis.

Therapeutic Uses

The active constituent in devil's claw is a compound called harpagoside.

LOWER-BACK PAIN. In a 6-week study at the University of Freiburg in Germany, researchers gave 44 people with back pain either the recommended daily dose of the arthritis drug Vioxx or devil's claw (60 milligrams of harpagoside per day). They found that compared with the drug-takers, those who used devil's claw were more likely to report a 50 percent decrease in pain, and more likely to become pain free.

Several other studies show similar results—with devil's claw generally causing few side effects. Another group of German researchers concluded that the herb "appears to be an effective alternative for the treatment of chronic back pain."

Commission E, the expert panel that evaluates herbal medicines for the German counterpart of the FDA, approves devil's claw for treating pain and inflammation.

OSTEOARTHRITIS. Beyond back pain, several studies show that devil's claw also relieves the aches, pain, and stiffness of osteoarthritis, the most common form of joint pain. French researchers gave 122 people with osteoarthritis of the knee or hip either a pharmaceutical pain reliever—a nonsteroidal anti-inflammatory drug—or devil's claw (6 capsules a day, 435 milligrams per capsule, 2,610 milligrams total, corresponding to approximately 54 milligrams of harpagoside per day). Four months later, both treatments produced the same relief, but the herb group reported significantly fewer side effects.

Intriguing Possibility

A South African animal study suggests that devil's claw reduces blood sugar. It's too early to call the herb a treatment for diabetes, but one day it might be.

Rx Recommendations

The studies showing relief of osteoarthritis and lower-back pain have used doses in the range of 50 to 60 milligrams per day of harpagoside, which corresponds to 2,400 to 2,900 milligrams of devil's claw extract. Follow label directions, or take 2,400 to 2,900 milligrams of extract per day divided into two or three doses.

The Safety Factor

Devil's claw causes no serious side effects, though mild stomach distress is possible.

Unlike the nonsteroidal anti-inflammatory drugs (NSAIDs) often prescribed for osteoarthritis and lower-back pain, devil's claw does not interfere with blood clotting, so it can be used safely by those taking blood-thinning drugs, or those with clotting disorders.

Devil's claw may stimulate secretion of stomach acid. People with stomach or duodenal ulcers should not use it.

Pregnant and nursing women should not use devil's claw.

Do not give this herb to children under 2. In older children, adjust the recommended dose based on the child's weight. For example, give a 50-pound child one-third of the dose a 150-pound adult would take.

If you're over 65, start with a low dose, and increase only if necessary.

Inform health care professionals of the herbs you use. Problematic herb-drug interactions are possible.

Devil's claw may cause allergic reactions or other unexpected side effects. If any develop, reduce your dose or stop taking it.

For more on herb safety, see Chapter 2.

If symptoms get worse or persist longer than 2 weeks, consult a health care professional promptly.

Growing Information

Devil's claw is not grown in the United States.

DILL

Beyond Pickles, a Potent Stomach Soother

Family: Umbelliferae; other members include carrot, parsley, celery, fennel, and angelica

Genus and species: *Anethum graveolens*

Also known as: No other common names

Parts used: Fruits (seeds); leaves are used in cooking

Dill does more for pickles than provide flavor. It's also a natural preservative. In fact, preserving food was the original purpose of pickling.

Dill has been used in herbal healing since the dawn of Egyptian civilization, and for good reason. In addition to its preservative action, the herb is an infection fighter and a soothing digestive aid.

Healing History

Records found in 3,000-year-old Egyptian tombs show that ancient physicians used fragrant dill as a digestive aid and a remedy for intestinal gas. The 1st-century Greek physician Dioscorides prescribed dill so frequently that it was known for centuries as "the herb of Dioscorides." The Romans chewed dill seeds to promote digestion, and they hung dill garlands in their dining halls, believing that the herb would prevent stomach upset.

Traditional Chinese physicians have used dill as a digestive aid for more than 1,000 years. They recommend it especially for children because its action is milder than that of other digestive herbs such as caraway, anise, and fennel.

The Vikings were well aware of dill's digestive benefits. The word *dill* comes from the Old Norse *dilla*, meaning to lull or soothe.

The 17th-century English herbalist Nicholas Culpeper claimed dill "stayeth the belly . . . and is a gallant expeller of wind." Culpeper also recommended the herb for hiccups and swelling and to "strengthen the brain."

Colonists brought dill to North America. Its seed infusion, known as dillwater, became a favorite among American folk healers for childhood ailments such as colic, cough, indigestion, gas, stomachache, and insomnia. In adults, the herb was used to treat hemorrhoids, jaundice, scurvy, and "dropsy" (congestive heart failure).

Contemporary herbalists still tout dill as the herb of choice for infant colic. They recommend chewing the seeds for bad breath and drinking dill tea both as a digestive aid and to stimulate milk production in nursing mothers.

Therapeutic Uses

If you use dill only in pickling spices or on salmon, you're missing out on a marvelous healer. While it won't cure hemorrhoids or increase milk production, some of its other traditional applications are supported by science.

DIGESTIVE PROBLEMS. Research has validated dill's 3,000 years of use as a digestive aid. The herb helps relax the smooth muscles of the digestive tract. One study found dill to be an antifoaming agent, meaning that it helps prevent the formation of intestinal gas bubbles. Dill seed oil also inhibits the growth of several types of bacteria that attack the intestinal tract, suggesting that it may help prevent infectious diarrhea caused by these microorganisms.

Commission E, the expert panel that evaluates herbal medicines for the German counterpart of the FDA, endorses dill for indigestion.

URINARY TRACT INFECTIONS. *Escherichia coli*, the bacteria that usually cause urinary tract infections, is one type of bacteria that is inhibited by dill.

Intriguing Possibilities

When injected into laboratory animals, dill extract stimulates respiration, slows heart rate, and opens blood vessels, all of which reduce blood pressure. Of course, people don't inject dill preparations, but these effects suggest that there's more to learn about dill's healing potential.

Rx Recommendations

To benefit from dill's breath-freshening effects, chew $1/2$ to 1 teaspoon of seeds.

If you're using the herb as a digestive aid, take it as an infusion or tincture. To make a pleasant-tasting infusion, use 2 teaspoons of crushed seeds per cup of boiling water, steep for 10 minutes, and strain. Drink up to 3 cups a day.

As a homemade tincture, take $1/2$ to 1 teaspoon up to three times a day.

When using commercial preparations, follow the package directions.

The Safety Factor

Never ingest dill seed oil. As little as a teaspoon may be toxic.

In people who are sensitive to it, dill may cause skin rash. In addition, dill may cause other allergic reactions or unexpected side effects. If any develop, reduce your dose or stop taking it. The leaves and seeds are generally considered nontoxic.

Inform health care professionals of the herbs you use. Problematic herb-drug interactions are possible.

For more on herb safety, see Chapter 2.

If symptoms get worse or persist longer than 2 weeks, consult a health care professional promptly.

Growing Information

Dill is an annual with a long taproot like its close relative, carrot. It has a delicate, fast-growing, spindly stem with lacy leaves. Yellow flowers appear in summer and produce great quantities of tiny ridged fruits (seeds).

Dill grows vigorously from seeds sown $1/4$ inch deep in early spring. Germination takes about 2 weeks. Thin seedlings to 12-inch spacing. The plants grow to 3 feet in rich, moist, slightly acidic soil under full sun, or in partial shade in the South. Shelter plants from the wind.

You may harvest the leaves once the plants have established themselves. Fresh dill leaves are much more aromatic than dried. To guarantee a supply of fresh leaves from late spring to late fall, plant seeds periodically throughout your growing season.

The seeds mature in about 2 months. Harvest them when they begin to turn brown.

Dill self-sows, so if you leave a few plants unharvested, you'll have this tasty healing herb every year.

ECHINACEA
A Major Immunity Booster

Family: Compositae; other members include daisy, dandelion, and marigold

Genus and species: *Echinacea angustifolia* and *E. purpurea*

Also known as: Purple coneflower

Parts used: Primarily roots; also leaves and flowers

Echinacea (pronounced *eh-kin-AY-sha*) has certainly had its ups and downs on its way to becoming one of the nation's best-selling herbal medicines. Since the 1870s, it has been reviled, then lionized, then forgotten, and finally resurrected.

Today, echinacea is widely accepted as an effective herbal remedy for colds and flu. Many—but not all—studies published in mainstream medical journals agree that it is a safe, effective immune stimulant that helps the body combat all manner of infections, particularly upper respiratory viruses.

Healing History

Echinacea is a tall, daisylike flower native to the American Great Plains. It was the primary medicine of the region's Native Americans. They applied root poultices to wounds, insect bites and stings, and snakebites. They used echinacea mouthwash for painful teeth and gums and drank echinacea tea to treat colds, smallpox, measles, mumps, and arthritis.

Plains settlers adopted the herb, but it remained a folk remedy until 1870, when a cantankerous patent-medicine purveyor, Dr. H. C. F. Meyer of Pawnee City, Nebraska, used it in his Meyer's Blood Purifier. He promoted the remedy as "an absolute cure" for rattlesnake bite, blood poisoning, and a host of other ills. Claims like Dr. Meyer's are what earned patent medicines the derisive name "snake oil."

Dr. Meyer truly believed that echinacea could cure rattlesnake bite, however, and he set out to prove it. In 1885, he sent a sample to John Uri Lloyd, professor at the Eclectic Medical Institute in Cincinnati. Lloyd was also one of the first presidents of the American Pharmaceutical Association and a cofounder (with his brothers) of Lloyd Brothers Pharmacists, a prominent 19th-century drug company. Lloyd identified the plant as echinacea, but after one look at Dr. Meyer's label with its claim of "absolute cure" for rattlesnake bite, he dismissed Dr. Meyer as a crackpot.

Dr. Meyer wrote back, insisting that echinacea was indeed a cure for rattlesnake bite. He was so confident that he offered to take a live rattlesnake to Cincinnati and let it bite him in Lloyd's presence to demonstrate his Blood Purifier's effectiveness. Lloyd declined the offer.

Undaunted, Dr. Meyer shipped some echinacea to Lloyd's Eclectic colleague, John King, who, in the 1850s, had mentioned the Native Americans' uses of the plant in the first edition of his pharmacological text, *King's American Dispensatory*. King tested the herb, and after successfully using it to treat bee stings, chronic nasal congestion, leg ulcers, and a variety of infections, he extolled the plant and included it in subsequent editions of his book.

Eventually, Lloyd also accepted echinacea, declaring it useful for treating wounds, venomous bites and stings, blood poisoning (septicemia), diphtheria, meningitis, measles, chickenpox, malaria, scarlet fever, influenza, syphilis, and gangrene.

Lloyd's enthusiasm was not simply academic. His family business, Lloyd Brothers Pharmacists, developed several echinacea products, which enjoyed tremendous national popularity as infection treatments from the 1890s well into the 1920s. During the early 20th century, it was a rare home medicine cabinet that didn't contain tincture of echinacea. (The Lloyd brothers also owned the New York Giants baseball team and founded the Lloyd Library in Cincinnati, which today houses one of the world's largest collections of botanical literature and publishes the *Journal of Natural Products*, formerly *Lloydia*.)

Unfortunately, echinacea became a casualty of the war between mainstream physicians (known prior to World War I as regulars), who favored the emerging laboratory-synthesized drugs, and the Eclectics, who were more herbally inclined. Each side was hostile to the medicines touted by the other. In 1909, the following statement appeared in the *Journal of the American Medical Association*: "Echinacea . . . has failed to sustain the reputation given it by its enthusiasts . . . [who] make use of early unverified reports to endow their nostrums with remarkable therapeutic properties."

By World War II, as modern antibiotics became available, echinacea's popularity waned. It was listed in the *National Formulary*, the pharmacists' reference, from 1916 until 1950. But from the 1940s on, it was largely forgotten— until the herbal revival of the 1970s.

Contemporary herbalists are as enthusiastic about echinacea as the Eclectics were. They tout it as a botanical antibiotic and immune-system stimulant for boils, colds and flu, bladder infections, tonsillitis, and other infectious diseases. Many recommend taking the herb daily as a tonic and immune-system enhancer.

Therapeutic Uses

Old Dr. Meyer would be tickled to learn how potent his favorite herb actually is. Echinacea has never been shown to cure rattlesnake bite, but from the 1950s through the 1980s, many studies (almost all of them German) concluded that echinacea possesses remarkable immune-stimulating and infection-fighting properties. By the 1990s, American researchers were studying the herb and coming to the same conclusion.

ENHANCED IMMUNITY. Echinacea helps treat infection by revving up the immune system. When disease-causing microorganisms attack, infected cells secrete chemicals that attract infection-fighting white blood cells, called macrophages, to the area. The macrophages

(literally, "big eaters") engulf and digest the invaders. Echinacea boosts their ability to destroy germs.

The herb also energizes other important white blood cells, the natural killer cells and T lymphocytes. And it increases secretion of interleukin-1, another component of the immune system.

Athletes who engage in ultra-strenuous activities, such as triathlons, often experience immune suppression. German researchers gave 42 triathletes one of three daily treatments: medically inactive placebos, mineral supplements, or echinacea. A month later, shortly after a triathlon, those who had taken the echinacea showed the least immune suppression.

INFECTIONS. In addition to its ability to stimulate the immune system, echinacea helps combat a broad range of disease-causing viruses, bacteria, fungi, and protozoa. This attribute lends support to the herb's traditional use for healing wounds and treating many infectious diseases.

Echinacea fights infection in several ways. First, the herb contains echinacoside, a natural antibiotic with broad-spectrum antimicrobial activity.

Second, it strengthens tissues against assault by invading microorganisms. Tissues contain hyaluronic acid (HA), a chemical that in part acts as a shield against germ attacks. Many germs produce the enzyme hyaluronidase to dissolve the HA shield so they can penetrate tissues and cause infection. But echinacea contains another substance, echinacein, that counteracts the germs' tissue-dissolving enzyme and keeps them out of the body's tissues.

Third, echinacea mimics interferon, the body's own virus-fighting compound. Before a virus-infected cell dies, it releases a tiny amount of interferon, which boosts the ability of surrounding cells to resist infection. Echinacea appears to do the same thing. Researchers bathed cells in echinacea extract, then exposed them to two potent viruses (influenza and herpes). Compared with untreated cells, only a small number of the treated cells became infected.

German researchers report success in using echinacea to treat tonsillitis, bronchitis, tuberculosis, meningitis, wounds, abscesses, whooping cough (pertussis), ear infections, and especially colds and flu.

COLDS AND FLU. By the late 1990s, more than a dozen studies had investigated echinacea as a cold treatment. While most showed significant benefit in the form of shorter, milder colds, there were enough that showed no benefit to keep critics carping that echinacea offered more hype than substance.

Then, in a 1999 report published in the *Journal of Family Practice*, two mainstream M.D.s from the University of Wisconsin at Madison and a naturopathic physician from Bastyr University, the naturopathic medical school near Seattle, teamed up to analyze every published study of echinacea for prevention and treatment of upper-respiratory infections.

On the treatment side, the researchers looked at eight studies involving a total of more than 1,000 people. All the studies were double-blind, meaning that neither the participants nor the researchers knew who was taking echinacea and who was taking a placebo. Those who received the herb were given various preparations: tablets, capsules, juices, and tinctures. All of the preparations contained the immune-boosting parts of the plant: the roots, leaves, and flowers.

Among the eight studies, this one was typical. In a large Swedish furniture factory, researchers identified 60 workers who were experiencing the initial stages of colds. Half of the workers were given placebos, and the rest were given tincture of echinacea (20 drops in water every 2 hours for the first day, then the same amount three times a day for up to 10 days). Among those taking placebos, the average recovery time was 8 days. Among those taking echinacea, however, recovery time was reduced by half, to just 4 days.

All eight studies showed similar results. Six were statistically significant. Two were not, but they showed a clear trend in the direction of benefit. The reviewers' verdict: Echinacea is a solid winner as a treatment for colds and flu. In all eight studies, compared with placebos, the herb produced an average 50 percent reduction in the severity of symptoms and a similar reduction in the number of days that people actually felt ill.

Commission E, the expert panel that evaluates herbal medicines for the German counterpart of the FDA, also endorses echinacea as a treatment for colds and flu.

On the prevention side, the researchers analyzed four studies with a total of 1,152 participants. Again, the studies were double-blind and used various preparations of all parts of the herb. None of these studies showed echinacea to have statistically significant preventive value. The reviewers concluded that the herb isn't useful in preventing colds and flu. (It should be noted that traditional herbalists have recommended echinacea only as a treatment for infectious illnesses, not as a preventive.)

The researchers concluded that treatment with echinacea should begin as soon as you feel the first twinges of a cold or flu coming on. Take it several times a day, then taper off as you begin to feel better.

Unfortunately, echinacea remains controversial. In 2005, a study by Austrian researchers published in the prestigious *New England Journal of Medicine* showed the herb useless against colds. The researchers squirted live cold virus up the noses of 399 college students and then treated them with echinacea or a placebo. The herb neither prevented colds nor reduced the severity of those that developed. This study was widely publicized. The article in the *New York Times* was headlined: "Study Says Echinacea Has No Effect on Colds." But the study had a fatal flaw. The researchers used a dose that many herbal medicine experts considered too low to have any effect.

In 2007, researchers at the University of Connecticut School of Pharmacy analyzed 14 studies of echinacea for prevention and treatment of colds. They found that the herb significantly reduces cold severity and reduces cold duration by 1.4 days. In addition, they found that contrary to traditional recommendations, echinacea also *prevents* colds, reducing risk by 58 percent.

No doubt, echinacea will continue to be a controversial cold remedy. But the weight of the evidence shows that it's an effective treatment.

WOUNDS. Science has confirmed echinacea's traditional use for wound healing. Echinacein—the same compound that prevents germs from penetrating tissues—also helps broken skin knit faster by spurring the cells that form new tissue (fibroblasts) to work more efficiently.

Echinacea preparations can be applied to cuts, burns, psoriasis, eczema, genital herpes sores, and cold sores. Commission E supports the use of echinacea for wound treatment.

YEAST INFECTIONS. In a German study, 203 women with recurrent vaginal yeast infections were treated with either a standard pharmaceutical anti-yeast cream or the cream plus oral echinacea. Within 6 months, 60 percent of the women who used just the antifungal cream experienced recurrences. Among those who also took echinacea, that figure was only 16 percent, a highly significant difference.

GASTROINTESTINAL INFECTIONS. University of Arkansas researchers analyzed 12 volunteers' stool samples for evidence of bacteria that cause food poisoning and other gastrointestinal infections. Then the participants took echinacea (1,000 milligrams per day for 10 days). Subsequent stool analysis showed significantly fewer bacteria, enough of a decrease to reduce risk of GI infections.

CANCER CHEMOTHERAPY AND RADIATION THERAPY. Cancer patients undergoing chemotherapy typically experience reductions in their white blood cell counts, which increases their risk of infection. German researchers gave 15 people with advanced esophageal and colorectal cancers chemotherapy treatment plus echinacea and an extract of the thymus gland, a component of the immune system. Instead of falling, as would be expected, their white blood cell counts increased.

Radiation treatments can also depress white blood cell counts, suggesting that echinacea may help. If you're receiving cancer chemotherapy or radiation therapy, ask your medical and radiation oncologists about incorporating echinacea into your treatment plan.

Intriguing Possibility

In animals, echinacea has demonstrated promising anticancer activity against leukemia and a few tumors. It would be premature to describe the herb as a cancer treatment, but that day may come.

Rx Recommendations

You can use either a decoction or a tincture to take advantage of echinacea's infection-fighting potential.

To make a decoction, use 2 teaspoons of root material per cup of water. Bring it to a boil, then simmer for 15 minutes; strain before drinking. Drink up to 3 cups a day. You'll find the taste initially sweet, then bitter.

As a homemade tincture, take 1 teaspoon up to three times a day.

When using commercial preparations, follow the package directions.

The Safety Factor

Echinacea tincture often causes numbing of the tongue or a tingling sensation. This is harmless and goes away in about 30 minutes.

AUTOIMMUNE DISEASES. Through the mid-1990s, herbal medicine authorities agreed that echinacea should not be used by people who are HIV-positive or those who have autoimmune conditions such as lupus, multiple sclerosis, and rheumatoid arthritis. The thinking was that stimulating the immune system might aggravate these conditions. But echinacea has become so popular that many people with HIV or autoimmune diseases have used it, and according to a 1999 report in the *European Journal of Herbal Medicine*, there have been no published reports that the herb causes exacerbations of AIDS or autoimmune conditions. If you are HIV-positive or have an autoimmune disease, ask your physi-

cian about the advisability of using echinacea to treat your colds.

PREGNANT AND NURSING WOMEN. Medical authorities advise pregnant and nursing women not to take any drugs or pharmacologically active herbs without consulting their physicians. This is sound advice. Drugs and medicinal herbs might harm the fetus, particularly during the first trimester. However, two studies of echinacea use by pregnant women have shown no increased risk of fetal damage or birth defects. One was a 2000 report in *Archives of Internal Medicine* that tracked 112 pregnant echinacea users. The other was a 2006 survey of case reports in the *Canadian Journal of Clinical Pharmacology*. Pregnant and nursing women should still consult their physicians before using echinacea, but these reports should provide some reassurance for pregnant women who use this herb.

LONG-TERM USE. Traditional herbalists recommended echinacea only for short-term treatment of wounds or acute illnesses (colds, flu, etc.), not for regular use over long periods. However, some people lump this herb together with vitamins and take it every day. No trials of daily, long-term echinacea use have been published. But herbal medicine authorities discourage regular long-term use and recommend echinacea only for short-term treatment of wounds or acute illnesses.

Do not give echinacea to children under 2. In older children, adjust the recommended dose based on the child's weight. For example, give a 50-pound child one-third of the dose a 150-pound adult would take.

If you're over 65, start with a low dose, and increase only if necessary.

Inform health care professionals of the herbs

you use. Problematic herb-drug interactions are possible.

Echinacea may cause allergic reactions or other unexpected side effects. If any develop, reduce your dose or stop taking it.

For more on herb safety, see Chapter 2.

If symptoms get worse or persist longer than 2 weeks, consult a health care professional promptly.

Growing Information

Echinacea is a 2- to 5-foot perennial whose flowers resemble black-eyed Susans, with purple rays radiating from a cone-shaped center (hence its common name, purple coneflower). The herb has black roots, a single stem covered with bristly hairs, and narrow leaves.

Echinacea grows from seeds or root cuttings taken in spring or fall. Don't cover the seeds. When the temperature is in the seventies, simply tamp them into moist, sandy soil.

Echinacea grows in poor, rocky, slightly acidic soil under full sun. It also thrives in richer soils.

It takes 3 to 4 years for the roots to grow large enough to harvest. Pull them in autumn after the plant has gone to seed. Roots larger than $1/2$ inch in diameter should be split before drying.

ELDERBERRY

Herbal Flu-Fighter—And More

Family: Caprifoliaceae; other members include honeysuckle

Genus and species: *Sambucus nigra* (European) and *S. canadensis* (American)

Also known as: Sweet elder, common elder, sambucus

Parts used: Berries, flower extract

An old Austrian saying goes: "Tip your hat to the elder." It refers not to older adults but to the elder tree, in honor of its many traditional medical uses.

Elder is two related plants, an American shrub that grows to 12 feet and a European tree that reaches 30 feet. Both plants produce dark purple berries.

Elderberry was used medicinally in the

ancient world, but fell into obscurity. In the early 1990s, it was resurrected when researchers discovered its remarkable flu-fighting action. Now the elderberry product Sambucol is widely marketed as an herbal flu treatment.

Healing History

As early as 400 B.C., Hippocrates called the elder his "medicine chest." Other noted ancient physician/herbalists—among them, the Greek physician/botanists Theophrastus and Dioscorides, and the Roman Galen—also considered elder to be a great healer. They recommended the flowers and leaves—but not the berries—to treat many maladies, including arthritis, asthma, colds, constipation, and even cancer.

From the Middle Ages into the 19th century, European and American herbalists used the berry as a laxative and diuretic, to treat diabetes, and to increase resistance to illness and treat infections, such as flu.

Beyond herbal medicine, elderberry has also been used for centuries to make preserves and wine.

Therapeutic Uses

FLU. In the early 1990s, fascinated by folk use of elderberry against flu, Israeli researchers discovered that the purple berry substantially reduces replication of flu viruses. The researchers processed the berries into a syrup. In 1993, they used it to treat a flu outbreak on an Israeli kibbutz. Those people who did not receive elderberry took 6 days to recover. But 90 percent of the group that received the herb recovered in just 3 days. The elderberry syrup used in this study is now marketed at health food stores and some pharmacies as Sambucol.

During the 1999–2000 flu season, the researchers who developed Sambucol journeyed to Norway and gave 60 Norwegian flu sufferers either a placebo or the herb syrup (2 teaspoons four times a day for 5 days). The Sambucol group recovered an average of 4 days faster.

Subsequent studies have shown that elderberry does not attack the flu virus. Instead, it boosts the immune system so the body can fight the flu virus more effectively. Elderberry increases production of an important class of immune compounds called cytokines.

PREVENTION OF DEGENERATIVE DISEASES. Dark-colored fruits, among them elderberry, have been shown to contain potent antioxidants called anthocyanins. Antioxidants help prevent and reverse the cell damage at the root of heart disease, cancer, and many other conditions associated with aging.

HEART ATTACK AND STROKE. At Tufts University, USDA researchers tested elderberry on the cells that line human arteries. Damage to these cells initiates a cascade of reactions that eventually leads to the arterial blockages that trigger heart attack and most strokes. The herb protected the arterial cells from damage. The researchers concluded that elderberry reduces risk of cardiovascular disease.

GUM DISEASE. Elderberry also boosts the immune system's ability to combat the bacteria responsible for gum disease. In a study reported in the *Journal of Periodontology*, researchers at Louisiana State University Health Sciences Center incubated infection-fighting white blood cells and gum-disease bacteria with or without elderberry extract. The white blood cells exposed to the herb "potently inhibited" the bacteria. Elderberry toothpaste and mouthwash can't be too far away.

Intriguing Possibilities

To date, no studies have shown that elderberry reduces cancer risk. But given the berries' antioxidant content, that's a good bet.

While elderberry is better known for deactivating flu virus, it also inhibits the herpes virus and HIV, the virus that causes AIDS. It's too early to call the herb a treatment for these conditions, but in the future, it's a possibility.

Rx Recommendations

The most popular elderberry product is Sambucol (produced in Israel, distributed in North America by Nature's Way). For general health and cardiovascular disease prevention, the recommended adult dose is 2 teaspoons a day, or 1 teaspoon for children. For flu symptoms—fever, aches, malaise—adults should take 2 teaspoons four times a day; children should be given 1 teaspoon four times a day.

The Safety Factor

No significant side effects have been reported among people using Sambucol.

If an elderberry bush or tree grows near you, the ripe berries are safe to eat. However, eating unripe, uncooked berries may produce nausea. Elderberry leaves and stems contain cyanide. Ingestion has caused poisonings.

Growing Information

The European tree has been naturalized to the United States, so both varieties are found here. Elder thrives in shady, moist, temperate locations. It tolerates marginal soils. Fragrant white flowers appear in early summer, and by autumn, they give rise to purple-black berries. The berries must be cooked before eating. Ingestion of uncooked berries may cause diarrhea and vomiting.

ELECAMPANE
Good-Bye, Intestinal Parasites

Family: Compositae; other members include daisy, dandelion, and marigold

Genus and species: *Inula helenium*

Also known as: Wild sunflower, velvet dock, scabwort, and horseheal

Parts used: Roots

Legend has it that Helen of Troy carried a handful of elecampane on the fateful day that the Trojan prince Paris abducted her from Sparta, igniting the Trojan War. Perhaps the woman whose face launched 1,000 ships had amoebic dysentery, pinworms, hookworms, or giardiasis.

We'll probably never know. We do know that elecampane, whose Latin name (*Inula helenium*) memorializes the Greek beauty, may help expel parasites from the intestine.

Healing History

According to Hippocrates, elecampane stimulates the brain, kidneys, stomach, and uterus. The ancient Romans used the herb to treat indigestion. The Roman naturalist Pliny wrote, "Let no day pass without eating some roots of elecampane to help digestion, expel melancholy, and cause mirth." And the Roman physician Galen recommended the herb as "good for passion of the hucklebone [sciatica]."

Traditional Chinese and Indian Ayurvedic physicians recommended elecampane as a treatment for respiratory problems, particularly bronchitis and asthma.

During the Middle Ages, European herbalists prescribed elecampane to treat coughs, bronchitis, and asthma, but the herb was more popular as a veterinary medicine. It was reputed to cure scab disease in sheep, hence one of its popular names, scabwort. It was also considered a panacea for horses, and for that reason, it was known as horseheal.

As time passed, elecampane regained its reputation as a human digestive aid. It was the main ingredient in a medieval elixir known as *potio Paulina*.

The 17th-century London herbalist Nicholas Culpeper touted elecampane "to relieve cough, shortness of breath, and wheezing in the lungs." Echoing Galen, he also endorsed the herb for sciatica and claimed that it restored vision and cured gout, sores, and "worms in the stomach."

In those days, elecampane root was candied and eaten as a confection. Lozenges combining elecampane and honey were a popular treatment for whooping cough (pertussis).

Early American colonists naturalized elecampane and used it as an expectorant, digestive aid, menstruation promoter, and diuretic for treating the water retention associated with dropsy (congestive heart failure). Native American tribes in the Northeast adopted the plant for respiratory problems.

America's 19th-century Eclectic physicians, forerunners of today's naturopaths, also used elecampane as a diuretic and menstruation promoter. Primarily, however, they prescribed the herb for "asthma, bronchial and chronic pulmonary [lung] affections, weakness of the digestive organs, itching, dyspepsia [indigestion], night sweats, and severe colds."

Present-day herbalists generally recommend elecampane only for respiratory ailments: cough, asthma, bronchitis, and emphysema. Some recommend it as a digestive aid, as a treatment for menstrual and skin problems, and to banish intestinal parasites.

Therapeutic Uses

Elecampane has not been well researched, but the few scientific studies that have been done suggest that for once, Nicholas Culpeper wasn't completely off the deep end.

INTESTINAL PARASITES. European scientists have discovered that elecampane contains a chemical called alantolactone that really does help expel intestinal parasites, as Culpeper claimed. The herb also kills some bacteria and fungi, adding to its potential therapeutic action in the intestine.

Infestation with intestinal parasites, especially pinworms and the protozoan *Giardia lamblia* (which causes giardiasis), is a growing problem in the United States. Families with children in day care are particularly susceptible. Intestinal parasites are quite common in the tropics. If you travel overseas, do what Helen of Troy did: Take some elecampane with you.

Intriguing Possibilities

In animal tests conducted in Europe, elecampane was found to lower blood pressure. People with high blood pressure might try it, in consultation with their physicians.

Elecampane has also been shown to have a sedative effect in experimental animals. People with insomnia might try taking some before bed.

Rx Recommendations

Elecampane's main use is to help prevent and treat intestinal parasites. To try it for this purpose or—in consultation with your physician—to keep your blood pressure down, take it as either a decoction or a tincture.

To prepare a decoction, gently boil 1 to 2 teaspoons of dried, powdered root in 3 cups of water for 30 minutes, then strain if you wish. The taste is bitter. Take 1 to 2 tablespoons at a time with honey, up to 2 cups a day.

As a homemade tincture, use 1/4 to 1/2 teaspoon up to three times a day.

When using commercial preparations, follow the package directions.

The Safety Factor

People who are sensitive to elecampane may develop a rash from skin contact with the herb or its oil. Otherwise, no harmful effects have been reported.

Pregnant and nursing women should not use elecampane.

Do not give elecampane to children under 2.

In older children, adjust the recommended dose based on the child's weight. For example, give a 50-pound child one-third of the dose a 150-pound adult would take.

If you're over 65, start with a low dose, and increase only if necessary.

Inform health care professionals of the herbs you use. Problematic herb-drug interactions are possible.

Elecampane may cause allergic reactions or other unexpected side effects. If any develop, reduce your dose or stop taking it.

For more on herb safety, see Chapter 2.

If symptoms get worse or persist longer than 2 weeks, consult a health care professional promptly.

Growing Information

Elecampane is a striking perennial that reaches 5 feet and produces a large flower (hence its common name, wild sunflower). The entire plant is covered with woolly hairs. The medicinal roots are large, branching, and fleshy.

Elecampane may be started from seeds sown indoors in late winter, then transplanted. Once plants have been established, however, the herb is best propagated from 2-inch root cuttings taken in fall from the buds (eyes) of 2-year-old roots. Cover the cuttings with moist, sandy soil and store them for the winter in a cool indoor room. Plant the cuttings 3 feet apart after the danger of frost has passed. Deeply cultivated soil produces the biggest roots.

Elecampane likes rich, moist, well-drained, slightly acid loam and full sun or partial shade. Harvest the roots during the fall of their second year. Older roots become too woody. To speed drying, slice roots into pieces.

ELEUTHERO
Ginseng's Siberian Cousin Offers Similar Benefits

Family: Araliaceae; other members include ginseng and English ivy

Genus and species: *Eleutherococcus senticosus*

Also known as: Siberian ginseng and eleuthero

Parts used: Primarily root, sometimes leaves and berries

Eleuthero, sometimes called eleutherococcus, looks nothing like ginseng. It's a deciduous shrub that grows to 6 feet. Ginseng is an ivylike ground cover. Eleuthero stems have thorns; ginseng does not. And eleuthero has a woody root, while ginseng's is fleshy. But both of these plants belong to the same botanical family, and they are both "adaptogens," medicinal herbs that offer a remarkable number of healing benefits. Their benefits are so similar that eleuthero is often called Siberian ginseng. The name is misleading. These plants are different, though they have similar benefits.

Healing History

Eleuthero is native to China, Japan, and Russia. But Asians, particularly Chinese and Koreans who have revered ginseng for thousands of years, largely ignored its shrubby relative.

That began to change in 1947, when Russian scientist N.V. Lazarev, Ph.D., of the Academy of Sciences of the former Soviet Union, became interested in drugs that helped the body adapt to physical and emotional stress, and coined the term *adaptogen* to describe them. Ginseng was the prime adaptogen, but Dr. Lazarev's student, Israel I. Brekhman, Ph.D., wondered if there might be a less expensive substitute and began looking into folk claims for eleuthero. He discovered that eleuthero had similar action. His research popularized this herb.

Adaptogens increase energy, counteract stress, increase resistance to many diseases, and have a normalizing effect on the body, improving many parameters of health while causing few, if any, side effects.

"Adaptogens give the body a tune-up," says Salt Lake City herb researcher Daniel Mowrey, Ph.D. "They help the cells produce energy and use it more efficiently. But adaptogens don't overpower the cells as drugs often do. Their effects are subtle, which accounts for the controversy these herbs arouse. Over time, adaptogenic herbs are very beneficial to health."

Therapeutic Uses

ENERGY AND STAMINA. Polish researchers evaluated the health and physical fitness of 50 men and women, and then gave them either the well-known immune booster echinacea or eleuthero (25 drops of tincture three times a day). After 1 month, the echinacea group showed no changes in fitness. But the eleuthero group showed enhanced muscle use of oxygen, which improves fitness and stamina.

While some eleuthero studies show no increase in stamina or reduced fatigue, a study at the University of Iowa showed promise for the herb. Researchers gave 96 people suffering chronic fatigue either a placebo or eleuthero. After 2 months, the severity of fatigue in the eleuthero group was significantly diminished.

Commission E, the expert panel that evaluates herbal medicines for the German counterpart of the FDA, approves eleuthero for invigoration during convalescence, and for fatigue and debility.

IMMUNE FUNCTION. German researchers measured the immune function of 36 people and then gave them eleuthero (10 milliliters of tincture three times a day). After 4 weeks, the herb increased the number of T-cells, a key component of the immune system. Eleuthero also increases production of interleukin-1 and -6, important immune proteins. A Russian report concludes that eleuthero "stimulates immunological vigor."

THE COMMON COLD. In a cell-culture study published in *Antiviral Research*, German scientists have documented eleuthero's "strong antiviral" action. In addition, Russian researchers gave 40 children with colds either conventional treatment or an herbal preparation that included eleuthero (as well as andrographis, see page 63). The herb group recovered faster.

DIABETES. Eleuthero lowers blood sugar, which may help prevent and treat diabetes.

PREVENTION OF DEGENERATIVE DISEASES. Russian researchers have identified six antioxidants in eleuthero. Antioxidants help prevent and repair the cell damage at the root of heart disease and cancer.

HEART DISEASE. A Polish study shows that eleuthero reduces LDL ("bad") cholesterol and triglycerides (blood fats), both risk factors for heart disease. It also helps prevent the internal blood clots that trigger heart attacks (and most strokes). Eleuthero's effects on blood sugar also help prevent heart disease because diabetes is a strong risk factor for heart attack. Finally, a Russian animal study shows that the herb helps normalize heart rhythm.

MEMORY AND VISUAL ACUITY. Eleuthero even improves short-term memory and visual acuity, according to Russian research. It increases the sensitivity of the retina, which improves color perception and the ability to see clearly in low light.

BONE STRENGTH. According to a Russian study at Vladivostok State Medical University, eleuthero treats osteoporosis as well as soy protein does.

RADIATION EXPOSURE. Bulgarian scientists have shown that eleuthero speeds recovery from radiation exposure.

QUALITY OF LIFE. Add up all of these effects, and like ginseng, eleuthero improves quality of life. In a study by Italian researchers at the University of Bologna published in *Archives of Gerontology and Geriatrics*, 20 elderly people completed a health status survey, and then took either a placebo or eleuthero. Four weeks later, the herb group scored higher on mental health and social functioning.

Intriguing Possibilities

A Korean animal study found that eleuthero improves liver function.

Eleuthero's effects on cancer have not been well studied. But one Russian study shows the herb contains four compounds with anticancer action. Another Russian report finds that in animals with drug-induced tumors, the herb extends survival. A third Russian study shows that eleuthero boosts the immune systems of people with cancer. These results suggest that eleuthero may help treat human cancers.

Rx Recommendations

Follow package directions. If using dry powdered root, the recommended dose is 2 to 3 grams (approximately 2 teaspoons) per day. To make a tea, steep 2 to 3 grams per cup of boiling water for 10 minutes, then strain. Drink up to 2 cups per day.

The Safety Factor

Studies to date suggest that eleuthero causes few side effects. But drowsiness, anxiety, irritability, headache, insomnia, and depressed mood are possible. Large doses have caused irritability, insomnia, and anxiety. Commission E says it should not be used by people running a fever or with high blood pressure.

Pregnant and nursing women should not use eleuthero.

Do not give eleuthero to children under 2. In older children, adjust the recommended dose based on the child's weight. For example, give a 50-pound child one-third of the dose a 150-pound adult would take.

If you're over 65, start with a low dose, and increase only if necessary.

Inform health care professionals of the herbs you use. Problematic herb-drug interactions are possible.

Eleuthero may cause allergic reactions or other unexpected side effects. If any develop, reduce your dose or stop taking it.

For more on herb safety, see Chapter 2.

If symptoms get worse or persist longer than 2 weeks, consult a health care professional promptly.

Growing Information

Eleuthero can be grown in the United States, though most medicinal root material is imported. This herb grows in coniferous and mixed mountain forests, forming shrubby undergrowth or thickets at forest edges. It prefers rich, well-drained soil, but grows in a variety of soils: sandy, loamy, and heavy clay with acid, neutral, or alkaline pH, including poor soils. It can tolerate sun or dappled shade, but grows best when protected from wind. It tolerates cold to 5°F. Seeds can be slow to germinate. Seedlings should be kept in a greenhouse or cold frame for at least the first winter. Plant out in late spring or summer.

EPHEDRA

An Ancient—And Controversial—Healer

Family: Ephedraceae; other members include broom and horsetail

Genus and species: *Ephedra sinica, E. vulgaris, E. nevadensis, E. antisyphilitica,* and other species

Also known as: Ma huang, Mormon tea, and whorehouse tea

Parts used: Stems and branches

Ephedra—or, in Chinese, ma huang—is a powerful bronchial decongestant and stimulant. Many herbalists view ephedra as the world's oldest medicine. It is certainly one of the oldest.

Sadly, few people who take over-the-counter cold remedies containing the herb's laboratory equivalent (pseudoephedrine) have any idea that they are part of an herbal healing tradition that's estimated to date back some 5,000 years. Even more sadly, a small but widely publicized group who've used irresponsibly large amounts of ephedra have experienced serious consequences, including death.

Healing History

The origins of Chinese medicine are lost in legend. Authorities generally agree, however, that Chinese physicians began prescribing a tea made from Chinese ephedra for colds, asthma, and hay fever around 3000 B.C. The Indian and Pakistani species of the herb have been used medicinally for almost as long.

When the Mormons reached Utah in 1847, local Native Americans introduced them to American ephedra, a piney-tasting tonic beverage. The Mormons adopted it as a substitute for coffee and tea, and around the West it became known as Mormon tea, a name that survives today.

American ephedra is a mild diuretic. In the Old West, it developed a reputation as a cure for syphilis and gonorrhea. It was served in many Western brothels, hence another of its common names, whorehouse tea, and the Latin name for one species, *E. antisyphilitica*.

Contemporary herbalists recommend ephedra just as the ancient Chinese did—to treat asthma, hay fever, and the nasal and chest congestion of colds and flu.

Therapeutic Uses

American ephedra is simply a refreshing beverage. It contains none of the pharmacologically active compounds (ephedrine, pseudoephedrine, and norpseudoephedrine) found in Chinese ephedra, which is the plant used in herbal medicine.

When people say "ephedra," they're usually referring to the Chinese variety, ma huang (*E. sinica*). However, some herb marketers mistakenly refer to American ephedra as ma huang and the Chinese herb as Mormon tea.

Worldwide, there are about 40 species of ephedra. If you're interested in using the herb medicinally, look for a product that's identified by species on the label and be sure that it says *Ephedra sinica* or *E. sinica*.

The active compounds in Chinese ephedra are strong central nervous system stimulants, more powerful than caffeine but less potent than amphetamine. All three open the bronchial passages (meaning that they're bronchodilators). They also stimulate the heart and uterine contractions; increase blood pressure, metabolic rate, and perspiration and urine production; and reduce the secretion of both saliva and stomach acid.

RESPIRATORY PROBLEMS. From the late 1920s through the 1940s, Chinese ephedra's active constituent, ephedrine, was added to cold, asthma, and hay fever products as a decongestant and bronchodilator. Ephedrine was generally effective and reasonably safe, but it was known to cause potentially hazardous side effects, including increased blood pressure and rapid heartbeat (palpitations). It was eventually replaced with a close chemical substitute, pseudoephedrine, which is also an active compound in ma huang.

Scientists consider pseudoephedrine as effective as ephedrine but with less likelihood of problematic side effects. Pseudoephedrine is the active ingredient in many over-the-counter cold and allergy products, most notably Sudafed, whose name is derived from its active ingredient.

Ephedra continues to be used in herbal cold,

flu, allergy, and decongestant products. Chinese physicians prescribe it to treat asthma. Commission E, the expert panel that evaluates herbal medicines for the German counterpart of the FDA, endorses ma huang for the treatment of bronchial congestion.

OBESITY. Ma huang increases metabolic rate, the speed at which the body burns calories. It also depresses appetite somewhat. This combination of effects led to studies of the herb (actually chemically isolated ephedrine) for weight control, usually in combination with another stimulant, caffeine.

In physician-supervised weight-loss programs that include a low-fat diet and regular exercise, treatment with a combination of ephedrine and caffeine has increased weight loss by about an additional 5 percent. In other words, a person who loses 100 pounds without ma huang might lose 105 pounds with the addition of the herb.

One 3-month study conducted by Danish researchers showed that compared with overweight women taking medically inactive placebos, those taking oral ephedrine (20 milligrams three times a day) lost somewhat more weight. And in a 2-month study, Italian researchers found that overweight women lost more weight if they supplemented their low-calorie diets with oral ephedrine (50 milligrams three times a day).

To experience ephedra's weight-reduction benefits, you must be clinically obese, that is, at least 20 percent heavier than your recommended weight. Ephedrine has shown no effect in moderately overweight people who simply want to lose 5 to 10 pounds.

Keep in mind that pounds lost with the help of ephedra may not be gone permanently, especially once you stop using the herb. What's more, routine use of ephedra for weight control typically causes side effects that may be unpleasant (more on this later).

Experts generally agree that the keys to permanent weight loss are a low-fat, low-calorie diet and daily exercise. Nonetheless, ephedra is an ingredient in many herbal weight-loss formulas sold in health food stores and drugstores.

WOMEN'S HEALTH CONCERNS. Ephedrine causes uterine contractions in laboratory animals. Women may want to try ephedra to initiate menstruation.

Medicinal Myths

Although American ephedra was popular in the Old West as a remedy for syphilis and gonorrhea, in reality, the herb has no effect on either disease. Anyone who develops a genital sore or discharge should consult a physician.

In addition, ephedra does not appear to benefit athletic performance. Some stimulants, such as coffee, increase stamina. Some athletes believe that ephedra offers performance-enhancing benefits, but there is little evidence of this.

Rx Recommendations

To take advantage of ephedra's potent healing benefits as a decongestant or a menstruation promoter, you'll want to use a decoction or tincture. You'll find the taste pleasantly piney.

For a decoction, use 1 teaspoon of dried herb per cup of water. Bring it to a boil, simmer for 10 to 15 minutes, and then strain. Drink up to 2 cups a day.

As a homemade tincture, take $1/4$ to 1 teaspoon up to three times a day.

When using commercial preparations, follow the package directions.

The Safety Factor

During the 1990s, very large doses of Chinese ephedra were included in products that promised a legal high similar to that of methamphetamine ("speed"). Brand names of these products included Herbal Ecstasy, Cloud 9, and Ultimate X-phoria.

Irresponsibly large doses of ephedra can indeed produce effects similar to those of methamphetamine. In such enormous doses, however, the herb may also cause serious—even fatal—heart problems and stroke in healthy people.

In one study, researchers at the New England Medical Center in Boston used data supplied by the FDA to document 14 cardiac arrests, 13 strokes, 9 heart attacks, and more than 900 other adverse reactions associated with high-dose ephedra. The people who suffered harm were typically either dieters using the herb to lose weight or young people seeking intoxication.

Subsequently, however, an audit of the FDA's ephedra database by the Government Accountability Office (GAO), the investigative arm of Congress, accused the FDA of using "questionable" science and unsubstantiated information to compile its statistics. The GAO concluded that the FDA's database of adverse reactions was "open to question."

Despite the GAO's criticism, in 2003 the FDA announced tough new labeling rules that critics charged amounted to banning the herb. In 2005, a federal judge struck down the FDA's rules. Since then, the U.S. government has taken no action to reduce the use of this herb.

Assuming that you steer clear of irresponsibly large doses of ephedra, it's important to understand that even recommended doses can have a powerful stimulant effect. They may also cause nervousness, jitters, irritability, anxiety, insomnia, dizziness, heart palpitations, and skin flushing.

Some compounds in ma huang have been shown to raise blood pressure and blood sugar levels. Other compounds have been shown to lower them. People with diabetes or high blood pressure should err on the side of caution and not use the herb. Nor is ephedra appropriate for people with heart disease, glaucoma, or kidney conditions, because of the risk of elevated blood pressure.

People with overactive thyroid (hyperthyroidism or Graves' disease) should avoid all stimulants, including ephedra.

Likewise, ephedra constricts the urethra and can lead to difficulty urinating. For this reason, men with benign prostate enlargement, which also causes urinary problems, should not use the herb.

Ephedra often causes insomnia. People who have difficulty sleeping should avoid taking the herb late in the day, or at all.

Ephedra may cause dry mouth. If you use the herb, be sure to increase your intake of nonalcoholic liquids.

If you're an Olympic athlete, don't use ephedra. It's on the United States Olympic Committee's list of banned substances.

Even if you're not an Olympian, you might think twice before using ephedra because it appears to increase risk of potentially fatal heatstroke. Heatstroke deaths of U.S. athletes decreased steadily from the mid-1960s through the mid-1990s, then began increasing. Some evidence links the uptick in heatstroke deaths to use of ephedra products.

Pregnant and nursing women should not use ephedra.

Do not give ephedra to children.

If you're over 65, start with a low dose, and increase only if necessary.

Inform health care professionals of the herbs you use. Problematic herb-drug interactions are possible.

Ephedra may cause allergic reactions or other unexpected side effects. If any develop, reduce your dose or stop taking it.

For more on herb safety, see Chapter 2.

If symptoms get worse or persist longer than 2 weeks, consult a health care professional promptly.

Growing Information

Ephedra is not a garden herb. It is an odd-looking, botanically primitive, almost leafless shrub that resembles horsetail. It has tough, jointed, barkless stems and branches, with small scalelike leaves and tiny yellow-green flowers that appear in summer. Male and female flowers appear on different plants. The seeds develop in cones.

EUCALYPTUS

The Australian Cold
and Flu Remedy

Family: Myrtaceae; other members include myrtle, tea tree, and clove

Genus and species: *Eucalyptus globulus*

Also known as: Gum tree, blue gum, and Australian fever tree

Parts used: Leaves

Eucalyptus is Australia's contribution to herbal healing. The herb has even won FDA approval as a treatment for colds and flu.

If you've ever used Listerine mouthwash or a decongestant such as Vicks VapoRub, you're familiar with the unique, refreshing scent of eucalyptus. And if you've ever seen a koala in a zoo, you've probably seen eucalyptus, because the plant's long, scythe-shaped leaves are the sole food source for the cute, furry marsupial.

Healing History

Eucalyptus roots hold an astonishing amount of water. Australia's aborigines chewed them for water in the dry outback. They also drank eucalyptus leaf tea for fevers.

In the 1780s, England declared Australia a penal colony and started shipping convicts to what is now Sydney. It took a while for the new immigrants to catch on to eucalyptus roots as a water source, however. Many early outback explorers died of thirst within sight of eucalyptus groves.

Around 1840, crew members on a French freighter anchored off Sydney developed a disease involving high fever. They were cured with eucalyptus tea. Reports of similar incidents slowly made their way back to Europe, and the herb became known as Australian fever tree.

By the 1860s, eucalyptus leaves and oil were being used around the Mediterranean area to treat "intermittent fever" (malaria), which had plagued the area since ancient times. Some physicians reported curing it with eucalyptus, but others dismissed the herb as worthless.

Today, we understand that eucalyptus has no direct effect on the protozoan that causes malaria. Ironically, however, the eucalyptus tree was responsible for virtually eradicating the devastating disease throughout much of Italy, Sicily, and Algeria, where it had raged unchecked for thousands of years. Malaria is transmitted by mosquitoes that live in swampy areas. Europeans planted eucalyptus trees in the marshlands bordering the Mediterranean, and as the trees grew, their roots soaked up water and drained the swamps, eliminating malarial mosquitoes' habitat—and the disease they carried.

Eucalyptus oil was used as an antiseptic on urinary catheters in 19th-century British hospitals, where it became known as catheter oil. In America, 19th-century Eclectic physicians, forerunners of today's naturopaths, used eucalyptus oil as an antiseptic on wounds and medical instruments. They also recommended inhaling the vapors in steam to treat bronchitis, asthma, whooping cough (pertussis), and emphysema.

Contemporary herbalists recommend eucalyptus as a topical antiseptic, a gargle for sore throat, and a treatment for the nasal and chest congestion of colds, flu, bronchitis, croup, and asthma.

Therapeutic Uses

Eucalyptus leaf oil contains eucalyptol, a compound that gives the herb its pleasant aroma and healing value.

COLDS AND FLU. Eucalyptol loosens phlegm in the chest so it's easier to cough up. That's why so many cough lozenges are flavored with eucalyptus.

Eucalyptus is one of the few traditional herbal medicines approved by the FDA. Commission E, the expert panel that evaluates herbal medicines for the German counterpart of the FDA, also endorses the herb as a cold and flu treatment.

In Russia, animal studies have shown that eucalyptol kills influenza A, the virus that causes the most serious form of flu. It also kills certain bacteria. Inhaling the vapors of a strong eucalyptus infusion may help prevent bacterial bronchitis, a possible complication of colds and flu.

WOUNDS. The antibacterial action of eucalyptol makes it an effective treatment for minor cuts and scrapes.

PERIODONTAL HEALTH. Japanese researchers gave 97 people with gum disease either a placebo chewing gum or a gum containing eucalyptus extract. After 12 weeks, those who chewed the eucalyptus gum showed significantly reduced symptoms of gum disease.

HEADACHES. In two very similar studies, German researchers treated people who were prone to tension headaches with either medically inactive placebos or different combinations of eucalyptus and peppermint oils. Participants rubbed the preparations on their foreheads and temples. The herb treatments produced more significant relief. The formula that was mostly eucalyptus oil produced the greatest muscle relaxation, while the formula that was mostly peppermint oil yielded the greatest pain relief. The researchers suggested trying an herbal treatment instead of or in addition to an over-the-counter pain reliever.

Intriguing Possibility

Eucalyptus could have value as a natural insect repellent. According to a report in *Science News*, eucalyptol repels cockroaches.

Rx Recommendations

To make a eucalyptus inhalant, boil a handful of leaves or a few drops of essential oil in water.

For minor cuts and scrapes, thoroughly wash the wound with soap and water, then apply a drop or two of eucalyptus oil.

To relieve headaches, rub the oil on your forehead and temples.

To prepare a eucalyptus bath, wrap a handful of leaves in a cloth and run the bathwater over it.

For a cool, spicy, refreshing infusion to treat colds and flu, use 1 to 2 teaspoons of dried, crushed leaves per cup of boiling water. Steep for 10 minutes, then strain. Drink up to 2 cups a day. You can also make an infusion by using 1 or 2 carefully measured drops (but no more) of eucalyptus oil.

When using commercial preparations, follow the package directions.

If your home is infested with cockroaches and you don't want to use insecticides, try soaking small cloths in eucalyptus oil and placing them around your cabinets.

The Safety Factor

Used externally, eucalyptus oil is considered nonirritating, but it may cause a rash in people who are unusually sensitive to it. Anyone who does not develop a rash may use eucalyptus preparations externally, although infants and children may rebel against the pungent aroma.

If you use eucalyptus oil, be very careful not to ingest more than a drop or two. It is highly poisonous, and fatalities have been reported from ingestion of as little as a teaspoon.

Pregnant and nursing women should not use eucalyptus.

Do not give eucalyptus to children under 2. In older children, adjust the recommended dose based on the child's weight. For example, give a 50-pound child one-third of the dose a 150-pound adult would take.

If you're over 65, start with a low dose, and increase only if necessary.

Inform health care professionals of the herbs you use. Problematic herb-drug interactions are possible.

Eucalyptus may cause allergic reactions or

other unexpected side effects. If any develop, reduce your dose or stop taking it.

For more on herb safety, see Chapter 2.

If symptoms get worse or persist longer than 2 weeks, consult a health care professional promptly.

Growing Information

The more than 500 species of eucalyptus account for three-quarters of the native vegetation in Australia. Eucalyptus varies from 5-foot shrubs to the tallest trees on Earth—up to 475 feet, the size of a 40-story building.

Eucalyptus grows anywhere with loamy soil and adequate water, as long as the temperature does not dip below freezing. Plant saplings obtained at a nursery. If the leaves begin to blister, cut back on watering.

Eucalyptus often kills surrounding vegetation (except other Australian plants), which is why the trees are usually found in stands with little between them. They grow extremely rapidly, up to several feet per year, and their trunks eventually attain enormous girth. If you plant a eucalyptus, be prepared for it to dominate your yard.

Horticulturists discourage planting eucalyptus. The plant's roots break up water and sewer lines, its trunks buckle sidewalks, and its limbs have a tendency to break off in gusting winds, damaging property and endangering lives.

EVENING PRIMROSE
Bursting with Therapeutic Power

Family: Onagraceae; other members include fuchsia

Genus and species: *Oenothera biennis*

Also known as: Evening star

Parts used: Seeds

Have you ever seen an evening primrose bloom? It's one of the most beautiful sights in the plant kingdom.

Each flower opens for only one night. Just before dusk, all that's visible is the ripe, unopened bud. As the light of day begins to fade, the bud starts quivering. All of a sudden, the four green sepals flick out perpendicular to the flower stem, revealing a tight bundle of dainty yellow petals. The petals tremble as they emerge from their tight cocoon. With jerky, dancing contortions that take about a minute, the golden petals spread out, 2 inches across, radiant in the sunset. By morning, the flower withers and dies.

Fortunately, the healing power of evening primrose's seed oil lasts much longer than the plant's flowers. Evening primrose oil (EPO) is a relative newcomer to herbal medicine. It began attracting research attention only in the 1970s. Since then, many studies have shown that it helps treat cardiovascular disease, premenstrual syndrome, rheumatoid arthritis, eczema, and possibly even breast cancer, multiple sclerosis, and a complication of diabetes.

Healing History

Evening primrose is native to North America. Native Americans used the plant as both a food and a medicine. Many tribes boiled the roots and ate them; others ate the young leaves and seeds.

Medicinally, Native Americans applied the whole evening primrose plant externally to control the swelling and inflammation of wounds. They also drank root tea to treat coughs.

Early colonists adopted evening primrose enthusiastically. They, too, boiled the roots as food and used the seeds to garnish breads. They also adopted the Native American practice of applying the plant to treat wounds.

The Shakers, whose enormous herb gardens supplied many early Americans with medicinal herbs, used a tea made from evening primrose seeds to treat indigestion and other digestive problems.

America's 19th-century Eclectic physicians, forerunners of today's naturopaths, picked up on the Native American and Shaker recommendations. They advised mixing a strong tea with lard and applying it to wounds and other skin conditions. They also prescribed the tea for digestive upsets and suggested evening primrose for "sallow skin when the patient's mentality is of a gloomy and despondent character."

Until the 1980s, evening primrose was a minor medicinal herb. Herbalists recommended it mostly for indigestion. But since researchers discovered a key essential fatty acid in the herb's seed oil, evening primrose has become much more widely studied and recommended.

Therapeutic Uses

Evening primrose seeds (and borage seeds, see page 112) contain an oil that has a high concentration of a compound rarely found in plants: gamma-linolenic acid (GLA), an essential fatty acid, or EFA. Essential fatty acids play many important roles in the body. They are involved in the synthesis of prostaglandins, compounds that regulate dozens of bodily functions. They also act as anti-inflammatory agents and help to regulate metabolism.

EFA cannot be synthesized by the body and must be obtained from diet. Fish—especially cold-water fish such as salmon—contain these fatty acids, most notably the omega-3s. People who eat meat-dominated diets tend to have low EFA intakes.

When laboratory animals have been placed on diets devoid of EFA, they develop a number of health problems: eczema-like skin conditions, immune suppression, cardiovascular disease, poor wound healing, liver abnormalities, and infertility. This finding led researchers to give EFA supplements to people with conditions linked to EFA deficiencies. The results have been remarkably positive.

The *Review of Natural Products*, a scientific publication that monitors research on herbal medicines, has concluded that for conditions related to EFA deficiencies, the value of evening primrose oil "cannot be overstated . . . [and it produces] excellent results."

HEART DISEASE AND STROKE. The GLA in evening primrose oil can lower cholesterol substantially. In one Scottish study, 79 people with high cholesterol took 4,000 milligrams of evening primrose oil daily for 3 months. Their average cholesterol levels fell 31.5 percent. Cardiologists have found that for every 1 percent decrease in total cholesterol, the risk of heart attack drops 2 percent. So in the Scottish study, the participants' risk of heart attack plummeted more than 60 percent.

Other research has shown that evening primrose oil lowers blood pressure and reduces the likelihood of formation of the blood clots that lead to heart attacks and most strokes.

PREMENSTRUAL SYNDROME (PMS). The current research goes both ways on evening primrose oil as a treatment for the mood swings, fluid retention, and breast tenderness of PMS. Some studies show benefit, while others do not. Those that show benefit generally are of longer duration, lasting five cycles or more. In one of these studies, 19 women took evening primrose oil for the 2 weeks before their menstrual periods for 5 months. Their PMS symptoms declined significantly, with the greatest benefit occurring during the final month.

BREAST PAIN. PMS may trigger breast pain or tenderness, but other conditions unrelated to the menstrual cycle may also cause it. In one study, which spanned 17 years and involved more than 400 women, researchers at the University of Wales prescribed either one of two standard drugs (Danazol or bromocriptine) or evening primrose oil. All three treatments produced similar results: significant relief for about 90 percent of the women whose pain came and went with their menstrual cycles as well as for 60 percent of the women with constant breast pain.

RHEUMATOID ARTHRITIS. Several studies have shown that evening primrose helps relieve the joint pain, swelling, and tenderness of rheumatoid arthritis. At the University of Pennsylvania, researchers gave 37 people with rheumatoid arthritis either GLA or medically inactive placebos. After 6 months, those receiving placebos experienced no change in their symptoms, while those taking GLA reported 36 percent fewer tender joints and 45 percent less joint pain. What's more, the GLA caused no side effects.

Two British studies came up with similar results. In one, 40 people with rheumatoid arthritis added either evening primrose oil or placebos to their routine drug regimens. After 6 months, those on the placebos reported no change in their symptoms, while those taking evening primrose oil noted significant improvement.

ECZEMA AND OTHER SKIN CONDITIONS. Finnish researchers gave 25 people with eczema either evening primrose oil or placebos for 3 months. The participants taking the evening primrose oil showed a significantly greater decrease in the amount and severity of their skin inflammation. Several other studies confirmed this finding, recording significant relief from inflammation and itching after treatment with evening primrose oil.

BREAST CANCER. Animal studies have shown that evening primrose oil, when injected under the skin, reduces the size of breast tumors. British researchers gave 38 women with breast cancer either a standard regimen of the drug tamoxifen, or tamoxifen plus GLA (8 capsules per day, totaling 2.8 grams). Biopsies before and after assessed changes in estrogen receptors. Those receiving the drug and herb oil showed a significant decrease in estrogen receptors, a sign of desired clinical response.

Intriguing Possibilities

Pilot trials hint that the oil may improve some symptoms of multiple sclerosis. If you have MS, discuss the herb with your physician. Evening primrose oil causes no significant side effects, so why not try it?

Evening primrose oil has also been used successfully to treat diabetic nerve damage (neuropathy) and alcohol-related liver damage.

Rx Recommendations

Evening primrose oil is sold commercially in 500-milligram capsules containing 320 to 480 milligrams of GLA. Studies showing benefit from evening primrose oil supplementation have used 3 to 12 capsules a day. Take the product you choose according to the package directions.

The Safety Factor

No significant side effects from evening primrose oil have been documented in the medical literature. Still, allergic reactions and mild digestive upsets are possible. If any problematic side effects develop, reduce your dose or stop taking it.

Pregnant women who would like to use eve-ning primrose oil should discuss it with their physicians.

Breast milk is rich in GLA, so nursing women may use evening primrose oil in consultation with their physicians.

Do not give evening primrose oil to children under 2. In older children, adjust the recommended dose based on the child's weight. For example, give a 50-pound child one-third of the dose a 150-pound adult would take.

If you're over 65, start with a low dose, and increase only if necessary.

Inform health care professionals of the herbs you use. Problematic herb-drug interactions are possible.

For more on herb safety, see Chapter 2.

If symptoms get worse or persist longer than 2 weeks (or, in the case of PMS, longer than 6 months), consult a health care professional promptly.

Growing Information

Evening primrose is an annual or biennial that grows throughout the United States and is very popular with gardeners. Botanically, it is not a true primrose.

Depending on conditions, the plants reach from 3 to 9 feet. Flowers bloom from June through September for one night each.

The medicinal uses of evening primrose have led to its commercial farming in the United States and Canada, which together produce about 400 tons of seed annually. In this country, most commercial production is centered in California, the Carolinas, Oregon, and Texas.

FENNEL
Great for Digestion

Family: Umbelliferae; other members include carrot, parsley, celery, dill, and angelica

Genus and species: *Foeniculum vulgare* and *F. vulgare dulce*

Also known as: Finocchio, carosella, and Florence fennel

Parts used: Fruits (seeds); stalks and bulbs are used in cooking

New England's Puritans referred to fennel as "meeting seeds." The meetings were their endless church services, and some experts believe that they used fennel as an appetite suppressant. Others theorize that many Puritans steeled themselves for church with whiskey and then chewed fennel seeds to mask the odor.

The Puritans also used fennel as a digestive aid. This has been the herb's primary purpose in herbal healing from the time of the Pharaohs to the present day.

Healing History

In Greek mythology, humanity received knowledge from Mount Olympus as a fiery coal encased in a fennel bulb.

The ancient Greeks had several different ideas about the medicinal value of fennel. During the 3rd century B.C., Hippocrates prescribed the herb as a stomach soother to treat infant colic. Four hundred years later, Dioscorides deemed it an appetite suppressant and recommended the seeds to nursing mothers to boost milk production. The Greeks also called fennel *maraino*, meaning "to grow thin." They thought the herb contributed to weight loss.

The Roman naturalist Pliny loved fennel and included the plant in 22 medicinal recipes. He noted that some snakes rubbed against the plant after shedding their skins and that soon after, their glazed eyes cleared. Pliny took this as a sign that fennel could cure human eye problems, including blindness.

Ancient India's Ayurvedic physicians revered fennel as a digestive aid.

Under the medieval Doctrine of Signatures—the notion that plants' physical characteristics revealed their medicinal value—fennel's yellow flowers were linked to the liver's yellow bile. Thus, the herb was recommended for jaundice.

The emperor Charlemagne ordered that fennel be cultivated in all of his imperial "physic" (medicinal) gardens. And the household of King Edward I of England consumed more than 8 pounds of the herb a month. The Church permitted the seeds to be nibbled on fast days as an appetite suppressant.

Fennel was one of Hildegard of Bingen's favorite herbs. The 12th-century German abbess/herbalist recommended it for colds, flu, the heart, and to "make us happy, [with] good digestion . . . and good body odor."

The Anglo-Saxons who settled England around the 5th century used fennel as both a spice and a digestive aid. They also hung fennel over their doors to protect against witchcraft.

By the 17th century, fennel was a mainstay of herbal healing and a standard seasoning for fish. Seventeenth-century English herbalist Nicholas Culpeper, apparently not a fish lover, wrote that fennel "consumes the phlegmatic humour which fish . . . annoys the body with." Culpeper also echoed the ancient recommendations, prescribing fennel to "break wind, increase milk, cleanse the eyes from mists that hinder sight, take away the loathings which oftentimes happen to stomachs of sick persons . . . [and] in drink or broth to make people lean that are too fat." He also claimed that it "brought women's courses" (menstruation).

Folk herbalists often mixed fennel with strong laxative herbs, such as buckthorn, senna, rhubarb, and aloe, to relieve the intestinal cramps that the laxatives often caused.

Colonists brought fennel to North America. Henry Wadsworth Longfellow alluded to Pliny when he wrote:

Above the lower plants it towers
The Fennel with its yellow flowers;
And in an earlier age than ours
Was gifted with wondrous powers
Lost vision to restore.

America's 19th-century Eclectic physicians, forerunners of today's naturopaths, prescribed fennel as a digestive aid, milk and menstruation promoter, and flavoring agent to "conceal the unpleasantness of other medicines." Latin Americans still boil the seeds in milk as a milk promoter for nursing mothers. Jamaicans use fennel to treat colds. And Africans take the herb for diarrhea and indigestion.

Contemporary herbalists recommend fennel as a digestive aid, milk promoter, expectorant, eyewash, and buffer in herbal laxative blends.

Therapeutic Uses

Fennel won't cure blindness, but science has supported some of its other traditional uses.

DIGESTIVE PROBLEMS. Like most other aromatic herbs, fennel relaxes the smooth muscle lining the digestive tract, meaning that it's an antispasmodic. It also expels gas and promotes the secretion of bile, which helps in the digestion of fats. And European research shows that fennel kills some bacteria, lending some support to its traditional role in treating diarrhea.

In Germany, where herbal medicine is more mainstream than it is in the United States, fennel is used like caraway as a treatment for indigestion, gas pains, irritable bowel syndrome, and infant colic. And many Indian restaurants keep a bowl of candied fennel seeds by the door as a digestive aid for departing diners.

German researchers gave either a standard pharmaceutical stomach-settler (metoclopramide) or a combination of herbs (fennel, peppermint, caraway, and wormwood) to 60 people ages 18 to 85, all of whom had complained of indigestion, heartburn, nausea, or unusual belching or fullness. The participants were instructed to take their medicine 20 minutes before meals. After 2 weeks of treatment, those taking the herbal combination reported significantly greater relief from their symptoms, and with fewer side effects.

Commission E, the expert panel that evaluates herbal medicines for the German counterpart of the FDA, endorses fennel for the treatment of digestive upsets.

INFANT COLIC. Russian researchers gave either a placebo or a fennel seed preparation to infants 2 to 12 weeks old who had symptoms of colic, notably persistent crying. Among the infants in the placebo group, 24 percent showed significantly reduced crying. But in the fennel group, the figure was 65 percent.

OVERWEIGHT. Animal studies show that fennel has diuretic action. This probably accounts for the herb's traditional role in weight control.

Keep in mind that diuretics of any kind eliminate only water weight. For this reason, weight-loss experts discourage the routine use of diuretics for weight management. The keys to permanent weight loss are a low-calorie, low-fat, high-fiber diet and regular exercise.

Intriguing Possibilities

Antispasmodics soothe not only the digestive tract but also other smooth muscles, including the uterus. Fennel, however, was traditionally used not to relax the uterus but to stimulate it into menstruation. Though this contradiction remains scientifically unresolved, one study has found that fennel might have a mild estrogenic effect, meaning that it acts like the female sex hormone estrogen. This action may have something to do with its traditional use as a milk and menstruation promoter.

Rx Recommendations

To use fennel as a digestive aid, either chew a handful of seeds or try an infusion or tincture. You can also use an infusion or tincture to attempt to bring on menstruation.

To make a pleasant, licorice-flavored infusion, steep 1 to 2 teaspoons of bruised seeds in 1 cup of boiling water for 10 minutes, then strain. Drink up to 3 cups a day.

As a homemade tincture, take $\frac{1}{2}$ to 1 teaspoon up to three times a day.

When using commercial preparations, follow the package directions.

The Safety Factor

At best, fennel has only a mild estrogenic effect. But estrogen, a key ingredient in birth control pills, has many effects on the body. Women advised by their doctors not to take the Pill should not use medicinal amounts of fennel. The same is true for anyone with a history of abnormal blood clotting or estrogen-dependent breast tumors.

Pregnant women should not use medicinal amounts of fennel.

Parents may give dilute fennel preparations to colicky infants in consultation with the child's physician.

Fennel seeds are safe, but fennel oil may cause skin rash in people who are sensitive to it. When taken internally, even small amounts of the oil—a teaspoon or so—may cause nausea, vomiting, and possibly seizures. Don't ingest it.

Inform health care professionals of the herbs you use. Problematic herb-drug interactions are possible.

For more on herb safety, see Chapter 2.

If symptoms get worse or persist longer than 2 weeks, consult a health care professional promptly.

Growing Information

Native to southern Europe and Asia Minor, fennel is a striking 6-foot perennial with feathery leaves and tall stalks capped by large umbrella-like clusters of tiny yellow flowers. The tiny oval-shaped fruits (seeds) are ribbed and greenish gray. All parts of the plant have the herb's characteristic anise/licorice fragrance.

Fennel grows easily from seeds sown in rich, moist soil in fall or after the danger of frost has passed. Germination takes about 2 weeks. Thin seedlings to 12-inch spacing. Do not overwater the seedlings, but as plants develop, extra water increases stem succulence. The leaves may be harvested once plants are established.

When the stems are about an inch thick, hill the soil over them to cause blanching, which results in milder flavor. Harvest about 10 days after hilling.

Harvest the seeds in late summer as they turn greenish gray.

Fennel may damage some neighboring plants, including bush beans, tomatoes, caraway, and kohlrabi. If coriander is planted nearby, fennel will not fruit.

Warning: In the wild, fennel may be easily confused with poison hemlock, which can be fatal when consumed. Don't eat wild fennel unless you're sure you've identified it correctly.

FENUGREEK

The Cholesterol Controller

Family: Leguminosae; other members include beans and peas

Genus and species: *Trigonella foenum-graecum*

Also known as: Greek hay, foenu greek, and fenigreek

Parts used: Seeds

In 1922, when the 3,000-year-old tomb of the Egyptian pharaoh King Tutankhamen (King Tut) was opened, fenugreek was found inside. From ancient times through the late 19th century, fenugreek played a major role in herbal healing. Then it fell by the wayside.

Lately, however, things are looking up for the herb with a taste that is an odd combination of bitter celery and maple syrup. Fenugreek helps reduce cholesterol levels, as well as blood sugar levels in people with diabetes.

Healing History

Fenugreek plants were used to help sick animals long before the seeds became a popular remedy for human ills. Early Greeks mixed the plant into moldy or insect-damaged animal forage to make it more palatable. In the process, they discovered that sick horses and cattle would eat fenugreek when they wouldn't eat anything else. The Egyptians and Romans subsequently adopted "Greek hay." The plant's Latin name, *foenum graecum*, evolved into "fenugreek."

Today fenugreek is widely used to flavor horse and cattle feed. Some veterinarians still rely on it to encourage sick livestock to eat.

As fenugreek spread around the Mediterranean, ancient physicians learned that its seeds contain a great deal of a special type of fiber called mucilage. When mixed with water, mucilage becomes gelatinous and soothes inflamed or irritated tissue. Egyptian physicians put fenugreek into ointments to treat wounds and abscesses. They also recommended using the herb internally to treat fevers and respiratory and intestinal complaints. Hippocrates and other ancient Greek and Roman physicians used the herb similarly.

Ancient Chinese healers recommended fenugreek to treat fevers, hernias, gallbladder problems, muscle aches, and even impotence.

In India, where the herb is an ingredient in curry spice blends, Ayurvedic physicians prescribed it to treat arthritis, bronchitis, and digestive upsets.

Indian women ate fenugreek seeds to increase their milk production. Arab women from Libya to Syria ate the roasted seeds to help them gain weight, enlarge their breasts, and attain the Rubenesque proportions that were synonymous with beauty from ancient times through the 19th century.

Fenugreek is the only healing herb ever used as a weapon of war. During the Roman siege of Jerusalem (A.D. 66–70), general and future emperor Vespasian ordered his troops to scale the city's imposing walls. The standard defense against this kind of attack was to pour boiling water or oil on the attackers and their ladders. According to *The History of the Jewish War* by Flavius Josephus, Jerusalem's defenders added fenugreek to their oil, making it more slippery and hindering the Romans as they tried to climb their ladders.

Around the 9th century, the Benedictine monks, who were avid herb gardeners and creators of fine liqueurs, popularized fenugreek throughout Europe. From that time on, the herb was widely used in folk medicine as it had been by the ancients—to treat wounds, fevers, and digestive and respiratory ailments.

Early settlers brought fenugreek to North America and used it as forage and in folk medicine, where it gained a reputation as a treatment for menstrual complaints and the discomforts of menopause. The herb became a key ingredient in Lydia E. Pinkham's Vegetable Compound, one of 19th-century America's most popular patent medicines for "female weakness" (menstrual cramps and menopausal discomforts). The manufacturer proclaimed her compound "the greatest medical discovery since the dawn of history." Health authorities were outraged, and their outcry played a part in creating the FDA, which regulates drug claims.

Modern herbalists recommend fenugreek poultices and plasters to treat wounds, boils, and rashes. They say that a warm fenugreek gargle soothes a sore throat. They also recommend using the herb internally to treat coughs, bronchitis, and menstrual and menopausal complaints. Some are even convinced that eating fenugreek—especially its sprouts—enlarges women's breasts.

Today, fenugreek is most widely used in the U.S. as a source of imitation maple flavor.

Therapeutic Uses

Some of fenugreek's traditional uses have been supported by modern science, but the herb's most important potential benefit has only recently come to light.

HIGH CHOLESTEROL. Indian researchers measured the cholesterol levels of 60 people who were not taking any cholesterol-lowering medications. Then the participants were instructed to eat a bowl of soup containing about 1 ounce of powdered fenugreek seed before lunch and dinner each day.

After 4 weeks of consuming about 2 ounces per day of powdered fenugreek seed in this way, the participants saw their cholesterol levels begin to decline. After 24 weeks, their average total cholesterol dropped 14 percent. For every 1 percent decrease in total cholesterol, the risk of heart attack risk drops about 2 percent, so in this study, the participants' risk of heart attack plummeted by about 28 percent.

In another study lasting 3 months, 2 teaspoons (5 grams) of powdered fenugreek seed a day produced no changes in the cholesterol levels of 30 people with normal readings. In 30 people with elevated cholesterol, however, the same dose for the same period of time reduced levels significantly.

DIABETES. In the same Indian study previously mentioned, all of the participants had type 2 (noninsulin-dependent) diabetes. In addition to lowering their cholesterol levels, daily consumption of about 2 ounces of powdered fenugreek seed also lowered their blood sugar levels. Another Indian study produced the same results. These trials corroborate animal research showing that fenugreek reduces blood sugar levels.

SORE THROAT. Fenugreek's soothing mucilage may help relieve sore throat pain and cough, as well as mild indigestion.

WOUNDS. Fenugreek's mucilage also soothes minor wounds. Commission E, the expert panel that evaluates herbal medicines for the German counterpart of the FDA, approves fenugreek as an external wound treatment.

WOMEN'S HEALTH CONCERNS. Fenugreek seeds contain diosgenin, a compound that's similar to the female sex hormone estrogen. Estrogen causes fluid retention and resulting weight gain, validating one of this herb's traditional uses. Likewise, just as many women who take estrogen-based birth control pills report breast swelling, the diosgenin in fenugreek has also been found to stimulate breast tissue growth.

ARTHRITIS. Belgian researchers have discovered that fenugreek has mild anti-inflammatory action. This lends some credence to the herb's traditional role in treating arthritis, wounds, and other inflammatory conditions.

Intriguing Possibilities

Antioxidant flavonoids have been isolated from fenugreek seeds. Antioxidants help prevent and reverse the cell damage that causes heart disease and most cancers.

Fenugreek might also help ease a major complaint of menopausal women. The discovery of a plant estrogen in fenugreek suggests that the herb may be used as a natural form of hormone replacement therapy to treat the hot flashes associated with menopause.

As for the herb's use as a breast enhancer, James A. Duke, Ph.D., retired USDA herbal medicine authority and author of several highly regarded herbal medicine references, has observed that fenugreek sprouts contain much more diosgenin than the unsprouted seeds. He has recommended the sprouts to women interested in nonsurgical breast augmentation, and he says that he has received several thank-you notes from satisfied users.

Only one study has been published on fenugreek's effects, if any, on breast size. It was an animal study, and the animals' breast weight increased, indicating increased size.

Rx Recommendations

Use a fenugreek decoction to take advantage of the herb's many potential healing benefits: to soothe a sore throat, relieve menstrual or menopausal discomforts, or possibly relieve arthritis pain. You might also try the herb to lower your cholesterol or to help control blood sugar levels, in conjunction with conventional therapy and under the supervision of your physician.

For a bitter, maple-flavored decoction, gently boil 2 teaspoons of crushed seeds in 1 cup of water, then simmer for 10 minutes and strain. Drink up to 3 cups a day. To improve the flavor,

add sugar, honey, lemon, anise, or peppermint.

As a homemade tincture, use $1/4$ to $1/2$ teaspoon up to three times a day.

When using commercial preparations, follow the package directions.

The Safety Factor

Because fenugreek may be a uterine stimulant, pregnant women should not take it. Nursing women should also avoid it—unless they want even larger breasts.

Do not give fenugreek to children under 2. In older children, adjust the recommended dose based on the child's weight. For example, give a 50-pound child one-third of the dose a 150-pound adult would take.

If you're over 65, start with a low dose, and increase only if necessary.

Inform health care professionals of the herbs you use. Problematic herb-drug interactions are possible.

Fenugreek may cause allergic reactions or other unexpected side effects. If any develop, reduce your dose or stop taking it.

For more on herb safety, see Chapter 2.

If symptoms get worse or persist longer than 2 weeks, consult a health care professional promptly.

Growing Information

Fenugreek is an annual that reaches 18 inches and resembles a large clover. It has three-lobed leaves and white, triangular, pealike flowers, which produce the long seed pods characteristic of the bean family. Fenugreek's seed pod is sickle-shaped and 2 inches long, containing 10 to

20 hard, smooth, oblong, somewhat flattened seeds.

After the danger of frost has passed and the soil temperature has reached 55°F, sow seeds in almost any soil in an area that receives full sun. Germination typically takes only a few days. To prevent root rot, do not overwater the plants.

The plants flower in about 3 weeks and produce seeds in another 3 weeks. Harvest the pods when they're fully formed but before they begin to crack. Remove the seeds and dry them in the sun.

FEVERFEW
A Potent Migraine Preventive

Family: Compositae; other members include daisy, dandelion, and marigold

Genus and species: *Chrysanthemum parthenium; Matricaria parthenium; Tanacetum parthenium*

Also known as: Febrifuge plant, wild quinine, and bachelor's button

Parts used: Leaves

From the 19th century well into the late 1970s, feverfew was largely washed up as a healing herb. In 1974, in *The Herb Book*, noted herbalist John Lust summarized most of his colleagues' feelings: "Feverfew has fallen into considerable disuse. It is also hard to find, even at herb outlets."

Shortly after Lust penned this obituary, however, feverfew experienced something of a renaissance. It became clear that the herb is remarkably effective at preventing migraines.

Healing History

Many sources claim that the herb's name comes from the Latin *febrifugia*, meaning "driver-out of fevers." They also say that the herb has been used since ancient times to treat fever.

They're wrong on both counts. The plant was never called febrifugia. Ancient physicians, including Dioscorides and Galen, referred to it by its Greek name, *parthenion*, and prescribed it for menstrual and childbirth-related problems, not fever.

During the Middle Ages, the name parthenion faded, and the plant was renamed featherfoil because of its feathery leaf borders. "Featherfoil" evolved into "featherfew" and eventually "feverfew."

Once the name feverfew became popular, herbalists decided that it was, in fact, a fever treatment. They planted the strong-smelling herb around their homes in hopes of purifying the air to ward off malaria, which they mistakenly believed was caused by bad air (the word *malaria* comes from the Italian *mala*, "foul," and *aria*, "air").

Malaria had plagued Europe since prehistoric times. It was untreatable until Spanish explorers returned from Peru with cinchona bark and early chemists isolated the bark's antimalarial constituent, quinine. Quinine proved so successful at curing malaria that for a brief period, other herbs prescribed for fever basked in its reflected glow. That's how feverfew became known as wild quinine. But the name didn't stick. Quinine proved so superior as a malaria treatment that feverfew was all but abandoned for this purpose.

For a while, some herbalists recommended feverfew for ailments other than fever, particularly for headache. In the 17th century, England's John Parkinson described feverfew as "very effectual for all paines in the head." More than 100 years later, John Hill wrote, "In the worst headache, this herb exceeds whatever else is known."

Most herbalists stuck with feverfew's traditional gynecological uses, however. Seventeenth-century English herbalist Nicholas Culpeper called it a "general strengthener of wombs" and prescribed it in tea form for colds and chest congestion. Culpeper also recognized the herb's decline, declaring it "not much used in present practice."

Early colonists introduced feverfew into North America, where malaria was also a major problem. But as the herb fell from fashion in England, it stopped being used here as well.

America's 19th-century Eclectic physicians, forerunners of today's naturopaths, prescribed feverfew mainly as a menstruation promoter and as a treatment for "female hysteria" (menstrual discomforts) and some fever-producing diseases.

Therapeutic Uses

In the late 1970s, a chance meeting between two migraine sufferers made earlier observations about feverfew's benefit for "paines in the head" appear prophetic.

MIGRAINES. The wife of the chief medical officer of Britain's National Coal Board was prone to chronic migraines. A miner heard about her problem. When she accompanied her husband on a visit to his mine, the miner told her that he'd also been a longtime migraine sufferer—until he started chewing a few feverfew leaves every day. Upon trying the herb, the woman noticed immediate improvement. Fourteen months later, she was free of her searing headaches.

The medical officer brought his wife's experience to the attention of Dr. E. Stewart Johnson of the City of London Migraine Clinic. In a pilot study, Dr. Johnson gave feverfew leaves to 10 of his patients. Three pronounced themselves cured, and the other seven reported significant improvement in their symptoms.

Next, Dr. Johnson gave feverfew to 270 of his migraine patients. Seventy percent reported significant relief—and for many of them, standard medical treatment had done nothing at all.

Finally, Dr. Johnson arranged a scientifically rigorous double-blind, placebo-controlled trial in which some of the participants took feverfew, while others took medically inactive placebos. Neither the participants nor the researchers knew who got what until after the trial had ended. (This is what's meant by "double-blind.") Feverfew significantly outperformed the placebos.

Soon after Dr. Johnson completed his research, the British medical journal *Lancet* reported the results of an even more rigorous experiment. Seventy-two people with chronic migraines were randomly assigned to take either placebos or capsules of powdered, freeze-dried feverfew (85 milligrams, the equivalent of two medium-size leaves) every day. Neither the participants nor the researchers knew who was using which treatment. After 2 months, the groups switched treatments, so those who had been taking placebos were given feverfew and vice versa (a "crossover trial"). The results were striking: Feverfew cut migraine episodes by 24 percent, and the headaches that did occur were comparatively mild, with significantly less nausea and vomiting.

Since then, several other studies have shown feverfew to be effective for migraine prevention. In 1996, however, one highly publicized study by Dutch researchers found that the herb had no benefit. As it turned out, this trial used a tincture (alcohol extract) of feverfew, not the leaves that had proven effective in all the other studies.

In 1998, British researchers reviewed five studies of feverfew for migraine prevention, using sophisticated statistical techniques to combine the studies as though they were all arms of one big trial (called a meta-analysis). The researchers' conclusion: Feverfew works.

DIGESTIVE PROBLEMS. Like chamomile, its close botanical relative, feverfew contains chemicals that calm the smooth muscles of the digestive tract, making the herb an antispasmodic. Try feverfew after meals to protect against digestive upset.

WOMEN'S HEALTH CONCERNS. Antispasmodic herbs soothe not only the digestive tract but also other smooth muscles, such as the uterus. In addition, feverfew has the ability to neutralize certain prostaglandins, substances that have been linked to pain and inflammation. (This may be another reason that feverfew helps prevent migraines.) Prostaglandins also play a role in menstrual cramps. Feverfew's possible antispasmodic and anti-prostaglandin actions support its traditional use in treating menstrual discomforts.

Intriguing Possibilities

One animal study suggests that feverfew has a mild tranquilizing effect. Taken before bedtime, the herb just might help bring on sleep.

Another report hints at feverfew's tumor-fighting properties. It's much too early to deem the herb a cancer treatment, but that day may come.

Rx Recommendations

To control the frequency and severity of migraine attacks, chew two fresh (or freeze-dried) leaves a day or take a pill or capsule containing 85 milligrams of whole-leaf material. Since feverfew is quite bitter, most people prefer taking the pills or capsules to chewing the leaves.

If feverfew doesn't seem to be helping within a few weeks, try changing brands before you decide to give up on the herb. A report in *Lancet* showed that some "feverfew" pills and capsules actually contain only trace amounts.

To improve digestion or promote menstruation, take feverfew as an infusion. Use $1/2$ to 1 teaspoon of herb per cup of boiling water, steep for 5 to 10 minutes, then strain. Drink up to 2 cups a day.

The Safety Factor

While feverfew suppresses migraines, it does not cure them. When treatment with the herb is suspended, the headaches typically return, which means that migraine sufferers might wind up taking feverfew for a long time. The herb has been used in migraine prevention for about 25 years with no reports of significant problems, but there is no research examining the herb's longer-term effects.

Feverfew has not been shown to cause uterine contractions, but it has a long folk history as a menstruation promoter. Pregnant women should err on the side of caution and not take it. Nursing women should also avoid it.

Chewing fresh feverfew leaves may cause mouth sores. Some people also report abdominal pain from using the herb.

Feverfew may inhibit blood clotting. People with clotting disorders and those who are taking anticoagulant (blood-thinning) medications or supplements (vitamin E, for example) should consult a physician before using it.

Do not give feverfew to children under 2. In older children, adjust the recommended dose based on the child's weight. For example, give a 50-pound child one-third of the dose a 150-pound adult would take.

If you're over 65, start with a low dose, and increase only if necessary.

Inform health care professionals of the herbs you use. Problematic herb-drug interactions are possible.

Feverfew may cause allergic reactions or other unexpected side effects. If any develop, reduce your dose or stop taking it.

For more on herb safety, see Chapter 2.

If symptoms get worse or persist longer than 2 weeks, consult a health care professional promptly.

Growing Information

Feverfew is a perennial that reaches 3 feet and has lovely daisylike flowers with yellow centers and up to 20 white rays. For personal migraine prevention, a few plants should suffice.

Feverfew grows from seeds, but most authorities recommend planting root cuttings when the temperature reaches 70°F. Space plants 18 inches apart.

Feverfew does best in partial shade. Compost stimulates better growth. Pinch back the flower buds to encourage bushiness. Harvest the leaves when they mature.

Bees dislike feverfew and generally avoid the plant, so don't plant it around other plants that require bee pollination. Feverfew can also be grown indoors year-round as a houseplant.

FLAX
From Linen to Healing

Family: Linaceae; other members include the more than 200 species of flax

Genus and species: *Linum usitatissimum*

Also known as: Flaxseed, linseed, linum

Parts used: Seeds

Ten thousand years ago, flax was one of the first plants farmed for purposes other than food. Flax has a fibrous stem, and the fibers were woven into cloth, eventually linen. But flax seeds also produce an oil (flaxseed or linseed oil) that has been used medicinally for almost as long.

Flax was among the most important crops to colonial American farmers. It was grown in almost every state east of the Mississippi River, and some beyond. Before the invention of the cotton gin in the early 1800s, most Americans wore clothing made from either wool or linen.

Even after cotton became affordable, linen remained an important fiber for clothes and other products.

Healing History

More than 1,000 years ago, French king Charlemagne decreed that all his subjects should eat flaxseed to stay healthy. In the 1600s, British herbalist Nicholas Culpeper hailed flaxseed as having "great use against inflammations and tumors."

Flaxseed is rich in mucilage, a soluble fiber that becomes spongy when immersed in water. In ancient Europe, flax mucilage and flaxseed oil were used topically to soothe irritated skin. Flaxseed oil was also used internally as a laxative and treatment for cough, colds, and urinary tract infections.

Therapeutic Uses

BREAST CANCER. Flaxseed is extraordinarily rich in plant estrogens (lignans), containing up to 800 times as much as other vegetable sources. But lignans are chemically weaker than the body's own hormones. Estrogen stimulates the growth of breast cancer. Lignans bind to cellular estrogen receptors and blunt the effects of the body's own estrogen, thus reducing risk of breast cancer.

In animal studies, flaxseed oil inhibits growth of mammary tumors. Finnish researchers compared lignan consumption (from flax and other foods) in 194 women with breast cancer and 208 controls. As lignan intake increased, breast cancer risk decreased. Compared with women who consumed little or no lignan, those who ate the most had 62 percent less risk of breast cancer.

Canadian researchers asked women newly diagnosed with breast cancer to eat one muffin a day containing about an ounce of flaxseed, while other recently diagnosed women were given a muffin without flaxseed. A month later, the flaxseed group showed biomarkers reflecting slower tumor growth. Swedish researchers conducted a similar study and came up with the same findings. "Our results suggest that flaxseed and its lignans may prove beneficial in breast cancer prevention," noted the researchers.

PROSTATE CANCER. Lignans have also shown benefit against prostate cancer. Duke University researchers drew blood from 25 men with prostate cancer who were awaiting prostate removal, then gave them 30 grams (about an ounce) of flaxseed daily. The men stayed on the diet about a month. After prostatectomy, their prostates were compared with those of similar men who had not eaten flaxseed. The tumors of men who had taken the herb showed less aggressive cancer.

CHOLESTEROL. Flaxseed is rich in soluble fiber. Many studies show that a diet high in soluble fiber—for example, a diet high in oatmeal—lowers cholesterol. Oklahoma State researchers gave 55 women with high cholesterol either a placebo or 30 grams of flaxseed per day. Three months later, the flaxseed group had significantly lower cholesterol. Several other studies have shown similar results.

HEART ATTACK. Harvard scientists assessed alpha-linolenic acid (ALA) intake (from flaxseed and foods) among 76,283 women nurses and then followed them for 10 years. As ALA intake increased, deaths from heart attack decreased. Compared with nurses who consumed the least ALA, those who ate the most had 45 percent lower risk of fatal heart attack.

DIABETES. Soluble fiber also reduces blood sugar levels. Studies by Chinese and Canadian researchers have shown that flaxseed lowers blood sugar levels, suggesting that it can be useful in preventing and treating diabetes.

HOT FLASHES. Lignans have an estrogenic effect, and estrogen minimizes hot flashes. Mayo Clinic researchers gave 40 grams of flaxseed daily to women complaining of hot flashes. The women kept diaries of their hot flash frequency and severity. After 6 weeks, the number and severity of hot flashes was reduced by about 50 percent.

In a similar study, Canadian researchers came up with similar findings. They reported, "Compared with placebo, hot flashes were significantly less severe with flaxseed."

Intriguing Possibilities

A pilot study at Oklahoma State University suggests that in postmenopausal women, flaxseed may prevent bone loss. If confirmed, flaxseed might help prevent osteoporosis.

Some research suggests that ALA may help treat attention deficit hyperactivity disorder (ADHD). Indian scientists gave flaxseed to children diagnosed with ADHD and reported significant improvement in their symptoms.

Rx Recommendations

Flax seeds can be found in bulk at most health food stores. They have a mild wheatlike flavor and can be sprinkled generously on cereals, baked into bread, or ground up and added to soups, casseroles, and many other dishes. Once ground,

flax seeds spoil quickly. Use them immediately.

Flaxseed oil supplements typically contain 1,000 milligrams of oil (500 to 600 milligrams of alpha-linolenic acid). Follow package directions.

The Safety Factor

Flaxseed contains a tiny amount of cyanide—not enough to harm an adult, but possibly enough to harm a fetus or infant. Pregnant and nursing women should not use it.

Do not give flaxseed to children under 2. In older children, adjust the recommended dose based on the child's weight. For example, give a 50-pound child one-third of the dose a 150-pound adult would take.

If you're over 65, start with a low dose, and increase only if necessary.

Inform health care professionals of the herbs you use. Problematic herb-drug interactions are possible.

Flaxseed may cause allergic reactions or other unexpected side effects. If any develop, reduce your dose or stop taking it.

For more on herb safety, see Chapter 2.

If symptoms get worse or persist longer than 2 weeks, consult a health care professional promptly.

Growing Information

Flax is a slender annual that reaches about 3 feet. It branches at the top and produces one or two delicate blue flowers that bloom from February to September. It likes well-drained soil. Yields suffer when flax is planted in the same field year after year. Plant in spring. Late frosts rarely damage flax seedlings.

GARLIC

The Wonder Herb

Family: Liliaceae; other members include lily, tulip, onion, and chive

Genus and species: *Allium sativum*

Also known as: Stinking rose, heal-all, and rustic's or poor man's treacle

Parts used: Bulbs

If the term *wonder drug* can be applied to any healing herb, garlic deserves the honor. It is one of the world's oldest medicines and is still among the best.

Within the genus *Allium*, garlic is the most powerful (and most thoroughly researched) healer. But traditional herbalists also valued garlic's close botanical relatives—onions, scallions, leeks, chives, and shallots—although they were considered less medicinally potent. Modern research bears this out. While onions have almost as much therapeutic value as garlic, scallions, leeks, chives, and shallots have less.

Healing History

Remains of garlic have been found in caves inhabited 10,000 years ago, but the first prescription for the herb, chiseled in cuneiform on a Sumerian clay tablet, dates from 3000 B.C.

Garlic also appears prominently in the world's oldest surviving medical text, the *Ebers Papyrus*, which dates to about 1500 B.C. The herb was an ingredient in 22 remedies for headache, insect and scorpion bites, menstrual discomforts, intestinal worms, tumors, and heart problems.

The entire ancient world from Spain to China loved garlic. No people enjoyed the herb more, however, than the Egyptians, who were called "the stinking ones" by Greek writers because of their garlic breath. Egyptians taking solemn oaths swore on garlic in the same way that we swear on the Bible. The herb was found in the tomb of King Tut. For 15 pounds of it, Egyptians could buy a healthy male slave.

Speaking of slavery, garlic played a major role in the lives of the slaves who built Egypt's pyramids. The Egyptians believed that the herb prevented illness and increased strength and endurance. They gave their slaves a daily ration, and over time, the slaves came to revere garlic just as their masters did.

Legend has it that during the construction of one pyramid, a garlic shortage forced the Egyptians to cut the slaves' ration. The result was a labor revolt that led to the world's first recorded strike.

Around 1200 B.C., soon after Moses led the Hebrew slaves out of Egypt, they complained of missing the finer things of life in bondage. As the Bible relates, "We remember the fish we ate in Egypt, and the cucumbers, melons, leeks, onions, and garlic" (Numbers 11:5).

For Combat and Competition

Greek athletes ate garlic before races, and Greek soldiers munched the herb before battle. In his play *Knights*, Aristophanes wrote: "Now bolt down garlic. You will have greater mettle for the fight."

In Homer's *Odyssey*, Ulysses needs to steel himself against the sorceress Circe, who had turned Ulysses' men into swine and planned to do the same to him. Hermes, the god of science (whose symbol, the serpent-wrapped staff, came to symbolize medicine), gives Ulysses garlic, which thwarts Circe's spells.

Greek midwives hung garlic cloves around birthing rooms to safeguard newborns from disease and witchcraft. As the centuries passed, Europeans fastened braided garlic plants to their doorposts to keep evil spirits at bay, a custom that survives today in the garlic braids hung in many kitchens.

Greek and Roman physicians loved garlic. Hippocrates recommended it for infections, wounds, cancer, leprosy, and digestive problems. Dioscorides prescribed it for heart problems. And Pliny listed it in 61 remedies for ailments ranging from the common cold to epilepsy and from leprosy to tapeworm. Many of these uses have been supported by modern science.

Upper-class Greeks and Romans came to hate the stinking rose, however. They viewed garlic breath as a sign of low social ranking. Antipathy to garlic breath is with us today.

Garlic may have been unfashionable among the well-to-do, but many Roman emperors couldn't eat enough. The ancients considered the herb to be an antidote to poisons, which were popular in ancient Rome, where political rivals were known to taint each other's food. In fact, many Roman herbalists specialized in poisons and in elaborate antidotes that usually included garlic.

Like the Greeks, ancient India's Ayurvedic healers prescribed garlic for leprosy, a practice that continued for thousands of years. In fact, when India became a British colony and adopted English, leprosy became known as "peelgarlic" because lepers spent so much time peeling cloves and eating them. The Indians also used garlic to treat cancer. Modern research supports garlic's ability to treat leprosy and prevent certain cancers.

Tenth-century Arab physicians inherited the Greco-Roman ambivalence toward garlic. One Persian herbal of that time said that the herb should be "despised because of its unpleasant odor," then affirmed that it "acts as an antidote to deadly poisons. It drives away toothache if you bruise it and lay it upon the tooth. We should not be without it in any kitchen."

The same ambivalence persisted in medieval Europe. While the well-to-do shunned garlic, the peasantry consumed huge amounts, viewing the herb as an all-purpose preventive medicine and cure-all—hence one of its names, heal-all. By the Elizabethan era, the Latin term for antidote, *theriaca*, had evolved into the English word *treacle*, meaning "panacea." Garlic was commonly called the poor man's treacle.

From Social Scourge
to Saving Grace

As the centuries passed, the upper class returned to using garlic, but only medicinally, and even then, they used it sparingly. The 17th-century English herbalist Nicholas Culpeper endorsed the herb as "a remedy for all diseases and hurts. . . . It helpeth the biting of mad dogs and other venomous creatures, killeth worms in children, cutteth tough phlegm, purgeth the head . . . and is a good remedy for any plague."

As an affluent, educated man, though, Culpeper also embraced upper-class disdain for garlic and criticized folk healers for "quoting many diseases this [herb] is good for, but concealing its vices." Culpeper warned against garlic's "offensiveness on the breath" and wrote, "Its heat is very vehement, [and it] sends up ill-favoured vapours to the brain. Therefore, let it be used inwardly with great moderation."

Culpeper's call for moderation fell on deaf ears. As a Welsh rhyme advised, "Eat leeks in March, and garlic in May / And all the year after, physicians may play."

During Culpeper's time, the typical breakfast for French peasants consisted of dark bread and garlic. French folk healers considered the herb a strengthener and cure-all.

In 1721, French reverence for garlic soared to new heights when a plague struck Marseilles, killing most of the city's inhabitants. Legend has it that convicted thieves were assigned to bury the dead, a task that was certain to infect them with the fatal disease and thus save the government the bother of executing them. But four enterprising thieves drank a mixture of garlic and wine and survived the plague. They not only escaped the guillotine, they grew rich robbing all the bodies. This tale is more myth than history, but to this day, southern Europeans drink a garlic/wine medicine called Four Thieves Vinegar (*Vinaigre des Quatre Voleurs*).

America's 19th-century Eclectic physicians,

forerunners of today's naturopaths, shared the Victorian prejudice against garlic's "strong, offensive smell . . . and acrimonious, almost caustic taste." But they conceded that the herb is effective in treating colds, coughs, whooping cough, and other respiratory ailments. They also believed that fresh garlic juice applied to the ear could cure deafness.

During World War I, British, French, and Russian army physicians used garlic juice to treat infected battle wounds. They also prescribed the herb to prevent and treat amoebic dysentery.

Alexander Fleming's discovery of penicillin in 1928 launched the age of antibiotics. By World War II, penicillin and sulfa drugs had largely replaced garlic as the treatment of choice for infected wounds. In Russia, however, the needs of more than 20 million World War II casualties overwhelmed its antibiotic supply. Red Army physicians relied heavily on garlic, which came to be called Russian penicillin.

Modern herbalists recommend garlic (as well as other *Allium* vegetables) for colds, coughs, flu, fever, bronchitis, ringworm, intestinal worms, and cardiovascular disease.

Therapeutic Uses

Garlic does not cure epilepsy or deafness, but an enormous amount of scientific evidence proves beyond doubt that the "poor man's treacle" is an herbal wonder drug.

INFECTIONS. During World War I, garlic's success in treating infected wounds and amoebic dysentery (caused by the protozoan *Entamoeba histolytica*) showed that the herb has potent antibacterial and anti-protozoan properties, validating thousands of years of healing tradition. But garlic's antibiotic constituent remained a mystery until the 1920s, when researchers at Sandoz Pharmaceuticals in Switzerland isolated a compound called alliin (pronounced AL-lee-in).

Alliin by itself has no medicinal value, but when garlic is chewed, chopped, bruised, or crushed, the alliin comes in contact with the enzyme allinase. This transforms alliin into allicin, a chemical that's a powerful antibiotic.

Since the 1920s, garlic's broad-spectrum antibiotic properties have been confirmed in dozens of animal and human studies. Garlic kills the bacteria that cause tuberculosis (*Mycobacterium tuberculosis*), food poisoning (salmonella), and women's bladder infections (*Escherichia coli*). The herb may also fend off the influenza virus.

Chinese researchers report success in using garlic to treat 21 cases of cryptococcal meningitis, an often fatal fungal infection. Several studies have also shown the herb to be effective in treating the fungi that cause athlete's foot (*Trichophyton mentagrophytes*) and vaginal yeast infections (*Candida albicans*).

Commission E, the expert panel that evaluates herbal medicines for the German counterpart of the FDA, recognizes garlic's antibiotic value.

THE COMMON COLD. In addition to its effects against bacteria and fungi, garlic also has antiviral action. British scientists gave 146 healthy volunteers either a daily placebo or a commercial garlic supplement rich in allicin. After 12 weeks, the garlic group reported significantly fewer colds, and the colds they developed resolved more quickly.

ULCERS. Most ulcers are caused by the bacterium *Helicobacter pylori*. In one study, garlic significantly inhibited the germ's growth. The researchers estimate that two cloves of garlic a day may provide significant protection against *H. pylori* infection.

HIGH CHOLESTEROL. More than a dozen journal reports document garlic's ability to reduce cholesterol levels. In one study published in the British medical journal *Lancet*, researchers had volunteers eat a meal containing about 4 ounces of butter, which raises cholesterol. Half of the volunteers also ate about nine cloves of garlic. After 3 hours, the average cholesterol level among those who didn't consume garlic increased by 7 percent. Among those who did consume garlic, average cholesterol decreased by 7 percent. The researchers concluded that "garlic has a very significant protective action [against high cholesterol]."

Two groups of researchers—one Australian, the other American—have published analyses of a selection of garlic-cholesterol studies. The Australian team reviewed 16 trials involving 952 people with high cholesterol. They concluded that a daily dose of either one fresh clove or 1 gram of a dried high-allicin preparation can reduce total cholesterol levels by about 12 percent.

Meanwhile, the American team reviewed five rigorous trials involving 365 people. They concluded that a daily dose of either one fresh clove or 1 gram of a dried high-allicin preparation can lower total cholesterol levels by about 9 percent.

Experts estimate that for every 1 percent decrease in total cholesterol, the risk of heart attack drops 2 percent. Going by the results of the Australian and American analyses, daily garlic consumption may reduce heart attack risk by as much as 24 percent.

Over the years, a few highly publicized

studies have found that garlic has no effect on cholesterol. These reports have been criticized for poor methodology. The scientific consensus is that garlic lowers cholesterol, and Commission E endorses it for that purpose.

Most recently (2007), British researchers analyzed 13 trials and found that garlic produces a "modest" reduction in cholesterol, less than that found in previous analyses. Nonetheless, it affirms that garlic does, indeed, lower cholesterol. So what if it does not work as well as the pharmaceuticals? Compared with drugs, it's safer and substantially less expensive. If you take cholesterol medication, ask your doctor about including garlic in your treatment program.

HIGH BLOOD PRESSURE. Several studies dating back to the Sandoz Pharmaceuticals experiments confirm garlic's ability to reduce blood pressure in animals and humans. The 2007 British report just mentioned analyzed 10 studies of garlic's effect on blood pressure. The researchers found that garlic reduces blood pressure significantly. In 2008, Australian researchers analyzed 11 studies. Their conclusion: Garlic reduces blood pressure significantly.

INTERNAL BLOOD CLOTS. These are the pernicious clots that trigger heart attacks and most strokes. Garlic has anticoagulant action that helps prevent them. One researcher describes the herb as "at least as potent as aspirin," a standard anti-clotting heart attack preventive.

HEART ATTACK AND STROKE. Garlic continues to be controversial for cardiovascular health. Every time a study shows that it reduces cholesterol only slightly or not at all, critics say: "See, it just doesn't work." But that's shortsighted. There's more to garlic than its ability to lower cholesterol, whatever that effect ultimately turns out to be. No medication simultaneously reduces cholesterol, blood pressure, and the risk of internal blood clot formation. Garlic does all three. If you want to reduce your risk of heart attack and stroke, eat more garlic.

In addition to reducing the risk of developing heart disease, garlic also helps treat the condition, even when it's advanced. German researchers gave 152 people with severe heart disease either medically inactive placebos or 900 milligrams of a standardized powdered garlic preparation (Kwai). Four years later, those taking the placebos had 16 percent more arterial narrowing. Among those taking the garlic, however, arterial blockages actually receded 3 percent.

CANCER. In addition to being an antibiotic, the allicin in garlic is a potent antioxidant. It helps prevent the cell damage that can set the stage for cancer. Many cell culture, animal, and human studies have shown that garlic helps protect against various cancers, especially those of the digestive tract, notably stomach and colon cancers.

In the Iowa Women's Health Study, researchers have been tracking the diet, lifestyle, and health status of 41,387 middle-aged Iowa women for many years. They have found that the women who eat the most garlic are the least likely to develop colon cancer. Eating just a few cloves a week has cut their risk by 35 percent. Greater consumption lowers their risk even more.

Generally, eating fruits and vegetables helps protect against cancer, but in this study, of all the plant foods analyzed, garlic yielded the greatest preventive benefits.

In the Netherlands Cohort Study, Dutch researchers have been following a group of more than 120,000 middle-aged men and women for many years. The research has shown that as the participants' consumption of garlic's close relative, onion, increases, their risk of stomach cancer significantly decreases.

Meanwhile, a study of 1,800 Chinese found that those most likely to develop stomach cancer eat the least garlic. The researchers concluded that a diet high in garlic "can significantly reduce risk of stomach cancer."

DIABETES. Garlic reduces blood sugar levels in both laboratory animals and humans. Diabetes is a serious condition that requires professional treatment, but if you have it, there's no harm in increasing your garlic consumption in combination with your standard therapy.

LEAD POISONING. European studies show that garlic helps eliminate lead and other toxic heavy metals from the body. Lead interferes with thinking and causes other serious medical problems. Children are particularly susceptible to its effects. Add liberal amounts of garlic to spaghetti sauces and other foods that kids enjoy.

Intriguing Possibilities

Alopecia areata is a condition that causes substantial hair loss. Iranian researchers gave 40 people with hair loss from this condition either a topical placebo gel or a garlic gel (applied twice daily). After 3 months, the garlic group experienced significantly greater hair regrowth.

Garlic may also help prevent a common male health problem. Italian scientists surveyed 2,820 middle-aged men, about half of whom had benign prostate enlargement. Those who ate the most garlic and onions had the lowest risk.

Modern research also reveals that ancient

Ayurvedic healers were on to something when they used garlic to treat leprosy, now called Hansen's disease. In one study, Indian researchers gave people with Hansen's an ointment made with garlic as well as foods containing large amounts of the herb. Compared with people in the study who did not receive garlic treatment, those who did showed significant improvement.

Finally, in addition to anti-HIV medications, garlic helps treat AIDS. In one study, people with AIDS who ate a clove of garlic a day for 3 months experienced significant increases in the immune functions normally destroyed by the disease. Some saw chronic herpes sores clear up during treatment, while others with chronic diarrhea, a common AIDS symptom, also reported improvement.

Rx Recommendations

For minor skin infections, garlic juice applied externally may prove sufficient. Unless you're working with an experienced herbalist, however, you shouldn't rely exclusively on garlic to treat infectious diseases. No antibiotic, including garlic, kills all disease-causing microorganisms.

The standard medical approach is to conduct a "sensitivity test," in which several antibiotics are tested against the germ. The doctor then prescribes the antibiotic that works best. You might ask your physician to include garlic in a sensitivity test, or simply take it in addition to standard medication.

Researchers have found that 1 medium garlic clove packs the antibacterial punch of about 100,000 units of penicillin. Depending on the type of infection, oral penicillin doses typically range from 600,000 to 1.2 million units. The equivalent in garlic would be about 6 to 12 cloves. It's best to chew 3 cloves at a time two to four times a day.

To help reduce blood pressure, cholesterol, and the likelihood of blood clots, experts recommend eating 3 to 10 fresh cloves of garlic a day. The herb must be chewed, chopped, bruised, or crushed to transform its medicinally inert alliin into antibiotic allicin. Using fresh garlic is most medicinally effective, but the herb does retain some of its healing benefits when lightly cooked.

Raw garlic has a sharp, biting flavor, which cooking eliminates. Use it in foods to taste. (The cloves' papery skins peel easily if you smash them with the flat side of a cleaver.)

To prepare an infusion, put six chopped cloves in 1 cup of cool water and steep for 6 hours.

For a tincture, soak 1 cup of crushed cloves in 1 quart of brandy. Shake the mixture daily for 2 weeks, then take up to 3 tablespoons a day.

When using commercial preparations, follow the package directions.

What about the Smell?

Since 3000 B.C., the main drawback to garlic has been its odor. The stinking rose continues to bother some people.

However, garlic-rich Italian and Asian cuisines are very popular. Some of the nation's finest restaurants now proudly serve dishes heavily flavored with garlic.

In Gilroy, California, near Monterey, garlic is already the height of fashion. Gilroy is the garlic capital of America, and every year garlic lovers gather for the annual Garlic Festival, which features delights such as garlic soup, garlic cake, and garlic ice cream. A popular festival bumper sticker proclaims "Fight Mouthwash. Eat Garlic."

Still, most of us are a long way from promoting garlic breath. To eliminate it, try chewing a traditional herbal breath freshener such as parsley, fennel, or fenugreek.

Today, deodorized medicinal garlic preparations are available in health food stores and some drugstores. Many scientists believe that the herb's medicinal value comes from its odor-causing sulfur compounds, which has raised doubts about the medicinal effectiveness of deodorized garlic. Still, some studies have shown that even without the stink, garlic retains its healing benefits.

The Safety Factor

Garlic's anti-clotting action may help prevent heart attacks and some types of stroke, but medicinal amounts could conceivably cause problems for people with clotting disorders. If you have this type of disorder, or if you take any anticoagulant (blood-thinning) medication or supplement (vitamin E, for example), consult your physician before using garlic in medicinal amounts.

Garlic's genus name, *Allium*, comes from the Celtic word *all*, meaning "burning." Fresh garlic can cause a burning sensation in the mouth that some people find unpleasant.

Garlic has been used as a food and medicine for thousands of years, by people of all ages, including pregnant women. It has never been implicated in miscarriage or birth defects. However, garlic enters the milk of nursing mothers and may cause colic in infants.

Inform health care professionals of the herbs you use. Problematic herb-drug interactions are possible, particularly given garlic's anti-clotting action.

Garlic may cause allergic reactions or other unexpected side effects. Some people have reported getting rashes from touching or eating the herb. If garlic gives you a rash, don't eat it. Garlic-induced stomach upset has also been reported. Depending on the severity of your symptoms, reduce your dose or stop taking it.

For more on herb safety, see Chapter 2.

If symptoms get worse or persist longer than 2 weeks, consult a health care professional promptly.

Growing Information

Garlic grows easily from seeds or cloves. It's easier to start with cloves. Plant them 2 inches deep and 6 inches apart in early spring for harvesting in fall.

Garlic is cold-tolerant and can be planted up to 6 weeks before the final frost date. It thrives best in rich, deeply cultivated, well-drained soil. Do not overwater. Full sun produces the largest bulbs, but garlic tolerates some shade. During summer, cut back the flower stalks so the plant devotes all its energy to producing fat, aromatic bulbs.

Harvest bulbs in late summer and store them in a cool, dark place.

Take care not to bruise the bulbs, as bruising invites mold and insects. You can braid the leaves into a wreath or rope and display it in your kitchen, removing bulbs as needed.

GENTIAN

Feel Better with Bitter Moxie

Family: Gentianaceae; other members include other gentians and marsh felwort

Genus and species: *Gentiana lutea*

Also known as: Yellow gentian, bitter root, and bitterwort

Parts used: Roots

In Depression-era slang, "moxie" meant courage tinged with recklessness. Teddy Roosevelt, Charles Lindbergh, Al Capone—they all had moxie. The term comes from Moxie, a bitter soft drink available only in New England since the 1890s.

Moxie owes its bite to gentian root, a healing herb with a 3,000-year history as a digestive "bitter." Modern research shows that gentian does indeed stimulate digestion.

Healing History

Gentian was used by the ancient Egyptians, Greeks, and Romans as an appetite stimulant and antiseptic wound wash. The herb also served as a treatment for intestinal worms, digestive disorders, liver ailments, and "female hysteria" (menstrual discomforts).

Sixth-century Arab physicians adopted gentian from the Greeks and introduced its medicinal uses to Asia. Since then, Chinese physicians have prescribed the herb to treat digestive disorders, sore throat, headache, and arthritis. India's Ayurvedic physicians have recommended it for fevers, venereal diseases, and jaundice and other liver problems.

During the Middle Ages, European herbalists prized gentian because it caused less intestinal irritation than other digestive bitters.

Seventeenth-century English herbalist Nicholas Culpeper wrote that gentian "strengthens the stomach exceedingly, helps digestion, comforts the heart, helps agues [fevers] of all sorts, kills worms, and preserves against fainting and swooning. It provokes urine and terms [menstruation] exceedingly; therefore, let it not be given to women with child."

When colonists arrived in Virginia and the Carolinas, they met Native Americans who applied a root decoction of American gentian (*Gentiana puberula*) to relieve back pain.

America's 19th-century Eclectic physicians, forerunners of today's naturopaths, considered gentian a powerful tonic and prescribed it to "improve appetite and stimulate digestion." But their text *King's American Dispensatory* (1898) warned, "When taken in large doses, it is apt to oppress the stomach, irritate the bowels, and produce nausea, vomiting, and headache."

Gentian was listed in the *U.S. Pharmacopoeia*, a standard drug reference, from 1820 to 1955 as a digestive stimulant.

Before the introduction of hops, gentian root was an ingredient in beer brewing. The herb is still used in liqueurs, vermouths, and many digestive bitters popular in Europe.

In 1885, Augustin Thompson of Union, Maine, introduced his beverage Moxie Nerve Food, made with gentian. The original label proclaimed that the bitter brew cured "brain and nervous exhaustion, loss of manhood, helplessness, imbecility, and insanity"—claims that took a lot of moxie even in the pre-FDA heyday of patent medicines.

Thompson peddled Moxie on the road in classic patent-medicine style, and eventually it caught on—not as a medicine but as a beverage. That was fine with Thompson, who backed off from his medicinal claims and repositioned Moxie as a soft drink. For years, Moxie outsold Coca-Cola in New England. It's still available there, and gentian is still one of its ingredients.

In the 1930s, in her *Modern Herbal*, Maude Grieve called gentian "one of our most useful bitter tonics, especially in general debility, weakness of the digestive organs, or want of appetite. It is one of the best strengtheners of the human system." Contemporary herbalists echo Grieve. One suggests chewing gentian root as a substitute for smoking cigarettes.

Therapeutic Uses

While you can forget gentian for "loss of manhood, helplessness, imbecility, and insanity," the bitter root lives up to its ancient reputation as a digestive aid.

DIGESTIVE PROBLEMS. Gentian contains gentianine, a bitter-tasting compound that stimulates salivation and the secretion of stomach acid and bile, lending credence to the herb's 3,000-year history as a digestive aid. Try some before meals.

Commission E, the expert panel that evaluates herbal medicines for the German counterpart of the FDA, endorses gentian for loss of appetite and digestive complaints.

ARTHRITIS. Several studies have shown that gentian has anti-inflammatory action, suggesting that traditional Chinese physicians may have been on the right track when they prescribed the herb for arthritis. Try it if you have arthritis or any other inflammatory condition.

WOMEN'S HEALTH CONCERNS. Gentian has never been shown to stimulate the uterus. In fact, it relaxes smooth muscle tissue, the type of tissue that forms the uterus. Nonetheless, for hundreds of years, herbalists have considered gentian a powerful menstruation promoter. Pregnant women should err on the side of caution and not use it.

Rx Recommendations

Use a decoction or tincture of gentian to stimulate digestion. Either form is also appropriate for treating arthritis or bringing on menstruation.

To make a decoction, boil 1 teaspoon of powdered root in 3 cups of water for 30 minutes, then strain if you wish and let cool. Take 1 tablespoon before meals. Gentian tastes very bitter, so you may want to add sugar or honey.

As a homemade tincture, take $1/4$ to 1 teaspoon before meals.

When using commercial preparations, follow the package directions.

The Safety Factor

Gentian digestive bitters are popular in Germany, where herbal medicine is considerably more mainstream than in the United States. German physicians discourage the herb's use by people with high blood pressure. They also echo the Eclectics' warning that large amounts may cause stomach irritation, with possible nausea and vomiting.

Pregnant and nursing women should not use gentian.

Do not give gentian to children under 2. It may taste too bitter for older children. But if they can tolerate it, adjust the recommended dose based on the child's weight. For example, give a 50-pound child one-third of the dose a 150-pound adult would take.

If you're over 65, start with a low dose, and increase only if necessary.

Inform health care professionals of the herbs you use. Problematic herb-drug interactions are possible.

Gentian may cause allergic reactions or other unexpected side effects. If any develop, reduce your dose or stop taking it.

For more on herb safety, see Chapter 2.

If symptoms get worse or persist longer than 2 weeks, consult a health care professional promptly.

Growing Information

Gentian is a striking 6-foot perennial with branching medicinal roots; deeply veined, pointed oval leaves; and large, beautiful yellow flowers.

Once established, the plant requires little care other than abundant water and shelter from wind and excessive sun. But establishing gentian can be a problem. The seeds need frost to germinate, and even with frost, germination may take a year, if it occurs at all. Most authorities recommend using root cuttings instead.

Gentian prefers rich, loamy, slightly acidic soil. An annual dressing of peat moss helps. Harvest the roots in late summer. Desirable roots are dark reddish brown, tough, and flexible, with a strong, unpleasant odor. They should taste rather sweet initially, then very bitter. Dry the roots, then powder them.

GINGER

Put a Stop to Motion Sickness and Morning Sickness

Family: Zingiberaceae; other members include turmeric and cardamom

Genus and species: *Zingiber officinale*

Also known as: Jamaican, African, and Cochin (Asian) ginger

Parts used: Rhizomes (commonly called roots)

An old Indian proverb says, "Every good quality is contained in ginger." That's not much of an exaggeration.

Fleshy and aromatic, ginger has played a role in cooking and healing since the dawn of history. Modern science has supported some of its traditional medicinal uses, most notably its remarkable ability to prevent the nausea of motion sickness and morning sickness.

Researchers have discovered that the herb has other therapeutic benefits as well.

Healing History

Ancient Indians used their native ginger in cooking, to preserve food, and to treat digestive problems. They also considered the herb a physical and spiritual cleanser. Indians shunned strong-smelling garlic and onions before religious celebrations for fear of offending their deities, but they ate lots of ginger because it left them smelling sweet and therefore presentable to the gods.

Ginger figured prominently in China's first great herbal, the *Pen Tsao Ching* (*Classic of Herbs*), which was reportedly compiled by the mythical emperor-sage Shen Nung around 3000 B.C. As the story goes, the wise herbalist tested hundreds of medicinal herbs on himself—until he took a little too much of a poisonous herb and died.

Shen Nung recommended ginger for colds, fever, chills, tetanus, and leprosy. The *Pen Tsao Ching* also echoed Indian practice, saying that fresh ginger "eliminates body odor and puts a person in touch with the spiritual [realm]."

Over time, Chinese women began taking ginger for menstrual discomforts. Then they noticed that the herb relieved the nausea of morning sickness. Chinese sailors adopted ginger to prevent seasickness by chewing the root while at sea. Chinese physicians prescribed it to treat arthritis, ulcers, and kidney problems.

The Chinese also consider ginger an antidote to shellfish poisoning. This is why Chinese fish and seafood dishes are often seasoned with the herb.

Ancient Greek traders learned of the Asian practice of using ginger as a nausea-preventing digestive aid. They brought the herb to Greece, where, after big meals, it was wrapped in sweetened bread and eaten as a stomach-settling dessert. Eventually, the Greeks began baking the herb into the sweet bread, and the herbal seasickness remedy evolved into the world's first cookie, gingerbread.

The Romans also used ginger as a digestive aid. After the fall of Rome, however, the herb became scarce in Europe and quite costly.

Once renewed Asian trade made ginger more available, European demand proved almost insatiable. The ancient Greeks' modest gingerbread cakes evolved into sugary gingerbread men and elaborate confections like the witch's gingerbread house in *Hansel and Gretel*.

In England and her American colonies, ginger was incorporated into a stomach-soothing drink called ginger beer, the forerunner of today's ginger ale. Ginger ale is still a popular home remedy for diarrhea, nausea, and vomiting.

America's 19th-century Eclectic physicians, forerunners of today's naturopaths, prescribed ginger powder, tea, wine, and beer for infant diarrhea, indigestion, nausea, dysentery, flatulence, fever, headache, toothache, and "female hysteria" (menstrual complaints).

Contemporary herbalists recommend ginger for colds, flu, and motion sickness and as a digestive aid.

Therapeutic Uses

Break out the gingerbread and ginger ale. Scientific research has lent support to some of ginger's traditional uses—and has revealed even more benefits.

MOTION SICKNESS AND MORNING SICKNESS. The ancient Chinese were right.

Ginger does indeed prevent the nausea associated with seasickness and other types of motion sickness, as well as the morning sickness of pregnancy.

Ginger's anti-nausea action first received scientific validation in 1982 in a study conducted by researchers at Brigham Young University and published in the British medical journal *Lancet*. The researchers gave 36 volunteers with a history of motion sickness either 100 milligrams of the popular anti–motion sickness drug dimenhydrinate (Dramamine) or 940 milligrams of ginger powder. A short time later, the participants were seated in a computerized rocking chair programmed to move in such a way that it would trigger motion sickness. The chair was equipped with a switch that allowed its riders to stop the movement when they began to feel nauseated.

Compared with the people who had taken Dramamine, those who had taken ginger were able to stay in the chair 57 percent longer. Based on their finding, the researchers also recommended ginger capsules, ginger tea, or ginger ale for morning sickness.

Since that study, many others have confirmed ginger's value for the prevention of motion and morning sickness. Here's a small sampling.

* Swedish Navy researchers gave ginger to 80 naval cadets who were sailing in turbulent seas. Compared with a group that took medically inactive placebos, those who took ginger experienced 72 percent less seasickness.

* British surgeons gave 60 women about to have gynecological surgery either ginger or the prescription anti-nausea drug metoclopramide (Reglan). Those who received ginger experienced significantly less postsurgical nausea and vomiting.

* Danish researchers gave 30 pregnant women, all battling morning sickness, either ginger or placebos for 4 days. Then the women switched treatments for 4 days. While taking ginger, 70 percent of the study participants reported significant relief from nausea. Doctors discourage moms-to-be from taking any drugs, including anti-nausea medications, but ginger is safe to use during pregnancy.

* Italian researchers asked all of the passengers boarding a cruise ship if they were prone to seasickness. Sixty reported a history of the condition. The ship's doctor gave these people either a standard dose of Dramamine or ginger (500 milligrams before embarking and 500 milligrams every 4 hours during 2 days of rough seas). Among those taking Dramamine, 50 percent reported "very good" or "excellent" results. Among those taking ginger, the figure rose to 70 percent.

* Another group of Italian researchers studied 28 children who took a 2-day class trip that involved travel by car, boat, and airplane. All were given either a standard children's dose of Dramamine or ginger (for those younger than 6, 250 milligrams before departure and every 4 hours thereafter; for those 6 and older, 500 milligrams). A physician rated their motion sickness symptoms. Among those who took Dramamine, 31 percent showed "good" benefits, while 69 percent demonstrated "modest" benefits. Among those who took ginger, 100 percent had "good" results.

Commission E, the expert panel that evaluates herbal medicines for the German counterpart of the FDA, endorses ginger for the prevention and treatment of motion sickness. In addition, many cancer specialists recommend it for the nausea associated with chemotherapy.

DIGESTIVE PROBLEMS. Ginger is a gastrointestinal antispasmodic. It prevents indigestion and abdominal cramping by soothing the muscles that line the intestines. It also contains some compounds similar to digestive enzymes that break down proteins. Commission E approves ginger to prevent and treat indigestion.

HEART DISEASE AND STROKE. Few people in the ancient world lived long enough— or combined a high-fat diet with a sedentary lifestyle—to develop heart disease or stroke. Today, these conditions account for half of all deaths in the United States.

Ginger may help prevent heart disease and stroke by controlling three key risk factors. The herb helps reduce cholesterol levels, according to a study published in the *New England Journal of Medicine*. It also helps lower blood pressure, and it prevents the blood clots that trigger heart attacks and most strokes.

ULCERS. Research confirms the ancient Chinese practice of using ginger to treat ulcers. In experiments involving animals that were given drugs known to produce ulcers, pre-treatment with a ginger preparation acted as a preventive.

Ginger does not cure ulcers, nor has it been well researched in humans. But a small pilot study, in which 10 people with ulcers took 6 grams of ginger a day, showed that the herb can help relieve symptoms.

ARTHRITIS. Studies have identified anti-inflammatory substances in ginger, lending support to the herb's traditional use in treating arthritis.

WOMEN'S HEALTH CONCERNS. Anti-spasmodics soothe not only the digestive tract but also other smooth muscles, such as the uterus. As an antispasmodic, ginger may help ease menstrual cramps.

COLDS AND FLU. Chinese studies show that ginger helps kill influenza virus, and an Indian report found that the herb increases the immune system's ability to fight infection. These findings lend some support to ginger's traditional role in treating colds, flu, and other infectious illnesses.

Intriguing Possibilities

In animal studies, ginger reduces blood sugar levels, suggesting that the herb may help control diabetes.

Other animal studies have shown that ginger promotes the shrinkage of tumors. While these findings don't necessarily apply to humans, ginger may someday find a role in the treatment of cancer. And if you have cancer, there's no harm in using ginger in consultation with your doctor.

Rx Recommendations

Use ginger to taste in cooking to create warm, spicy, aromatic dishes.

For motion sickness, the recommended dose of ginger is 1,000 milligrams approximately 30 minutes before travel. Commercial capsules are usually most convenient, but you'll easily get that amount from a 12-ounce container of ginger ale, provided that it's made with real ginger and not artificial flavor. Check the label to be sure.

You can also drink 2 cups of ginger infusion. To make it, use 2 teaspoons of powdered or fresh grated root per cup of boiling water, steep for 10 minutes, and strain if you wish.

To ease other digestive upsets or to treat colds or flu, make an infusion. To help relieve arthritis or prevent heart disease and stroke, use the herb in cooking or drink ginger ale or ginger tea.

You may give weak ginger preparations to children under age 2 for colic.

The Safety Factor

Ginger's anti-nausea effects may prevent morning sickness, but the herb has a long history as a menstruation promoter. Might it cause miscarriage? One study suggests that its uterine effects depend on the amount used.

In the study published in *Lancet* that was previously mentioned, less than 1 gram of ginger was needed to prevent nausea. To trigger menstruation, Chinese physicians recommend 20 to 28 grams. A strong cup of ginger tea contains about 500 milligrams, and an 8-ounce glass of ginger ale contains approximately 1,000 milligrams. None of these come close to the amount that promotes menstruation.

There have been no reports in the scientific literature of ginger triggering abortion or causing birth defects. Pregnant women with no history of miscarriage should feel free to try modest amounts of ginger tea or ginger ale to treat morning sickness.

Ginger is on the FDA list of herbs generally regarded as safe. For adults, ginger is safe when used in the amounts typically recommended.

You should use medicinal amounts of ginger only in consultation with your physician.

Although ginger generally relieves indigestion, some people who take it to prevent motion sickness report heartburn. If you experience heartburn or other minor discomfort after taking the herb, reduce the dosage or stop using it altogether. Let your doctor know if you experience any unpleasant effects or if the symptoms for which you're taking the herb do not improve significantly within 2 weeks.

Growing Information

Ginger is a tropical perennial that grows from a tuberous underground stem, or rhizome. Each year, the plant produces a round, 3-foot stem with thin, pointed, lance-shaped, 6-inch leaves and a single, large, yellow and purple flower.

Ginger grows outdoors in Hawaii, Florida, southern California, New Mexico, Arizona, and Texas. It does best when well-watered in partial shade in raised beds deeply cultivated with composted manure and kelp.

Ginger is propagated from young fresh roots, which contain eyes similar to those in potatoes. The ginger root sold in most supermarkets, with tough, tan skin, is neither young nor fresh, so its propagation potential is low. The best place to obtain growable ginger root is at an Asian specialty market, although some nurseries carry it as well. Look for roots with light green skin.

Plant the roots about 3 inches deep and 12 inches apart. After 12 months, uproot the plant, harvest some roots, and replant the rest.

You can also grow ginger indoors in deep pots with a soil mixture of loam, sand, compost, and peat moss. Indoors, it needs warmth, plenty of water, and high humidity. A greenhouse environment is best.

GINKGO

For Alzheimer's Disease and Many Other Conditions

Family: Ginkgoaceae; no other members

Genus and species: *Ginkgo biloba*

Also known as: Maidenhair tree

Parts used: Leaves

Ginkgo is the oldest surviving tree on Earth, a relic of the dinosaur age that first appeared some 200 million years ago. Individual trees can survive for up to 1,000 years.

Appropriately enough, as a healing herb, ginkgo aids the oldest surviving people. It helps prevent and treat many conditions associated with aging, including Alzheimer's disease, stroke, heart disease, deafness, blindness, memory loss, and erectile dysfunction.

Healing History

The ginkgo tree is considered sacred throughout Asia, where it is often planted around Buddhist temples. Ginkgo was deemed "good for the heart and lungs" in China's first great herbal, the *Pen Tsao Ching* (*The Classic of Herbs*), attributed to the mythical emperor-sage Shen Nung around 3000 B.C.

Traditional Chinese physicians used ginkgo to treat asthma and chilblains, swelling of the hands and feet due to damp cold. The ancient Chinese and Japanese ate roasted ginkgo seeds as a digestive aid and to prevent drunkenness. Even today, some bars in Japan serve the roasted seeds to prevent intoxication.

India's traditional Ayurvedic healers associated ginkgo with long life. They reportedly used the herb as an ingredient in soma, a longevity elixir.

Ginkgo trees were introduced into Europe in 1730. Today, they're popular street and park trees throughout the temperate world. But even though 18th-century horticulturists planted them throughout Europe, herbalists of that time ignored them. As a result, ginkgo's fan-shaped leaves have no history in Western herbal medicine.

Thanks to recent research, however, ginkgo has become one of the top-selling medicinal herbs in the United States and Europe, with sales approaching $1 billion annually. It is particularly popular in Europe, where it ranks among the most widely prescribed medications. An increasing number of older Americans take it as well.

Therapeutic Uses

There are two reasons for the medical excitement over ginkgo. First, the herb contains potent antioxidant compounds (ginkgo flavone glycosides and terpene lactones). Antioxidants help prevent and reverse the cell damage at the root of many degenerative conditions associated with aging, including heart disease, stroke, many cancers, and Alzheimer's disease.

In addition, ginkgo interferes with the action of a compound produced by the body, platelet activation factor (PAF). Discovered in 1972, PAF is involved in an enormous number of biological processes, including arterial bloodflow, asthma attacks, organ graft rejection, and the blood clots involved in heart attacks and most strokes.

ALZHEIMER'S DISEASE AND MULTI-INFARCT DEMENTIA (MID). In the United States, ginkgo made its biggest splash in 1997, when the *Journal of the American Medical Association* published a study by researchers at Albert Einstein College of Medicine in the Bronx, New York. It showed that ginkgo not only slows mental deterioration in people with Alzheimer's disease but, in some cases, actually improves their cognitive abilities.

The researchers gave 202 people in various stages of Alzheimer's either a medically inactive placebo or 120 milligrams per day of a standardized ginkgo extract. After 1 year, compared with those who received the placebo, participants who took ginkgo retained significantly more mental function.

Many other studies have corroborated ginkgo's effectiveness for slowing the progression of Alzheimer's. Here's a sampling of the research to date:

♣ European researchers gave 60 people with Alzheimer's disease either a placebo or 120-milligram or 240-milligram doses of ginkgo per day. After 3 months, compared with the placebo-takers, both ginkgo groups performed significantly better on cognitive function tests.

♣ Another European team gave 156 people with either Alzheimer's or multi-infarct dementia (MID, an Alzheimer's-like condition caused by mini-strokes) either a placebo or 240 milligrams of ginkgo per day. Six months later, the group taking ginkgo retained greater cognitive function.

♣ German researchers gave 404 people with mild to moderate Alzheimer's or MID either a placebo or 240 milligrams of ginkgo a day. After 6 months, the ginkgo group showed better cognitive function, fewer behavior problems (wandering, anxiety, angry outbursts, etc.), and greater ability to perform activities of daily living.

In all of these studies, the response to ginkgo was similar to what physicians would expect from the pharmaceuticals currently approved to slow the progression of Alzheimer's or MID. It's still not entirely clear how ginkgo ameliorates these conditions, but the fact that the herb is a powerful antioxidant and it improves bloodflow through the brain could play a role.

Commission E, the expert panel that evaluates herbal medicines for the German counterpart of the FDA, approves ginkgo for the treatment of Alzheimer's disease and MID.

Currently, no treatment, either pharmaceutical or herbal, permanently halts or reverses the progression of Alzheimer's disease or MID. But ginkgo slows the progression of these conditions as well as pharmaceuticals and causes few, if any, side effects.

CEREBRAL INSUFFICIENCY. As people get older, bloodflow through the brain tends to decline, a condition known as cerebral insufficiency. This slows reaction time and impairs memory, concentration, and problem-solving ability—effects called "senior moments." Many studies show that ginkgo improves bloodflow through the brain and, as a result, reduces symptoms of cerebral insufficiency.

MEMORY LOSS. Animal studies have found that ginkgo improves memory. Human trials have shown similar results.

- A team of European researchers gave 241 otherwise healthy elderly people who had memory problems either a placebo or ginkgo. After 6 months, those taking the herb showed memory improvement.

- British researchers gave 31 middle-aged people who reported memory problems either a placebo or 120 milligrams of ginkgo per day. After 6 months, the ginkgo group showed significant improvement in memory and reaction time.

- In another English study, researchers tested the short-term memory skills and reaction times of eight women in their twenties and thirties before and after they were given either a placebo or 600 milligrams of ginkgo. Both memory and reaction time improved "very significantly" after the women took the herb.

Commission E approves ginkgo as a treatment for memory problems.

STROKE. As bloodflow through the brain decreases with age, the blood delivers less food and oxygen to brain cells. If bloodflow becomes blocked, the result is a stroke, the third leading cause of death in the United States. In Europe, ginkgo is widely prescribed to support recovery from stroke. Commission E approves the herb for stroke treatment and rehabilitation.

HEART DISEASE. Ginkgo improves bloodflow not only through the brain but also through the heart muscle, according to Chinese researchers. It contains antioxidants that help prevent heart disease. It reduces blood pressure. And it helps prevent the blood clots that trigger heart attacks. These findings add up to reducing the risk of heart disease. A French study hints that treating heart patients with ginkgo may speed their recovery from coronary artery bypass surgery.

INTERMITTENT CLAUDICATION (IC). When cholesterol deposits narrow the arteries in the legs, the result is intermittent claudication, which causes pain, cramping, and weakness, particularly in the calves. Ginkgo improves bloodflow through the legs, thus relieving IC symptoms.

German researchers gave a standard medication or ginkgo to 36 people with IC. After a year, the herb produced significantly greater pain relief. Another German team measured how far people with IC could walk before developing leg pain. Then the participants began taking either a placebo or ginkgo. After 6 months, the placebo group showed scant improvement, while those taking ginkgo were able to walk 50 percent farther.

Commission E approves ginkgo as a treatment for intermittent claudication.

ERECTILE DYSFUNCTION (ED). A study published in the *Journal of Urology* shows that ginkgo helps relieve ED caused by narrowing of the arteries that supply blood to the penis. In the study, 60 men with ED caused by impaired penile bloodflow were instructed to take 60 milligrams of ginkgo per day. After 1 year, half of the men reported significant erection improvement.

ANTIDEPRESSANT-RELATED SEXUAL PROBLEMS. Pharmaceutical antidepressants work. Unfortunately, some often cause sex problems: ED in men, loss of vaginal lubrication in women, and in both sexes, loss of libido and difficulty with orgasm. At the University of California, San Francisco, an elderly man taking antidepressants who also used ginkgo for his memory told his doctor that the herb seemed to give him a sexual boost. This comment led to a study of ginkgo's effects in 63 people who were experiencing antidepressant-related sex problems. In addition to their medications, the patients took 207 milligrams of ginkgo daily. Ninety-one percent of the women and 76 percent of the men reported significant improvement: enhanced sexual desire, greater ability to have erections or produce lubrication, and generally more pleasurable sex.

In this study, the researchers didn't test ginkgo against a placebo, so the study was not scientifically rigorous. Placebos usually benefit about one-third of those who use them. But the response rate in this study was much greater than a typical placebo response, strongly suggesting that ginkgo has real ability to relieve antidepressant-related sexual problems.

ANXIETY. Because ginkgo reduces anxiety in people with Alzheimer's, German researchers wondered if it might do the same for nondemented older adults with anxiety problems. They gave 107 anxious elders either a placebo or 240 milligrams or 480 milligrams of ginkgo per day. After 4 weeks, both ginkgo groups showed significantly less anxiety.

MACULAR DEGENERATION. Macular degeneration is a leading cause of adult blindness. It involves the deterioration of the macula, the part of the eye's nerve-rich retina responsible for central vision (what you see when you look straight ahead). In a French study, people with macular degeneration who took ginkgo experienced "significant vision improvement."

DIABETIC RETINOPATHY. Another leading cause of adult blindness, this complication of diabetes involves substantially reduced bloodflow through the retina. Researchers in Taiwan gave 25 people with retinopathy from type 2 diabetes either a placebo or 240 milligrams of ginkgo daily. After 3 months, the ginkgo group showed improved retinal bloodflow.

COCHLEAR DEAFNESS. Researchers believe that cochlear deafness results from decreased bloodflow to the nerves involved in hearing. A French study that compared ginkgo with standard therapy showed significant improvement in both groups, but greater benefit in the ginkgo group.

CHRONIC DIZZINESS (VERTIGO). French researchers gave 70 people with vertigo either a placebo or ginkgo. After 3 months, 18 percent of the placebo group no longer felt dizzy, compared with 47 percent of the ginkgo group. Statistically, this is a highly significant difference. Commission E approves ginkgo as a treatment for vertigo.

MENTAL FUNCTION IN HEALTHY ADULTS? In one study mentioned on page 246, ginkgo improved memory in healthy young adults. A few other studies also show that ginkgo provides cognitive benefits in healthy adults, including one German report of a 30 percent decrease in errors among middle-aged people who worked on computers. However, British researchers analyzed 15 studies of ginkgo in healthy—that is, nondemented—adults and found little evidence of benefit. This issue remains unresolved. But ginkgo causes few side effects. If you'd like to try it, feel free.

CHRONIC RINGING IN THE EARS (TINNITUS)? A 13-month French study involving 103 people deemed ginkgo "conclusively effective" for chronic tinnitus. According to the researchers, the herb improved the condition in all of the patients who took it. Commission E approves ginkgo as a treatment for tinnitus. However, other studies have shown no benefit. Ginkgo's effect on tinnitus remains to be determined. But if you have this condition, it can't hurt to try the herb.

Intriguing Possibilities

There may be some truth to the age-old Asian belief that ginkgo helps prevent drunkenness. Japanese researchers have discovered an enzyme in ginkgo seeds that accelerates the body's metabolism of alcohol. Faster metabolism means less alcohol in the bloodstream and less likelihood of intoxication. Some bars in Japan serve roasted ginkgo seeds with drinks to minimize intoxication. Of course, consuming roasted ginkgo seeds is no substitute for responsible drinking.

In other research, ginkgo has shown possible benefit in relieving symptoms of multiple sclerosis. In a pilot study, researchers at the University of North Carolina, at Charlotte, gave either a placebo or 240 milligrams of ginkgo daily to 22 people with MS. After 4 weeks, the ginkgo group showed "significant" decreases in fatigue and symptom severity, and improved ability to perform activities of daily living.

Finally, preliminary reports also suggest that ginkgo may improve immune function. It may also be effective against allergies, high blood pressure, migraines, kidney problems, and dyslexia in children.

Rx Recommendations

The medicinal compounds in ginkgo leaves occur in concentrations too small for infusions or tinctures to provide any benefit. Commercial preparations use a concentrated 50:1 extract; in other words, 50 pounds of leaves are processed into 1 pound of standardized extract containing 24 percent ginkgo flavone glycosides and 6 percent terpene lactones.

Buy a standardized ginkgo product and take it according to the package directions. Most studies have used doses of 120 or 240 milligrams a day, typically divided into three doses—40 or 80 milligrams three times a day.

The Safety Factor

Bleeding hazard? Platelet activation factor plays a role in blood clotting. Ginkgo's PAF-inhibiting action may cause problems for people with clotting disorders and those taking anticoagulant (blood-thinning) medications. Several cases of hemorrhage have been reported in people taking ginkgo. As a result, surgeons have placed it on the list of herbs that should not be taken for at least 2 weeks before scheduled surgery.

But how much of a bleeding hazard is ginkgo? Not much, it turns out. British researchers analyzed 12 case reports and called the case for ginkgo as a hemorrhage risk "far from compelling."

The most convincing evidence that ginkgo is not a bleeding hazard, however, comes from a German analysis of a database that has tracked reactions among 5 million Germans who have filled 75 million prescriptions, including 320,644 who took ginkgo from 1999 to 2002. The researchers calculated the number of problematic bleeding episodes per 100 years of observation. When taking no medication at all, this group experienced 1.63 bleeding episodes per 100 years. When taking any medication, the figure was 3.51. When taking other Alzheimer's drugs, 1.44. When taking ginkgo, less than 1.0. In other words, ginkgo is *less* of a bleeding hazard than drugs in general and specifically other Alzheimer's medications. The authors suggest that ginkgo has been falsely accused of causing bleeding problems. Unfortunately, once erroneous information gets into the medical literature, it's very difficult to correct. Undoubtedly, ginkgo will continue to be called a bleeding hazard and surgeons will continue to urge people to stop taking it before surgery. But the best evidence shows that ginkgo is not a significant bleeding hazard.

No serious side effects have been associated with ginkgo in any study to date, but mild side effects such as stomach upset, headache, and rash are possible. Some people who take large doses have reported irritability, restlessness, diarrhea, nausea, and vomiting. Allergic reactions or other unexpected side effects are also possible. If any develop, reduce your dose or stop taking this herb.

Pregnant and nursing women should not use ginkgo.

There is no reason to give ginkgo to children, except as a treatment for dyslexia.

Inform health care professionals of the herbs you use. Problematic herb-drug interactions are possible.

For more on herb safety, see Chapter 2.

Growing Information

Ginkgo is a stately, deciduous tree that reaches 100 feet with a 20-foot girth. Its flat, fan-shaped leaves have two lobes, hence its Latin species name, *biloba*. Ginkgoes are dioecious—that is, male and female flowers appear on different trees. The females produce apricot-size, orange-yellow fruits that contain edible seeds.

Ginkgoes are attractive street or yard trees that can be grown throughout much of the United States. If you'd like to plant them for ornamental purposes, obtain saplings from a nursery in your area. Plant only males, however, since the fruits produced by female trees are messy and foul-smelling.

Plant saplings in well-drained soil and stake them to ensure straight growth. Young trees are oddly proportioned and often look gawky, but they become stately with age. Water regularly until the trees are about 20 feet tall. After that, they are self-sufficient.

Ginkgoes are resistant to insects and disease and grow up to 2 feet per year. In autumn, the leaves turn a beautiful gold color before they fall.

GINSENG

Asia's Revered Adaptogen

Family: Araliaceae; other members include ivy

Genus and species: *Panax ginseng*
(Chinese/Korean/Japanese); *Panax
quinquefolius* (American)

Also known as: Man root, life root, root of
immortality, Tartar root, heal-all, 'seng, and
'sang

Parts used: Roots

Ginseng is fascinating—and controversial. The
root of an unassuming, ivylike ground cover,
this herb has been the subject of more than
1,500 books and scientific papers, yet its effects
continue to be debated.

Herbalists call ginseng the ultimate tonic, a
Chinese medical term that means a general
body strengthener. Western scientific supporters
call it an adaptogen, an herb that helps the
entire body resist physical and emotional challenges, combat illness, and stay healthy.

Critics have countered that no drug provides
the enormous variety of benefits claimed for ginseng, therefore advocates must be overstating
the herb's value. But in the 21st century, as an
increasing number of rigorous scientific studies
have confirmed ginseng's many benefits, blanket
dismissals of the herb—and other adaptogens,
notably, eleuthero (see page 201) and rhodiola
(see page 397)—have diminished. Still, critics
continue to take shots at ginseng, and not every
study supports it. But the weight of the evidence
clearly shows that this herb is among the most
powerful medicinal plants.

Healing History

Ginseng is not one herb but two: Chinese,
Korean, or Japanese (*Panax ginseng*) and American (*P. quinquefolius*). Chinese physicians make
distinctions between the two plants' effects, but
Western scientists generally consider them
equivalent.

Ginseng has a fleshy, multibranched root. If
you stretch your imagination, some roots
resemble the human form, with limblike
branches suggesting arms and legs. The ancient
Chinese called the plant man root, or *jen shen*,
which eventually entered English as "ginseng."

Ginseng figured prominently in the first
great Chinese herbal, the *Pen Tsao Ching* (*The
Classic of Herbs*), purportedly compiled by the
mythical emperor-sage Shen Nung around
3000 B.C. Shen Nung recommended the herb
for "enlightening the mind and increasing
wisdom," and noted that "continuous use leads
to longevity."

Ginseng's fancied resemblance to the human

form led to the belief in ancient China that it was a whole-body tonic. The Chinese were not alone in this type of thinking. In medieval Europe, doctors believed wholeheartedly in a medical philosophy called the Doctrine of Signatures, the belief that a plant's physical characteristics revealed its healing virtues.

Since ancient times, Chinese physicians have revered ginseng, particularly for the elderly. It was widely used to treat infirmities of old age, such as lethargy, arthritis, senility, menopausal complaints, and loss of sexual interest and ability. The Chinese, Koreans, and Japanese still consider ginseng among the best health promoters, though one of its common names, "root of immortality," stretches things a bit.

As the popularity of ginseng spread throughout ancient Asia, demand soared and rapacious collection decimated the wild supply. Chinese ginseng became increasingly rare and more valuable than gold. Unscrupulous merchants sold other roots as ginseng. (Adulteration is still a problem today.)

Unlike other Asian herbs that became favorites in the West (for example, ginger, cinnamon, and ephedra), ginseng remained relatively unknown in Europe until the 18th century, when missionaries in China informed early European botanists of its reputation as a longevity promoter. Europeans scoffed at this claim, but those familiar with Asia, particularly the Jesuits, who had missions in China, appreciated the herb's great value there.

In 1704, a French explorer returned to Paris with a sample of what turned out to be American ginseng from southern Canada. Jesuits in France alerted their brethren in Canada to its enormous value in China. Jesuits in Montreal shipped a boatload to Canton, where other Jesuits sold it to the Chinese for what was then a king's ransom, $5 a pound.

Immediately, Jesuits in Canada asked their Native American acolytes to find as much ginseng as they could. Soon tons of the herb were being shipped to China, and the Jesuits made a fortune while keeping the lucrative trade a secret for many years. Eventually, word leaked out that the celibate fathers seemed to take an unusual interest in a certain low-growing herb that was rumored to be an aphrodisiac in far-off Cathay.

Once ginseng's reputation spread, the herb was discovered growing wild as far south as Georgia. It enjoyed a brief burst of popularity among American colonists who were interested in sexual stimulation. Most were disappointed. Virginia plantation owner William Byrd sniffed that ginseng "frisks the spirits" but causes none "of those naughty effects that might make men too troublesome and impertinent to their wives."

America's "Ginseng Rush"

By the 1740s, few Americans were consuming ginseng, but news of the herb's incredible value in China hit the 13 colonies like news of the California gold strike 100 years later. Shipping agents circulated handbills offering to buy the herb for the then-fabulous sum of $1 a pound. Foragers scoured the countryside, and frontier scouts, surveyors, and fur trappers collected ginseng as a sideline to their other work. Ginseng quickly became the colonies' most valuable export—more precious pound for pound than even the rarest furs.

By the 1770s, ginseng fever had wiped out the plant along the Eastern seaboard, forcing collectors into the trackless wilderness across the Appalachians. The search for ginseng played a significant role in the exploration of western Pennsylvania, West Virginia, Kentucky, and Tennessee. One intrepid pioneer who combined trapping and scouting with ginseng collecting was none other than Daniel Boone. According to Scott Persons, author of *American Ginseng: Green Gold*, in 1788, a boat owned by Boone capsized in the Ohio River—and 12 tons of ginseng were lost.

Native Americans learned about ginseng from the Jesuits and used it to combat fatigue, stimulate appetite, and aid digestion. Some tribes mixed it into love potions.

America's 19th-century Eclectic physicians, forerunners of today's naturopaths, called ginseng a stimulant for "mental exhaustion from overwork" and prescribed it for loss of appetite, indigestion, asthma, laryngitis, bronchitis, and tuberculosis. The Eclectic textbook *King's American Dispensatory* (1898) added that the herb "invigorates the virile powers."

Contemporary herbalists echo the Chinese, recommending ginseng as a tonic stimulant that promotes vitality, longevity, virility, and resistance to stress and illness. Various experts estimate that Americans currently spend $500 million a year on ginseng products.

Wild American ginseng is officially an endangered species, but in Appalachia, collectors still forage for it. According to a *New York Times* report, wild American ginseng roots sell for $100 apiece and around $300 per pound. Most collectors never use the herb themselves. In the words of Georgia ginseng trader Jake Plott, "I never found it worth a damn for anything but to get money out of." Well, Jake, if you read the research, you'd feel differently.

"Tonic" in the East, "Adaptogen" in the West

The scientific literature shows that ginseng is reasonably safe and beneficial for many ailments, thanks to several compounds collectively known as ginsenosides. The ginsenosides' actions are not fully understood, and their effects can be downright confusing. For example, some stimulate the central nervous system, while others depress it. Some raise blood pressure, while others lower it. These observations need to be clarified through additional study, but researchers have already learned a great deal about the herb and its many effects.

Among the first Western scientists to seriously investigate ginseng were two Russian pharmacologists, N.V. Lazarev, Ph.D., and his student, Israel I. Brekhman, Ph.D., of the Academy of Sciences of the former Soviet Union. In 1947, they coined the term *adaptogen* to describe ginseng and other herbs that help the body resist physical and emotional stresses. They discovered that ginseng increases resistance to disease and exerts subtle but real generalized strengthening effects, while causing few, if any, side effects.

Dr. Brekhman and researchers in China, Korea, and Japan conducted hundreds of studies on ginseng; the results showed that ginseng combats fatigue (without caffeine), improves physical stamina, counteracts the damage caused by physical and emotional stress, prevents the depletion of stress-fighting adrenal hormones, and enhances memory. Dr. Brekhman came to concur with what traditional Asian herbalists had been saying for more than 1,000 years—that ginseng is a tonic. Eventually, the work of Dr. Brekhman and Asian ginseng researchers piqued the interest of Western scientists. Today, scientists around the world study ginseng. (Dr. Brekhman eventually focused on another plant, eleuthero, or *Eleutherococcus senticosus*, a less expensive adaptogen sometimes called Siberian ginseng. Eleuthero is *not* a ginseng, but it offers similar benefits. See page 201.)

"Adaptogens give the body a tune-up," says Salt Lake City herb researcher Daniel Mowrey, Ph.D.-"They help the cells produce energy and use it more efficiently. But adaptogens don't overpower the cells as drugs often do. Their effects are subtle, which accounts for the controversy these herbs arouse. Over time, adaptogenic herbs are very beneficial to health."

Adaptogenic Value

INCREASED ENERGY. Ginseng is a noncaffeine stimulant that helps counteract fatigue. European researchers studied 232 people between the ages of 25 and 60 who complained of persistent fatigue. Half were given a daily placebo, while the rest received a formula containing nine vitamins, eight minerals, and 80 milligrams of ginseng per day. After 7 weeks, all the participants were evaluated using standard tests of fatigue. The group taking the ginseng formula showed significantly less lethargy. The researchers concluded that ginseng combats fatigue by supporting the adrenal glands.

ENHANCED ATHLETIC PERFOR-MANCE. For decades, Russian, Chinese, and Korean Olympic athletes have used ginseng in their training. They take the herb before events in the belief that it improves stamina and performance, much like coffee (see page 164). Some American athletes have also adopted ginseng. Research shows that the herb does indeed enhance athletic performance.

Italian researchers gave 50 male physical education teachers between the ages of 21 and 47 either placebos or a combination of ginseng, vitamins, and minerals. Then they had the men run on treadmills. Subsequently, the two groups switched treatments, so the men who had taken the placebos received the ginseng formula, and vice versa. While they were using the ginseng, the men's stamina increased significantly because their hearts and lungs worked more efficiently.

IMPROVED MENTAL FUNCTION. Danish researchers gave 112 healthy middle-aged adults a battery of tests that assessed their memory, reaction times, and ability to learn, concentrate, and perform abstract reasoning. Then they gave the participants either a placebo or 400 milligrams of ginseng daily. After 9 weeks, those taking the ginseng showed significant improvement in two of the tests: reaction time and abstract thinking. In a similar Italian study, ginseng significantly improved attention, reaction time, and ability to do mental arithmetic.

ENHANCED IMMUNITY. In animal studies, Chinese researchers have found that ginseng revs up the white blood cells (macrophages and natural killer cells) that devour disease-causing microorganisms. Meanwhile, researchers at the University of Southern California in Los Angeles have demonstrated that ginseng spurs the production of interferon, the body's own virus-fighting compound. It also increases the synthesis of immune-boosting antibodies.

German researchers demonstrated ginseng's immune-enhancing action in a study involving 36 healthy volunteers who took either a placebo or ginseng (about 2 teaspoons of tincture three times a day). After 4 weeks, the ginseng group showed significantly more activated T-lympho-cytes (T-cells), another type of infection-fighting white blood cell.

Italian researchers gave people with chronic bronchitis either a placebo or 100 milligrams of ginseng every 12 hours for 8 weeks. The researchers periodically took respiratory mucus samples and analyzed them for macrophages, the white blood cells that engulf and devour invading germs. By the end of the study, the white blood cells of the people taking ginseng were signifi-cantly more active and killed more germs.

The same Italian team gave flu (influenza) shots to 227 adults. In addition, some took a pla-cebo while others took 100 milligrams of ginseng per day. Flu shots do not act directly on the flu virus. Rather, they stimulate an immune response that prevents the virus from causing infection. The researchers reasoned that if gin-seng enhances immune function, the herb should boost the effectivenesss of the flu vaccine. That's exactly what they found. After 3 months, the ginseng group was significantly less likely to develop flu. These results were confirmed by researchers at Eastern Virginia Medical School in Norfolk, who gave flu shots plus either a pla-cebo or 200 milligrams per day of ginseng to 198 nursing home residents, average age 82. After 12 weeks, the ginseng group was 89 percent less likely to develop flu.

Enhanced immune function means greater resistance to illness, speedier recovery, and improved general well-being, all of which sup-port the Chinese belief that ginseng is a tonic. Commission E, the expert panel that evaluates herbal medicines for the German counterpart of the FDA, approves ginseng for invigoration, con-valescence, and support of work capacity and concentration.

IMPROVED GENERAL WELL-BEING. At the Medical School of the National Autono-mous University of Mexico, researchers gave 500 people questionnaires asking about their health, well-being, occurrence of pain, mood, energy level, sex life, sleep quality, and personal satisfaction. Then 162 members of the group were given a daily multivitamin/mineral supple-ment, while 338 were given the same supple-ment plus 80 milligrams of a standardized extract of ginseng daily. Four months later, the participants completed the questionnaires again. Both groups reported better quality of life, but those taking ginseng claimed signifi-cantly greater improvement.

Several other similar studies have also shown that ginseng improves quality of life. Researchers at Hartford Hospital in Connecticut analyzed nine studies of ginseng's effects on quality of life. Their conclusion: "Nearly every study (eight of the nine) demonstrated some degree of quality of life improvement."

Therapeutic Uses

In addition to its tonic-adaptogen benefits, gin-seng's immune-enhancing action has been shown to help prevent and treat several specific conditions.

CANCER. Korean researchers surveyed 4,634 Korean adults over the age of 40 about their diet and lifestyle, including their use of ginseng. Five years later, some of the group had developed cancer. Compared with those who did not use ginseng, those who took it regularly had an astonishing 60 percent lower risk of all can-cers. Another Korean study involving 1,467 par-ticipants showed similar results—in the ginseng users, there was a 44 percent lower risk of cancer. A third Korean study showed 50 percent less risk of all cancers in regular ginseng users compared with nonusers.

In addition, study at the Mayo Clinic in Rochester, Minnesota, shows that ginseng helps treat the fatigue cancer patients typically develop while taking chemotherapy. The researchers gave either a placebo or 1,000 to 2,000 milligrams of ginseng per day to 175 people with breast, lung, or colon cancer. After 8 weeks, those taking ginseng reported significantly less fatigue.

Finally, a study at Vanderbilt University in Nashville shows that in women with breast cancer, ginseng improves survival and quality of life. The researchers tracked 1,455 participants in the Shanghai, China, Breast Cancer Study for 2 years. Compared with those who did not use ginseng regularly, those who did had a 29 percent lower risk of death, and reported significantly greater quality of life.

COLDS. In the Italian flu-shot study mentioned on page 254, the ginseng group also gained some protection against colds. Other studies have confirmed this.

University of Connecticut researchers asked 43 people over age 65 to take either a placebo or 400 milligrams of ginseng daily. For the first 2 months (September and October), both groups experienced the same number of colds. But during the second 2 months (November and December), the ginseng group developed only half as many colds. In addition, colds in the ginseng users cleared up faster. In the placebo group, colds lasted an average of 13 days; in the ginseng group, 6 days.

In another study, Canadian scientists gave 323 adults, ages 18 to 65, either a placebo or 400 milligrams of ginseng per day. After 4 months, 23 percent of the placebo group developed two or more colds, but in the ginseng group, that figure was just 10 percent. In addition, colds in the ginseng group were milder and briefer.

HIGH BLOOD PRESSURE. According to studies at Yale University, ginseng increases the body's synthesis of a compound (nitric oxide) that opens (dilates) blood vessels. As the arteries dilate, blood pressure drops.

At Seoul National University College of Medicine, Korean researchers gave 34 middle-aged men and women with high blood pressure either a placebo or ginseng (1.5 grams three times a day). Eight weeks later, those taking the placebo showed no change in blood pressure, but the ginseng group registered a significant decrease in their readings.

Some of the study participants took the ginseng in combination with a mainstream blood pressure medication (a beta-blocker or calcium channel-blocker). Compared with ginseng alone, the addition of the pharmaceutical did not produce greater declines in blood pressure.

Despite this study, there have been scattered reports of ginseng *raising* blood pressure. If you have high blood pressure and want to include ginseng in your treatment program, work closely with your physician and monitor your pressure regularly. If it rises, stop taking ginseng.

DIABETES. In a Finnish study, 36 people newly diagnosed with type 2 diabetes were treated with either a placebo or 100 or 200 milligrams of ginseng daily. Compared with those in the placebo group, the people in both ginseng groups showed lower blood sugar levels—and greater improvement in mood and enhanced performance on physical and psychological tests. The high-dose group showed the greatest benefit. Korean and Canadian studies confirm these results.

Diabetes is a serious condition that requires professional treatment. If you'd like to try ginseng in addition to your standard treatment regimen, consult your physician.

EMPHYSEMA. Israeli researchers asked 15 people with emphysema (average age, 67) to undergo tests of lung function and then walk as far as they could in 6 minutes. Subsequently, all 15 patients were instructed to take 200 milligrams of ginseng per day. Three months later, the participants' lung function improved significantly, meaning that more oxygen entered their bloodstreams. This increased their work capacity, as demonstrated by the fact that the distance they could walk in 6 minutes increased by 42 percent, from 600 meters to 854 meters.

ERECTILE DYSFUNCTION (ED) AND LOW SEXUAL DESIRE. Ginseng dilates the arteries, including the ones that carry blood into the penis. More blood available to the penis means greater likelihood of erection. Korean researchers gave 90 men with ED one of three treatments: a placebo, an antidepressant (trazodone), or ginseng. Those in the placebo and antidepressant groups showed 30 percent improvement in erection rigidity and girth and sexual desire, but those in the ginseng group experienced 60 percent improvement. This study supports the traditional Chinese belief that ginseng is a mild aphrodisiac.

Other Korean scientists repeated this study. They gave a placebo or 2,700 milligrams of ginseng per day to 45 men with ED. After 8 weeks, the men taking ginseng reported significantly firmer, longer-lasting erections. "Ginseng," the researchers concluded, "can be an effective alternative for treating male erectile dysfunction."

MALE INFERTILITY. At the University of Rome, Italian researchers gave 4,000 milligrams of ginseng a day to 30 men, ages 26 to 41, who had very low sperm counts, and to 20 men with normal counts. After 3 months, the sperm counts in the infertile men rose 93 percent, from 15 million to 29 million per milliliter. The men with initially normal sperm counts showed a 9 percent increase, from 85 million to 93 million per milliliter.

MENOPAUSAL SYMPTOMS. Japanese scientists surveyed 20 women about their menopausal discomforts and then gave them 6,000 milligrams of ginseng per day. A month later, their symptoms had declined significantly.

LIVER DAMAGE. Ginseng protects the liver from the harmful effects of drugs, alcohol, and other toxic substances. In one experiment, researchers gave what should have been fatal doses of various narcotics to experimental animals pretreated with ginseng extract. Most of the animals survived. And in a pilot human study, ginseng improved liver function in 24 elderly people with alcohol-induced cirrhosis.

APPETITE LOSS. Asians have long considered ginseng particularly helpful for the elderly. As people age, their senses of taste and smell deteriorate, leading to reduced appetite. In addition, the intestine's ability to absorb nutrients declines. As a result, some older people suffer malnutrition, which reduces their energy and alertness, increases their risk of illness, and may even become life-threatening. Ginseng enjoys a thousand-year-old reputation as an appetite stimulant. One study showed that it increases the ability of the intestine to absorb nutrients, thus helping to prevent malnutrition.

Intriguing Possibilities

Ginseng can minimize the cell damage from radiation therapy. In two studies, experimental animals were injected with various protective agents, then subjected to doses of radiation similar to those used in treating cancer. Ginseng did the best job of protecting healthy cells against harm, suggesting that the herb may be beneficial during cancer radiation therapy.

In addition, pilot studies in Italy show that ginseng speeds recovery from bronchitis and liver disease.

Adulteration and Maturity

Many studies have produced impressive evidence of ginseng's therapeutic benefits. But critics cite other studies that have shown no benefit at all. Why such disparate results? Adulteration appears to be a big part of the answer. Because of ginseng's rarity and enormous value, adulteration has been a problem for centuries—and to some extent, still is. It's quite possible that some researchers have used "ginseng" that in fact contained little or none of the herb.

One study from the mid-1980s evaluated 54 ginseng products sold in health food stores in the United States. The researchers judged 60 percent of the products worthless because they contained too little of the herb to have any biological effect. Twenty-five percent contained no ginseng at all.

The health food industry denounced the study, and the health food trade journal *Whole Foods* commissioned an independent test. It produced essentially the same results.

The most notorious of the nonginseng "ginsengs" was wild red American ginseng or wild desert ginseng, which appeared in health food stores from the late 1970s into the 1980s. Ginseng is a shade-loving, moisture-demanding plant, which means that desert ginseng is a botanical impossibility. Nonetheless, many consumers fell for the fraud. The phony ginseng was actually red dock, a laxative plant.

An outcry from responsible herbalists forced wild desert ginseng off health food store shelves, but problems with adulteration and fraud have persisted. That's why the American Herbal Products Association, an herb trade group, and the American Botanical Council, the nation's leading nonprofit herb research and education organization, both periodically analyze ginseng products to help ensure quality, a program that's rarely undertaken with other herbs.

Meanwhile, even if you start with real ginseng, it may not provide medicinal benefits if it's not mature. Ginseng roots should not be harvested until they are 6 years old, but sometimes, younger roots are mixed in to stretch the amount—a form of adulteration that may render a ginseng product useless.

Unfortunately, the only way to be absolutely certain of ginseng's purity and age is to grow it yourself, which is much easier said than done. If you buy ginseng, read labels carefully. Look for products that are identified by species and made with 6-year-old roots.

Rx Recommendations

Ginseng tastes sweetish and slightly aromatic. To take advantage of its many therapeutic powers, use root powder, teas, tinctures, capsules, or tablets. All of these forms are available in health food stores, herb shops, supplement centers, and some drugstores. You can even buy soft drinks that contain ginseng and promise a lift similar to that of caffeinated sodas.

To prepare a tea, use $1/2$ to 1 teaspoon of powdered root per cup of boiling water, simmer for about 15 minutes, and strain if you wish. Drink up to 2 cups a day.

When using a tincture or any other commercial preparation, follow the package directions.

The Safety Factor

Ginseng is a stimulant. People taking large doses have reported nervousness and restlessness, symptoms similar to those experienced by people who drink more coffee than they're accustomed to. Ginseng may also enhance the effects of other stimulants, such as ephedra and caffeine, causing overstimulation.

Other problems with ginseng are rare, but the medical literature contains a few dozen reports of adverse reactions. The herb may cause insomnia, breast soreness, allergy symptoms, asthma attacks, increased blood pressure, and heart rhythm disturbances (cardiac arrhythmias). People with insomnia, fibrocystic breasts, or hay fever should use ginseng with caution. Anyone with asthma, high blood pressure, cardiac arrhythmia, or fever should use ginseng only in consultation with their doctor, if at all.

Because of ginseng's anti-clotting action, it should be considered off-limits to people who have clotting problems or are taking anticoagulant (blood-thinning) medications. Stop using ginseng 2 weeks before scheduled surgery.

Studies performed at Harvard University and in Korea and Hong Kong show that like soy, ginseng has weakly estrogenic action. This helps prevent breast cancer. But it may cause problems for those advised to avoid exposure to this hormone. Talk to your doctor.

In Asia, ginseng has been considered an herb for the elderly. In traditional Chinese medical practice, it was not given to children. Likewise, don't give it to children.

While Asian studies have concluded that ginseng does not cause birth defects in the offspring of rats, rabbits, or lambs, women who are pregnant or nursing should err on the side of caution and not use it. Nursing women should also avoid it.

A 1979 article in the *Journal of the American Medical Association* documented a condition its authors dubbed "ginseng abuse syndrome," with symptoms including diarrhea. This study was seriously flawed. Real ginseng does not cause diarrhea, but red dock—the plant fraudulently called wild desert ginseng—does. It's a laxative. In other words, the study documenting purported ginseng abuse syndrome *did not use ginseng*. Herb authorities immediately pointed this out, but herb critics cited ginseng abuse syndrome as a reason to shun herbs in general and ginseng in particular well into the 1990s. Then the controversy pretty much died. If you ever see a reference to ginseng abuse syndrome, ignore it. No such syndrome exists.

Inform health care professionals of the herbs you use. Problematic herb-drug interactions are possible.

For more on herb safety, see Chapter 2.

If symptoms get worse or persist longer than 2 weeks, consult a health care professional promptly.

Growing Information

Ginseng is extremely difficult and expensive to grow. Prospective ginseng gardeners should heed the words of one frustrated horticulturist: "God and the growers know what they're doing, but neither one is talking."

Back in 1992, almost all cultivated American ginseng was grown in Wisconsin—2.4 million pounds valued at $125 million per year. Today, however, competition from Chinese and Canadian (British Columbian) growers has taken a serious toll. Wisconsin's growers now produce only about 500,000 pounds a year.

Ginseng requires shade, so growers drape nylon mesh over frames constructed along their rows. The plant is prone to several fungal infections. It's a struggle to keep young plants alive. Also, since the roots should be 6 years old at harvest, growers must be extremely patient.

When it's time to harvest the roots, the process is painstaking. Their value in the Orient depends in part on the arrangement of their limbs. The more humanlike the root, the higher the price. Breaking off an "arm" or "leg" during harvesting or drying lowers the price.

Root cuttings are often diseased, so most growers start with seeds, which are costly. Before planting, the seeds must be disinfected in a solution of one part chlorine bleach and nine parts water for 10 minutes.

If you want to try your hand at growing ginseng, plant the seeds in early autumn in well-prepared, humus-rich beds at a depth of $1/2$ inch and using 6-inch spacing. Ginseng grows poorly in sandy or clay soils. Maintain soil pH in the range of 5.0 to 6.0.

Germination of the seeds can take up to a year. The plants must be shaded, ideally under trees, although the covered frames work, too.

Harvest roots after 6 years, digging carefully to avoid breaking the root limbs. Dry them for 1 month.

GOLDENSEAL
A Potent Antibiotic

Family: Ranunculaceae; other members include buttercup, larkspur, and peony

Genus and species: *Hydrastis canadensis*

Also known as: Yellow root, yellow puccoon, Indian turmeric, Indian dye, Indian paint, jaundice root, eye balm, eye root, golden root, and poor man's ginseng

Parts used: Rhizomes and roots

Goldenseal is both popular and powerful. This combination virtually guarantees controversy. Thus, it should come as no surprise that many contemporary herbalists view goldenseal as one of our most useful herbs, while several scientific authorities continue to quote a pharmacologist who, in 1948, wrote that the herb has "few, if any, rational indications" and may cause "death from respiratory paralysis or cardiac arrest."

On balance, there's no cause for alarm. Goldenseal can definitely be beneficial, though harmful side effects are also possible. Informed home herbalists who use it safely and carefully can take advantage of its many therapeutic powers.

Healing History

The Native Americans of the northeastern United States pounded goldenseal's yellow roots (the source of most of its names) and used the yellow juice as a dye. They also used the herb medicinally as an eyewash (hence the names eye balm and eye root), as a treatment for skin wounds, sore throat, and digestive complaints, and as an aid to recovery from childbirth. The Cherokees mixed the herb with bear grease to make an insect repellent.

American colonists adopted the plant but didn't do much with it until the early 19th century, when Samuel Thomson, founder of Thomsonian herbal medicine, popularized it as an antiseptic. Thomson disliked the herb's Indian name, yellow root. So he changed it to goldenseal, combining "golden" from its color and "seal" from the circular scars left on the plant's root by each year's stems. Thomson thought the scars resembled the circular wax seals that were used to keep correspondence private in the days before glued envelopes.

Thomsonian medicine fell from fashion by the time of the Civil War, but America's 19th-century Eclectic physicians, forerunners of today's naturopaths, adopted goldenseal. They called it hydrastis, after its Latin name, and greatly expanded its uses. They prescribed it externally to relieve hemorrhoids, rectal fissures, pinkeye (conjunctivitis), eczema, boils, and wounds. They also recommended it internally as a treatment for tonsillitis, diphtheria, uterine problems, postpartum hemorrhage, and digestive ailments and as a tonic during convalescence from any major illness.

After the Civil War, the golden herb enjoyed a golden age. Goldenseal was an ingredient in many patent medicines, notably Dr. Pierce's Golden Medical Discovery, a popular tonic. Demand for the herb soared. Its price jumped to $1 a pound, making it almost as costly as America's most expensive healing herb, ginseng. But while most American ginseng was exported to China, goldenseal remained in the United States. And like ginseng, goldenseal was collected to the point of near extinction.

Over time, goldenseal acquired some of ginseng's medicinal reputation as a panacea and longevity tonic, hence another of its popular names, poor man's ginseng. The herb was listed as an astringent and antiseptic in the *U.S. Pharmacopoeia*, a standard drug reference, from 1831 to 1936, and in the *National Formulary*, the pharmacists' reference, from 1936 to 1960, when modern antibiotics pushed it aside.

Still, goldenseal has remained a favorite among herbalists. In the late 1940s, Jethro Kloss, in his early modern herb guide, *Back to Eden*, described the herb as "one of the most wonderful remedies in the entire herb kingdom. . . . A real cure-all."

Modern herbalists recommend goldenseal externally as an antiseptic to clean wounds and as a treatment for eczema, ringworm, athlete's foot, itching, and conjunctivitis. They prescribe it internally for digestive upset and colds, as a douche, and to stop excessive menstrual flow and postpartum uterine bleeding—although most also caution that the herb may trigger uterine contractions and "overstimulate the nervous system."

Goldenseal is a favorite of homeopaths, who prescribe microdoses for alcoholism, asthma, indigestion, cancer, hemorrhoids, and liver ailments. The herb remains a popular folk medicine as well. In *Hoosier Home Remedies*, a 1985 survey of Indiana folk medicine, the late herb expert Varro E. Tyler, Ph.D., reported that goldenseal was used extensively as an astringent and antiseptic to treat canker sores, chapped lips, and many other external problems.

Therapeutic Uses

In the late 1970s, heroin addicts came to believe that goldenseal tea could prevent the detection of opiates in urine specimens. Much to their chagrin, they were wrong. Goldenseal absolutely does not prevent the detection of opiates, or any other drugs, in urine. Nor is it a cure-all.

Scientists have determined that goldenseal contains two active constituents: berberine and hydrastine. Berberine, the more important, is also the active chemical in barberry. As a result, barberry and goldenseal have similar uses (and similar hazards), though goldenseal is more popular—and more expensive. Those interested in a "poor person's goldenseal" should try barberry.

INFECTIONS. The berberine in goldenseal kills many of the bacteria that cause diarrhea (*Escherichia coli,* salmonella, shigella, klebsiella, and even *Vibrio cholerae*, which causes cholera). In one study, 165 adults with diarrhea resulting from either *E. coli* or cholera were given either a placebo or 400 milligrams of berberine. After 24 hours, among those with *E. coli* diarrhea, 20 percent of the placebo group was cured. But in the berberine group, the figure was 43 percent. Among those with cholera, berberine also produced significant benefit. These results support goldenseal's long history as a treatment for infectious diarrhea.

Goldenseal has also shown benefit against the protozoa that cause amoebic dysentery (*Entamoeba histolytica*) and giardiasis (*Giardia lamblia*). In addition, it kills the protozoan that causes trichomoniasis (*Trichomonas vaginalis*) and the fungus that causes yeast infections *(Candida albicans)*. This lends credence to goldenseal's traditional use as a treatment for fungal infections.

ENHANCED IMMUNITY. In addition to killing germs, some research shows that berberine boosts the immune system by revving up macrophages, the white blood cells that devour disease-causing microorganisms.

WOMEN'S HEALTH CONCERNS. In some animal studies, berberine has been shown to calm the uterus, supporting its traditional use in stopping excessive menstrual flow and postpartum hemorrhage. Other studies, however, show that it stimulates uterine contractions. For this reason, women who are pregnant or trying to conceive should not use it. Women troubled by heavy menstrual flow might try the herb to see if it helps.

Postpartum hemorrhage is a potentially serious condition that requires prompt professional attention. If you'd like to try goldenseal in addition to standard therapy, discuss it with your obstetrician or midwife.

DIGESTIVE PROBLEMS. Goldenseal stimulates bile secretion in humans, which means that it helps digest fats.

Intriguing Possibilities

Some naturopaths claim that goldenseal helps restore digestive and liver function in people with alcoholism.

Several cell culture studies have shown that the herb helps kill tumor cells, lending support to its traditional role as a cancer treatment. In the future, it may serve as a complement to cancer chemotherapy.

A Chinese report suggests that berberine lowers cholesterol.

A laboratory study by researchers at the University of Illinois at Chicago shows that goldenseal combats *Helicobacter pylori*, the bacteria that causes ulcers.

Medical Myth

Some people consider goldenseal a treatment for all manner of infectious diseases, including colds and flu, because it is often paired with echinacea in commercial preparations. However, there is no evidence that goldenseal is effective against the viruses that cause colds and flu. In traditional herbal folklore, goldenseal was used almost exclusively as an oral treatment for digestive tract infections or topically for bacterial and fungal infections. Modern research validates these benefits, but goldenseal should not be expected to shorten the duration of colds or flu.

Rx Recommendations

To take advantage of goldenseal's possible antibiotic or immune-stimulating properties or to help ease heavy menstrual flow, prepare the herb as an infusion or tincture.

For an infusion, use $1/2$ to 1 teaspoon of powdered root per cup of boiling water, steep for 10 minutes, and strain if you wish. Drink up to 2 cups a day. Goldenseal tastes bitter; you may add honey, sugar, or lemon or mix it with a beverage tea to improve its flavor.

As a homemade tincture, take $1/2$ to 1 teaspoon up to twice a day.

When using a commercial preparation, follow the package directions.

The Safety Factor

The active compounds in goldenseal have opposite effects on blood pressure: Berberine may lower it, but hydrastine may raise it. People with high blood pressure, heart disease, diabetes, glaucoma, kidney disease, or history of stroke should exercise caution and not take goldenseal. If you have a home blood pressure monitor, though, you might try goldenseal to see how it affects you. If it doesn't raise your blood pressure, feel free to use it in recommended amounts in consultation with your physician.

Because of goldenseal's high cost and scarcity, adulteration has been a problem for more than 100 years. One traditional adulterant is bloodroot (*Sanguinaria canadensis*). When fresh, bloodroot is red, but when dried, it turns yellow like goldenseal and tastes equally bitter. Bloodroot is a powerful laxative. In high doses, it also causes dizziness, gastrointestinal burning, intense thirst, and vomiting. If your "goldenseal" causes purging or any of these other symptoms, stop using it. It's probably bloodroot.

Large doses of goldenseal may irritate the skin, mouth, and throat and cause nausea and vomiting. Goldenseal douches may cause vaginal irritation.

The medical literature contains no reports of serious harm resulting from goldenseal, but hydrastine stimulates the central nervous system, and in animals, unusually large doses have caused death from respiratory paralysis and cardiac arrest. Do not use more than recommended amounts.

Pregnant and nursing women should not use goldenseal.

Do not give goldenseal to children under 2. In older children, adjust the recommended dose based on the child's weight. For example, give a 50-pound child one-third of the dose a 150-pound adult would take.

If you're over 65, start with a low dose, and increase only if necessary.

Inform health care professionals of the herbs you use. Problematic herb-drug interactions are possible.

Goldenseal may cause allergic reactions or other unexpected side effects. If any develop, reduce your dose or stop taking it.

For more on herb safety, see Chapter 2.

If symptoms get worse or persist longer than 2 weeks, consult a health care professional promptly.

Growing Information

A report in *Endangered Species Bulletin* described wild goldenseal as critically imperiled. Today, the herb is farmed but still costly, and adulteration continues to be a problem.

Goldenseal is a small, erect perennial with a hairy, purplish, annual stem that rises from a short, knotty rhizome with yellow-brown bark and bright yellow pulp. The herb has lobed leaves somewhat similar to raspberry leaves and small, greenish white flowers that bloom in spring and produce orange-red berries. It grows wild from Vermont to Arkansas, if you're fortunate enough to find it.

Goldenseal is difficult to raise in a garden. Plants may be started from seeds, but it takes 5 years for the roots to become medicinally mature. Most authorities recommend buying 2-year-old rhizomes from specialty nurseries so you can harvest the roots 3 years later.

Viable rhizomes should have a sweet, licorice-like aroma. Plant them in early fall at a depth of 1 inch with 8-inch spacing. The soil should be amended with compost, leaf mold, sand, and bonemeal. Frequently, top-growth will not appear until the second summer.

Goldenseal requires moisture with good drainage and about 70 percent shade. It grows best under tree cover or shade frames.

Harvest the rhizome and roots in late fall, after frost has killed the top-growth. Clean the roots and dry them until they become brittle, then powder them and store the powder in airtight containers.

GOTU KOLA

Soothes Skin Problems and More

Family: Umbelliferae; other members include carrot, parsley, celery, fennel, dill, and angelica

Genus and species: *Centella asiatica* or *Hydrocotyle asiatica*

Also known as: Sheep rot, Indian pennywort, marsh penny, water pennywort, and hydrocotyle

Parts used: Leaves

Long ago, the native Sinhalese of Ceylon (now Sri Lanka) noticed that elephants, renowned for their longevity, loved the rounded leaves of the diminutive gotu kola. The herb gained a reputation as a longevity promoter, and a Sinhalese proverb advised, "Two leaves a day keeps old age away."

While you can't expect gotu kola to add years to your life, it has been shown to accelerate wound healing, relieve psoriasis, prevent varicose veins, and possbily even improve memory.

Healing History

India's Ayurvedic herbalists first used gotu kola in the same way the Chinese used ginseng—to promote longevity and mental acuity and to treat problems associated with aging. Over time, however, the herb also became popular as an internal and external treatment for skin diseases, including leprosy.

Philippine healers prescribed gotu kola to treat wounds and gonorrhea. Chinese physicians recommended it for fever and colds.

Gotu kola got a bum rap in Europe, where several species grow. Europeans believed that the herb caused foot rot in sheep (hence its once-popular name, sheep rot). There's no evidence to support this claim.

Close relatives of gotu kola also grow in the United States. America's 19th-century Eclectic physicians, forerunners of today's naturopaths, were well aware of the herb's use as a treatment for leprosy in Asia. According to one report, "In 1852, Dr. Boileau of India, having been for many years afflicted with leprosy . . . experimented with [it] and recovered."

The Eclectics considered gotu kola safe and effective when used externally to treat skin problems. But they deemed the herb a poison when taken internally, asserting that large doses produce "headache, dizziness, stupor, itching, and bloody passages from bowels."

Gotu kola went into eclipse during the early 20th century. But after World War II, it surfaced in an herbal tea blend called Fo-Ti-Tieng, which was touted to boost longevity, a claim that revived the ancient Sinhalese belief. The legend was that one Li Ching Yun, an ancient Chinese herbalist, had taken the blend regularly and lived for 256 years, surviving 23 wives. The tea caught on, and gotu kola reemerged from obscurity as an herbal tonic.

Contemporary herbalists recommend gotu kola externally as a poultice for wounds. For internal use, they prescribe small doses as a tonic stimulant and large doses as a sedative.

Therapeutic Uses

Any longevity claims for gotu kola are as far-fetched as the tale of Li Ching Yun. But modern science has found support for other traditional therapeutic powers of this ancient herb.

WOUNDS. One compound in gotu kola, asiaticoside, speeds wound healing. Another, madecassoside, is an anti-inflammatory. According to a study published in *Annals of Plastic Surgery*, gotu kola accelerates the healing of burns and minimizes scarring. Other studies have shown that the herb accelerates the healing of skin grafts and surgical enlargement of the vagina during childbirth (episiotomy).

STRETCH MARKS. Pregnancy-related stretch marks are not wounds, but they are disfiguring and bother many women. British researchers gave 100 pregnant women either a placebo cream or one containing extract of gotu kola. Those using the gotu kola cream were less than half as likely to develop stretch marks.

PSORIASIS. Validating gotu kola's traditional role as a treatment for skin diseases, one study showed that a cream made with the herb can help relieve the painful, scaly red welts of psoriasis. For the study, seven people with psoriasis were instructed to apply the cream. In five of the participants, the welts healed within 2 months. Only one of the five experienced any recurrence within 4 months after the treatment ended. The gotu kola cream used in this study is not available commercially, but if you have psoriasis, you might try compresses of gotu kola infusion.

HIGH BLOOD PRESSURE. In one study, researchers gave either placebos or gotu kola extract to 89 people with high blood pressure. Those taking the herb experienced a significant drop in their blood pressures.

ANXIETY. Canadian researchers gave anxiety sufferers either a placebo or 12 grams of gotu kola daily and then subjected them to sudden loud noises. The gotu kola group reacted with significantly less physiological anxiety.

DIABETES. Diabetes impairs circulation through the smallest blood vessels, which over time causes most of the complications of the disease. In several studies, British researchers have shown that gotu kola improves circulation through these blood vessels. In one, 40 people with diabetes were treated with either a placebo or 60 milligrams of gotu kola extract twice a day. After 8 weeks, the herb group had significantly better circulation.

VARICOSE VEINS. Speaking of circulation, gotu kola improves bloodflow through the lower limbs, helping to prevent varicose veins. In one study, 94 people with swelling, heaviness, and pain from poor circulation in the legs (known as venous insufficiency) were given either 60 milligrams of gotu kola or medically inactive placebos. After 2 months, those taking the herb showed significantly improved circulation and less swelling. The researchers concluded that the herb strengthened veins.

LEPROSY. Gotu kola's traditional use in treating leprosy (now called Hansen's disease) was supported by a study published in the British journal *Nature*. The bacteria that cause leprosy have a waxy coating that protects them against attack by the immune system. The asiaticoside in gotu kola dissolves the waxy coating, allowing the immune system to destroy the bacteria.

Intriguing Possibilities

There may be something to the ancient Ayurvedic belief that gotu kola improves memory. Animal studies show improvement in learning and memory. And an Indian study found that treatment with the herb improves the intellectual performance of mentally challenged children.

In coming years, gotu kola may also have potential as a cancer treatment. A cell-culture study, also by Indian researchers, concluded that gotu kola extract destroys cancer cells without toxic effects on other cells. While the results of laboratory studies don't always apply to humans, at some time in the future, gotu kola may be included in cancer treatment regimens.

Rx Recommendations

Use an infusion of gotu kola to improve circulation in your legs. To prepare it, steep $1/2$ teaspoon of herb in a cup of boiling water for 10 to 20 minutes, then strain. Drink up to 2 cups a day. Gotu kola tastes bitter and astringent; adding sugar or honey and lemon or mixing it into an herbal beverage blend will improve its flavor.

To help treat wounds or psoriasis topically, apply compresses made from a gotu kola infusion. If the results are disappointing, try a stronger infusion.

When using commercial preparations, follow the package directions.

The Safety Factor

The only confirmed side effect of gotu kola is skin rash in people who are sensitive to it.

In laboratory animals, gotu kola acts as a sedative. Large doses are narcotic, causing stupor and possibly coma. Sedation has never been reported in humans, but some scientists claim that it's possible. They echo the Eclectics, who advised against ingesting the herb.

Ironically, reports have appeared claiming that gotu kola causes restlessness and insomnia, which is rather odd for a purported "narcotic." Apparently, these cases involved the caffeine-containing herb kola, which was mislabeled as gotu kola.

Pregnant women may use gotu kola topically to prevent stretch marks. But pregnant and nursing women should not ingest it.

Anyone may use gotu kola externally, but do not give it internally to children under age 2. In older children, adjust the recommended dose based on the child's weight. For example, give a 50-pound child one-third of the dose a 150-pound adult would take.

If you're over 65, start with a low dose, and increase only if necessary.

Inform health care professionals of the herbs you use. Problematic herb-drug interactions are possible.

Gotu kola may cause allergic reactions or other unexpected side effects. If any develop, reduce your dose or stop taking it.

For more on herb safety, see Chapter 2.

If symptoms get worse or persist longer than 2 weeks, consult a health care professional promptly.

Growing Information

Gotu kola is not related to true kola (*Cola nitida*), the caffeine-containing nut used in cola drinks. Nor is it cultivated in North America, although several related species grow wild.

As a member of the Umbelliferae family, gotu kola is related to carrot, parsley, dill, and fennel, but it has neither the characteristic feathery leaves nor the umbrella arrangement (umbel) of tiny flowers. Instead, gotu kola's creeping stem grows in marshy areas and produces fan-shaped leaves about the size of an old British penny—hence its names Indian pennywort, marsh penny, and water pennywort. A cuplike clutch of inconspicuous flowers develops near the ground. Leaves are harvested throughout the year.

HAWTHORN

Mayflower for Heart Disease

Family: Rosaceae; other members include rose, peach, almond, apple, and strawberry

Genus and species: *Crataegus oxycantha*

Also known as: Hawthorne, haw, may, mayblossom, and mayflower

Parts used: Flowers, leaves, and fruits

Every American schoolchild learns that the Pilgrims' ship was called the *Mayflower*. Few if any Americans, however, know that the name refers to hawthorn, which, in England, flowers in May. Even fewer know that the herb is very beneficial to the heart.

Today, hawthorn is widely used in Europe as a treatment for heart disease, especially congestive heart failure, which involves chronic fatigue of the heart muscle, shortness of breath after mild exertion, and fluid buildup around the body, notably in the ankles and lungs. Now hawthorn is starting to catch on in this country as well.

Healing History

Archeologists have discovered the seeds of hawthorn fruits at Neolithic sites, suggesting that the fruits were used for food.

To the ancient Greeks and Romans, hawthorn was rich in symbolism, linked to hope, marriage, and fertility. Greek bridesmaids wore fragrant hawthorn blossoms, and brides carried a hawthorn bough. The Romans placed hawthorn leaves in babies' cradles to ward off evil spirits.

The arrival of Christianity changed hawthorn's image dramatically. Christ's crown of thorns was reputedly made of hawthorn, and as a result, the herb became a symbol of bad luck and death.

The hawthorn-death association was bolstered by the unpleasant aroma of the flowers of some European species. These trees are pollinated by carrion-eating insects, and to attract them, their flowers emit the odor of rotting meat. A similar odor was associated with bubonic plague. (Because the disease killed so many so quickly, bodies often remained unburied for quite a while.) As a result, hawthorn came to be associated with plague, and it was shunned.

As time passed, hawthorn shed its bad reputation and was embraced as a medicinal herb. Seventeenth-century English herbalist Nicholas Culpeper praised it as "a singular remedy for the stone [kidney stones], and no less effectual for dropsy [congestive heart failure]."

Despite the influential Culpeper's endorse-ment, hawthorn was not widely recommended to treat heart problems until the very end of the 19th century, when it was popularized by an Irish doctor who used it to treat congestive heart failure. In 1896, an article touting the Irish physician's work appeared in a medical journal for Eclectic physicians, forerunners of today's naturopaths. The Eclectics began prescribing the herb for congestive heart failure and the chest pain of angina.

Modern herbals echo these recommendations. Most would agree with David Hoffmann's *Holistic Herbal*: "Hawthorn [is] one of the best tonic remedies for the heart. . . . It may be used safely in long-term treatment for heart weakness or failure . . . palpitations . . . angina pectoris . . . and high blood pressure."

Therapeutic Uses

A great deal of research supports the traditional role of hawthorn as a heart stimulant.

CONGESTIVE HEART FAILURE. Hawthorn supports the heart in several ways. It opens (dilates) the coronary arteries, improving the blood supply to the heart muscle. This strengthens the heart so it beats more forcefully and efficiently. As a result, the herb boosts the heart's blood-pumping force, which is vital in people with congestive heart failure. Many studies provide important evidence of hawthorn's benefits in treating congestive heart failure. Here's a sampling of the research to date.

❧German researchers gave heart function tests to 3,664 people with congestive heart failure. Then everyone was instructed to take hawthorn (one 300-milligram tablet, standardized to contain 2.2 percent flavonoids, three times a day). After 2 months, the participants were tested again. Their heart function improved significantly, about as much as would be expected from standard pharmaceuticals. In addition, the proportion of participants experiencing heart palpitations dropped from 40 percent to 18 percent. Leg swelling declined by 37 percent. And work capacity, measured as the ability to expend effort by riding a stationary cycle, increased by 15 percent.

* Another group of German scientists gave 136 people with congestive heart failure either medically inactive placebos or 80 milligrams of hawthorn twice a day. After 8 weeks, those taking the placebos had gotten worse, while those taking hawthorn had improved significantly.

* A third German trial involved 78 people with congestive heart failure. They took work-capacity tests on a stationary cycle and then began taking either a placebo or 600 milligrams of hawthorn a day. After 2 months, the work capacity of those in the placebo group improved slightly. Among those in the hawthorn group, work capacity increased almost *six times* as much.

Hawthorn caused no significant side effects in any of these studies.

In 2008, British researchers analyzed 14 trials of hawthorn for congestive heart failure. The studies included a total of 1,110 participants, who took the herb at dosages of 160 to 1,800 milligrams per day for 3 to 16 weeks, typically in addition to standard medications. The researchers concluded that hawthorn has "significant benefit" in treating heart failure.

Commission E, the expert panel that evaluates herbal medicines for the German counterpart of the FDA, approves hawthorn as a treatment for congestive heart failure. German doctors are permitted to prescribe any of several hawthorn-based heart medicines. According to noted German medical herbalist Rudolph Fritz Weiss, M.D., the herb "has become one of [our] most widely used heart remedies." German physicians rely on hawthorn to normalize heart rhythm, reduce the likelihood and severity of angina attacks, and prevent cardiac complications in elderly patients with influenza and pneumonia.

Dr. Weiss cautions, however, that hawthorn is no quick fix. "One cannot expect rapid improvement in cardiac function," he states. "[Hawthorn] has a long-term, sustained effect. . . . Hawthorn is not for cutting short angina attacks—nitroglycerin continues to be the drug of choice here."

Although hawthorn is considered safe and may be effective in the treatment of congestive heart failure, angina, and cardiac arrhythmias, these are serious, potentially life-threatening conditions that require professional medical care. Consult your physician if you'd like to use hawthorn as part of your overall treatment plan.

BLOOD PRESSURE. Part of the reason hawthorn treats congestive heart failure is that it lowers blood pressure, which allows blood to circulate more freely with less strain on the heart. Iranian researchers gave either a placebo or hawthorn to 92 men and women with high blood pressure. After 4 months, the herb group's blood pressure was significantly lower. A British study confirms these results.

CHOLESTEROL AND HEART RHYTHM. Some evidence also shows that hawthorn helps reduce cholesterol levels and corrects some types of heart rhythm disturbances (arrhythmias).

Intriguing Possibility

A pilot study by French researchers suggests that hawthorn may help treat anxiety.

Rx Recommendations

If you use a homemade tincture, German physicians recommend taking 1 teaspoon upon waking and at bedtime for periods of up to several weeks. To mask its bitter taste, you can sweeten it with sugar, honey, or lemon, or mix it with an herbal beverage blend.

To prepare an infusion, herbalists recommend using 2 teaspoons of crushed leaves or fruits per cup of boiling water. Steep for 20 minutes, then strain. Drink up to 2 cups a day.

When using commercial preparations, follow the package directions.

The Safety Factor

In the 14-study analysis of hawthorn for congestive heart failure, one-third of the trials reported no side effects at all. Two-thirds reported some dizziness, vertigo, and upset stomach.

Large amounts of hawthorn may cause sedation and/or a significant drop in blood pressure, possibly resulting in faintness.

Pregnant and nursing women should not use hawthorn.

Do not give hawthorn to children.

If you're over 65, start with a low dose, and increase only if necessary.

Inform health care professionals of the herbs you use. Problematic herb-drug interactions are possible.

Hawthorn may cause allergic reactions or other unexpected side effects. If any develop, reduce your dose or stop taking it.

For more on herb safety, see Chapter 2.

If symptoms get worse or persist longer than 2 weeks, consult a health care professional promptly.

Growing Information

Hawthorn is a small deciduous tree with white bark, extremely hard wood, sharp thorns, clusters of white, aromatic flowers, and brilliant red fruits that look like small apples. It blooms from April to June, depending on latitude. In England, blossoms appear in May; hence the herb's other names: may, mayblossom, and mayflower.

With approximately 900 North American species, hawthorn is well adapted to many environments, from urban areas to windswept hillsides. The tree tolerates a variety of soils but prefers somewhat alkaline, rich, moist loam. Some species prefer full sun, while others grow well in partial shade. Consult a nursery for the species best suited to your area.

HIBISCUS

This Beautiful Tropical Flower Lowers Blood Pressure

Family: Malvaceae; other members include cotton and mallow

Genus and species: *Hibiscus sabdariffa*

Also known as: Red tea, sour tea, red sorrel, Jamaica sorrel, and roselle

Parts used: Flowers

Have you ever enjoyed a cup of Red Zinger tea? Its red color comes from hibiscus flowers, hence the "red" in some of its common names. (But don't confuse hibiscus with African red bush tea, also known as rooibos, which is a different plant.) Native to Africa, hibiscus now grows around the world.

The hibiscus plant is remarkably versatile. For centuries, its leaves have been eaten like spinach. Its fibrous stems can be used to make rope. And its fragrant flowers have been used in perfumes and teas. But hibiscus was rarely used in Western herbal medicine until the 21st century, when it was shown to lower blood pressure.

Healing History

In tropical Africa, hibiscus leaves were used topically as a skin soother for bites, stings, and wounds, and internally as a laxative. In Egypt, hibiscus is a popular folk treatment for heart disease. In Iran, it's used to treat high blood pressure. Iranian researchers wondered if this use was medically valid. In 1999, they published the first study showing that hibiscus lowers blood pressure.

Therapeutic Uses

BLOOD PRESSURE. In the original Iranian study, the researchers took blood pressure readings from 54 adults with high blood pressure, and then had them drink either tea or hibiscus tea daily. After 15 days, the hibiscus group showed significantly lower blood pressure. Since then, several other studies by Iranian and Mexican researchers have confirmed this effect. In the most recent report, Mexican scientists gave 193 people with high blood pressure either a standard blood pressure medication (Zestril) or hibiscus. After 4 weeks, the drug produced a greater reduction, but the herb also reduced blood pressure significantly.

Intriguing Possibilities

An Indian animal study suggests that hibiscus has immune-stimulating action.

Rx Recommendations

Use 1 to 3 teaspoons of chopped or powdered flowers per cup of boiling water. Steep for 2 to 5 minutes, then strain. Drink up to 3 cups a day.

The Safety Factor

No significant side effects have been shown.

Hibiscus may cause allergic reactions or other unexpected side effects. If any develop, reduce your dose or stop taking it.

Growing Information

Hibiscus grows outdoors in the southern United States and Hawaii. Hibiscus is an annual that grows to 5 feet. It needs full sun. It tolerates many conditions, but thrives in sandy soil with some organic content and slight acidity. Water frequently until the plant is established. Mulching helps.

Propagate using seed or cuttings. In colder areas, this herb can be grown indoors in containers with many drainage holes. For best results, soil should be 80 percent potting mix and 20 percent sand, then add some compost. Water frequently.

HOP
Not Just for Beer

Family: Cannabaceae; other members include hemp and marijuana

Genus and species: *Humulus lupulus*

Also known as: Humulus

Parts used: Strobiles (glandular hairs of female fruits)

Hop, also known as hops, is best known as the bitter, aromatic ingredient in beer. Today, 98 percent of the world's hop harvest is used to make it. But hop also has a long history in herbal healing, and some of its traditional uses have been supported by modern science.

Our word "hop" comes from the Anglo-Saxon term *hoppan*, meaning "to climb," a reference to the climbing vine.

Healing History

Chinese physicians have prescribed hop for centuries as a digestive aid and a treatment for leprosy, tuberculosis, and dysentery.

Ancient Greek and Roman physicians also recommended the herb as a digestive aid and as a treatment for intestinal ailments. The Roman naturalist Pliny touted hop as a garden vegetable, the young shoots of which could be eaten in spring before they matured and grew tough and bitter. (People still eat the shoots, prepared like asparagus.)

Hop was a minor herb until about 1,000 years ago. That's when brewers began using it to preserve the fermented barley beverage that we know as beer.

Actually, beer was an accidental offshoot of bread baking. As agriculture developed, late-prehistoric homemakers noticed that bread made from raw grain did not keep as well as bread made from sprouted grain. So before pounding their grain into flour, they soaked it in water to sprout it. If the water happened to become contaminated with yeast microorganisms from the skins of fruit, it fermented into a crude, sweet beer.

Ancient beers, probably undrinkable by modern standards, were nonetheless amazingly popular. Around 2500 B.C., an estimated 40 percent of the Sumerian grain crop was used in brewing. And the world's first written legal code, Babylonia's Code of Hammurabi (1750 B.C.), described punishments for ale houses that sold beer that was understrength or overpriced.

As the centuries passed, brewers used herbs such as marjoram, yarrow, and wormwood to flavor their beers. Around the 9th century, the Germans began adding hop, both for its pleasantly bitter flavor and because it preserved the brew, extending shelf life in an age before refrigeration. By the 14th century, most European beers contained hop.

A Battle Brews in England

Hop was well known in England. The vine grew wild there, and in folk medicine, hop was a popular appetite-stimulating digestive bitter.

England's fermented beverage of choice was ale, a sweet beer that contained some other herbs, but not hop. Around 1500, British brewers began making European-style bitter beer with hop. This move was a boon to brewers and innkeepers because hop's preservative action extended the beer's shelf life, so they could keep batches longer and have less go bad. But the addition of hop to English beer also provoked national outrage.

Legions of hop haters petitioned Parliament to ban the herb from beer. Henry VIII, an ale traditionalist, supported banning hop as "a wicked weed that would endanger the people." Hop remained illegal in English beer until Henry's son, Edward VI, rescinded the ban in 1552.

But the furor refused to die. A century later, English writer John Evelyn declared, "Hop transmuted our wholesome ale into beer. This one ingredient preserves the drink indeed, but repays the pleasure in tormenting diseases and a shorter life."

Beer brewing transformed hop from a spring vegetable into a cash crop, but hop farmers noticed that the herb had two odd effects on those who harvested it. They fatigued easily, and the women got their periods early. Over time, the herb gained a reputation as a sedative and menstruation promoter.

Hop has been used ever since as a sedative, not only in tea but also in pillows. The herb's warm fragrance is supposed to induce sleep.

Seventeenth-century English herbalist Nicholas Culpeper recommended hop "in opening obstructions of the liver and spleen . . . cleansing the blood . . . helping cure the French disease [syphilis], and bringing down women's courses [menstruation]." Culpeper also added his twopence to the lingering beer-ale controversy, writing that hop's medicinal uses made beer "better than ale."

More Than a Sedative

Meanwhile, in North America, Native Americans were using the American species of hop as a sedative and digestive aid. America's 19th-century Eclectics, forerunners of today's naturopaths, deemed hop a digestive aid and a treatment for the "morbid excitement of delirium tremens." They were unimpressed with its reputation as a sedative, however, warning that it "often failed."

Still, hop was listed as a sedative in the *U.S. Pharmacopoeia*, a standard drug reference, from 1831 to 1916. Throughout the 19th century, it was a popular ingredient in many patent medicines, including Hop Bitters, a popular herbal tonic with a 30 percent alcohol base. Its advertising slogan typified patent-medicine claims in the era before the FDA: "Take Hop Bitters three times a day, and you will have no doctor bills to pay."

During the 1950s, jazz musicians who smoked marijuana were called hopheads, and marijuana was said to make its users "hopped up." Hop is, indeed, botanically related to marijuana, but smoking the herb does not produce intoxication.

Contemporary herbalists recommend hop primarily as a sedative, tranquilizer, and digestive aid.

Therapeutic Uses

Those old brewers knew what they were doing when they added hop to beer as a preservative. It contains two chemicals, humulone and lupulone, that kill the bacteria that make food—and beer—spoil.

INFECTIONS. The bacteria fighters in hop may help prevent infection in humans. Hop is not a major herbal antibiotic, but it's effective first aid in the garden. If you cut yourself near a hop vine, grab some leaves, crush them, and press them into the wound until you can wash it with soap and water. One laboratory study has shown hop to be effective against the bacteria that cause tuberculosis, lending some credence to one of the herb's traditional Chinese uses.

INSOMNIA AND ANXIETY. For decades, scientists were skeptical about hop's age-old reputation as a sedative. Then, in 1983, they discovered a sedative compound in the plant (2-methyl-3-butene-2-ol). This chemical is present in only trace amounts in the fresh leaves, but its concentration increases as the herb dries and ages. If you want to try hop as a sedative, stick with the dried, aged herb. Hop is often an ingredient in herbal sleep aids, along with valerian (see page 469).

Commission E, the expert panel that evaluates herbal medicines for the German counterpart of the FDA, approves hop for treatment of anxiety and sleep disturbances.

DIGESTIVE PROBLEMS. Hop appears to relax the smooth muscle lining the digestive tract, according to French researchers. This finding supports the herb's traditional role as an antispasmodic digestive herb.

Intriguing Possibility

German researchers have concluded that hop contains chemicals similar to the female sex hormone estrogen, which may explain some of the menstrual changes reported in women who picked it. Other studies dispute this. Currently, the issue remains unresolved. But one French study suggests that hop helps relieve hot flashes.

Rx Recommendations

To help protect against infection and avoid digestive upset, use the freshest hop you can find. For insomnia, use hop that has been dried and aged.

To make an infusion, use 2 teaspoons of herb per cup of boiling water and steep for 5 minutes, then strain. Drink up to 3 cups a day. Hop tastes warm and pleasantly bitter.

When using commercial preparations, follow the package directions.

The Safety Factor

Some hop pickers develop a rash called hop dermatitis. Otherwise, there are no reports of harm from using the herb.

In case hop does contain chemicals similar to estrogen, women who are pregnant or who have estrogen-dependent breast cancer should not use it.

Do not give hop to children under 2. In older children, adjust the recommended dose based on the child's weight. For example, give a 50-pound child one-third of the dose a 150-pound adult would take.

If you're over 65, start with a low dose, and increase only if necessary.

Inform health care professionals of the herbs you use. Problematic herb-drug interactions are possible.

Hop may cause allergic reactions or other unexpected side effects. If any develop, reduce your dose or stop taking it.

For more on herb safety, see Chapter 2.

If symptoms get worse or persist longer than 2 weeks, consult a health care professional promptly.

Growing Information

Hop is a resinous, hairy, climbing perennial vine that resembles grape. Grown commercially in Bavaria, Germany, and in the Pacific Northwest in pole-studded fields called hop yards, mature vines often reach 25 feet.

Hop can be raised from seeds, but most growers use root cuttings taken in spring or fall. Plant the cuttings in hills, three roots per hill, with hills 18 inches apart.

Hop needs deeply cultivated, rich, moist soil; full sun; and frequent watering.

Harvest the female flowers in fall when they feel firm, turn amber-colored, and are covered with yellow dust. Dry them immediately in an oven no hotter than 150°F.

HOREHOUND

For Coughs, Colds, and Flu

Family: Labiatae; other members include mints

Genus and species: *Marrubium vulgare*

Also known as: Hoarhound, white horehound, and marrubium

Parts used: Leaves and flowers

Horehound was a popular herbal expectorant and cough remedy for almost 2,000 years. Even skeptics of herbal medicine acknowledged its safety and effectiveness.

Then, in 1989, completely out of the blue, the FDA banned horehound from over-the-counter cough remedies, claiming that it was ineffective. The action left herbalists shaking their heads. Worse yet, the FDA decreed that another expectorant, guaifenesin, was effective, over the objections of many scientists.

Healing History

Horehound was first used medicinally in ancient Rome as an ingredient in the multi-ingredient (and ineffective) poison antidotes known as theriaca. Medieval Europeans generalized this application and came up with the belief that the herb provided protection from witches' spells.

The Roman physician Galen was the first to prescribe horehound for coughs and respiratory problems. It's been used as an expectorant ever since. The ancients also relied on it to calm upset stomachs.

The medieval German abbess/herbalist Hildegard of Bingen considered horehound one of the best herbs for colds. And England's John Gerard wrote, "Syrup made of the greene fresh leaves and sugar is a most singular remedie against cough and wheezings of the lungs."

Seventeenth-century English herbalist Nicholas Culpeper wrote that in addition to curing "those that have taken poison . . . a decoction of the dried herb taken with honey is a remedy for those that are short-winded, have a cough, or are fallen into consumption. . . . It helpeth to expectorate tough phlegm from the chest."

Early settlers introduced horehound into North America, where it became a popular cough, cold, and tuberculosis remedy. Folk herbalists also considered it to be a digestive aid, laxative, and treatment for hepatitis, malaria, intestinal worms, and menstrual problems.

America's 19th-century Eclectic physicians, forerunners of today's naturopaths, prescribed horehound for coughs, colds, asthma, intestinal worms, and menstrual complaints.

Most contemporary American herbalists recommend horehound only for minor respiratory problems such as coughs, colds, and bronchitis.

In Europe, it is also used as a digestive aid.

Therapeutic Uses

The FDA order to remove horehound from cough and cold remedies says more about the watchdog agency's shortcomings than it does about the herb's.

COUGHS. Horehound contains a compound called marrubiin that Russian and German studies have found to have phlegm-loosening (expectorant) properties. In Europe, the herb has been used for decades in a large number of cough syrups and lozenges. It has been widely used in the United States as well. Even the late herb conservative Varro Tyler, Ph.D., author of *Tyler's Honest Herbal*, describes horehound as an effective expectorant.

The FDA's horehound ban followed the recommendation of an agency advisory panel, which decreed that only one expectorant, guaifenesin, is safe and effective. Ironically, many lung experts question guaifenesin's effectiveness.

The FDA order applies only to horehound preparations marketed as cough remedies. The herb is still available in bulk and in some sore throat products.

DIGESTIVE PROBLEMS. Commission E, the expert panel that evaluates herbal medicines for the German counterpart of the FDA, approves horehound for the treatment of indigestion, bloating, and flatulence.

Intriguing Possibilities

European animal studies show that horehound opens (dilates) blood vessels, a finding that hints at the herb's possible value in treating high blood pressure.

Other animal studies show that in small amounts, horehound helps normalize irregular heart rhythm (arrhythmia), but in large amounts, the herb can cause them.

Rx Recommendations

For an infusion to treat cough or upset stomach, use $1/2$ to 1 teaspoon of dried leaves per cup of boiling water. Steep for 10 minutes, then strain. Drink up to 3 cups a day. To offset horehound's bitter taste, sweeten it with sugar or honey.

As a homemade tincture, take $1/4$ to $1/2$ teaspoon up to three times a day.

When using commercial preparations, follow the package directions.

The Safety Factor

There have been no reports of adverse reactions to horehound in humans. In light of the animal studies showing that large doses of the herb may cause cardiac arrhythmias, however, people with this condition should avoid it.

Horehound's traditional use as a menstruation promoter has not been confirmed scientifically. Still, pregnant women should exercise caution and not take it. Nursing women should also avoid horehound.

Do not give horehound to children under 2. In older children, adjust the recommended dose based on the child's weight. For example, give a 50-pound child one-third of the dose a 150-pound adult would take.

If you're over 65, start with a low dose, and increase only if necessary.

Inform health care professionals of the herbs you use. Problematic herb-drug interactions are possible.

Horehound may cause allergic reactions or other unexpected side effects. If any develop, reduce your dose or stop taking it.

For more on herb safety, see Chapter 2.

If symptoms get worse or persist longer than 2 weeks, consult a health care professional promptly.

Growing Information

Horehound is a spreading, pleasantly aromatic perennial with square annual stems that reach about 18 inches. The leaves are rounded, wrinkled, and deeply veined, and tiny white flowers develop at the stem-leaf stalk junctions. The entire plant is covered with soft hairs, giving it a woolly appearance and a grayish white cast.

A self-seeder, horehound grows so easily that it may become a pest. It needs little water and tolerates poor soil. It thrives in full sun but tolerates partial shade.

Plant seeds just under the soil surface in either spring or fall. Thin seedlings to 9-inch spacing. Horehound does not bloom until its second year, but you can harvest the leaves and top-growth after one growing season.

In the soil, the herb exudes a musky odor that some people dislike. As the plant dries, the odor disappears.

HORSE CHESTNUT

Very Good for Varicose Veins

Family: Hippocastanaceae; other members include Ohio buckeye

Genus and species: *Aesculus hippocastanum*

Also known as: Chestnut and buckeye

Parts used: Seeds

Horse chestnut owes its name to the fact that the ancients thought the large seeds resembled a horse's eyes. The seeds also resembled the eyes of stags, hence buckeye, one of the herb's common names.

Healing History

Since ancient times, horse chestnut has been used in many ways. The wood was popular in construction and furniture-making. Bark extracts produce a yellow dye that was used in weaving. Seed preparations were applied topically to treat joint aches and pains.

In 1615, a French traveler returned from a trip to Constantinople (now Istanbul) with some horse chestnut seeds. He planted them in Paris, and within 100 years, the tree had spread throughout Europe.

All parts of the horse chestnut plant are poisonous when ingested—especially the seeds, which are the parts used in herbal medicine. Fortunately, the seeds can be detoxified. Native Americans did this in several ways, including burying the seeds in the ground for many months so the soil would absorb the poisonous compounds. Then they unearthed the detoxified seeds, boiled them, and ate them as food. Some tribes combined crushed seeds with bear fat and applied the mixture to treat hemorrhoids, one type of varicose vein condition.

Native Americans in California used the fresh seeds as a poison. They crushed them and scattered them in lakes and streams to stupefy fish, making them easier to catch.

In 1896, a French researcher reported that horse chestnut seed extract helped relieve hemorrhoids. America's 19th-century Eclectic physicians, forerunners of today's naturopaths, incorporated the herb into their treatment of hemorrhoids. The Eclectic textbook *King's American Dispensatory* (1898) noted that horse chestnut helps treat "vascular fullness and capillary engorgement," in other words, varicose veins.

The Eclectics also used horse chestnut topically to relieve joint pain, and they detoxified the seed extract for internal use to treat fevers, including malaria.

Contemporary herbalists recommend horse chestnut seed almost exclusively for varicose veins and hemorrhoids.

Therapeutic Uses

Horse chestnut seed contains aescin, a compound that helps strengthen the walls of veins and increases their elasticity. This promotes normal bloodflow and helps prevent the pooling of blood that contributes to varicose veins and hemorrhoids.

VARICOSE VEINS. In a German study, 22 people with leaky veins (venous insufficiency), an early sign of varicose veins, were given either a medically inactive placebo or horse chestnut (600 milligrams of extract containing 50 milligrams of aescin). Three hours later, fluid leakage increased in those who had taken the placebo but decreased 22 percent in those who had taken horse chestnut, demonstrating that the herb strengthened their veins.

Another German research team gave 240 people with venous insufficiency one of three treatments: a placebo, compression therapy (support stockings, a standard mainstream medical treatment), or horse chestnut seed extract (50 milligrams of aescin twice a day). After 3 months, leg swelling increased slightly among those taking the placebos, but it decreased significantly (by about 25 percent) in both the people wearing support stockings and those taking horse chestnut. The researchers concluded that compression therapy and herbal therapy produced equivalent benefits. Several other studies have shown that horse chestnut and support hose offer similar benefits.

British researchers analyzed 13 studies of horse chestnut for venous insufficiency. Their conclusion: It works. For varicose veins, they called horse chestnut seed extract "an option worth considering."

Commission E, the expert panel that evaluates herbal medicines for the German counterpart of the FDA, endorses horse chestnut extract as a treatment for varicose veins.

HEMORRHOIDS. While more recent studies have focused on horse chestnut's effectiveness in relieving varicose veins in the legs, the herb's vein-strengthening action was first described as a treatment for hemorrhoids. Horse chestnut seed extract should help heal varicosities in the anal area.

HEARING PROBLEMS. Poor blood circulation in the inner ear is associated with hearing loss and ringing in the ears (tinnitus). German researchers gave either a standard medication (pentoxyfyllin) or a treatment that included horse chestnut (125 milligrams of aescin a day) to 68 people with hearing difficulties. After 44 days, those taking the horse chestnut preparation experienced significantly greater hearing restoration.

ARTHRITIS. Horse chestnut seed has anti-inflammatory action, lending credence to its traditional use as a treatment for joint pain.

Rx Recommendations

In the varicose vein studies, the typical dose has been 50 milligrams of aescin two or three times a day.

The Safety Factor

Warning: All parts of the horse chestnut plant are poisonous unless they're detoxified. Poisoning from the fresh, unprocessed herb causes muscle weakness and spasms, loss of coordination, pupil dilation, vomiting, diarrhea, and paralysis. Adults have become quite ill from drinking tea made from fresh leaves and twigs. Children have died. Never ingest any part of the horse chestnut tree. Commercial medicinal preparations are detoxified, so buy one and follow the label directions.

Aescin is not recommended for internal use by women who are pregnant. If you are pregnant and you develop varicose veins, try a topical cream made with horse chestnut seed extract. Likewise, nursing women should not take horse chestnut internally, but may use it topically.

Do not give horse chestnut to children under 2. In older children, adjust the recommended dose based on the child's weight. For example, give a 50-pound child one-third of the dose a 150-pound adult would take.

If you're over 65, start with a low dose, and increase only if necessary.

Inform health care professionals of the herbs you use. Problematic herb-drug interactions are possible.

Horse chestnut may cause allergic reactions or other unexpected side effects. If any develop, reduce your dose or stop taking it.

For more on herb safety, see Chapter 2.

If symptoms get worse or persist longer than 2 weeks, consult a health care professional promptly.

Growing Information

Native to the Balkans and the Middle East, horse chestnut trees now grow worldwide. They are majestic, climbing as high as 75 feet and producing large leaves and attractive pink and white flowers in spring or summer, depending on latitude. The fruit has a thick, leathery husk that contains from one to six seeds, or nuts.

HORSETAIL

An Herbal Gold Mine

Family: Equisetaceae; the family is extinct except for horsetail

Genus and species: *Equisetum arvense*

Also known as: Equisetum, scouring rush, pewterwort, shave grass, corncob plant, and bottle brush

Parts used: Stems

All that's gold does not necessarily glitter. Take horsetail. The bamboolike marsh dweller is capable of absorbing gold dissolved in water. What makes this of interest to herbalists is that doctors often prescribe preparations containing gold for rheumatoid arthritis, and horsetail has a long history as an herbal remedy for joint pain.

Healing History

Centuries before anyone realized that horsetail contains gold, the ancients discovered its value as an abrasive cleanser. Over time, the herb was used to scour pots, polish pewter, and sand or "shave" wood—hence its popular names scouring rush, shave grass, and pewterwort (*wort* is Old English for "plant").

During ancient famines, Romans ate horsetail shoots, which look like asparagus but are neither as tasty nor as nutritious. (Backpacking guides still recommend the tough, stringy shoots for wilderness foragers.) The Roman physician Galen claimed that horsetail healed severed tendons and ligaments and helped stop nosebleeds.

Ancient Chinese physicians recommended horsetail as a treatment for wounds, hemorrhoids, arthritis, and dysentery.

Seventeenth-century English herbalist Nicholas Culpeper called horsetail "very powerful to stop bleeding . . . [and] heal ulcers . . . the juice or decoction being drunk . . . or applied outwardly. . . . It solders together wounds and cures all ruptures."

Over the years, horsetail gained a reputation as a diuretic. America's 19th-century Eclectic physicians, forerunners of today's naturopaths, prescribed the herb for incontinence, gonorrhea, kidney stones, kidney infections, urinary complaints, and congestive heart failure, which causes fluid retention and swelling.

Contemporary herbalists recommend horsetail externally for wounds and internally for urinary and prostate problems. Homeopaths prescribe microdoses of the herb for urinary problems: bladder infections, bed-wetting, incontinence, and urethritis.

Therapeutic Uses

Horsetail is not a major medicinal herb and has not been well researched. But the available evidence suggests that it lives up to its traditional reputation.

WOUNDS. Commission E, the expert panel that evaluates herbal medicines for the German counterpart of the FDA, approves horsetail compresses as a wound treatment.

URINARY PROBLEMS. Horsetail contains a weak diuretic chemical called equisetonin, which lends support to the herb's traditional use as a urinary stimulant. Commission E approves horsetail as a treatment for urinary tract infections and kidney stones.

ARTHRITIS. Horsetail absorbs gold dissolved in water better than most plants, as much as 4 ounces per ton of fresh stalks. Of course, the amount of gold in a cup of horsetail tea is tiny, but only small amounts of the mineral have been given in the past as a treatment for rheumatoid arthritis. For this disease, the Chinese rely on horsetail. If you'd like to try the herb as part of an overall rheumatoid arthritis treatment plan, discuss it with your physician. However, be aware that mainstream physicians in the United States no longer use gold to treat rheumatoid arthritis. Drugs that work better have been developed.

Medicinal Myth

Because horsetail contains nicotine, some herbalists recommend the herb as a nicotine substitute for smokers attempting to quit. But compared with cigarettes, horsetail's nicotine content is minute, only about 0.00004 percent. It's unlikely to satisfy a smoker's craving. Prescription nicotine gum (Nicorette) would be a better alternative.

Rx Recommendations

To treat a urinary tract condition, take either an infusion or a tincture. For wounds, try a topical application of either form.

To prepare an infusion, use 1 to 2 teaspoons of dried herb per cup of boiling water, steep for 10 minutes, and strain. Drink up to 2 cups a day. Horsetail has little taste.

As a homemade tincture, use $1/2$ to 1 teaspoon up to twice a day.

When using commercial preparations, follow the package directions.

The Safety Factor

Horsetail may cause rashes in people who are sensitive to it.

In addition to absorbing an unusually large amount of gold, horsetail also absorbs relatively large amounts of selenium. Selenium is an important nutrient, a potent antioxidant that has been shown to help prevent several types of cancer. But too much selenium may cause birth defects. In marshes downstream from heavily fertilized agricultural areas, horsetail may have hazardously high selenium levels. Pregnant women should not use the herb. Nursing women should also avoid it.

Horsetail contains a chemical called equisetine that in large amounts is a nerve poison. Animals that were fed the herb have experienced fever, weight loss, muscle weakness, and abnormal pulse rate. Some have even died. Children have reportedly suffered nonfatal reactions after using the hollow stems as toy blowguns and ingesting the juice. Don't let children play with this herb.

If you're over 65, start with a low dose, and increase only if necessary.

Inform health care professionals of the herbs you use. Problematic herb-drug interactions are possible.

Horsetail may cause allergic reactions or other unexpected side effects. If any develop, reduce your dose or stop taking it.

For more on herb safety, see Chapter 2.

If symptoms get worse or persist longer than 2 weeks, consult a health care professional promptly.

Growing Information

Horsetail is the sole surviving descendant of the giant fernlike plants that covered the Earth some 200 million years ago. The herb's creeping rhizome sends up hollow, jointed, virtually leafless, bamboolike stalks that reach 6 feet. At the ends of the stalks, spore-bearing structures (catkins) develop. These resemble horse tails, corncobs, or bottle brushes, hence some of the herb's names.

Horsetails may be purchased from specialty nurseries, or root cuttings may be taken from wild plants in the spring when the spearlike stems have reached a few inches in length. Set plants or cuttings just under the surface of marshy soil. Keep it wet. If you do not want the plant to spread, contain it by embedding sheet metal in the soil to a depth of 18 inches. Harvest the stalks in the fall. Make sure that children do not suck on the hollow stems.

HYSSOP

The Biblical Antiseptic

Family: Labiatae; other members include mints

Genus and species: *Hyssopus officinalis*

Also known as: No other names, but many other plants are called hyssop

Parts used: Leaves and flowers

The Book of Psalms (51:9) says, "Purge me with hyssop and I shall be clean." But this biblical herb does more than clean. It may work as an antiseptic for infections such as cold sores and genital herpes.

Healing History

Some 2,500 years ago, Jewish priests used strong-smelling hyssop to clean the temple in Jerusalem and other places of worship. Unfortunately, so many plants were called hyssop back then that we have no way of knowing if the cleanser and the medicinal herb (*Hyssopus officinalis*) were one and the same.

Despite the confusion, the Greeks adopted hyssop. The noted Greek physician Dioscorides prescribed the herb as a tea for cough, wheezing, and shortness of breath; in plasters and chest rubs; and as an aromatic nasal and chest decongestant.

The medieval German abbess/herbalist Hildegard of Bingen wrote that hyssop "cleanses the lungs." She also recommended a meal of chicken cooked in hyssop and wine as a treatment for sadness (depression).

In 17th-century Europe, hyssop was a popular air freshener or "strewing herb." At the time, people rarely bathed, and farm animals often shared human living quarters. To mask odors, crushed hyssop leaves and flowers were scattered (strewn) around homes. When bathing became popular and strewing ceased, hyssop was placed in scent baskets in sickrooms.

Seventeenth-century English herbalist Nicholas Culpeper echoed Dioscorides' endorsement of hyssop for chest ailments: "It expelleth tough phlegm and is effectual for all griefs of the chest and lungs." He also claimed, "It killeth worms in the belly. . . . Boiled with figs, it makes an excellent gargle for quinsey [tonsillitis]. . . . Boiled in wine, it is good to wash inflammations . . . the head being anointed with the oil, it killeth lice."

Colonists introduced hyssop into North America and continued using the herb to treat chest congestion. It developed a reputation as a means of promoting menstruation and inducing abortions. (It doesn't do either.)

As time passed, hyssop's popularity waned.

America's 19th-century Eclectic physicians, forerunners of today's naturopaths, prescribed the herb externally to relieve the pain of bruises and internally as a gargle for sore throat and tonsillitis and as a treatment for asthma and coughing.

Contemporary herbalists recommend hyssop compresses and poultices for bruises, burns, and wounds, and suggest infusions for colds, coughs, bronchitis, flatulence, indigestion, and even epileptic seizures. Some also still mistakenly recommend it for menstruation promotion. As proof of the herb's effectiveness for wounds and respiratory infections, some herbalists point to the fact that the microorganism that produces penicillin (*Penicillium*) grows on hyssop leaves.

Therapeutic Uses

Hyssop won't whiten your toilet bowl as modern cleansers do, but its main traditional uses have some scientific support.

COUGHS. Hyssop is a member of the aromatic mint family, and its volatile oil contains several soothing camphorlike constituents, plus one expectorant chemical (marrubiin) that loosens phlegm so it's easier to cough up. Scientific sources agree that hyssop is a "reasonably effective" treatment for the cough and respiratory irritation of colds and flu.

HERPES. Hyssop inhibits the growth of herpes simplex virus, which causes genital herpes and cold sores. Try the infusion in a compress if you have this chronic, recurring infection.

VARICOSE VEINS. Hyssop contains diosmin, a compound that helps strengthen veins. The herb can be up to 6 percent diosmin (by dry weight). It takes only about 5 grams of hyssop (approximately 2 teaspoons) to provide the 300 milligrams of diosmin considered necessary to have vein-strengthening action.

HEMORRHOIDS. Hemorrhoids are a type of varicose vein and thus may benefit from treatment with hyssop.

Intriguing Possibility

A few laboratory studies have shown that hyssop extract exhibits potent activity against HIV, the virus that causes AIDS. It's too early to call hyssop an AIDS treatment, but in time it just might become one.

Medicinal Myth

Penicillium does indeed grow on hyssop. But the assertion that hyssop heals because it carries this microorganism is nonsense.

Rx Recommendations

To make a compress for treating herpes, use 1 ounce of dried herb per pint of boiling water. Steep for 15 minutes and let cool. Soak a clean cloth in the infusion and apply it to cold sores and genital herpes sores as needed.

For an infusion to treat cough, varicose veins, or hemorrhoids, use 2 teaspoons of herb per cup of boiling water, steep for 10 minutes, and strain. Drink up to 3 cups a day. Hyssop has a strong, camphorlike smell and tastes bitter. Add sugar, honey, or lemon or mix it with an herbal beverage blend to improve the flavor.

As a homemade tincture, take 1 teaspoon up to three times a day.

When using commercial preparations, follow the package directions.

The Safety Factor

Make sure that the hyssop you're taking is *Hyssopus officinalis*. Several other North American plants are also called hyssop, including hedge hyssop (*Gratiola officinalis*), the giant hyssops (several species of the genus *Agastache*), and the water hyssops (several species of *Bacopa*). Except for one species of bacopa (*Bacopa monnieri*, see page 84), these plants should not be ingested. Buy hyssop only from sources that identify it by botanical name.

Hyssop has not been shown to stimulate the uterus, but its traditional use to induce abortion should discourage pregnant women from taking it. Nursing women should also avoid it.

No reports of harm from hyssop appear in the world medical literature. Recently, however, laboratory animals injected with the herb's essential oil developed convulsions that caused some deaths. Do not exceed recommended amounts.

Do not give hyssop to children under 2. In older children, adjust the recommended dose based on the child's weight. For example, give a 50-pound child one-third of the dose a 150-pound adult would take.

If you're over 65, start with a low dose, and increase only if necessary.

Inform health care professionals of the herbs you use. Problematic herb-drug interactions are possible.

Hyssop may cause allergic reactions or other unexpected side effects. If any develop, reduce your dose or stop taking it.

For more on herb safety, see Chapter 2.

If symptoms get worse or persist longer than 2 weeks, consult a health care professional promptly.

Growing Information

If you want bees in your garden, plant this pretty, hardy, shrubby perennial. Hyssop also has a reputation for enhancing the flavor of grapes and increasing the yield of cabbages planted nearby.

Hyssop has small, lance-shaped leaves, as well as the square stems characteristic of the mints. The plant reaches 2 feet and has a medicinal odor that becomes more mintlike when the leaves are crushed. Dense clusters of blue or violet flowers form on 6-inch spikes atop the stems in summer and early fall.

Hyssop enjoys dry, sunny locations and tolerates most soils. In partial shade, it tends to become leggy. It may be propagated from seeds, cuttings, or root divisions. Seeds should be sown $^1/_4$ inch deep after the danger of frost has passed. Cuttings and divisions may be rooted either indoors or outdoors in a cool, shady place.

Thin established plants to 12-inch spacing. Add compost each spring, and water seedlings every few days. Mature plants prefer a drier environment and require little care.

Once the plant reaches about 18 inches and exudes its characteristic aroma, cut back the tops to stimulate leaf growth. The leaves may be harvested at any time. If you don't plan to use the flowers, cut back the entire plant to 4 inches aboveground just before it blooms. Dry the herb and store it in airtight containers.

JUNIPER
The Gin-Flavored Healer

Family: Cupressaceae; other members include cypress

Genus and species: *Juniperus communis*

Also known as: Genvrier and geneva

Parts used: Berries (actually miniature female cones)

If you've ever had a martini, you've had juniper. Aromatic juniper berries are the flavoring agent in gin. Juniper also increases urine production, making the herb a possible treatment for premenstrual syndrome, high blood pressure, and congestive heart failure.

Healing History

During the Middle Ages, Europeans believed that planting a juniper beside the front door kept witches out. Unfortunately, it did not provide complete protection. A witch could still enter if she correctly guessed the number of needles on the tree.

As time passed, juniper's protective reputation evolved into the belief that its smoke prevented leprosy and bubonic plague. As recently as World War II, French nurses burned juniper in hospital rooms to fumigate them.

By the 17th century, juniper was a popular diuretic. English herbalist Nicholas Culpeper wrote that the herb "provokes urine exceedingly. . . . [juniper] is so powerful a remedy against dropsy [congestive heart failure], it cures the disease." In addition, Culpeper prescribed juniper for "cough, shortness of breath, consumption [tuberculosis] . . . to provoke terms [menstruation] . . . and give safe and speedy delivery to women with child."

Native Americans independently discovered juniper's childbirth-assisting properties. In 1540, when the Spanish explorer Coronado entered what is now New Mexico looking for the mythical, gold-encrusted Seven Cities of Cibola, he found Zuni women using juniper berries to promote uterine recovery after childbirth. They also used the herb to treat wound infections and arthritis.

America's 19th-century Eclectic physicians, forerunners of today's naturopaths, dismissed juniper as a childbirth aid but strongly endorsed it for congestive heart failure. The Eclectics also prescribed juniper externally for eczema and psoriasis and internally for gonorrhea, bladder and kidney infections, and other genital and urinary problems.

Contemporary herbalists recommend juniper externally as an antiseptic and internally for bladder infections, arthritis, intestinal cramps, and gout. One herbalist suggests using the herb as a urinary deodorant in cases of chronic incontinence because it gives urine the fragrance of violets.

The medicinal claims for juniper take a back seat to its use in gin, invented in the 17th century by a Dutch professor of medicine, Franciscus Sylvius, who was interested in creating a diuretic tincture. Our word *gin* comes from the Dutch word for juniper, *geniver*. The English took to gin so enthusiastically that references to its native land still pepper the English language. Drink a little gin, and you obtain "Dutch courage." Drink too much, and you get in trouble, or "in Dutch."

Therapeutic Uses

Juniper's aromatic oil contains terpinen-4-ol, a diuretic compound that increases the fluid-filtering rate of the kidneys. This supports the herb's traditional role as a diuretic.

HIGH BLOOD PRESSURE. Physicians often prescribe diuretics to treat high blood pressure (hypertension). This is a serious condition requiring professional care. If you'd like to use juniper as part of your treatment plan, discuss it with your physician.

CONGESTIVE HEART FAILURE. Culpeper exaggerated when he said that juniper "cures" congestive heart failure. As a diuretic, however, the herb can be part of an overall treatment plan. Congestive heart failure is a serious condition requiring professional care. If you'd like to try juniper, discuss it with your physician.

WOMEN'S HEALTH CONCERNS. In animal studies, juniper stimulates uterine contractions. For this reason, pregnant women should not take it (except at term under the supervision of a physician, when it may help stimulate labor). Other women might try it to help start their menstrual periods.

PREMENSTRUAL SYNDROME. Diuretics can help relieve the bloated feeling caused by premenstrual fluid retention. Women bothered by premenstrual syndrome might try juniper during the uncomfortable days right before their periods.

ARTHRITIS. Juniper has anti-inflammatory properties, suggesting that it may be of value in treating arthritis. Native Americans used the herb for this purpose. Likewise, in Germany, where herbal medicine is considerably more mainstream than in the United States, physicians prescribe juniper preparations for arthritis and gout.

Intriguing Possibility

Animal studies show that juniper reduces blood sugar levels. It's too early to call it a treatment for diabetes, but it may play that role in the future.

Medicinal Myth

Juniper has never been shown to be effective for gonorrhea or for bladder or kidney infections.

Rx Recommendations

If you want to take advantage of juniper's diuretic properties or to try it to relieve arthritis pain or bring on your period, take it as an infusion. Use 1 teaspoon of crushed berries per cup of boiling water. Steep for 10 to 20 minutes, then strain. Drink up to 2 cups a day for no more than 6 weeks. Juniper has a strong, pleasantly aromatic taste.

When using commercial preparations, follow the package directions.

The Safety Factor

Diuretics deplete the body of potassium, an essential mineral. If you use juniper, be sure to eat foods rich in potassium, such as bananas and fresh vegetables.

In large doses, the diuretic compound in juniper irritates the kidneys. It may cause kidney damage in people who are particularly sensitive to it and in those who have kidney disease. For this reason, people with kidney infections or a history of kidney impairment should not take it. Even low doses taken over long periods may cause problems. "The rule," notes distinguished German medical herbalist Rudolph Fritz Weiss, M.D., "is never take juniper for longer than 6 weeks."

Symptoms of overdose include diarrhea, intestinal pain, kidney pain, protein in the urine (albuminuria), blood in the urine (hematuria), purplish urine, rapid heartbeat, and elevated blood pressure. If you notice any of these symptoms while taking juniper, stop using it.

Many elderly people have kidney impairment. Those over age 65 should have their kidney function checked by a physician before taking juniper, and then start with a low dose, increasing it only if necessary.

Up to one-third of people with hay fever develop allergy symptoms from exposure to juniper, according to a study in *Clinical Allergy*. If you have hay fever, you may want to avoid the herb. It may trigger other allergic reactions as well, notably rash.

Pregnant and nursing women should not use juniper.

Do not give juniper to children under 2. In older children, adjust the recommended dose based on the child's weight. For example, give a

50-pound child one-third of the dose a 150-pound adult would take.

Inform health care professionals of the herbs you use. Problematic herb-drug interactions are possible.

Juniper may cause allergic reactions or other unexpected side effects. If any develop, reduce your dose or stop taking it.

For more on herb safety, see Chapter 2.

If symptoms get worse or persist longer than 2 weeks, consult a health care professional promptly.

Growing Information

The genus *Juniperus* contains more than 70 species of aromatic evergreens. Most are small trees, but some grow to 40 feet.

The species most widely used in herbal healing, common juniper (*J. communis*) reaches 6 to 20 feet, depending on locale. Its close, tangled, spreading branches are covered with reddish brown bark, sticky gum, and pointed $^1/_2$-inch needles. Males produce yellow flowers and females have green flowers. The females also produce scaly, green, aromatic $^1/_4$-inch cones (berries) that turn blue-black during their 2-year maturation. If you want berries, be sure to plant both male and female junipers, or the females will not fruit.

Junipers usually prefer sandy soil and full sun, but they adapt to many soil and climate conditions. Consult a nursery for advice specific to your locale.

Females produce immature (green) and mature (blue-black) berries simultaneously. Harvest only the mature berries in fall. Dry them in the sun. When dried, they turn a dull black. Store them in airtight containers to preserve their volatile oil.

KAVA
The South Pacific Soother

Family: Piperaceae; other members include black pepper

Genus and species: *Piper methysticum*

Also known as: Kava kava, awa, kew, tonga

Parts used: Rhizomes and roots

For centuries, the people of the South Pacific have used kava the way Americans use beer—socially, as a mild intoxicant. In the mid-1990s, kava became popular in the United States as a treatment for stress and anxiety. But during 2000 and 2001, almost 100 people who had taken kava developed liver damage. Some suffered liver failure and died. Headlines proclaimed the herb "a killer," and its popularity plummeted. Since then, scientists have done extensive research to determine the herb's safety. Their conclusion: Kava root is not a killer, and it's not toxic to the liver.

Healing History

Polynesians from New Guinea to Tahiti have a longstanding tradition of enjoying this herb in "kava circles." The circle begins with one or more participants placing powdered kava root in half of a coconut shell and adding about a cup of water to form a milky solution. Then everyone claps as the drinker downs the brew in one big gulp. The shell is passed to the next person in the circle, and the ceremony is repeated until each participant has taken several gulps. As the festivities continue, the conversation and laughter flow more easily, as they might after a few beers.

In the South Pacific, kava has been used as a treatment for headache, colds, and arthritis and as a sedative and aphrodisiac. Native Hawaiians took the herb to control asthma.

The 18th-century British explorer Captain James Cook and his crew were offered kava during their voyage among the islands of the South Pacific (1768–1771). They enjoyed its peppery taste and mild intoxicating effect. They also noticed that elderly kava drinkers who had consumed large amounts of the herb over the course of many decades had oddly scaly skin; this is the main sign of kava dermopathy (more on this later).

Around 1990, kava began attracting the attention of American herbalists. European (mostly German) studies had shown that at doses lower than those used in the South Pacific, the root produces little or no euphoria but instead acts as a mild tranquilizer.

Therapeutic Uses

The active compounds in kava, called kavalactones, have a mild tranquilizing effect similar to a low dose of diazepam (Valium). But unlike the drug, kava is much less likely to cause sedation, and it's not addictive. (The combination of kava and alcohol or other depressants is powerfully sedative, however.)

ANXIETY AND STRESS. Many recent studies, almost all German, show that kava is an effective treatment for stress and anxiety. Here's a brief overview of the research.

❧ German researchers gave 100 people who were complaining of nervous anxiety, agoraphobia, or social phobia either a placebo or 300 milligrams of kava a day. After 8 weeks, those taking kava showed measurably less anxiety and depression. The benefits continued for the 6-month duration of the study. Side effects were mild and minor, reported by only 5 of the 50 who used kava.

❧ In another German study, 58 people with anxiety disorders took either a placebo or 100 milligrams of kava three times a day. In the kava group, anxiety symptoms began to decline after just 1 week of treatment and continued to diminish throughout the month-long study. The kava takers reported no side effects.

❧ At the Medical College of Virginia, researchers gave either a placebo or 240 milligrams of kava per day to 60 adults dealing with stress and anxiety. After 4 weeks, those taking the placebo showed no significant change in anxiety symptoms, but those taking kava reported fewer interpersonal problems, fewer anxiety symptoms, and less stress—without side effects.

❧ In another study involving 172 participants, German scientists compared kava (taken in a dose of 100 milligrams three times a day) with standard doses of two drugs in the Valium family of tranquilizers. After 6 weeks, all three treatments were equally effective.

❧ Italian researchers gave one of three treatments to 68 women complaining of menopause-induced anxiety: a placebo, low-dose kava (100 milligrams per day), or high-dose kava (200 milligrams per day). Both kava treatments were significantly more effective than the placebo.

❧ Two research teams, one British and the other German, performed sophisticated statistical tests (meta-analyses) on studies of kava for anxiety. The English group reviewed seven trials, the Germans six. In both analyses, kava proved an effective treatment for anxiety.

Commission E, the expert panel that evaluates herbal medicines for the German counterpart of the FDA, endorses kava as a treatment for stress and anxiety problems. The herb is best used short-term, for periods of up to a few months. If you feel that you still need anti-anxiety medication after a few months, consult your physician.

Rx Recommendations

You may be able to buy powdered bulk kava root, particularly in Hawaii, but most Americans take commercial capsules.

Look for a standardized extract that contains 60 to 75 milligrams of kavalactones per capsule. The dose used in most studies is 300 milligrams of standardized extract (the equivalent of about 200 milligrams of kavalactones), taken in divided doses. Follow the package directions.

The Liver Toxicity Scare of 2000 and 2001—And Its Resolution

In 2000, a 14-year-old American girl developed persistent nausea, vomiting, fatigue, weight loss, and loss of appetite, a constellation of symptoms that suggests acute hepatitis. She saw a doctor, who prescribed rest and liver-function tests. The test results showed much more liver damage than hepatitis typically causes. The girl was hospitalized with liver failure and received an emergency liver transplant.

Liver failure is extremely rare in otherwise healthy teenagers. This girl did not use alcohol, which, in large amounts, is toxic to the liver, and she took no medication implicated in liver damage, just ibuprofen (Motrin, Advil) occasionally. However, she'd taken kava for 44 days to treat anxiety.

This was just one of an estimated 82 reports from around the world of kava users developing liver disease ranging from mild liver impairment (elevated liver enzymes) to jaundice, to hepatitis, to acute liver failure requiring an estimated dozen transplants. Nine of these people died.

By early 2001, these reports generated headlines around the world. *USA Today* declared, "Herb Kava Linked to Liver Problems." The *New York Times* ran an article entitled, "Questions about Kava's Safety." They also prompted several countries—Germany, Austria, Canada,

France, Ireland, Singapore, Switzerland, and the United Kingdom—to ban the herb. Kava was not banned in the United States, but the FDA warned consumers about the possibility of life-threatening liver damage.

Kava sales plummeted. As sales fell, so did reports of kava-induced liver damage. The controversy became old news—but not to herb researchers. Studies continued. Some suggested that the herb is toxic. Others made the safety scare look more like a tempest in a teapot—or in a traditional Polynesian kava bowl. In 2005, the German counterpart of the FDA repealed its kava ban. But soon after, the United Kingdom decided to uphold its ban on kava products.

Kava cannot be called completely safe. Like virtually all pharmacologically active substances, it has benefits and risks. But by the same token, it's an overstatement to call this herb hazardous. Most people can use kava safely in recommended amounts. But kava consumers should be well informed about this herb because its downside, liver damage, though rare, is potentially life-threatening.

According to distinguished German herb researcher Mathias Schmidt, Ph.D., an expert on kava, the herb is reasonably safe. Many of the case reports of kava-related liver damage turn out to be much less than compelling. Researchers at the University of Munster, Germany, analyzed 78 European case reports of alleged kava toxicity. Only four could be persuasively linked to kava alone. Dr. Schmidt's own analysis knocked that number down to three. The tiny number of European kava-related problems, Dr. Schmidt says, "stand against 450 million doses of kava taken in Europe during the 10 years before the German ban." An analysis by University of Sydney, Australia, researchers agrees: "Only a negligible fraction of the case reports are attributable to kava."

Even if every case were attributable to kava, its rate of serious side effects would be comparable to that of many FDA-approved drugs.

In most case reports of kava toxicity, the herb was just one of many drugs the people used that might harm the liver, including alcohol, aspirin, Prozac, Paxil, and birth control pills.

Furthermore, according to a report in the *German Pharmacists Journal*, kava has been used throughout Polynesia for at least 1,500 years with few reports of significant side effects and no reports in the ethnopharmacological literature of liver damage, such as jaundice.

Finally, various research reports show that the traditional water extract of the herb (powdered kava root mixed with water) is not toxic to the liver in rats, and causes no toxicity in isolated human liver cells.

Many drugs considered safe in recommended amounts can cause liver damage when taken in large amounts, however. One example of this is acetaminophen (Tylenol). Two studies have looked at kava use among Australia's aboriginal population. Heavy users have developed elevated liver enzymes, the first sign of liver damage. But none developed liver failure—and the native Australians were using at least *4 ounces of kava a week for decades*, thousands of times more than the typical American users.

If kava is reasonably safe when typical amounts are ingested, why did several dozen people around the world develop serious liver disease while taking it? Researchers have identified four possible reasons.

1. As already mentioned, most of those who developed liver disease were also taking other drugs that can cause liver toxicity. It's possible that kava increases the likelihood of such damage.

2. Kava is a fairly slow-growing herb. It takes 4 to 5 years for the root/rhizome to mature enough to be harvested for sale. Kava's popularity as an herbal tranquilizer dates from the late 1990s. At that time, demand for the herb grew much faster than its supply. There were reports that some growers stretched their supply by including not just root material but also the aerial parts of the plant. The aerial parts contain an alkaloid, pipermethystin, that is toxic to the liver. It's possible that contamination of the root with stem material containing pipermethystin was responsible for the liver toxicity.

   The contamination theory dovetails with the timeline of problems with kava. The first report of liver toxicity was published in 1998. The story became news in 2001. Since then, reports have fallen off. Part of the reason is that kava consumption has fallen. As that happened, there was less pressure to stretch supply, so it's likely that there was less contamination of root material with the liver-toxic aerial parts of the plant.

3. Traditionally, Polynesians pound kava root into a powder and mix it with water, then drink the cloudy white liquid. Western commercial extracts do not use water, but alcohol, acetone, or methanol. This results in different concentrations of the herb's active constituents (kavalactones). It's possible that the difference between traditional and commercial kava preparations plays a role in liver damage. In addition, water extracts of kava contain glutathione, a potent antioxidant that helps prevent liver toxicity. Commercial preparations don't contain glutathione, which might increase risk of liver problems.

4. Kava is one of a great many drugs and herbs that affect the body's cytochrome P450 system. This system, little known outside of professional medicine, involves a group of 50 enzymes, six of which are involved in the metabolism of 90 percent of drugs, including medicinal herbs. When drugs and herbs that both affect the cytochrome P450 enzyme system are taken simultaneously, liver damage or potentially problematic interactions are possible. Cytochrome P450 problems are most likely in those with a genetic deficiency in a certain enzyme, CYP2D6.

   This deficiency is rare in Polynesians. But an estimated 8 percent of people of European descent have it. A CYP2D6 deficiency might increase susceptibility to liver damage, and at the same time, explain why it has not been observed in traditional kava-using cultures.

   The situation is confusing, Dr. Schmidt concedes. But he believes there is "a high probability" that the problem was caused by kava root material adulterated with material from aerial parts of the plant that are liver-toxic.

   Compared with pharmaceuticals with similar action, such as Valium, kava is *safer*. German researchers estimate that kava produces 0.008 adverse event reports (AERs) per million doses. Valium produces 2.12. But Valium does not cause liver failure.

The American Botanical Council (ABC) in Austin, Texas, the nation's leading herb education organization, has developed a series of guidelines for safe use of kava.

🍀 Don't use kava if you have been diagnosed with liver disease, or have a history of liver disease.

🍀 Don't use it if you take drugs with potential liver toxicity, including alcohol. Take a list of your medications to your physician or pharmacist and ask if any might cause liver toxicity. If so, do not take kava.

🍀 Kava-related liver damage is associated with long-term use of the herb. Don't take it daily for more than 4 weeks without consulting a medical professional for a liver-function test. "Periodic liver-function tests are required for those who take statin drugs to lower cholesterol," ABC executive director Mark Blumenthal says. "I'd recommend them for long-term kava users."

🍀 Stop taking kava if you notice nausea, vomiting, unusual fatigue, loss of appetite, darkening of urine, or yellowing of the eyes. These are all symptoms of liver disease. If you develop these symptoms, consult a physician promptly.

In addition, here are other prudent suggestions.

🍀 Look for products that specify only root/rhizome material. This is no guarantee that you'll get only root/rhizome material. But care in labeling often indicates care in harvesting.

🍀 If you have had unusual reactions to other drugs, you might have a CYP2D6 enzyme deficiency. Recently, a test became available that can identify this deficiency, but it costs $500 and most health insurers do not cover it. At this price, it's probably more cost effective to use other herbal tranquilizers instead of kava, such as chamomile, hop, and passionflower.

If Dr. Schmidt developed anxiety, would he use kava? Would he encourage a family member to use it? "Absolutely yes," he says, "provided that I know the quality of the raw material."

The Safety Factor

In unusually large doses—considerably larger than those necessary to relieve anxiety—kava causes inebriation similar to that caused by alcohol. Thinking and coordination become impaired. Walking becomes difficult, and stumbling and falling are likely. The eyes become bloodshot.

Taking unusually large doses for many years leads to the development of scaly skin, a condition called kava dermopathy. This side effect is highly unlikely in the doses recommended for anxiety. To treat kava dermopathy, experts recommend terminating use of kava.

Do not use kava at the same time as alcohol or other tranquilizing, sedative, or psychoactive medications, including antidepressants. The herb intensifies the sedative effect of other drugs.

Kava may cause some numbness of the mouth, which is harmless. Allergic reactions are also possible.

People who have conditions that impair coordination, such as Parkinson's disease, and those taking sedative or antidepressant medications should not use kava.

Pregnant and nursing women should not use kava.

Do not give kava to children under 2. In older children, adjust the recommended dose based on the child's weight. For example, give a 50-pound child one-third of the dose a 150-pound adult would take.

If you're over 65, start with a low dose, and increase only if necessary.

Inform health care professionals of the herbs you use. Problematic herb-drug interactions are possible.

Kava may cause allergic reactions or other unexpected side effects. If any develop, reduce your dose or stop taking it.

For more on herb safety, see Chapter 2.

If symptoms get worse or persist longer than 2 weeks, consult a health care professional promptly.

Growing Information

Kava is not a garden herb in the continental United States, though cultivation in Hawaii is possible. A botanical relative of black pepper, kava is a perennial shrub with heart-shaped leaves that grows throughout the South Pacific at altitudes of 500 to 1,000 feet. It does best in stony ground with full sun exposure. Plants can climb to 20 feet, but the roots are usually harvested when the shrub reaches about 8 feet.

KOLA

Sip It for Easy Breathing

Family: Sterculiaceae; other members include cocoa

Genus and species: *Cola nitida*, *C. vera*, and *C. acurninata*

Also known as: Cola

Parts used: Nuts (actually seed leaves, or cotyledons)

Cola drinks account for a whopping 70 percent of the enormous U.S. soft drink market. Americans might consume even more if they knew that the tropical nut responsible for colas' flavor can help relieve asthma.

Healing History

West Africans have used kola since prehistoric times. They chewed the seeds for their stimulant effect and as a treatment for fever.

West African slaves introduced the kola tree into Brazil and the Caribbean. Among Caribbean natives, the herb became a favorite diuretic for water retention as well as a digestive aid and a folk remedy for diarrhea, fatigue, and heart problems. Over time, kola's stimulant properties led to the belief that it was an aphrodisiac.

Kola arrived in the United States after the Civil War. Nineteenth-century Eclectic physicians, forerunners of today's naturopaths, noted that the Caribbean people ascribed "innumerable fabulous virtues" to the herb.

The Eclectics correctly identified the stimulants in kola—notably caffeine—as the same ones in cocoa, coffee, and tea. They prescribed kola to "overcome mental depression" and prepare for "severe physical and mental exertion." They also recommended it to relieve diarrhea, pneumonia, typhoid fever, migraines, seasickness, and morning sickness and for anyone who "attempts to break the tobacco habit."

Because kola was used medicinally, it was kept in stock by 19th-century pharmacists. Legend has it that on May 8, 1886, Atlanta pharmacist John Styth Pemberton was toying with herbs for a new headache remedy. He mixed some sugar with extracts of kola and coca (the source of cocaine) in a three-legged brass pot in his backyard. He added carbonated water to his sweet syrup and created a refreshing drink that his bookkeeper dubbed Coca-Cola.

Two years later, Pemberton sold all rights to his beverage to Atlanta businessman Asa Candler for $2,300. Candler was an imaginative marketer, and by 1895, Coca-Cola had become America's first national soft drink.

Today, Coca-Cola is among the best-known products in the world. People request it 250 million times a day in 80 languages and in 135 countries.

Since its development, Coca-Cola's formula has been a closely guarded secret, although it has evolved over the years. When the United States outlawed cocaine, the drug was removed from the formula. Today, Coca-Cola is known to contain decocainized coca leaf extract and a small amount of kola.

Modern herbalists recommend kola for its "marked stimulating effect on human consciousness," according to medical herbalist David Hoffmann's *Holistic Herbal*.

It's also prescribed as a treatment for diarrhea, depression, nervous debility, migraines, and loss of appetite.

Therapeutic Uses

STIMULANT ACTION. Some herbals claim that kola contains more caffeine than coffee. Not so. A 6-ounce cup of brewed coffee contains 100 to 150 milligrams of caffeine. A cup of instant coffee has 65 milligrams. By comparison, a 12-ounce can of a cola soft drink contains about 50 milligrams of caffeine. Most of this amount comes not from the kola nut but from added caffeine. (For more information on the health benefits and downsides of caffeine, see Coffee on page 164.)

ASTHMA. Coffee can help control asthma, but many children don't like the taste. That's why an article in the *Journal of the American Medical Association* recommended using cola beverages when kids start wheezing without their medicine handy or as tasty adjuncts to standard asthma medication.

Rx Recommendations

Cola beverages are the most convenient way to enjoy small amounts of this pleasant-tasting herb.

If you prefer to make a decoction, place 1 to 2 teaspoons of powdered kola nuts in 1 cup of water.

Bring to a boil and simmer for 10 minutes, then strain if you wish. Drink up to 3 cups a day.

You may give small amounts of dilute cola beverages cautiously to children under age 2.

The Safety Factor

Women hoping to become pregnant should avoid herbs containing caffeine because they reduce the likelihood of conception. However, this fertility-impairing effect is not reliable enough to be considered a contraceptive.

Pregnant and nursing women should not use kola.

People with any of the conditions mentioned in the discussion on the safety of coffee on page 169 should also avoid using kola.

Inform health care professionals of the herbs you use. Problematic herb-drug interactions are possible.

Kola may cause allergic reactions or other unexpected side effects. If any develop, reduce your dose or stop taking it.

For more on herb safety, see Chapter 2.

If symptoms get worse or persist longer than 2 weeks, consult a health care professional promptly.

Growing Information

Kola is a 40-foot tree that grows in West Africa, the Caribbean, Brazil, Sri Lanka, and Indonesia. Kolas have beautiful, purple-spotted yellow flowers that produce chocolate-colored seed pods in spring and fall.

For most plants, *nut* refers to the whole seed, but the kola nut is only part of the seed, specifically the embryonic leaves (or cotyledons) inside the seed coat. These are dried and powdered.

KUDZU VINE

From Miracle, to Pest, to Medicine

Family: Fabaceae; other members include beans, peas, and alfalfa

Genus and species: *Pueraria montana* (formerly *P. lobata*)

Also known as: Kuzu, gat gun, ge gan, miracle vine, foot-a-night vine, mile-a-minute vine, and the vine that ate the South

Parts used: Primarily the root, also flowers

Our word *kudzu* comes from the Japanese name of this fragrant-flowered vine, *kuzu*. It arrived in the United States in 1876 and was touted as a farmer's and gardener's dream come true. Then during the 1930s, it became a nightmare in the Southeast, where it still causes major environmental problems. But slowly, the much-reviled vine is starting to become appreciated as an herbal medicine. It contains compounds that can help treat menopausal discomforts, high cholesterol, heart disease, and stroke. It might even help alcoholics stop drinking.

Healing History

Kudzu is native to southern Japan and southeast China, where it is known as *gat gun* and *ge gan*. In Asia, it has been used for centuries as a food, animal feed, and treatment for a variety of conditions, including vertigo, tinnitus, and hangover.

Kudzu was introduced into the United States in 1876 at the Philadelphia Centennial Exposition, where it was touted as "miracle vine," a forage crop that could be a boon to farmers and ranchers, and a lovely ornamental for gardeners. It never caught on as a livestock feed, but as a garden plant, it was well suited to the Southeast, where it became popular because of its large, attractive leaves and spikes of fragrant purple flowers.

Kudzu also has an extensive root system, the kind that can be used to stabilize soil and prevent erosion. Starting in 1935, the federal Soil Conservation Service encouraged farmers from Virginia to Arkansas to Texas to plant it near streambeds to prevent loss of topsoil. The Depression-era Civilian Conservation Corps joined in this effort, planting the vine all over the South.

This turned out to be a huge mistake. The Southeast has perfect conditions for kudzu: lots of rain, hot summers, no hard freezes in winter, and no natural kudzu predators. As a result, the vine's runners ran amok. Kudzu grew out of control throughout the Southeast, earning such names as foot-a-night vine, mile-a-minute vine, and the vine that ate the South. Kudzu choked streambeds and strangled an enormous number of crops and shrubs, often completely covering full-grown trees and multistory buildings. In 1953, the U.S. Department of Agriculture dubbed it a pest. Kudzu now covers 12,000 square miles of the United States and costs an estimated $500 million a year in lost cropland and removal costs.

Therapeutic Uses

Kudzu research is still in its infancy. It may be the vine that ate the South, but it's also an herb with a surprisingly large number of medicinal uses.

MENOPAUSAL COMPLAINTS. Kudzu root contains two powerful plant estrogens (phytoestrogens), puerarin and daidzin. Treatment of menopausal discomforts with phytoestrogens does not involve the same potential for serious side effects as hormone replacement therapy, so the use of herbs containing phytoestrogens has emerged as an effective but safer alternative for treating menopausal complaints.

Researchers in Thailand assessed the menopausal symptoms of 48 women and then gave them either 50 or 100 milligrams of kudzu root per day. After 6 months, both groups reported significantly reduced symptoms. The researchers concluded that kudzu shows "great promise" for treatment of menopausal complaints.

HIGH CHOLESTEROL. Chinese researchers gave 120 people with high cholesterol one of three treatments: a standard pharmaceutical (pravastatin), kudzu, or a combination of the two. The drug and herb produced virtually the same benefit—on the drug, 81 percent of participants' cholesterol fell significantly; on the herb, 80 percent. The combination of the two worked best—97 percent showed significantly reduced cholesterol.

ANGINA. This form of heart disease causes severe chest pain with little or no exertion. Asian doctors often treat angina with injections of puerarin. Chinese researchers analyzed 20 studies of this practice involving 1,240 people with angina.

The results were published in *Cochrane Systematic Database Reviews*, a project of researchers worldwide whose conclusions are considered authoritative. Puerarin controlled angina as well as standard pharmaceuticals. And combinations of the herbal extract and drugs controlled it better than any standard drug by itself.

STROKE. Chinese animal studies show that puerarin improves bloodflow through the brain and spurs recovery from stroke.

In a Chinese study, cerebral hemorrhage survivors were treated with a standard pharmaceutical (nimodipine) or kudzu root (2 milligrams per kilogram of body weight per day, or 136 milligrams per day for a person weighing 150 pounds). For restoration of memory and spatial judgment, the herb was more beneficial than the drug. This is just one of 14 Asian studies of kudzu for stroke recovery. A review of all of them, totaling 1,141 people, shows that the herb improves memory and reasoning ability.

Intriguing Possibilities

Kudzu's use in Asia as a hangover treatment piqued the curiosity of Western researchers. A major contributor to hangover misery is the compound acetaldehyde. It slowly accumulates in drinkers' bloodstreams, causing "the moaning after." Kudzu contains compounds that make acetaldehyde build up in the blood more quickly, so you develop hangover symptoms not the next morning, but *while drinking*.

Now, a hangover is still a hangover no matter when it occurs, but animal studies have suggested that a hangover while drinking reduces alcohol consumption. Two studies have tested kudzu for deterrence of drinking in alcoholics. One showed no benefit, but the other produced intriguing results. Researchers at McLean Hospital in Belmont, Massachusetts, monitored 14 alcoholics as they drank at a bar, counting the number of drinks and the time it took them to drink them during a specified interval. Then the researchers gave the participants either a placebo or 1,000 milligrams of kudzu root three times a day. After 1 week, the participants returned to the bar. Those in the placebo group consumed just as many drinks just as quickly. The kudzu group, however, consumed significantly fewer drinks more slowly.

Kudzu is no miracle cure for alcoholism, and one beneficial study doesn't prove that it works. But alcoholism is a major public health problem that's notoriously difficult to treat medically. Kudzu offers real possibilities.

In addition, animal studies showing that kudzu reduces alcohol cravings also show that the herb protects the liver from alcohol-induced damage, and may even reverse that damage.

Kudzu may also be of benefit in osteoporosis prevention. Premenopausal blood levels of estrogen help protect women's bones. But with menopause, estrogen declines, and osteoporosis becomes a major issue. Several animal studies show that kudzu helps prevent bone loss.

Finally, animal studies suggest that kudzu lowers blood sugar levels, which means it might one day be used to help treat diabetes.

Rx Recommendations

At this writing, there is no standard dosage for kudzu. Human trials have used from 50 to 136 milligrams per day.

The Safety Factor

Kudzu root is starchy, like a potato. For centuries, it has been used in cooking in Asia, with no reports of harm. Kudzu is considered safe.

However, this herb affects the cytochrome P450 system. Kudzu's action on this metabolic pathway means that the herb might cause harmful interactions if used in combination with drugs that also affect this system. If you want to try kudzu, first check with your doctor to make sure that you are not taking other drugs that affect the cytochrome P450 system.

Pregnant and nursing women should not use kudzu.

Do not give kudzu to children.

If you're over 65, start with a low dose, and increase only if necessary.

Inform health care professionals of the herbs you use. Problematic herb-drug interactions are possible.

Kudzu may cause allergic reactions or other unexpected side effects. If any develop, reduce your dose or stop taking it.

For more on herb safety, see Chapter 2.

If symptoms get worse or persist longer than 2 weeks, consult a health care professional promptly.

Growing Information

Kudzu can be grown in pots indoors from seed or cuttings. It likes rich, moist soil, full sun, and heat.

Outdoors, kudzu grows in the arc from southern New Jersey to the middle of Texas. Because it so readily becomes a pest, gardening authorities recommend against growing it. One cautions, "If you plant it, do it only at night. If you plant it during the day and anyone sees you, they're likely to throw rocks."

LAVENDER

The First Herb of Aromatherapy

Family: Labiatae; other members include mints

Genus and species: *Lavandula angustifolia*; also known as *L. officinalis* and *L. spica*

Also known as: True lavender, spike lavender, lavandin, and aspic

Parts used: Flowers

Lavender grew in abundance around the ancient Syrian city of Nardus, near the Euphrates River. As a result, the ancient Greeks called the plant *nard*. The Bible refers to it as spikenard, a reference to the spikes on which the flowers form.

Our word *lavender* comes from the Latin *lavare*, meaning "to wash." Lavender was a frequent addition to baths and was also considered a purifier for the body and mind.

Healing History

Since ancient times, lavender has been used as a digestive aid, sleep aid, and tranquilizer for people who are anxious, restless, or emotionally troubled. Because of its mood-altering effects, lavender was also considered an antidepressant.

English farmers wore spikes of lavender flowers under their hats to prevent headache and sunstroke. The flowers were dried, powdered, and sewn into pillows as a fragrant treatment for insomnia. The herb was also considered a remedy for acne, migraines, diabetes, faintness, headache, and muscle spasms. Until World War I, lavender infusions and tinctures were used to disinfect wounds.

For centuries, lavender has been an ingredient in sachets and potpourris to freshen the air, especially in sickrooms. Sprigs were placed in wardrobes and closets to add fragrance to clothing and to repel moths.

During the Middle Ages, sprinkling lavender water on a lover's head was said to keep the person faithful, a reputed effect that generated great demand for the herb.

There was also a persistent rumor that the asp, a poisonous snake, nested in lavender bushes, which made people think twice about gathering the herb. This was pure fiction, apparently promoted by herbalists because it drove up lavender's price.

In his *Herball* or *Generall Historie of Plantes*, 16th-century British herbalist John Gerard wrote of lavender's use in treating palsy (tremors or paralysis): "It profiteth them much that have the palsy if they be washed with water of lavender flowers, or are anointed with the oil made from the flowers and olive oil."

Fifty years later, Nicholas Culpeper prescribed lavender for "all the grief and pains of the head . . . it strengthens the stomach . . . two spoonfuls of the distilled water of the flowers help them that have lost their voice. . . . "

America's 19th-century Eclectic physicians, forerunners of today's naturopaths, recommended lavender as a digestive aid. They cautioned, however, that immoderate use of lavender infusions might cause stomach upset.

The Birth of Aromatherapy

During the 1920s, French fragrance chemist Rene-Maurice Gattefosse was toiling in his laboratory, developing a new perfume. Lost in thought while blending essential oils from various herbs, he set off an explosion that burned his arm. Frantic with pain, he plunged his arm into the nearest cold liquid, which happened to be a bowl of lavender oil.

Immediately, Gattefosse felt surprising relief from his pain. In addition, instead of the extended healing process he'd known from previous burns—accompanied by redness, heat, inflammation, blisters, and scarring—this burn healed remarkably quickly, with little pain and no scarring. Perhaps, the perfumer thought, he had discovered a powerful healer that had literally been right under his nose.

Gattefosse devoted the rest of his life to studying the role of essential oils in health and healing. In 1928, he published the book *Aromatherapie*, coining the term that's now used to describe the healing discipline that involves inhaling aromatic plant oils or massaging them into the skin for physical or emotional benefits.

Today, aromatherapists use dozens of essential oils, but they still consider lavender one of the best for treating anger, anxiety, burns, depression, indigestion, infection, insomnia, irritability, muscle aches, and wounds.

Therapeutic Uses

Exposure to lavender is no guarantee of a lover's faithfulness. But modern research has validated many of the herb's traditional medicinal uses.

The essential oil extracted from lavender flowers is chemically very complex, containing more than 150 compounds. When rubbed on the skin, the oil penetrates quickly and can be detected in the blood in as little as 5 minutes.

ANXIETY AND STRESS. After exposure to the scent of lavender, mice become calmer. Studies at the Smell and Taste Research Foundation in Chicago have found that some scents, including lavender, increase the type of brain waves associated with relaxation. This lends support to the age-old practice of using lavender to treat restlessness, anxiety, and insomnia.

At a British hospital, researchers divided more than 90 patients in intensive care units into three groups. One group received standard care, another got standard care plus up to three massages, and the third was treated with standard care plus massages with lavender oil. All three groups experienced similar reductions in blood levels of stress-related hormones, but the people who received aromatherapy massages reported the greatest mood elevation and anxiety relief.

At the University of Miami, mothers of fussy, crying infants bathed their babies in water with or without lavender-scented bath oil. In the lavender oil group, the infants cried less, and the mothers reported less stress.

Many people with dementia become so agitated that they are difficult to control. At a nursing home where 15 severely demented and agitated people lived, British researchers released either water vapor or lavender oil into the day room. When exposed to the herb oil, 60 percent of the residents became calmer.

Commission E, the expert panel that evaluates herbal medicines for the German counterpart of the FDA, approves lavender as a treatment for anxiety and restlessness.

INSOMNIA. In the baby study just mentioned, the infants exposed to lavender bath oil slept better.

At the University of Leicester in England, researchers monitored the sleep habits of nursing home residents who had been taking sleeping pills for several years. For the first 2 weeks, the residents took their medications as usual. For the next 2 weeks, they stopped using their medications and lost sleep. For the last 2 weeks, they took no medications, but the fragrance of lavender oil was infused into the air during the overnight hours. The participants slept just as long as they had while taking medication. What's more, they slept more soundly. This study involved only four people, but it lends credence to lavender's traditional role as a sleep aid—especially because another small English study in younger people corroborates these results.

Commission E endorses lavender for treating insomnia. Several British hospitals reportedly offer lavender baths or lavender pillows to help patients sleep.

WOUNDS. Like most aromatic herb oils, lavender oil has antimicrobial action. This means that it can protect wounds from infection and help them heal.

DIGESTIVE PROBLEMS. Like its close botanical relatives, the mints, lavender helps calm the smooth muscle lining the digestive tract. It also promotes the secretion of bile, which helps digest fats.

Commission E endorses lavender as a digestive aid and antiflatulent.

MENSTRUAL CRAMPS. Herbs that soothe the digestive tract may also calm another smooth muscle, the uterus. Korean researchers asked 67 young women with severe cramps to massage their abdomens with either almond oil or almond oil plus lavender oil and a little rose and clary sage oil. The herb oil group reported significantly less painful cramps.

RECOVERY FROM CHILDBIRTH. In a study of lavender as an aid to recovery from childbirth, British researchers divided 635 new mothers who had normal, uncomplicated deliveries into three groups. One group added true lavender oil to their baths, another used synthetic lavender oil, and the third was given a placebo. During the 10-day study, all three groups experienced reduced pain in the genital area, and the differences in their recovery rates were not statistically significant. Nonetheless, those who used true lavender oil reported the speediest recoveries.

INSECT REPELLENT. Modern research has shown that some of the compounds in lavender oil repel insects. This validates the centuries-old practice of strewing lavender flowers for insect control.

Intriguing Possibility

According to a report in the *Journal of the National Cancer Institute*, a compound in lavender oil (perillyl alcohol) has been shown to exert remarkable action against a variety of cancerous tumors in animals, notably, cancers of the breast, lung, liver, colon, and pancreas.

Perillyl alcohol is being tested in clinical trials as a possible cancer preventive and treatment.

Rx Recommendations

To prepare an infusion, use 1 to 3 teaspoons of lavender flowers per cup of boiling water, steep for 10 minutes, and strain. Drink up to 3 cups a day.

To treat a minor wound or burn, wash it with soap and water, then apply a compress made with a lavender infusion.

As a homemade tincture, take 1 teaspoon up to three times a day. You may also apply the tincture topically to wounds and burns.

When using commercial preparations, follow the package directions.

For a relaxing bath, place a handful of lavender flowers in a cloth bag and run water over it, or add lavender infusion, tincture, or oil to your bath.

For an aromatherapy massage, apply a few drops of lavender oil directly to the skin or blend it into a commercial massage lotion (10 drops of oil per ounce of lotion).

To make a lavender pillow, put powdered flowers into a cloth bag and place the bag inside your pillowcase.

The Safety Factor

Do not ingest lavender oil. A drop or two is probably harmless, but as little as a teaspoon can be toxic, especially to children and the elderly.

Researchers at the National Institute of Environmental Health Sciences in North Carolina investigated three preteen boys who had inexplicably developed enlarged breasts (gynecomastia). All three had been using a skin lotion that contained lavender and tea tree oil. Shortly after discontinuing the lotion, their breasts reverted to normal. Lavender and tea tree oils have effects that mimic the female sex hormone estrogen. If you use lavender oil regularly, inform your doctor of its estrogenic action and discuss the implications based on your personal medical situation.

Inform health care professionals of the herbs you use. Problematic herb-drug interactions are possible.

Lavender may cause allergic reactions or other unexpected side effects. If any develop, reduce your dose or stop taking it.

For more on herb safety, see Chapter 2.

If symptoms get worse or persist longer than 2 weeks, consult a health care professional promptly.

Growing Information

Lavender is grown as an ornamental all over the temperate world, but almost all of the commercial crop is used in perfumes, soaps, cosmetics, and hair care products. Some is used to flavor foods such as vinegars, vegetable oils, cheeses, and honey. Lavender scones are popular in England, and in France, lavender sorbet is considered a summer treat.

Native to the Mediterranean, lavender is a pleasantly aromatic, woody, branching perennial shrub that grows to about 3 feet. Its narrow, fuzzy leaves change color from gray to green as they mature. In summer, lavender produces small blue or purple flowers that develop on spikes 6 to 8 inches long, creating beautiful, aromatic bouquets.

There are more than 25 species of lavender, all of which grow easily in sunny locations. The plants prefer sandy soil but will tolerate a wide range of soil conditions.

If you'd like to grow lavender for medicinal purposes, *Lavandula angustifolia* is considered the best species. Other species presumably have comparable benefits, because the oil they produce is the same or very similar. Consult a nursery for the species that grows best in your area.

The fragrance of lavender remains potent long after the flowers are dried.

LEMON BALM

For Insomnia and Herpes

Family: Labiatae; other members include mints

Genus and species: *Melissa officinalis*

Also known as: Balm, bee balm, melissa, sweet balm, and cure-all

Parts used: Leaves

Bees love lemon balm, which has been a favorite among beekeepers for more than 2,000 years. It's not surprising that its genus name, *Melissa*, is Greek for "bee."

Lemon balm is also a honey of a healer. It calms the stomach, soothes the nerves, promotes restful sleep, and helps treat herpes.

Healing History

The ancient Greek physician Dioscorides applied lemon balm leaves to skin wounds and added the herb to wine to treat a variety of illnesses. The Roman naturalist Pliny recommended lemon balm to stop bleeding.

During the 10th century, Arab doctors recommended lemon balm for nervousness and anxiety. The great 11th-century Arab physician Avicenna wrote, "Balm causeth the mind and heart to become merry."

Medieval Europeans adopted the Arabs' practice of using lemon balm for nervousness and anxiety. Melissa water, or eau de Melisse, became so popular as a tranquilizer and sedative that the emperor Charlemagne ordered the plant grown in every medicinal herb garden, or "physic garden," in his realm to guarantee an adequate supply.

During the Middle Ages, European herbalists greatly expanded on lemon balm's earlier uses, prescribing it for just about everything: insomnia, arthritis, headache, toothache, sores, digestive problems, and cramps and other menstrual problems. In fact, they recommended the herb for so many ailments that lemon balm was referred to as cure-all.

In his influential herbal, 17th-century English herbalist Nicholas Culpeper echoed Avicenna, commenting, "[Lemon balm] causeth the mind and heart to become merry, and driveth away all troublesome cares and thoughts arising from melancholy. . . ." Culpeper also recommended lemon balm for "faintings and swoonings . . . to help digestion . . . open obstructions of the brain . . . [and] procure women's courses [menstruation]."

In North America, colonists had surprisingly little regard for the bees' favorite herb. They used lemon balm primarily to relieve menstrual cramps and to induce sweating, a traditional treatment for fever.

America's 19th-century Eclectic physicians, forerunners of today's naturopaths, also had few uses for lemon balm. Despite the herb's long history as a tranquilizer, it was considered only a moderate stimulant.

Contemporary herbalists tout lemon balm's traditional roles as a tranquilizer, digestive aid, and treatment for wounds and viral infections.

Therapeutic Uses

Culpeper was way off base when he reported that lemon balm "opens obstructions of the brain," but many of the plant's other traditional uses have stood up to scientific scrutiny. Researchers have even determined that lemon balm is a potent antiviral, a benefit that the ancients knew nothing about.

WOUNDS. Dioscorides was right about at least one of lemon balm's therapeutic properties. The herb contains chemicals called polyphenols that help fight several infection-causing bacteria, among them streptococcus and mycobacteria. Lemon balm also contains eugenol, a natural anesthetic that may help relieve wound pain.

HERPES AND OTHER VIRAL INFECTIONS. Research has shown that lemon balm has antiviral action. In one German study, 116 people with herpes lesions (cold sores or genital herpes) were given either a placebo cream or a cream containing 1 percent lemon balm extract. The participants applied the creams two to four times a day for up to 10 days. By the second day, those using the lemon balm showed greater healing, and by the fifth, their sores were 50 percent more likely to have cleared entirely. The researchers concluded: "Melissa was judged conclusively superior to the placebo by physician and patient alike." To be effective, however, treatment with lemon balm must begin as soon as a sore begins to erupt.

In Germany, where herbal medicine is more mainstream than in the United States, lemon balm extract is an active ingredient in ointments intended for the treatment of cold sores and genital herpes. Experts say that compresses of lemon balm infusion should also help.

ANXIETY. Lemon balm won't "driveth away all troublesome cares and thoughts arising from melancholy," but a British study shows that it relieves anxiety. The researchers gave 24 volunteers mental challenges that produced stress. After treating them with varying doses of lemon balm (600, 1,200, or 1,800 milligrams along with 120 milligrams of valerian), the participants were subjected to similar challenges. The 600-milligram dose reduced their anxiety. (But the 1,800-milligram dose increased it.)

INSOMNIA. Animal studies have found that several compounds in fragrant lemon balm oil have tranquilizing properties. This supports lemon balm's traditional role as a relaxant.

In Germany, lemon balm is widely used as a tranquilizer and sedative. In one German study, a combination of lemon balm and valerian provided significant relief to 68 people with insomnia. In another study, the same herb combination proved as effective as the pharmaceutical tranquilizer/sedative triazolam (Halcion), but unlike the drug, it caused no morning "hangover." A third German study shows that this herb relieves insomnia in children.

Commission E, the expert panel that evaluates herbal medicines for the German counterpart of the FDA, approves lemon balm as a treatment for insomnia.

DIGESTIVE PROBLEMS. German researchers have discovered that lemon balm relaxes the smooth muscle tissue of the digestive tract, thus supporting the herb's age-old reputation as a digestive aid. Many other herbs in the mint family, notably peppermint, are also traditional digestive aids.

Commission E endorses lemon balm for treating indigestion.

WOMEN'S HEALTH CONCERNS. Herbs that relax the digestive tract may also calm another smooth muscle, the uterus. This potential effect could explain lemon balm's traditional role in treating menstrual cramps.

Curiously, lemon balm has also been recommended as a uterine stimulant to promote menstruation. No contemporary research clarifies this confusing situation. For this reason, pregnant women should not take the herb.

Intriguing Possibility

Animal studies have found that lemon balm interferes with thyroid-stimulating hormone activity, suggesting that it may prove useful as a treatment for an overactive thyroid gland (hyperthyroidism or Graves' disease).

Rx Recommendations

For a relaxing bath, tie a handful of balm into a cloth and run the bathwater over it. In addition to feeling the tranquilizing effect, you'll love the lemony aroma.

To treat wounds or herpes sores, make a hot compress using 2 teaspoons of leaves per cup of water. Boil for 10 minutes, strain, and apply with a clean cloth.

To treat a minor cut, crush some fresh lemon balm leaves and apply them directly to the wound.

For a light, lemony-tasting infusion that helps soothe the stomach, relieve anxiety, or promote sleep, use 2 teaspoons of leaves per cup of water. Steep for 10 to 20 minutes, then strain. Drink up to 3 cups a day.

As a homemade tincture, take $1/2$ to $1^1/2$ teaspoons up to three times a day.

When using commercial preparations, follow the package directions.

The Safety Factor

Because lemon balm interferes with thyroid-stimulating hormone, it may aggravate problems associated with an underactive thyroid (hypothyroidism). Although there are no published reports of the herb having this effect, anyone with hypothyroidism should consult a physician before taking lemon balm.

At high doses, lemon balm may aggravate anxiety. Do not exceed recommended amounts.

Pregnant and nursing women should not use lemon balm.

Do not give lemon balm to children under 2. In older children, adjust the recommended dose based on the child's weight. For example, give a 50-pound child one-third of the dose a 150-pound adult would take.

If you're over 65, start with a low dose, and increase only if necessary.

Inform health care professionals of the herbs you use. Problematic herb-drug interactions are possible.

Lemon balm may cause allergic reactions or other unexpected side effects. If any develop, reduce your dose or stop taking it.

For more on herb safety, see Chapter 2.

If symptoms get worse or persist longer than 2 weeks, consult a health care professional promptly.

Growing Information

Lemon balm is an erect, branching perennial that grows to 2 feet. It has the mint family's characteristic square stems and small, two-lipped white or yellow flowers, which bloom in bunches throughout the summer. The above-ground parts die back each winter, but the root is perennial.

Lemon balm grows easily from seeds sown in spring or from cuttings or root divisions. Seeds germinate indoors or out and often do best when left uncovered. Simply keep them moist. Germination typically takes 3 to 4 weeks.

Lemon balm likes well-drained soil with a pH near neutral. Thin seedlings to 12-inch spacing. The herb prefers partial shade; it wilts in full sun and loses some aroma.

For medicinal use, the leaves should be harvested before the plant flowers. Cut the entire plant back to a few inches above the ground. Dry the leaves quickly, or they may turn black.

Lemon balm loses much of its fragrance when dried. After drying, powder the leaves, then store them in tightly sealed opaque containers to preserve the volatile oil.

LICORICE
Safe When Used Sensibly

Family: Leguminosae; other members include beans and peas

Genus and species: *Glycyrrhiza glabra*

Also known as: No other names

Parts used: Rhizomes and roots

Licorice is both beneficial and controversial. Advocates point out that the herb has been used around the world for thousands of years to treat coughs, colds, rashes, arthritis, ulcers, hepatitis, cirrhosis, and infections. Critics concede the herb's effectiveness but insist that its "potentially life-threatening side effects" make it too dangerous to use.

In a small number of cases, the concentrated licorice extracts that flavor candies have caused some harm when eaten in enormous amounts. But for healthy adults who ingest the herb in recommended amounts, licorice's benefits greatly outweigh its risks.

Healing History

Licorice appears prominently in the first great Chinese herbal, the *Pen Tsao Ching* (*Classic of Herbs*) attributed to the mythical emperor-sage Shen Nung around 3000 B.C. According to legend, the emperor tested dozens of herbs on himself and died after taking a bit too much of a poison plant. Since Shen Nung's time, licorice has remained one of China's most popular healing herbs.

Licorice also has a long history in Western herbalism. Amid the treasures of King Tut's tomb, archeologists found a bundle of licorice sticks.

During the 3rd century B.C., Hippocrates extolled licorice for coughs, asthma, and other respiratory complaints. He called it sweet root—in Greek, *glukos riza*, which evolved into the herb's genus name, *Glycyrrhiza.*

The Romans changed *glycyrrhiza* to *liquiritia*, which evolved into "licorice." The noted 1st-century Roman naturalist Pliny recommended it as an expectorant and stomach soother. The Greek physician Dioscorides, who served in the Roman army, prescribed licorice juice for colds, sore throats, and chest and gastrointestinal complaints.

India's ancient Ayurvedic physicians extolled licorice as an expectorant, diuretic, and menstruation promoter.

The 12th-century medieval German abbess/herbalist Hildegard of Bingen prescribed the herb for stomach and heart problems. It was mentioned frequently in 14th- and 15th-century German and Italian herbals as a cough and respiratory remedy.

The 17th-century English herbalist Nicholas Culpeper described licorice as "a fine medicine . . . for those that have dry cough or hoarseness, wheezing or shortness of breath, phthisis [tuberculosis], heat of urine [burning], and griefs of the breast and lungs."

North American colonists found Native Americans drinking a tea brewed from American licorice as a cough remedy, laxative, earache treatment, and mask for the bitter flavor of other herbs.

America's 19th-century Eclectic physicians, forerunners of today's naturopaths, prescribed licorice for urinary problems, coughs, colds, and other "bronchial and pectoral [chest] affections."

Among American folk herbalists, licorice was considered a treatment for menstrual discomforts. It was included in Lydia E. Pinkham's Vegetable Compound, the popular 19th-century patent medicine for "female hysteria," that era's term for menstrual and menopausal complaints.

Many cultures around the world have used licorice to treat a variety of cancers.

In contemporary Chinese medicine, licorice is known as the great harmonizer. Its sweetness masks the bitter taste of many other medicinal herbs. Chinese physicians believe that in their multi-herb formulas, licorice improves the ability of the ingredients to work together. It is found in a variety of formulas, including those for indigestion, asthma, depression, varicose veins, and conditions that cause inflammation.

Contemporary American herbalists recommend licorice for its soothing effects on the respiratory, urinary, and gastrointestinal tracts, especially as a treatment for ulcers. They also follow the Chinese example of using licorice to mask the bitter taste of other healing herbs.

A few herbalists believe that licorice has

hormonelike action. They recommend it as a treatment for Addison's disease, a condition in which the adrenal glands produce abnormally low amounts of certain hormones.

Therapeutic Uses

True to its Greek name, sweet root, licorice is 50 times sweeter than sugar. The herb contains a remarkable chemical, called glycyrrhetinic acid (GA), that has a broad range of healing powers. But a bitter battle has erupted over the sweet root's hazards.

COLDS, COUGHS, AND SORE THROATS. Several studies support licorice's traditional role as a cough remedy. Glycyrrhetinic acid has some cough-suppressant properties. In Europe, licorice is quite common in cough and cold formulas. Commission E, the expert panel that evaluates herbal medicines for the German counterpart of the FDA, approves the herb as a cold and cough treatment.

ULCERS. Back in 1946, a Dutch pharmacist noticed that licorice candies and cough remedies were unusually popular with customers who had gastrointestinal ulcers. They told him that licorice provided better, longer-lasting relief than other ulcer medicines. Intrigued, the pharmacist published a report in a Dutch medical journal.

Soon after, the British medical journal *Lancet* and the *Journal of the American Medical Association* published studies showing that concentrated GA extracted from licorice heals ulcers in both animals and people. Unfortunately, it also causes swollen ankles, a classic sign of water retention.

Water retention is potentially serious. It can lead to elevated blood pressure, which can be dangerous for women who are pregnant or nursing and for anyone with diabetes, glaucoma, high blood pressure, heart disease, or a history of stroke.

By the late 1970s, mainstream medicine had developed an effective ulcer drug called cimetidine (Tagamet). Several studies compared licorice head-to-head against Tagamet. Overall, while the pharmaceutical was more effective for stomach ulcers, the two treatments were equally effective for duodenal (small intestine) ulcers— and licorice provided better protection against recurrences. However, water retention related to glycyrrhetinic acid continued to be a problem.

Eventually, researchers figured out why GA causes water retention. The chemical acts like the adrenal hormone aldosterone, which is involved in salt and water metabolism. Large amounts of aldosterone can cause a potentially serious condition called pseudoaldosteronism, with symptoms that include water retention as well as headache, lethargy, elevated blood pressure, and possibly heart failure.

Fortunately, scientists also discovered that they could retain licorice's ulcer-healing benefits but eliminate its hormonal side effects by removing 97 percent of its glycyrrhetinic acid. This led to the creation of a new semi-herbal medicine, deglycyrrhizinated licorice (DGL).

European and British journals published research demonstrating DGL's anti-ulcer effectiveness and lack of serious side effects. In one 12-week study of 874 people with duodenal ulcers, published in the *Irish Medical Journal*, DGL healed ulcers faster than Tagamet.

American scientists, who had dismissed glycyrrhetinic acid as too hazardous, decided to take a second look. They conducted several studies, but they unknowingly used improperly prepared DGL. It produced such poor results that the scientists deemed DGL to be totally ineffective against ulcers.

These unfortunate findings crushed any interest in licorice as an ulcer treatment in the United States. As it turned out, the improperly prepared DGL had released very little medicine (in other words, it had poor bio-availability).

In the late 1980s, research revealed that most ulcers are caused by bacteria and can be treated with antibiotics. As a result, DGL is of little use to most American physicians, but it remains a popular ulcer remedy in Europe. Commission E endorses licorice as a treatment for ulcers.

People with ulcers who are interested in incorporating licorice into their treatment regimens should discuss the herb with their physicians.

CANKER SORES. Canker sores are painful mouth sores that can last a week before clearing up. In one study, Indian researchers asked 20 people with canker sores to use a DGL mouthwash. Fifteen of them (75 percent) experienced substantial relief after 1 day, with complete healing by the third day.

HERPES. According to a study published in *Microbiology and Immunology*, licorice stimulates cell production of interferon, the body's own antiviral compound. Herpes sores (genital herpes and cold sores) are caused by the herpes simplex virus. Some studies have shown that licorice inhibits its replication. Sprinkling some powdered licorice root on sores may speed their healing.

HEPATITIS. Chinese physicians have used licorice for centuries to treat liver problems including hepatitis, a viral infection that can cause liver failure and liver cancer. Japanese researchers injected 453 people who had hepatitis C with a licorice preparation (100 milliliters

a day for 8 weeks, then several times a week for 10 years). Within 15 years, 25 percent of the untreated control group had developed liver cancer. By comparison, only 12 percent of those in the licorice group had developed cancer.

In a similar study, Indian researchers injected 18 people who had hepatitis with the same licorice preparation (40 milliliters a day for 30 days, then 100 milliliters three times a week for 8 weeks). Among those who didn't receive injections, the survival rate was 31 percent. Among those treated with licorice, the survival rate jumped to 72 percent.

The injectable licorice preparation used in these studies (Stronger Neo-Minophagen C) is not available in the United States. Nonetheless, the studies provide convincing evidence that licorice is a potent antiviral. The herb has also shown liver-protecting ability in people with cirrhosis as well as some action against influenza viruses and HIV, the virus that causes AIDS.

People who want to take advantage of licorice's possible healing action against liver disease or HIV should discuss the herb with their physicians.

OTHER INFECTIONS. Many laboratory studies have found that licorice fights disease-causing bacteria (staphylococcus and streptococcus) and the fungus responsible for vaginal yeast infections (*Candida albicans*). Sprinkling some powdered licorice root on clean wounds may help prevent infection.

Streptococcus mutans is a major cause of dental cavities. A study by UCLA researchers shows that licorice inhibits this bacterium. Rinsing the mouth with licorice tea might help prevent cavities.

MENOPAUSAL COMPLAINTS. Lydia Pinkham was on the right track when she included licorice in her Vegetable Compound. In a pilot study, naturopathic researchers in Portland and Seattle gave 13 women who were experiencing hot flashes either medically inactive placebos or an herbal formula containing equal parts of licorice and four other herbs used to treat menopausal complaints: Chinese angelica, motherwort, burdock, and wild yam root. The women took 1,500-milligram capsules of the formula three times a day. After 3 months, 6 percent of the women in the placebo group reported significant relief from their hot flashes. Among those using the herb formula, that figure rose to 100 percent.

Intriguing Possibilities

Immune stimulation may help explain licorice's anti-tumor activity against cancerous melanomas in experimental animals. It's too early to deem the herb a treatment for such tumors, but that day may come.

Licorice also has anti-inflammatory and anti-arthritis properties. One study found that GA could be applied like hydrocortisone cream to treat skin inflammations such as eczema. These findings led to several animal studies, which concluded that licorice taken internally has anti-inflammatory, and specifically anti-arthritis, effects. People with arthritis who want to try licorice should discuss it with their physicians.

Rx Recommendations

To help keep a minor wound from becoming infected, first wash it with soap and water, then sprinkle it with powdered licorice. The herb can also be used in this way on herpes sores, but check with your physician before doing so.

To help soothe a cough or sore throat, add a pinch of sweet-tasting licorice to any herbal beverage tea.

To make a decoction for canker sores, gently boil $1/2$ teaspoon of powdered herb per cup of water for 10 minutes, then strain if you wish. Drink up to 2 cups a day, holding the liquid in your mouth for a while so it washes over the sores.

As a homemade tincture, take $1/2$ to 1 teaspoon up to twice a day.

When using commercial preparations, follow the package directions.

The Safety Factor

In the United States, medical journals have been slow to pick up on licorice's therapeutic benefits, but they've jumped all over its potential to cause pseudoaldosteronism. The problem is real, and some people should not take the herb. In moderation, however, most people can use it safely.

There have been no reports of licorice sticks or powdered herb causing adverse reactions. According to the few dozen reports that have appeared in the world medical literature, problems have been caused by the highly concentrated licorice extracts used in some candies, laxatives, and tobacco products. The vast majority of these problems have resulted from overindulgence in licorice candies.

The *Journal of the American Medical Association* recounted the case of a man who ate 2 to 4 ounces of real licorice candies every day for 7 years. He developed weakness and hormone disturbances and required hospitalization. Another man ate more than a pound of licorice candy a day for 9 days. He, too, required hospital treatment. And a 15-year-old boy developed severely high blood pressure after eating more than a pound of licorice candy.

Clearly, consuming unusually large amounts of licorice can have adverse effects. For this reason, women who are pregnant or nursing and anyone with a history of diabetes, glaucoma, high blood pressure, stroke, or heart disease should avoid the herb. It may raise blood pressure and cause potentially serious problems.

Healthy adults may take licorice, but they should familiarize themselves with overdose symptoms, which include headache, facial puffiness, ankle swelling, weakness, and lethargy.

Remember, though, that in the United States, most "licorice" candies are made with anise, not licorice. Real licorice is available in specialty shops.

Italian researchers have found that licorice reduces male sex hormone (androgen) levels in women. Androgens are responsible for libido. Women bothered by low libido should avoid licorice.

Do not give licorice to children under 2. In older children, adjust the recommended dose based on the child's weight. For example, give a 50-pound child one-third of the dose a 150-pound adult would take.

If you're over 65, start with a low dose, and increase only if necessary.

Inform health care professionals of the herbs you use. Problematic herb-drug interactions are possible.

Licorice may cause allergic reactions or other unexpected side effects. If any develop, reduce your dose or stop taking it.

For more on herb safety, see Chapter 2.

If symptoms get worse or persist longer than 2 weeks, consult a health care professional promptly.

Growing Information

Licorice is an erect, hardy perennial that reaches 3 to 7 feet. Small, alternate, inch-long leaflets and $1/2$-inch purple midsummer flowers give the plant a graceful beauty.

Mature plants have long taproots that send out creeping horizontal rhizomes (stolons), which are the source of other shoots and more branching roots. This creates a tangled mass of underground growth. Licorice roots have brown bark and sweet, juicy, yellow pulp.

Hard freezes kill licorice. It grows best in warm, sunny climates or in greenhouses in pots 48 inches deep. Greenhouse licorice often requires artificial light.

Licorice is usually propagated from root cuttings containing eyes. Plant them vertically about an inch below the soil surface, with 18-inch spacing. Beds should be rich, well-dug, well-manured, and well-drained. Once established, the herb can become extremely invasive, so be sure to keep it contained.

Licorice requires little care other than weeding. Expect slow growth the first year or two, then harvest rhizomes and roots during the fall of the third or fourth year. The year that you plan to harvest, pinch the flowers back. Flowering drains some of the roots' sweet sap.

Thick roots should be split to dry. Shade-dry the roots for 6 months. Licorice root keeps for a long time. Scientists who analyzed a sample from A.D. 756 found that even after 1,250 years, it still contained active compounds.

MACA

It Stimulates More Than Just the Imagination

Family: Brassicaceae; other members include mustards, cabbage, and broccoli

Genus and species: *Lepidium meyenii*

Also known as: Peruvian ginseng

Part used: Root

Maca is a perennial ground cover that produces matlike creeping stems, scalloped leaves, small white flowers, and a turniplike tuber. It grows high in the Andes at altitudes of 11,000 to 14,500 feet, where few plants can survive the poor soil, freezing temperatures, and gale-force winds. Clearly, maca is a hardy herb. It makes livestock and people hardier, too—and possibly sexier.

Healing History

Before the Incas, ancient Andean shepherds ate the fleshy maca root as a vegetable and fed it to their livestock. They noticed that maca made herds healthier and appeared to increase their fertility. As a result, maca gained a reputation as a nutritious food and sex stimulant.

The Incas domesticated maca 2,000 years ago. They fed maca root to their livestock and cooked the tubers in water to make a sweet, aromatic porridge for themselves known today as *mazamorra*. The Incas believed that in addition to nourishment, maca boosted energy, elevated mood, strengthened resistance to disease, enhanced memory, had laxative action, improved fertility, treated menstrual problems and meno-pausal complaints, and enhanced sex. Inca warriors ate maca before battle, believing it increased their strength and ferocity. After conquering cities, Incan commanders forbid their men to eat it to minimize rapes among vanquished women.

When the Spanish conquered the Incas, they had trouble keeping their horses healthy and reproducing high in the Andes. Local people advised them to feed maca to the horses. The Spaniards did, and when the health and fertility of their horses improved, they embraced maca as a food and sex booster. They also required Andeans to supply them with several tons a year.

Maca's many healing actions resemble those of ginseng. As a result, maca has been called Peruvian ginseng. It is botanically unrelated to ginseng, however.

Therapeutic Uses

APHRODISIAC? In the world's traditional medical systems, any plant that increases energy was believed to boost sexual energy as well. Research on maca's sexual effects is scant, but that hasn't stopped supplement companies from marketing it as a libido-enhancer. It just might be one.

Animal studies show that maca significantly increases sperm production, copulation, and impregnation. Peruvian researchers gave adult men either a placebo or 3 grams of the herb daily. After 8 weeks, maca had no effect on male sex hormones, but it "improved sexual desire." This is the only human trial of maca as a sex-booster. Researchers do not consider it sufficient evidence to pronounce the herb an aphrodisiac. But a report in the *Journal of Sex and Marital Therapy* concludes: "While evidence for a pro-sexual effect of maca is currently minimal, an effect on libido is plausible."

HOT FLASHES. The Incas were right about maca for women's health. Australian researchers gave menopausal women either a placebo or 2 grams of maca a day. After 2 months, the herb provided significant relief of hot flashes and night sweats.

Rx Recommendations

Human studies to date have used 2 to 3 grams per day in divided doses. Some sources recommend up to 5 grams per day. Follow package directions.

The Safety Factor

There have been no reports of significant side effects or toxicity. Maca has been used as a food for at least 2,000 years, which suggests safety.

Pregnant and nursing women should not use maca.

Do not give maca to children under 2. In older children, adjust the recommended dose based on the child's weight. For example, give a 50-pound child one-third of the dose a 150-pound adult would take.

If you're over 65, start with a low dose, and increase only if necessary.

Inform health care professionals of the herbs you use. Problematic herb-drug interactions are possible.

Maca may cause allergic reactions or other unexpected side effects. If any develop, reduce your dose or stop taking it.

For more on herb safety, see Chapter 2.

If symptoms get worse or persist longer than 2 weeks, consult a health care professional promptly.

Growing Information

Maca is not grown in the United States.

MAITAKE

Many Reasons to Call It "King of Mushrooms"

Family: Polyporaceae; other members include other mushrooms

Genus and species: *Grifola frondosa*

Also known as: King of mushrooms, sheep's head, ram's head, hen of the woods, and dancing mushroom

Parts used: Whole fungus

Maitake mushrooms (pronounced *my-TAH-key*) are native to northern Japan, Europe, and the eastern United States from the Gulf Coast to Canada. They grow in temperate deciduous forests in clusters at the foot of trees, especially oaks. Clusters can weigh up to 100 pounds, hence the name king of mushrooms.

Unlike many mushrooms, maitakes have no cap. Instead, the fruiting body has a frilly, wooly, feathery appearance that earned it such common names as sheep's head, ram's head, and hen of the woods. Maitake has also been called dancing mushroom. Some sources say that those who found the valuable delicacy danced for joy. Others say that in a breeze, the frilly fruiting bodies appear to dance.

The Japanese have prized maitake mushrooms as a culinary delicacy for centuries. In fact, hundreds of years ago, the mushrooms were worth their weight in silver. Hunters kept the mushroom's locations a secret, whispering their discoveries to their sons on their deathbeds. Regional lords offered the mushroom as tribute to the shogun.

In 1979, Japanese mycologists figured out how to cultivate maitake commercially, making the mushroom much more widely available and less expensive.

Healing History

Traditional Japanese healers recommended maitake to treat high blood pressure and cancer.

The mushroom became prized as medicine in China. In a Chinese medical text from 210 A.D., it was recommended to treat digestive upsets and hemorrhoids, and to calm the nerves.

In the 1980s, Japanese scientists discovered that like shiitake and reishi mushrooms, maitake is a potent immune stimulant. Since then, maitake has been the focus of a great deal of research.

Therapeutic Uses

Maitake research is still in its infancy. Only a few human trials have been published. But they confirm the many animal studies showing that maitake is a healer.

IMMUNE STIMULANT. Maitake activates several components of the immune system. It increases the activity of T-cells, natural killer cells, and germ-devouring macrophages. It boosts production of interleukin-1, an important immune protein. It's rich in beta-glucan, a compound that supports the body's defenses against cancer. And it increases synthesis of cytokines, which help the various components of the immune system coordinate their efforts.

CANCER. In laboratory experiments, maitake extract has inhibited the growth and reproduction of several cancer cell types. In animals, the mushroom has substantially reduced the spread of metastatic cancers.

In a Chinese clinical trial, 63 people with various cancers were treated with radiation and chemotherapy. Some of them also received maitake (amount unspecified). In the maitake group, treatment was more successful. Japanese researchers have produced similar findings using a daily maitake dose of 4 to 6 grams.

Finally, a Chinese researcher has shown that a close relative of maitake, *Grifola umbellata*, improves treatment of bladder cancer. In the study, 313 bladder cancer survivors were given either a placebo or *Grifola umbellata* (amount unspecified). After an average of 7.6 years, cancer had recurred in 65 percent of the control group. But in the mushroom group, the figure was only 35 percent.

WEIGHT CONTROL. Japanese researchers gave some animals high-fat, high-cholesterol feed, while others received the same feed with maitake added (making up 5 to 20 percent of the feed). As expected, the control animals gained weight, but the maitake group did not.

By the end of the study, the control animals weighed 25 percent more than the animals fed maitake.

Tokyo researchers told 30 overweight adults to continue eating as they had, except that in addition, they should take maitake tablets, the equivalent of 7 ounces of the mushroom a day. Two months later, all of them had lost weight, ranging from 12 to 26 pounds.

HEPATITIS AND OTHER LIVER DISEASE. Chinese researchers treated 32 people with chronic hepatitis B with either standard medication or maitake. Liver enzymes returned to near normal in 57 percent of the drug group. But in the maitake group, the figure was 73 percent.

In addition, in the weight control animal study just mentioned, the control animals also developed precursors of fatty liver disease. The maitake group did not.

VITAMIN D. Until recently, scientists believed that vitamin D could be obtained only by exposing the skin to sunlight, or from fish liver oils, fortified milk, or supplements. However, maitake contains significant amounts of vitamin D, approximately 100 IU per 100 grams (roughly 25 IU per ounce).

No wonder that like ginseng and eleuthero, maitake is considered an adaptogen, an herb that strengthens the entire body.

Intriguing Possibilities

Animal studies conducted in Japan show that compared with regular feed, feed containing 5 percent maitake extract lowers blood pressure. Similar animal studies at Georgetown University Medical Center have confirmed these results.

Animal research also shows that the mushroom lowers cholesterol.

Further, animal studies suggest that maitake lowers blood sugar, hinting that it may help treat diabetes.

Finally, laboratory studies at Washington State University suggest that maitake may help treat malaria.

Rx Recommendations

Take 3 to 7 grams per day in capsules, tablets, or mixed into food. Increasingly, maitakes can be found dried in Asian and gourmet food stores.

The Safety Factor

No side effects from maitake mushrooms have been reported. However, some wild mushrooms are poisonous. Mushroom hunters should be sure of what they've picked before eating.

Growing Information

Maitake can be grown indoors from kits marketed by Fungi Perfecti. Visit www.fungi.com.

MARSHMALLOW

A Confection with Healing Roots

Family: Malvaceae; other members include cotton, hollyhock, and hibiscus

Genus and species: *Althaea officinalis*

Also known as: Althaea and cheeses

Parts used: Roots; sometimes leaves and flowers

Yes, marshmallow is the plant that inspired the pillowy white confections toasted over campfires. But today's marshmallows contain none of their namesake herb and bear no resemblance to the marshmallow sweets of old.

It's a shame that so few people know marshmallow as anything other than a candy. The herb has a healing tradition that dates back some 2,500 years.

Healing History

Marshmallow was a food before it became a medicine. The Book of Job (30:4) refers to a plant whose name translates as mallow that was eaten during famines. And during the Middle Ages, when crops failed, people boiled marshmallow roots, then fried them with onions in butter. Even today, backpacking guides suggest the plant for wilderness foragers.

Marshmallow's history as a healing herb goes back to Hippocrates, who prescribed a root decoction to treat bruises and blood loss from wounds. Four hundred years later, the Greek physician Dioscorides recommended marshmallow root poultices for insect bites and stings. He also prescribed a decoction for toothache and vomiting and as an antidote to poisons.

The Romans loved marshmallow. The Roman naturalist Pliny enthused, "Whosoever shall take a spoonful of the mallows shall that day be free from all diseases." This thinking led to the herb's genus name, *Althaea*, from the Greek *altho*, to cure.

Ancient India's Ayurvedic physicians used marshmallow to treat coughs and bronchitis.

Tenth-century Arab physicians applied marshmallow leaf poultices as a treatment for inflammation. Early European folk healers used marshmallow root both internally and externally to relieve toothache, sore throat, digestive upset, and urinary irritation.

Marshmallow was a special favorite of 17th-century English herbalist Nicholas Culpeper. "You may remember that not long since, there was a raging disease called the bloody flux . . . the college of physicians not knowing what to make of it," he wrote. "My son was taken with [it] and . . . the only thing I gave him was mallows bruised and boiled in milk and drunk. In two days (the blessing of God be upon it), it cured him. And I here, to show my thankfulness to God in communicating it to his creatures, leave it to posterity."

Culpeper recommended marshmallow roots, leaves, and seeds for their soothing action in treating "agues [fever] . . . torments of the belly . . . pleurisy, phthisis [tuberculosis], and other diseases of the chest . . . coughs, hoarseness . . . shortness of breath, wheezing, cramps . . . and swellings in women's breasts . . . and other offensive humors."

Early colonists introduced marshmallow into North America, and by the mid-19th century, it had found its way into the *U.S. Pharmacopoeia*, a standard drug reference. The Eclectic physicians of that time, the forerunners of today's naturopaths, prescribed the herb externally for "wounds, bruises, burns, scalds, and swellings of every kind." They also recommended a root decoction internally for colds, hoarseness, diarrhea, gonorrhea, gastrointestinal problems, and "nearly every affection of the kidney and bladder."

Contemporary herbalists generally limit their recommendations of marshmallow to respiratory and gastrointestinal irritation. Some tout the herb for urinary complaints.

Incidentally, you can thank the French for the spongy confection that bears the herb's name. They made the first candied marshmallow roots centuries ago. They peeled the root bark to expose the white pulp and boiled it to soften it and release its sweetness. Then they added sugar. The result: sweet, white, somewhat spongy sticks that over time evolved into today's campfire treat.

Therapeutic Uses

The spongy material in marshmallow roots is a fiber called mucilage. When mucilage comes in contact with water, it absorbs the liquid, swells, and forms a soothing, protective gel.

WOUNDS. Applied topically, the mucilage gel from marshmallow helps soothe and protect cuts, scrapes, wounds, and burns.

RESPIRATORY PROBLEMS. Taken internally, marshmallow helps relieve stomach upset and the respiratory rawness associated with sore throats, coughs, colds, flu, and bronchitis. Slovakian researchers used irritant chemicals to induce coughing in animals and then treated them with a variety of herbs with reputations as cough suppressants. Marshmallow root worked best.

ACE inhibitors, a group of standard blood pressure medications, have an annoying side effect—cough. Iranian scientists gave 60 people with ACE inhibitor cough either a placebo or 20 drops of marshmallow tincture every 8 hours. After 4 weeks, coughs in the placebo group remained unchanged. But in the marshmallow group, they were significantly reduced.

Commission E, the expert panel that evaluates herbal medicines for the German counterpart of the FDA, approves marshmallow for treating coughs.

ENHANCED IMMUNITY. In one experiment, marshmallow improved the ability of white blood cells to devour disease microbes, a process called phagocytosis. This suggests that marshmallow's traditional role in treating wounds and gastrointestinal infections may have been therapeutic as well as soothing.

Intriguing Possibility

One animal study has found that marshmallow root reduces blood sugar levels, so the herb may have value in managing diabetes.

Rx Recommendations

Prepare a sweet decoction to take advantage of marshmallow's soothing powers and possible infection-fighting abilities. Gently boil $^1/_2$ to 1 teaspoon of chopped or crushed root per cup of water for 10 to 15 minutes. Drink up to 3 cups a day.

When using commercial preparations, follow the package directions.

For external use, chop the root very fine and add enough water to produce a gooey gel. Apply the gel directly to superficial wounds or sunburn. If you have a serious wound or blistering sunburn, however, see a physician.

The Safety Factor

The medical literature contains no reports of any harm from marshmallow.

Because the safety of marshmallow has not been studied in pregnant and nursing women, they should not use it.

Marshmallow may cause allergic reactions or other unexpected side effects. If any develop, reduce your dose or stop taking it.

For more on herb safety, see Chapter 2.

If symptoms get worse or persist longer than 2 weeks, consult a health care professional promptly.

Growing Information

You can guess from its name where marshmallow grows: in marshes, bogs, and damp meadows and along stream banks. The plant is a downy, erect, 5-foot perennial with a long taproot. The stems, which die back each autumn, are hairy and branching. The roundish, gray-green leaves, 1 to 3 inches long, are lobed, toothed, and covered with velvety hairs. Pink or white flowers bloom in summer. They are up to 2 inches across and give rise to round fruits called cheeses, which is one of the herb's names.

In moist soil under full sun, marshmallow is a hardy plant that grows easily from seeds, cuttings, or root divisions. Seeds should be planted in spring and root divisions in autumn. Thin them to 2-foot spacing.

Do not harvest roots from plants less than 2 years old. In autumn, when the top-growth has died back, dig out mature roots and remove the lateral rootlets. Wash, peel, and dry them whole or in slices.

MATÉ
The High-C Stimulant

Family: Aquifoliaceae; other members include holly

Genus and species: *Ilex paraguayensis* or *I. paraguariensis*

Also known as: Yerba maté, Paraguay tea, and Jesuit tea

Parts used: Leaves

More than 300 years ago, Jesuit missionaries noticed that a group of South American Indians ate a virtually all-meat diet. In spite of this, however, they didn't develop "sailor's sickness" (scurvy), which decimated European mariners who ate similar diets while at sea.

The Jesuits concluded that the Indians must be protected by the tea they drank out of cups made from calabash gourds. The missionaries dubbed it *maté*, from the Spanish for "gourd."

They began cultivating the hollylike shrub and using its leathery leaves to produce the bitter tea.

Maté (pronounced *MAH-tay*), also called yerba maté or Paraguay tea, was introduced into the United States in the 1970s as a coffee substitute. It contains caffeine and a rather large amount of vitamin C, which does, indeed, prevent scurvy.

Healing History

The Jesuits introduced maté to European colonists. Today, the herb is one of South America's most popular stimulants. In Argentina, Paraguay, and Uruguay, it's more popular than coffee or tea. More than 200 brands of maté are currently marketed in Argentina alone.

Argentinians consume 11 pounds of maté per capita annually. In Uruguay, that figure is 22 pounds. South American breads often have maté added. The herb is also a key ingredient in a popular South American soft drink.

South Americans consider maté not only a pleasant stimulant but also an appetite suppressant and a diuretic. Although there has been no scientific research to back it up, maté has a long-standing reputation as a digestive aid. Argentinian cowboys (gauchos) sometimes live on just meat and maté, like the Indians of old.

Therapeutic Uses

A 6-ounce cup of maté contains about 50 milligrams of caffeine, about as much as a cup of tea or a can of cola. By comparison, a cup of instant coffee has about 65 milligrams of caffeine. A cup of brewed coffee has 100 to 150 milligrams. (For details on caffeine's health benefits, see Coffee on page 164.)

FATIGUE. Because maté contains only one-third to one-half as much caffeine as a compa-rable-size cup of brewed coffee, its effects would be only a fraction as stimulating. But it's still a stimulant.

Commission E, the expert panel that evaluates herbal medicines for the German counterpart of the FDA, approves maté as a treatment for fatigue.

COLDS. The Jesuits were right about maté's ability to prevent scurvy. The herb is fairly high in vitamin C, which also helps treat the common cold. Drinking maté when you have a cold gives you an extra dose of C.

PREMENSTRUAL SYNDROME (PMS). Diuretics help relieve the bloated feeling caused by premenstrual fluid retention. Women bothered by PMS might try maté during the uncomfortable days just before their periods.

Rx Recommendations

Maté has a distinctive odor that some people find offensive.

For a pleasantly bitter infusion, use 1 teaspoon of dried crushed herb per cup of boiling water and steep for 10 minutes. Add honey and lemon to taste, if you like. Drink up to 3 cups a day.

When using commercial preparations, follow the package directions.

The Safety Factor

Caffeine is classically addictive. Large amounts may cause significant harm. Because, cup for cup, maté contains less caffeine than coffee, however, it should cause fewer problems. (For a more detailed discussion of caffeine's safety, see page 169.)

Maté also contains tannins, which have both pro- and anti-cancer action. A Uruguayan study, published in the *Journal of the National Cancer*

Institute, found that heavy maté users have an increased risk of esophageal cancer. The average Uruguayan consumes 22 pounds of the herb a year, so it's anyone's guess how much heavy users consume. This finding, if confirmed, has no real significance to Americans who drink only an occasional cup of maté tea. Nevertheless, people who have been diagnosed with esophageal cancer should avoid this herb.

Pregnant and nursing women should not use maté.

Do not give maté to children under 2. In older children, adjust the recommended dose based on the child's weight. For example, give a 50-pound child one-third of the dose a 150-pound adult would take.

If you're over 65, start with a low dose, and increase only if necessary.

Inform health care professionals of the herbs you use. Problematic herb-drug interactions are possible.

Maté may cause allergic reactions or other unexpected side effects. If any develop, reduce your dose or stop taking it.

For more on herb safety, see Chapter 2.

If symptoms get worse or persist longer than 2 weeks, consult a health care professional promptly.

Growing Information

Maté is not cultivated in the United States. In South America, the plant grows wild near streams, but it is also extensively cultivated, especially in Argentina.

Maté is a perennial shrub with spineless, oval, toothed, leathery leaves. Its fruits (berries) are red, black, or yellow and about the size of black peppercorns.

MEADOWSWEET
Herbal Aspirin

Family: Rosaceae; other members include rose, peach, almond, apple, and strawberry

Genus and species: *Filipendula ulmaria*, formerly *Spiraea ulmaria*

Also known as: Spiraea, bridewort, meadwort, dropwort, and queen-of-the-meadow

Parts used: Leaves and flowers

It's rare to find a medicine cabinet that doesn't contain aspirin. It's even rarer to find anyone who knows that we owe the word *aspirin* to the beautiful, aromatic meadowsweet.

Healing History

During the Middle Ages, meadowsweet's delicate almond fragrance made it a popular air freshener, or "strewing herb." It was scattered around homes to minimize odors at a time when people rarely bathed and when farm animals often shared human living quarters.

Early British herbalist John Gerard wrote of the herb, "The leaves and floures of Meadowsweet farre excell all other strowing herbs for to decke up houses . . . for the smell thereof delighteth the senses." One fan of meadowsweet as a strewing herb was none other than Queen Elizabeth I, who had the flowers spread around her living quarters.

The herb's sweet aroma and lovely blossoms earned it a place in bridal bouquets, hence its name bridewort (*wort* is Old English for "plant"). Meadowsweet was also used to flavor mead, a fermented beverage made from honey and fruit juices, hence another of its names, meadwort.

Gerard documented meadowsweet's contributions to healing: "The floures boiled in wine and drunke do take away fits of ague [fever]. The distilled water of the floures dropped into the eies taketh away burning and itching thereof and cleareth the sight." Later, herbalists recommended meadowsweet to treat diarrhea, fevers, arthritis, "falling sickness" (epilepsy), and respiratory ailments.

Colonists introduced the herb into the Western Hemisphere. America's 19th-century Eclectic physicians, forerunners of today's naturopaths, considered meadowsweet "an excellent astringent . . . in diarrhea. [It] is less offensive to the stomach than other agents of its kind." They also prescribed it for menstrual cramps and vaginal discharge.

Contemporary herbalists recommend meadowsweet for colds and flu; nausea, heartburn, childhood diarrhea, and other digestive ailments; muscle aches; and congestive heart failure.

From Salicin to Aspirin

In 1839, a German chemist discovered that meadowsweet flower buds contain salicin, the same chemical that had been isolated from white willow bark 11 years earlier. Salicin has powerful pain-relieving (analgesic), fever-reducing, and anti-inflammatory properties.

Unfortunately, salicin (and its close chemical relatives, notably salicylic acid) can also cause potentially serious side effects, including stomach upset, nausea, diarrhea, bleeding in the stomach, and ringing in the ears (tinnitus). In high doses, it can even cause respiratory paralysis and death.

Chemists began tinkering with salicin and salicylic acid, hoping to preserve the benefits while minimizing the hazards. In 1853, German chemists added a molecular acetyl group to a meadowsweet extract and synthesized acetylsalicylic acid.

"Acetylsalicylic acid" proved to be quite a mouthful, so the scientists who created the compound combined the "a-" from *acetyl* with "-spirin," a variation of meadowsweet's former Latin name, *Spiraea*, to create *aspirin*.

The new compound provided greater relief from fever, pain, and inflammation than either salicin or salicylic acid. Unfortunately, it still had its predecessors' side effects, which disappointed its creators. They published news of aspirin's development in an obscure German medical journal, and the drug was promptly forgotten for almost 50 years.

In the late 1890s, a German chemist, Felix Hoffman, became upset that his father's rheumatoid arthritis medication provided so little relief and so much stomach upset. Hoffman worked at the Fredrich Bayer pharmaceutical company. He began combing the journals for leads on a better arthritis treatment. He came across the old report about aspirin and decided to make a batch himself. As the story goes, he gave some to his father, who pronounced aspirin effective, with fewer side effects than the medications he'd been taking.

At first, Hoffman had a tough time selling aspirin to his superiors at Bayer. Eventually, though, they saw its potential. In 1899, they introduced acetylsalicylic acid in Europe and North America under the brand name Aspirin.

Aspirin quickly became the household drug of choice for relief of pain, fever, and inflammation. Later, in one of the earliest U.S. trademark-protection battles, Bayer lost its trademark to the name Aspirin. The court ruled that the word had passed into general usage. Ever since, the company has promoted its product as Bayer Aspirin.

Therapeutic Uses

While meadowsweet gave us aspirin, the herb can't match all of the pharmaceutical's therapeutic effects. Still, it has some impressive benefits of its own.

PAIN, FEVER, AND INFLAMMATION. Meadowsweet does not pack aspirin's pain-relieving, fever-reducing, and anti-inflammatory punch. The herb has a small amount of salicylate, so even strong infusions may not have much effect. Tinctures provide more salicylate and greater relief.

On the other hand, meadowsweet is less likely to produce aspirin's major side effect, stomach upset. In fact, a few laboratory trials have shown that the herb protects experimental animals from aspirin-induced stomach ulcers. This finding supports the Eclectics' observation that meadowsweet is gentle on the stomach. At least one animal study, however, suggests that meadowsweet increases the risk of ulcers when given with drugs that cause them.

If you'd rather take an herbal preparation than a pharmaceutical, especially if aspirin upsets your stomach, you can try meadowsweet for headache, arthritis, menstrual cramps, low-grade fever, and other types of pain and inflammation. The herb may help. And if it's taken in combination with aspirin or another pain reliever, it may let you reduce your dose of the drug.

ARTHRITIS. Meadowsweet's aspirin effect can help treat the pain and inflammation of arthritis.

COLDS. Because meadowsweet helps relieve pain, inflammation, and fever, Commission E, the expert panel that evaluates herbal medicines for the German counterpart of the FDA, approves the herb as a treatment for the common cold.

DIARRHEA. Meadowsweet contains astringent tannins that can help relieve diarrhea. In addition, a European study found the herb to be effective against *Shigella dysenteriae*, one of the bacteria that cause infectious diarrhea. This finding lends some credence to the herb's traditional use for this condition.

URINARY TRACT INFECTIONS. Meadowsweet is active against *Escherichia coli*, the bacteria most likely to cause urinary tract infections. One report describes the herb as a urinary antiseptic.

Intriguing Possibilities

A great deal of research has shown that low-dose aspirin (one-half to one standard tablet a day) helps prevent the blood clots that trigger heart attack and most strokes. Meadowsweet's effect on heart disease and stroke has not been well researched, but animal studies have shown that the herb has anticoagulant (blood-thinning) properties, so it's likely that it provides similar cardiovascular protection.

Aspirin has also been shown to reduce the risk of digestive tract cancers, notably colon cancer. To date, no studies have linked meadowsweet to reduced risk of these conditions, but again, it seems reasonable to assume that the herb may offer similar benefits.

One study revealed that salicin reduces blood sugar (glucose) levels, suggesting that meadowsweet may be of value in managing diabetes.

Rx Recommendations

To prepare a pleasantly astringent infusion, use 1 to 2 teaspoons of dried, powdered herb per cup of boiling water. Steep for 10 minutes, then strain if you wish. Drink up to 3 cups a day.

As a homemade tincture, take $\frac{1}{2}$ to 1 teaspoon up to three times a day.

When using commercial preparations, follow the package directions.

Do not give meadowsweet to children under age 2 or to children under age 16 who have colds, flu, or chickenpox. For other children and adults over age 65, start with low-strength preparations and increase the strength if necessary.

The Safety Factor

Aspirin is a well-documented asthma trigger. Research has shown that meadowsweet has the same effect. For this reason, people with asthma or any aspirin sensitivity should not take meadowsweet.

In children under age 16 who have fevers from colds, flu, or chickenpox, aspirin is associated with Reye's syndrome, a rare but potentially fatal condition. Meadowsweet has never been linked to Reye's syndrome, but because it's related to aspirin, children who have fevers from those illnesses should not take it.

Do not give meadowsweet to children under 2. In older children, adjust the recommended dose based on the child's weight. For example, give a 50-pound child one-third of the dose a 150-pound adult would take.

European animal studies suggest that meadowsweet may stimulate uterine contractions. The herb has no history of use as a menstruation promoter, but because aspirin has been associated with an increased risk of birth defects, women who are pregnant or trying to conceive should not take meadowsweet.

Pregnant and nursing women should not use meadowsweet.

If you're over 65, start with a low dose, and increase only if necessary.

Inform health care professionals of the herbs you use. Problematic herb-drug interactions are possible.

Meadowsweet may cause allergic reactions or other unexpected side effects. If any develop, reduce your dose or stop taking it.

For more on herb safety, see Chapter 2.

If symptoms get worse or persist longer than 2 weeks, consult a health care professional promptly.

Growing Information

Meadowsweet is an eye-catching perennial with stems that reach 2 to 6 feet. It has elmlike leaves and large clusters of small, coiled white or pink flowers that bloom throughout summer and have a fragrant, sweet almond aroma. The flower clusters droop, hence the common name dropwort. The plant stands taller and has more striking flowers than most other meadow plants, hence another of its common names, queen-of-the-meadow.

Meadowsweet grows wild from Newfoundland to Ohio in marshes, along stream banks, and in moist forests and meadows. It is best propagated from cuttings of its creeping underground perennial stem (rhizome).

Meadowsweet does best in rich, moist, well-drained soil under partial shade. Harvest the leaves and flowers when the plant is in bloom.

MILK THISTLE
A Potent Liver Protector

Family: Compositae; other members include daisy, dandelion, and marigold

Genus and species: *Silybum marianum*

Also known as: Silybum and holy thistle

Parts used: Seeds

Milk thistle is the single most important liver-protecting herb. Once again modern science has confirmed what the ancients believed. Milk thistle has been used to treat liver conditions for more than 2,000 years.

Healing History

Ancient herbalists recognized the herb's value as a liver tonic. The 1st-century Roman naturalist Pliny wrote that the herb's juice helped "carry off bile." And influential 17th-century

British herbalist Nicholas Culpeper endorsed milk thistle as a treatment for jaundice, the yellowing of the skin and eyes caused by liver disease.

America's 19th-century Eclectic physicians, forerunners of today's naturopaths, prescribed milk thistle to treat liver conditions as well as varicose veins, menstrual complaints, and kidney problems.

Homeopaths use a microdose of the herb to treat liver disorders, gallstones, and varicose veins.

Therapeutic Uses

In 1968, German researchers isolated three liver-protective compounds from milk thistle seeds: silibinin, silidianin, and silicristin. Collectively, these compounds are known as silymarin.

Silymarin benefits the liver in several ways. It binds tightly to the receptors on liver cell membranes that allow toxins in, thus locking them out. It's a powerful antioxidant, protecting liver cells from the chemical process responsible for a great deal of harm in the body. It spurs the repair of damaged liver cells. And it stimulates the immune system.

Medicine needs a good liver protector. Many conditions attack the liver, notably cirrhosis, mushroom poisoning, and hepatitis A, B, and C. Unfortunately, mainstream medicine doesn't have much to offer people with liver disease.

For hepatitis, doctors advise resting and refraining from behavior that could further damage the liver, such as drinking alcohol or taking drugs. For mushroom poisoning, conventional treatment often fails, with fatal consequences. For cirrhosis, doctors can only offer relief from complications. Research has shown

that milk thistle extract can help treat all of these conditions safely and effectively. In fact, Commission E, the expert panel that evaluates herbal medicines for the German counterpart of the FDA, approves milk thistle extract as a treatment for liver conditions.

HEPATITIS. Several European studies have shown that compared with hepatitis patients who did not receive silymarin, those who did recovered more quickly. In an Italian study, 20 people with hepatitis were given either medically inactive placebos or silymarin. Those taking the herb showed greater normalization of liver function.

MUSHROOM POISONING. Amanita mushrooms are called death caps for good reason: They contain a potent liver poison. Every year, the news media issue reports of serious illness and death among people who pick wild mushrooms without knowing how to distinguish the Amanita from edible species.

Without treatment, the death rate from Amanita poisoning is around 50 percent. Standard medical treatment (activated charcoal) saves some lives, but the death rate may still be as high as 40 percent. In 2007, six members of a California family accidentally ate death caps. They were treated with intravenous milk thistle. Five (83 percent) survived.

Silymarin works by blocking the Amanita poison from entering liver cells. In one German study, 60 people were treated with silymarin after accidentally eating death caps, and none died. In another German study, this one involving 205 people with Amanita poisoning, 189 received standard medical care and 16 received silymarin. Of those given standard care, 24 percent died. Of those given silymarin, none died.

In a multicenter European study, researchers

looked at 220 cases of Amanita poisoning in which the patients had been treated with silymarin. The death rate was 13 percent, well below the rate associated with conventional medical treatment.

CIRRHOSIS. Several studies have determined that milk thistle helps stabilize liver function in people with cirrhosis. One study included 170 people—91 with alcoholic cirrhosis, the rest with cirrhosis from other causes. They were given either placebos or 200 milligrams of milk thistle extract three times a day. Four years later, 31 members of the placebo group had died of liver disease. In the milk thistle group, there were only 18 deaths.

For another study, Scandinavian researchers recruited 97 heavy drinkers who had liver damage but not cirrhosis. Forty-seven participants were given silymarin for 4 weeks. Compared with those taking placebos, the silymarin group showed significant decreases in several liver enzymes that had been abnormally high. The researchers concluded that the people taking silymarin had greater potential for regaining normal liver function.

DRUG-INDUCED LIVER DAMAGE. Alcohol is not the only drug that can harm the liver. In large enough doses, even everyday medications like acetaminophen (Tylenol) can cause liver damage. In one laboratory trial, silymarin protected the livers of animals that were given large doses of acetaminophen. In other studies, the compound has prevented the liver damage associated with antibiotics, antidepressants, and antipsychotic medications.

TOXIN-INDUCED LIVER DAMAGE. Research has shown that silymarin can minimize the damage associated with long-term exposure to several toxic industrial chemicals. In one study, workers with liver damage from the chemicals toluene and xylene took 140 milligrams of silymarin three times a day for a month. The treatment produced substantial reductions in liver enzymes that had been at abnormally high levels.

DIABETES. Iraqi researchers gave one of three treatments to 59 people with diabetes who had been taking the standard diabetes medication glibenclamide (Glyburide): continued Glyburide, the drug plus a placebo, or the drug plus 200 milligrams of milk thistle per day. The herb treatment resulted in the greatest reductions in blood sugar.

Intriguing Possibilities

Some research suggests that silymarin lowers cholesterol and may reduce the risk of complications from diabetes.

Rx Recommendations

Silymarin is not very soluble in water, so infusions and decoctions don't supply very high doses of the compound. Neither does wild milk thistle.

German plant scientists have bred a high-silymarin variety of milk thistle that produces a standardized extract. A 200-milligram dose of the extract contains 140 milligrams of silymarin. This dose, taken in tablets or capsules three or four times a day, has become the standard in milk thistle research.

Look for a standardized extract containing 70 percent silymarin and use it according to the package directions.

The Safety Factor

If you suspect that you have mushroom poisoning, seek emergency medical care immediately.

If you have liver disease, talk to your doctor before taking milk thistle. While the herb is generally regarded as safe, there have been a few reports linking it with stomach upset or a laxative effect.

Pregnant and nursing women should not use milk thistle.

Do not give milk thistle to children under 2. In older children, adjust the recommended dose based on the child's weight. For example, give a 50-pound child one-third of the dose a 150-pound adult would take.

If you're over 65, start with a low dose, and increase only if necessary.

Inform health care professionals of the herbs you use. Problematic herb-drug interactions are possible.

Milk thistle may cause allergic reactions or other unexpected side effects. If any develop, reduce your dose or stop taking it.

For more on herb safety, see Chapter 2.

If symptoms get worse or persist longer than 2 weeks, consult a health care professional promptly.

Growing Information

Native to Kashmir in India-Pakistan, milk thistle is a weedy plant that now grows throughout the temperate world. It typically reaches 5 to 10 feet and produces large, prickly leaves. When broken, the leaves and stems exude milky sap, hence the name milk thistle. The plant produces reddish purple flowers that are ringed with sharp spines. The flowers resemble miniature artichokes.

Like its close botanical relative, artichoke, milk thistle was once grown in Europe as a vegetable. Backpacking guides still suggest that back-country foragers steam the prickly young leaves and stalks, which taste similar to spinach. Young leaves may also be eaten in salads.

MISTLETOE

A Christmas Gift for People with Cancer

Family: Loranthaceae; all members are called mistletoe

Genus and species: *Viscum album* (European); *Phoradendron serotinum* or *P. tomentosum* (American)

Also known as: Viscum, *herbe de la croix*, and *lignum crucis*

Parts used: Leaves, fruits (berries), and young twigs

Mistletoe is best known for the sprigs under which people kiss at Christmas, a custom with an ironically gruesome origin. As a healing herb, mistletoe is also fraught with irony. One scientific authority calls it "gentle . . . [and] nontoxic." Others insist that "all parts of the plant should be regarded as toxic."

The fact is, mistletoe's purported toxicity has been greatly overstated. Europeans use it extensively—and safely—to help treat cancer. Unfortunately, American oncologists have not adopted this healing herb.

Healing History

We owe mistletoe's association with kissing to Norse mythology. Balder, god of peace, was slain by an arrow made from mistletoe. When his parents, god-king Odin and goddess-queen Frigga, restored him to life, they gave the plant to the goddess of love and decreed that anyone who passed under it should receive a kiss.

Early Christians believed that mistletoe was a freestanding tree during Jesus' time and that its wood was used to make the cross of the Crucifixion. God punished the plant for its role in the Crucifixion by turning it into a parasite. It was because of this story that mistletoe came to be called *lignum crucis* ("wood of the cross") in Latin and *herbe de la croix* in French.

Hippocrates prescribed mistletoe for disorders of the spleen. Most other ancient physicians, particularly Dioscorides and Galen, advised limiting the herb to external use, foreshadowing the current controversy over its safety.

Roman soldiers reported that England's ancient Druid priests cut mistletoe from oak trees and used the plant in elaborate fertility rituals.

A French medical text from 1682 recommended mistletoe for "falling sickness" (epilepsy). Some herbals still prescribe it for convulsions (ironically, high doses may cause convulsions).

Seventeenth-century English herbalist Nicholas Culpeper reiterated Hippocrates' recommendation, asserting that mistletoe "doth mollify hardness of the spleen, and helpeth old sores." He also advocated mistletoe for "falling sickness and apoplexy [stroke]," and advised wearing a sprig around the neck to "remedy witchcraft."

In the United States, several Native American tribes used American mistletoe to induce abortion and to stimulate contractions during childbirth.

America's 19th-century Eclectic physicians, forerunners of today's naturopaths, recommended both European and American mistletoe for epilepsy, typhoid fever, and "dropsy" (congestive heart failure). They also prescribed the herb for "hysterical" (gynecological) complaints, recommending it for relief of menstrual cramps, menstruation promotion, and treatment of postpartum hemorrhage. But the Eclectic text *King's American Dispensatory* (1898) warned that large amounts "possess toxic properties. Vomiting, catharsis, muscular spasms, coma, convulsions, and death have been reported from eating the leaves and berries."

Koreans use mistletoe tea to treat colds, muscle weakness, and arthritis. Chinese physicians prescribe the dried inner stems as a laxative, digestive aid, sedative, and uterine relaxant during pregnancy.

Somewhere along the line, herbalists came to believe that European and American mistletoe had opposite effects. European mistletoe was reputed to reduce blood pressure and soothe the digestive tract, while the American variety was said to raise blood pressure and stimulate uterine and intestinal contractions.

Therapeutic Uses

Despite the traditional belief that European and American mistletoe have opposite actions, science has determined that the plants contain similar active chemicals and have similar effects. Mistletoe has the ability to slow the pulse, stimulate gastrointestinal and uterine contractions, and lower blood pressure.

ENHANCED IMMUNITY. Studies from around the world show that mistletoe preparations, notably the Swiss mistletoe-based drug Iscador, enhance immune function, boosting the activity of several immune cells: macrophages, T-cells, and natural killer cells. The studies have also shown that mistletoe preparations increase production of cytokines, proteins that help regulate immune function.

Injected preparations of mistletoe improve immune function in people with AIDS.

CANCER. European studies going back 30 years show that Iscador, which is administered by injection, enhances immune activity against various types of cancer, slowing tumor growth and sometimes reversing it. A sampling of recent studies:

❧ Swiss researchers analyzed six studies of surgery, radiation, and chemotherapy for breast cancer versus standard therapies plus Iscador. The Iscador group survived longer and reported better quality of life—improved feelings of well-being, increased appetite, reduced pain, and normalized sleep.

❧ German scientists gave 253 women with uterine endometrial cancer either standard therapies or standard treatments plus Iscador. The Iscador group survived longer and reported better quality of life.

❧ A different group of German researchers gave 148 women with ovarian cancer either standard therapies or standard therapies plus Iscador. For women with early, localized tumors, the herb provided no benefit. But among those with metastatic cancer—and most ovarian cancer is metastatic—Iscador showed significant benefit, and those who used it reported significantly better quality of life.

Distinguished German medical herbalist Rudolph Fritz Weiss, M.D., notes, "The great advantage offered by mistletoe extracts is that unlike [other chemotherapeutic] drugs, its . . . immunostimulant and tonic effects are nontoxic and well tolerated."

Commission E, the expert panel that evaluates herbal medicines for the German counterpart of the FDA, approves mistletoe as a complementary cancer therapy to be used in combination with mainstream treatments.

In the United States, mistletoe has not been seriously studied as a cancer treatment because of the herb's reputation as a poison. Ironically, many approved cancer drugs are also toxic. It's a shame American oncologists do not use this herb.

BLOOD PRESSURE REGULATION. While mistletoe contains substances that both raise and lower blood pressure, those that have a lowering effect predominate. In Germany, where herbal medicine is considerably more mainstream than in the United States, mistletoe extract is an ingredient in many medications prescribed to reduce blood pressure. Dr. Weiss writes, "Anyone who treats hypertension [high blood pressure] will confirm that mistletoe by mouth has definite benefit. . . . For a gentle antihypertensive drug that is well tolerated . . . and nontoxic in the usual dosage . . . mistletoe is the drug of choice."

High blood pressure is a serious condition that requires medical supervision. Use the herb only in consultation with your doctor.

Rx Recommendations

You should take mistletoe only under the close supervision of a physician who has knowledge of herbs.

To treat high blood pressure, Dr. Weiss recommends a tea made from equal parts of mistletoe, hawthorn, and lemon balm. "Infuse 2 teaspoons of the mixture for 5 to 10 minutes," he writes. After straining it, "take 1 cup in the morning and 1 at night."

Other herbalists recommend 1 cup a day of an infusion made with 1 teaspoon of freshly dried plant material steeped in 1 cup of boiling water for 10 minutes, then strained.

As a homemade tincture, the recommended dose for blood pressure control is five drops daily.

When using commercial preparations, follow the package directions.

The Safety Factor

How toxic is mistletoe? The Eclectics reported coma, convulsions, and death from the ingestion of large doses of leaves and berries. Since then, there have been scattered reports of fatalities from consuming the berries or beverages made from them.

On the other hand, a review of more than 300 cases of mistletoe ingestion, published in *Annals of Emergency Medicine*, found no deaths associated with the herb. A majority of those who consumed the plant—typically its berries—developed no symptoms of poisoning.

In a 1996 review of 11 cases of mistletoe ingestion (amounts up to 20 berries), researchers affiliated with the Kentucky Regional Poison Control Center reported generally minor stomach upset, except in two infants who suffered more severe reactions. There were no deaths. The researchers concluded that ingesting mistletoe causes "infrequent symptoms, and in all but one case would not require direct medical supervision."

Based on these findings, it would appear that mistletoe's reputation for toxicity is undeserved. Nonetheless, keep the herb away from young children.

Mistletoe contains a chemical called tyramine that may stimulate uterine contractions. For this reason, pregnant women should not use the herb, except possibly at term and only under the supervision of a physician to induce labor.

Mistletoe's abortion-inducing dose is close to its fatal dose. It should never be used to terminate pregnancy.

Nursing women should not use mistletoe.

People with heart disease or a history of stroke should not take mistletoe, as the herb may slow the heart rate.

Do not give mistletoe to children under 2. In older children, give it only under a doctor's direction. Adjust the recommended dose based on the child's weight. For example, give a 50-pound child one-third of the dose a 150-pound adult would take.

If you're over 65, start with a low dose, and increase only if necessary.

Inform health care professionals of the herbs you use. Problematic herb-drug interactions are possible.

Mistletoe may cause allergic reactions or other unexpected side effects. If any develop, reduce your dose or stop taking it.

For more on herb safety, see Chapter 2.

If symptoms get worse or persist longer than 2 weeks, consult a health care professional promptly.

Growing Information

Mistletoe is a parasitic shrub that grows in trees, rooting into their bark. Both European and American mistletoe are branching, woody evergreens that live on a large number of trees. The European herb has thin, leathery, tongue-shaped 2-inch leaves. The American variety also has leathery leaves, but they are broader and up to 3 inches long. Both plants produce small, sticky white berries, which contain single seeds.

Mistletoe is well adapted to its aerial existence. Its sticky white berries attract birds, which carry them to perches in other trees. The birds eat some but drop others, which stick to the tree bark. Within a few days, the seeds inside newly "planted" mistletoe berries produce tiny roots, which bore their way into the host tree and establish new plants.

Mistletoe is gathered from the wild, not cultivated, although some crafters of mistletoe Christmas products reportedly "plant" the sticky seeds by inserting them into the bark of host trees.

MOTHERWORT

A Potential Heart Helper

Family: Labiatae; other members include mints

Genus and species: *Leonurus cardiaca*

Also known as: Lion's tail and heartwort

Parts used: Leaves, flowers, and stems

The word *wort* is Old English for "plant," but the name motherwort is somewhat misleading. The herb is more likely to prevent motherhood than to promote it.

Also, despite one of the herb's popular names, lion's tail, motherwort won't strengthen the lion-hearted. In fact, it's more apt to turn lions into lambs.

Healing History

The ancient Greeks and Romans used motherwort to treat both physical and emotional problems of the heart—namely, palpitations and depression.

In ancient China, motherwort was reputed to promote longevity. According to legend, a youth who had committed a minor crime was banished from his village to a remote valley with a spring surrounded by motherwort. Supposedly, he lived to be 300.

In Europe, motherwort first gained prominence as a treatment for cattle diseases. Sixteenth-century British herbalist John Gerard called it "a remedy against certain diseases in cattell . . . and for that husbandmen much desire it." Gerard also recommended the herb for "infirmities of the heart."

Seventeenth-century English herbalist Nicholas Culpeper wrote, "There is no better herb to take melancholy vapors from the heart . . . and make a merry, cheerful soul." While Culpeper viewed motherwort primarily as an antidepressant, he also said, "It is . . . of much use in trembling of the heart [palpitations], and faintings, and swoonings, from whence it took the name cardiaca. . . . It took the name motherwort [because] it settles mothers' wombs . . . and is a wonderful help to women in their sore travail [labor]. . . . It also provoketh women's courses [menstruation]."

As the centuries passed, herbalists used motherwort in contradictory ways, both to relax the uterus during pregnancy and after childbirth and to stimulate menstruation and labor. Eventually, it came to be known as a uterine stimulant.

Colonists introduced motherwort into North America. The 19th-century Eclectic physicians, forerunners of today's naturopaths, recommended the herb as a menstruation promoter and an aid to expelling the afterbirth. They also prescribed it as a tranquilizer for "morbid nervous excitement, and all diseases with rest-lessness [and] disturbed sleep." The Eclectics did not consider motherwort a heart remedy.

Contemporary herbalists recommend motherwort as a tranquilizer, a women's health tonic, and a remedy for heart palpitations and delayed or suppressed menstruation.

Therapeutic Uses

Until recently, scientists dismissed motherwort as useless. Studies have indicated, however, that the ancients who named the herb cardiaca may have been on to something.

HEART DISEASE. In China, laboratory studies have shown that motherwort helps relax heart cells. Other Chinese research suggests that it helps prevent the blood clots that trigger heart attack. Russian researchers have also found that the herb contains compounds that reduce blood pressure. These findings are preliminary, but they lend credence to the ancient view that motherwort has a general tonic effect on the heart.

Commission E, the expert panel that evaluates herbal medicines for the German counterpart of the FDA, approves motherwort as a treatment for "nervous cardiac disorders."

In generally healthy adults, occasional heart palpitations are usually no cause for alarm. If the palpitations are frequent and persistent, however, they may be a sign of a heart rhythm disturbance (cardiac arrhythmia), a potentially serious condition that requires professional care. If you experience frequent palpitations, consult your physician.

If you have high blood pressure or heart disease and would like to incorporate motherwort into your treatment plan, do so only in consultation with your physician.

INSOMNIA AND ANXIETY. German studies have determined that motherwort has mild sedative action. It may be effective in relieving insomnia and anxiety.

WOMEN'S HEALTH CONCERNS. Not many tranquilizers are also uterine stimulants, but motherwort contains a compound called leonurine that encourages uterine contractions. This lends support to the herb's traditional role in childbirth and menstruation promotion.

Women who are trying to conceive or are pregnant should not take motherwort, except possibly at term and only under the supervision of a physician to help stimulate labor. For other women, the herb may help induce periods.

Rx Recommendations

To make a possibly tranquilizing, uterine-stimulating, blood-pressure-lowering infusion, use 1 to 2 teaspoons of dried herb per cup of boiling water. Steep for 10 minutes, then strain. Drink up to 2 cups a day, a tablespoon at a time. Motherwort tastes very bitter; you can add sugar, honey, and lemon, or mix it into an herbal beverage tea to improve the flavor.

As a homemade tincture, take $\frac{1}{2}$ to 1 teaspoon up to twice a day.

When using commercial preparations, follow the package directions.

The Safety Factor

Because of motherwort's possible anti-clotting effect, people who are taking anticoagulants (blood thinners)—whether medications (including aspirin), herbs (garlic and willow bark), or supplements (vitamin E)—should not use it. People with clotting disorders should also avoid motherwort.

Some people develop rashes from contact with the plant.

Pregnant and nursing women should not use motherwort.

Do not give motherwort to children under 2. In older children, adjust the recommended dose based on the child's weight. For example, give a 50-pound child one-third of the dose a 150-pound adult would take.

If you're over 65, start with a low dose, and increase only if necessary.

Inform health care professionals of the herbs you use. Problematic herb-drug interactions are possible.

Motherwort may cause allergic reactions or other unexpected side effects. If any develop, reduce your dose or stop taking it.

For more on herb safety, see Chapter 2.

If symptoms get worse or persist longer than 2 weeks, consult a health care professional promptly.

Growing Information

Motherwort's perennial root gives rise to stout, square stems that are tinged with red or violet and grow to 4 feet. The plant's lower leaves are sharply lobed, like maple leaves. Its upper leaves are narrow and toothed. It also produces whorls of small white, pink, or red flowers, which bloom in summer.

This herb grows so easily that it may become a pest. Plant seeds in spring and thin seedlings to 12-inch spacing. Motherwort prefers rich, moist, well-drained soil and full sun, but it tolerates considerably less ideal conditions. Harvest the entire plant after the flowers blossom.

MUIRA PUAMA

Herbal Viagra?

Family: Olacaceae; other members include various tropical trees

Genus and species: *Ptychopetalum olacoides*

Also known as: Marapuama and potency wood

Part used: Root

Muira puama is a shrubby Amazonian tree that grows to 15 feet. In recent years, it has become popular as a male sex stimulant. Ironically, research to date suggests that it works better for women.

Healing History

For centuries, indigenous people in the Amazon rain forest considered muira puama a "nerve tonic," meaning a stimulant. They used its root to treat fatigue, depression, and the confusion that often develops during old age. Through the years, all stimulants—among them, coffee and ginseng—have also been considered sex stimulants. The same has been true for muira puama, hence the name potency wood.

Muira puama has also been used traditionally to treat indigestion, menstrual irregularity, and muscle aches.

Therapeutic Uses

Brazilian researchers have confirmed that muira puama is a stimulant, but that it does not contain caffeine.

SEX STIMULANT? Muira puama does not contain yohimbine, the erection-boosting compound in yohimbe bark (see page 487). However, French researchers have demonstrated that it has sex-stimulating action. They surveyed 202 healthy women complaining of low libido on various aspects of their sexuality, including frequency and intensity of sexual desire, sexual fantasies, intercourse, and orgasm, plus overall sexual satisfaction. Then the researchers gave the women a combination of muira puama and ginkgo. After 1 month, two-thirds of them reported significantly greater sexual desire, more frequent and more intense fantasies, more frequent intercourse, more orgasms, and more intense orgasms.

In Brazil, an over-the-counter product, Catuama, is marketed as an energy-booster and sex stimulant. It contains muira puama plus caffeine, ginger, and a few other herbs.

PREVENTION OF DEGENERATIVE DISEASES. Antioxidant nutrients help prevent and reverse the cell damage at the root of heart disease, many cancers, and other conditions, such as Alzheimer's disease. Brazilian researchers have identified antioxidants in muira puama.

Intriguing Possibilities

Stimulants such as caffeine have mild antidepressant action. In animal models of depression, Brazilian scientists have shown that muira puama is mood-elevating.

The herb may also have potential as a treatment for Alzheimer's disease. In addition to containing antioxidants, muira puama also inhibits the action of an enzyme (acetylcholinesterase) that plays an important role in learning and memory. Drugs used to treat Alzheimer's disease are acetylcholinesterase inhibitors. Muira puama has similar action. Animal studies show that the herb improves memory and learning. It's too soon to call muira puama a treatment for Alzheimer's, but one day it might be.

Rx Recommendations

The typical dose is 1 to 2 milliliters (about 1 teaspoon) of extract in water two to three times a day. Or follow package directions.

The Safety Factor

No significant side effects have been reported.

Pregnant and nursing women should not use muira puama.

Do not give this herb to children. If you're over 65, start with a low dose, and increase only if necessary.

Inform health care professionals of the herbs you use. Problematic herb-drug interactions are possible.

Muira puama may cause allergic reactions or other unexpected side effects. If any develop, reduce your dose or stop taking it.

For more on herb safety, see Chapter 2.

If symptoms get worse or persist longer than 2 weeks, consult a health care professional promptly.

Growing Information

Muira puama is not grown in the United States.

MULLEIN

A Velvety Soother

Family: Scrophulariaceae; other members include figwort, foxglove, and eyebright

Genus and species: *Verbascum thapsus*

Also known as: Candlewick plant, torches, velvet dock, flannel plant, feltwort, Aaron's rod, shepherd's staff, and lungwort

Parts used: Leaves, flowers, and roots

Mullein (its name rhymes with *sullen*) grows everywhere and is hard to miss. Despite this, however, few who encounter the velvet-leafed weed with its rodlike stem and striking yellow flowers appreciate its place in herbal healing as a treatment for cough.

Healing History

When dried, mullein burns vigorously. Before the introduction of cotton, mullein's leaves and stems were used by the ancients as candlewicks, earning the herb the name candlewick plant. The dried stems and flowers were dipped in suet to make them burn longer, hence another of the herb's popular names, torches.

Ancient cultures around the world considered mullein a magical protector against witchcraft and evil spirits. Like other herbs used in magic, mullein has a long history as a healer. Its botanical family name, Scrophulariaceae, is derived from *scrofula*, an old term for chronically swollen lymph glands. The condition was later identified as a form of tuberculosis.

The 1st-century Greek physician Dioscorides prescribed a decoction of mullein root in wine as a treatment for "fluxes of the belly" (diarrhea). During the Middle Ages, the French used the herb to treat malandre, an animal disease that causes boils on horses' necks. *Malandre* eventually became *malen* and finally, *mullein*.

Early on, the herb gained a reputation as a respiratory remedy, which endures to this day. In ancient India, Ayurvedic physicians prescribed mullein for cough. Seventeenth-century English herbalist Nicholas Culpeper wrote that gargling a mullein decoction "easeth toothache . . . and old cough." His contemporary, herbalist William Coles, wrote that farmers "give it [to] their cattle against cough."

Colonists introduced mullein into North America, and Native Americans quickly adopted the herb for coughs, bronchitis, and asthma. The accepted way of taking mullein in early America seems ridiculous today: People smoked it.

America's 19th-century Eclectic physicians, forerunners of today's naturopaths, viewed mullein as a diuretic to treat water retention and as a stomach and respiratory soother, with mild pain-relieving and tranquilizing action. The Eclectic text *King's American Dispensatory* (1898) asserted, "Upon the upper portion of the respiratory tract, its influence is pronounced." The Eclectics recommended mullein for colds, coughs, asthma, and tonsillitis, as well as diarrhea, hemorrhoids, and urinary tract infections.

During the late 19th and early 20th centuries, mullein was listed in the *National Formulary*, the pharmacists' reference, as a cough remedy. It was deleted in 1936 for lack of proof of effectiveness. Nonetheless, in his 1986 survey of folk medicine in Indiana, the late herb expert Varro E. Tyler, Ph.D., found mullein "a very popular Hoosier remedy for all types of respiratory complaints."

Contemporary herbalists recommend mullein as an internal treatment for coughs, colds, sore throat, and other respiratory complaints and as an external treatment (in compresses) for hemorrhoids.

Therapeutic Uses

In laboratory studies, at least, mullein inhibits the growth of the bacteria that cause tuberculosis, so perhaps it was of some value against scrofula. Today, the herb is used mostly to soothe minor respiratory irritations.

COUGHS AND SORE THROATS. Mullein contains a soluble fiber called mucilage that swells and turns into a slippery gel when it absorbs water. This accounts for the herb's soothing action on the throat and skin. Distinguished German medical herbalist Rudolph Fritz Weiss, M.D., writes that mullein has a "well-founded reputation as a cough remedy."

Commission E, the expert panel that evaluates herbal medicines for the German counterpart of the FDA, endorses mullein as a soothing treatment for colds.

HEMORRHOIDS. Its mucilage is not the only reason that mullein soothes hemorrhoids. The herb also contains astringent tannins, which are widely used to treat hemorrhoids and other skin conditions. One study showed that mullein has anti-inflammatory properties as well.

DIARRHEA. The astringent tannins probably account for mullein's traditional role in treating diarrhea.

Intriguing Possibility

In a laboratory study, mullein infusion helped to combat the virus that causes genital herpes and cold sores. If you develop either of these conditions, you might apply a compress made from a strong mullein infusion.

Rx Recommendations

For an infusion that can soothe cough and sore throat and may help relieve diarrhea, use 1 to 2 teaspoons of dried leaves, flowers, or roots per cup of boiling water. Steep for 10 minutes, then strain. Drink up to 3 cups a day.

Mullein has a bitter taste. To improve its flavor, you can add sugar, honey, and lemon to the tea, or mix it into an herbal beverage blend.

To help treat hemorrhoids, apply a compress made with a strong, cool infusion.

As a homemade tincture, take $1/2$ to 1 teaspoon up to three times a day.

When using commercial preparations, follow the package directions.

The Safety Factor

Mullein seeds are toxic and may cause poisoning. There have been no reports of adverse effects from the herb's leaves, flowers, and roots.

Pregnant and nursing women should not use mullein.

Do not give mullein to children under 2. In older children, adjust the recommended dose based on the child's weight. For example, give a 50-pound child one-third of the dose a 150-pound adult would take.

If you're over 65, start with a low dose, and increase only if necessary.

Inform health care professionals of the herbs you use. Problematic herb-drug interactions are possible.

Mullein may cause allergic reactions or other unexpected side effects. If any develop, reduce your dose or stop taking it.

For more on herb safety, see Chapter 2.

If symptoms get worse or persist longer than 2 weeks, consult a health care professional promptly.

Growing Information

Mullein is a hardy biennial that grows almost anywhere in temperate climates. During its first year, the plant produces a rosette of 6- to 15-inch leaves that are greenish white, tongue-shaped, and hairy—hence its common names velvet dock, flannel plant, and feltwort. In its second year, mullein sends up a solitary, fibrous stem that reaches 3 to 6 feet, the source of common names such as Aaron's rod and shepherd's staff. In summer, a striking, cylindrical spike of small, dense, yellow, honey-scented flowers develops atop the stem.

Mullein grows easily from seed in light sandy soil under full sun, but it tolerates other conditions. Sow seeds in spring after the danger of frost has passed.

Harvest up to one-third of the leaves during the plant's first year and the rest the following year, before the flowers bloom. Pick the flowers as they open. Harvest the roots in autumn.

Mullein is a prolific self-sower. Many authorities recommend removing the flower heads before the seeds ripen to keep it under control.

MYRRH

A Thoroughly Modern Mouthwash— And Anti-Parasitic

Family: Burseraceae; other members include balm of Gilead

Genus and species: *Commiphora abyssinica* or *C. myrrha*

Also known as: Balsamodendron

Part used: Gum-resin from incisions in bark

In the biblical account, Joseph's jealous brothers decide to sell him into slavery. Egypt was the place to sell slaves, but who would take him there? The answer soon appeared on the horizon: "And looking up, they saw a caravan of Ishmaelites coming from Gilead [Jordan], with their camels bearing gum, balm, and myrrh on their way to carry it down to Egypt" (Genesis 37:25). They sold Joseph to the Ishmaelites.

This is just the first of a dozen biblical references to myrrh, the hardened, tear-shaped nuggets of clear or reddish brown aromatic resin that exude from incisions in the bark of a small Middle Eastern tree. Of course, the Bible's best-known mention of myrrh involves the three Magi offering the rare and costly herb to the newborn Jesus (Matthew 2:11).

Healing History

The world's oldest surviving medical text, the *Ebers Papyrus* (1500 B.C.), discusses myrrh. The ancient Egyptians used the herb as an ingredient in embalming mixtures and as a treatment for wounds. From these humble beginnings, myrrh emerged in the Bible as an all-purpose aromatic for perfumes and insect repellents.

The Arabs called the herb *murr*, meaning "bitter." When the ancient Greeks adopted the herb, they attributed its teardrop shape to Myrrha, daughter of the Syrian king Thesis. Myrrha refused to worship Aphrodite, the goddess of love. Angered by this blasphemy, Aphrodite tricked Myrrha into committing incest with her father. When Thesis realized what he had done, he threatened to kill his daughter. To save her, the gods transformed her into a myrrh tree, whose teardrop resin recalls the girl's sorrow.

Hippocrates recommended myrrh to treat mouth sores, and the Greeks also considered the herb an antidote to poisons.

As the centuries passed, myrrh became valued primarily as a mouthwash to treat bleeding gums, mouth ulcers, and sore throats. The 12th-century German abbess/herbalist Hildegard of Bingen prescribed a mixture of powdered myrrh and aloe for dental problems. Later herbalists recommended myrrh as an expectorant for colds and chest congestion, and as a menstruation promoter.

By the Middle Ages, the belief that myrrh protected against poisons grew to encompass infectious disease. In 1665, when the Black Plague struck London, however, myrrh offered no benefit, and belief in its protective powers faded. Nonetheless, the powdered resin continued to be used to treat sores in the mouth and on the skin.

America's 19th-century Eclectic physicians, forerunners of today's naturopaths, considered myrrh an antiseptic for the external treatment of "indolent sores and gangrenous ulcers." They prescribed the herb internally for colds, laryngitis, asthma, bronchitis, indigestion, gonorrhea, menstruation promotion, sore throat, dental cavities, and bad breath. The Eclectics also cautioned that large doses of myrrh could have violent laxative action and cause sweating, nausea, vomiting, and accelerated heartbeat.

Contemporary herbalists recommend using powdered myrrh on well-washed wounds as an antiseptic. They also consider a gargle made from the herb to be effective against sore throats, colds, sore teeth and gums, coughs, asthma, and chest congestion.

Therapeutic Uses

Today, myrrh continues to be used for oral hygiene, just as it has been for 1,000 years.

MOUTHWASH. Myrrh contains tannins, which have an astringent, drawing effect on tissues. Chinese researchers have identified other substances in the herb that fight bacteria, and Indian scientists have discovered that the herb has anti-inflammatory action. All of these factors make myrrh an effective mouthwash.

Myrrh tastes bitter but refreshing. It may help relieve the inflammation and destroy the bacteria involved in gingivitis, the early form of gum disease. Commission E, the expert panel that evaluates herbal medicines for the German counterpart of the FDA, approves myrrh as a treatment for mouth sores.

TOOTHPASTE. Myrrh is a common ingredient in European toothpastes. It's used to help fight the bacteria that cause tooth decay and gum disease.

PARASITES. Several veterinary studies show that myrrh kills intestinal parasites. These reports led to studies of the herb as a treatment for human schistosomiasis, a life-threatening parasite that infests some 150 million people in Asia and Africa. The parasite can be difficult to treat with conventional drugs. Egyptian researchers gave 600 milligrams of myrrh daily for 6 days to 67 people with schistosomiasis. Three months later, the researchers judged more than 90 percent cured. They called myrrh "safe and very effective."

In another Egyptian study, 204 people with schistosomiasis were treated with myrrh. Again, more than 90 percent were cured. Side effects were mild and brief.

Intriguing Possibilities

In an Italian study, treatment with myrrh appeared to raise the pain threshold of laboratory mice. The herb's pain-blocking action would enhance its effectiveness in treating mouth problems.

Myrrh may also help prevent heart disease. Preliminary Indian studies suggest that the herb reduces cholesterol. It may also protect against the blood clots that trigger heart attack.

Rx Recommendations

To prepare a mouthwash, steep 1 teaspoon of powdered herb and 1 teaspoon of powdered boric acid in 1 pint of boiling water. Let stand for 30 minutes, then strain if you wish. Be sure the rinse is cool before using it. Do not swallow it.

For an infusion that may help prevent heart disease, use 1 teaspoon of powdered herb per cup of boiling water. Steep for 10 minutes, then strain if you wish. Drink up to 2 cups a day. Myrrh has an unpleasant, bitter taste; to improve its flavor, you can add sugar, honey, and lemon, or mix it into an herbal beverage blend.

If you return from travel to rural areas of Asia and Africa feeling ill and fatigued, consult a tropical medicine specialist. If you test positive for schistosomiasis, ask your doctor to try treating you with 600 milligrams of myrrh per day.

As a homemade tincture, take $1/4$ to 1 teaspoon up to three times a day.

When using commercial preparations, follow the package directions.

The Safety Factor

Myrrh has not been shown to stimulate uterine contractions, but its traditional use as a menstruation promoter should serve as a red flag to pregnant women. Nursing women should also avoid it.

Large doses of the herb may produce a violent laxative action. They could also cause other symptoms described by the Eclectics, including sweating, nausea, vomiting, and rapid heartbeat.

Do not give myrrh to children under 2. In older children, adjust the recommended dose based on the child's weight. For example, give a 50-pound child one-third of the dose a 150-pound adult would take.

If you're over 65, start with a low dose, and increase only if necessary.

Inform health care professionals of the herbs you use. Problematic herb-drug interactions are possible.

Myrrh may cause allergic reactions or other unexpected side effects. If any develop, reduce your dose or stop taking it.

For more on herb safety, see Chapter 2.

If symptoms get worse or persist longer than 2 weeks, consult a health care professional promptly.

Growing Information

Myrrh is not grown in the United States. It's a large shrub or small tree that grows in the Middle East, Ethiopia, and Somalia. Pale yellow oil drips from cuts in its dull gray bark and hardens to form teardrop-shaped nuggets, which are powdered for medicinal purposes.

NEEM

The Indian Bug and Germ Killer

Family: Meliaceae; other members include mahogany

Genus and species: *Azadrichta indica*

Also known as: Margosa

Parts used: Leaf and bark extract

Recently, one of my houseplants became bug-infested. I sprayed it with diluted neem oil. After two applications, the bugs were gone. Oil of neem is a widely marketed natural pesticide. But neem is far more than just a nonpetrochemical bug killer. This Indian tree has been a mainstay of India's traditional Ayurvedic medicine for more than 1,000 years.

Healing History

The word *neem* comes from the Sanskrit *nimba*, meaning "bestower of good health." Its medical use dates back to India's ancient religious texts, the *Vedas*, which called the tree *sarva roga niva-rini*, meaning the "one that cures all ailments."

According to the Neem Foundation, based in Mumbai (Bombay), India, which promotes the tree's medical and commercial uses, neem is an ingredient in an estimated 75 percent of traditional Ayurvedic medical formulas. For example, neem has been used for centuries in India to treat all manner of skin conditions, including acne, eczema, psoriasis, warts, herpes, athlete's foot, chickenpox, and skin cancer.

Therapeutic Uses

The Vedic promise that neem "cures all ailments" is a stretch, but modern Indian researchers continue to gush over it. One Indian researcher has extolled the tree as "omnipotent . . . a wonder tree because of its diverse utility." Diverse is right:

PESTICIDE. Many studies show that neem repels, kills, or disrupts reproduction of a large number of agricultural pests, among them the boll weevil, which infests cotton, and the beetles that threaten Florida citrus groves.

Neem may also help worldwide efforts to eradicate malaria. Though rare in the United States, malaria is the fourth leading cause of childhood death in the developing world, killing more than 700,000 people a year. Korean researchers have shown that at concentrations as low as one part per million, the neem constituent, azadirachtin, kills 100 percent of the larvae of mosquitoes that transmit malaria. But unlike petrochemical pesticides, neem-based pesticides apparently carry no risk to nonpest animals.

DENTAL HEALTH. Neem extract kills the bacteria that cause plaque, tooth decay, and gum disease. In a study described in the *Interna-tional Dental Journal*, Indian researchers assessed the amount of dental plaque and gum inflammation in 48 volunteers, and then asked them to use one of three products after breakfast and before bed: toothpaste containing neem extract, toothpaste with a pharmaceutical anti-plaque ingredient, or a pharmaceutical mouthwash. After 6 weeks, the neem product was found to be as effective as the pharmaceuticals.

ULCERS. Several studies show that neem reduces secretion of stomach acid and treats ulcers. One group of Indian researchers induced ulcers in animals and then gave them either neem leaf extract or the popular anti-ulcer drug Zantac. The herb was as effective as the drug.

Other Indian researchers measured stomach acid secretion in people with ulcers and then gave them 30 milligrams of neem bark extract twice a day. After 10 days, they showed a highly significant decrease in acid secretion. When the participants took 30 to 60 milligrams of neem bark extract twice a day for 10 weeks, their ulcers "almost completely healed." There were no significant side effects.

Intriguing Possibilities

Several animal studies show that neem leaf extract is spermicidal, raising the possibility that it could be used as a contraceptive.

Neem could also have potential as a deterrent to AIDS transmission. In a laboratory study at Howard University in Washington, D.C., researchers exposed white blood cells to HIV, the virus that causes AIDS. All of them became infected. Then they treated different white blood cells with neem leaf extract and subsequently exposed them to HIV. Only 25 percent became infected.

Combine neem's anti-HIV and spermicidal actions, and the herb might be used by women intravaginally as a spermicide that helps prevent the spread of HIV. Indian researchers recently tested the safety of such a spermicide in 20 women free of AIDS. The neem preparation caused some genital irritation, itching, and burning, but no medically worrisome side effects. The next step would be a larger study to test neem's effectiveness in the battle against AIDS transmission.

Rx Recommendations

Neem oil is sold as a pesticide at garden supply stores. Follow package directions.

Neem toothpaste and neem leaf and bark extracts are available at some health food stores. Or search "neem toothpaste" or "neem extract" on the Internet. Follow label directions.

The Safety Factor

Neem oil is toxic. It has poisoned infants and children. Keep it away from children, and do not ingest it. Because of potential toxicity, do not self-treat with neem oil. If not using products such as toothpaste that contain it, use it only in consultation with a professional practitioner.

Pregnant and nursing women and children should not use neem.

If you're over 65, start with a low dose, and increase only if necessary.

Inform health care professionals of the herbs you use. Problematic herb-drug interactions are possible.

Neem may cause allergic reactions or other unexpected side effects. If any develop, reduce your dose or stop taking it.

For more on herb safety, see Chapter 2.

If symptoms get worse or persist longer than 2 weeks, consult a health care professional promptly.

Growing Information

Neem is a broad-leafed evergreen tree native to India that can grow as tall as 100 feet with a trunk girth of 8 feet. It produces large, honey-scented flowers. It prefers tropical or subtropical conditions, but can survive temperatures that fall as low as 35°F for brief periods. It prefers rich soil, but can thrive in just about any soil that is not marshy or waterlogged. Migrating Indians have introduced it from Fiji to Africa, Australia to Latin America and the southwestern United States.

The neem tree can also thrive indoors as a potted plant. The best location is a south-facing window with full sun. Plant seeds in well-drained potting mix. Water regularly. Fertilize periodically.

NETTLE

Good News for Men with Enlarged Prostates

Family: Urticaceae; other members include other nettles

Genus and species: *Urtica dioica*

Also known as: Stinging nettle, common nettle, and greater nettle

Parts used: Leaves, stems, and roots

Nettle stings hurt, but this herb can also help men over age 50 who have noncancerous prostate enlargement, known as benign prostatic hypertrophy (BPH).

Healing History

Around the 3rd century B.C., Hippocrates' Greek contemporaries prescribed nettle juice externally to treat snakebite and scorpion stings and internally as an antidote to plant poisons such as hemlock and henbane. (Science has shown that nettle is not an antidote to these poisons.)

When in cold climates, Roman soldiers flailed themselves with nettle branches because the herb's sting warmed their skin. This practice, called urtication, evolved into a treatment for the joint stiffness of arthritis that is still in use today.

Early European herbalists touted nettle tea to combat cough and tuberculosis. Strange as it seems today, they recommended smoking the herb as a treatment for asthma. Herbalists also prescribed nettle to cure scurvy and stop bleeding, particularly nosebleeds.

Somewhere along the way, nettle juice gained a reputation as a hair-growth stimulant. It remained an ingredient in hair-growth nostrums well into the 19th century.

Seventeenth-century English herbalist Nicholas Culpeper endorsed all of the nettle prescriptions that preceded him. He also added one of his own: "The decoction of the leaves in wine is singularly good to provoke women's courses [menstruation]."

Native American women believed that drinking nettle tea during pregnancy strengthened the fetus and eased delivery. They also used the herb to stop uterine bleeding after childbirth, an application that early settlers adopted. Nursing mothers took nettle to increase their milk production.

America's 19th-century Eclectic physicians, forerunners of today's naturopaths, recommended nettle primarily as a diuretic to treat urinary, bladder, and kidney problems. The Eclectic text *King's American Dispensatory* (1898) describes the herb as an excellent styptic (bleeding stopper) and as a treatment for infant diarrhea, hemorrhoids, and eczema.

Contemporary herbalists recommend nettle mostly for treatment of BPH, but also as a diuretic.

Therapeutic Uses

BENIGN PROSTATIC HYPERTROPHY. Traditionally, doctors have prescribed diuretics to treat BPH. In 1950, a German researcher tried nettle root, with some success: increased urine volume and less need to get up at night to urinate. But nettle was largely forgotten as a BPH treatment until the 1970s and did not become widely used in the United States until the 1990s.

Nettle works by inhibiting 5-alpha-reductase, an enzyme that plays a key role in the overgrowth of prostate tissue that's characteristic of BPH. (The pharmaceuticals used to treat BPH are also 5-alpha-reductase inhibitors.)

Iranian researchers gave 620 men with BPH either a placebo or 120 milligrams of nettle per day. After 6 months, 16 percent of the placebo group reported benefits using standard measures of BPH. But in the nettle group, the figure was 81 percent.

In most studies, nettle has been paired with saw palmetto. Russian researchers gave 257 men with BPH either a placebo or a combination of nettle (120 milligrams twice a day) and saw palmetto (160 milligrams twice a day) for 6 months, then stopped treatment and followed the men for another year. Compared with the placebo group, urine flow in the herb group improved 19 percent, and overall BPH symptom scores were reduced by half.

German researchers gave 140 men with BPH either a standard dose of a popular pharmaceutical BPH treatment (Flomax) or a combination of nettle (120 milligrams twice a day) and saw palmetto (160 milligrams twice a day). After more than a year, both treatments showed the same benefit; the herb combination worked as well as the drug.

Commission E, the expert panel that evaluates herbal medicines for the German counterpart of the FDA, endorses nettle root preparations for mild to moderate BPH.

URINARY TRACT INFECTIONS. As a diuretic, nettle can help flush the bladder of the bacteria that cause urinary tract infections (UTIs). Commission E approves nettle leaf preparations for the prevention of UTIs and kidney stones.

HIGH BLOOD PRESSURE. Diuretics are often used to treat high blood pressure. In the United States, physicians prescribe pharmaceutical diuretics. In Germany, where herbal medicine is more mainstream, doctors may prescribe nettle instead of drugs. According to noted German medical herbalist Rudolph Fritz Weiss, M.D., "Nettle juice is definitely useful [in] diuretic therapy. It has the advantage of being well tolerated and safe, as distinct from the [pharmaceutical] thiazides."

High blood pressure is a serious condition that requires professional care. If you'd like to include nettle in your overall treatment plan, do so only under the supervision of your physician.

CONGESTIVE HEART FAILURE. Physicians often prescribe diuretics to combat the fluid accumulation associated with congestive heart failure. This condition demands professional care. If you'd like to include nettle in your overall treatment plan, do so only with the approval and supervision of your physician.

PREMENSTRUAL SYNDROME (PMS). Diuretics help relieve the bloating caused by premenstrual fluid buildup. Women who are bothered by PMS may want to try taking nettle in the days before their periods.

HAY FEVER. A study at the National College of Naturopathic Medicine in Portland, Oregon, found that freeze-dried nettle capsules (300 milligrams twice a day) provide significant relief from hay fever symptoms.

ARTHRITIS. At the University of Frankfurt in Germany, researchers assessed the pain of 40 people with various forms of arthritis, including osteoarthritis, rheumatoid arthritis, and gout. Then they gave 20 of them a standard dose of the prescription arthritis medication diclofenac (Voltaren, 200 milligrams per day). The rest of the volunteers took just 50 milligrams of the drug plus about 2 ounces of stewed nettle leaves. (Cooking removes the nettle hairs and their sting, making the leaves a vegetable similar to spinach.) After 2 weeks, both the drug-only group and the drug-nettle group reported about 70 percent improvement in their pain scores.

Diclofenac is a nonsteroidal anti-inflammatory drug (NSAID). NSAIDs are notorious for causing abdominal distress and gastrointestinal bleeding, which can become serious. Combining diclofenac with nettle provided equivalent pain relief while allowing a substantial decrease in the NSAID dose—meaning less risk of NSAID side effects. (Since this study, a new class of NSAIDs, the COX-2 inhibitors, was introduced that caused less abdominal distress. But the most popular of these drugs, Vioxx, was withdrawn when researchers found that it increased risk of heart attack.)

SCURVY. Nettle is a good source of vitamin C. This validates the herb's traditional role in treating scurvy, which is caused by a vitamin C deficiency.

Intriguing Possibility

Nettle has some antioxidant action, suggesting that it might help prevent and treat cancer. German researchers have discovered that nettle root extract impairs the growth of prostate cancer cells. In the future, it's possible that this herb may treat not just BPH, but also prostate cancer.

Rx Recommendations

To prepare a pleasant-tasting diuretic infusion, use 1 to 2 teaspoons of dried herb per cup of boiling water. Steep for 10 minutes, then strain. Drink up to 3 cups a day.

As a tincture, use $1/4$ to 1 teaspoon up to twice a day.

To treat hay fever, look for freeze-dried nettle capsules in health food stores. If you can't find them, try an infusion or a tincture.

For arthritis, harvest nettle leaves (wearing gloves and protective clothing), then steam the leaves until they are wilted. If you don't have access to nettle leaves, try an infusion or a tincture.

To treat BPH, buy a commercial root preparation and follow the package directions.

The Safety Factor

Nettle's main safety issue is its sting. The hairs that give the herb a downy appearance are actually hollow needles attached to sacs filled with irritant chemicals, notably histamine. Brushing against the plant bends the hairs, squeezing the irritants onto the skin. The pain can last for 12 hours or longer.

Herbal folklore is filled with remedies for nettle stings. One age-old recommendation is to rub the affected area with nettle juice. Rubbing with other herbs—notably peppermint and other plants of the mint family, such as rosemary—also reportedly helps. This makes some sense, since the menthol in peppermint has some anesthetic action.

The most famous remedy for nettle stings is dock, immortalized in this old British rhyme: "Nettle in, dock out / Dock rub nettle out." Nonherbal treatments include washing the affected skin with soap and water, applying topical hydrocortisone cream (such as Cort-Aid), and taking oral antihistamines.

Diuretics deplete the body of potassium, an essential nutrient. If you take nettle frequently, be sure to eat potassium-rich foods such as bananas and fresh vegetables.

Some weight-loss programs tout diuretics to eliminate water weight, but weight-loss experts advise against taking diuretics. Any pounds lost this way almost invariably return. The key to permanent weight control is a low-fat, high-fiber diet and regular, moderate exercise.

Nettle has been shown to stimulate uterine contractions in rabbits. For this reason, and because of its diuretic action, pregnant women should not take the herb internally. Nursing women should also avoid diuretics.

Do not give nettle to children under 2. In older children, adjust the recommended dose based on the child's weight. For example, give a 50-pound child one-third of the dose a 150-pound adult would take.

If you're over 65, start with a low dose, and increase only if necessary.

Inform health care professionals of the herbs you use. Problematic herb-drug interactions are possible.

Nettle may cause allergic reactions or other unexpected side effects. If any develop, reduce your dose or stop taking it.

For more on herb safety, see Chapter 2.

If symptoms get worse or persist longer than 2 weeks, consult a health care professional promptly.

Growing Information

Nettle is only one of 500 species of *Urtica*, a name derived from the Latin *uro*, meaning "to burn." And burn they do. Just be thankful that the Javanese species, *U. urentissima*, doesn't grow in North America. Its burning sting is said to last a year.

Nettle's erect stem grows from a creeping underground rhizome. It has opposite, serrated, heart-shaped, dark green leaves. It is dioecious, meaning that male and female flowers grow on separate plants. If you harvest nettle, wear heavy gloves, a long-sleeved shirt, and long pants to avoid contact with the hairs and the irritants they transmit.

Nettle grows very easily from seeds or root divisions in just about any soil. Plant seeds in spring. Take root divisions in autumn after the leaves have died back.

Harvest the leaves (wearing gloves and protective clothing) before the plants flower in late spring or early summer. You may boil or steam young leaves like spinach and eat them as a vegetable. Boiling or drying eliminates the sting. The fresh, tender shoots do not sting and may be used in salads.

Nettle has a reputation for increasing the aromatic oil content of angelica, marjoram, oregano, peppermint, sage, valerian, and other fragrant herbs. Nettle also reputedly speeds decomposition in compost.

PAPAYA

A Tropical Digestive Aid

Family: Caricaceae; other members include custard apple

Genus and species: *Carica papaya*

Also known as: Pawpaw and melon tree

Parts used: Fruits, leaves, and latex

Cookbooks caution that gelatin won't gel if you add pineapple. The same is true if you add papaya, only more so. Both fruits contain digestive enzymes that prevent the proteins in gelatin from solidifying. Those powerful enzymes are key to papaya's therapeutic powers.

Healing History

Centuries ago, the indigenous peoples of the Caribbean noticed that meat wrapped in papaya's broad leaves became more tender. Today, papaya extract is the active ingredient in most commercial meat tenderizers.

The Caribbean natives also cut incisions into mature but unripe papayas, collected the milky fluid (latex), and applied it to their skin to treat psoriasis, ringworm, wounds, and infections. Caribbean women ate unripe papayas to trigger menstruation, abortion, and labor.

After Europeans introduced papaya into tropical Asia, it quickly became incorporated into local healing practices. Filipinos used a root decoction to treat hemorrhoids. The Javanese believed that eating papaya fruit prevented arthritis. The Japanese used the latex to treat digestive disorders. Throughout Asia, the leaves were applied to wounds, and the latex was dabbed onto the cervix at term to stimulate labor.

Papaya did not play a role in traditional American herbal medicine. Over the past 25 years, however, as tropical fruits have become more widely available in this country, papaya has grown in popularity. The plant's leaves and latex are commonly sold in specialty herb shops.

Contemporary herbalists recommend papaya fruit and leaf infusions to aid digestion, ease stomach upset, and eliminate intestinal worms. They also suggest applying the leaves and latex externally to wounds.

Therapeutic Uses

Papaya fruits, leaves, and latex contain several enzymes that account for the herb's action as a digestive aid and its ability to tenderize—that is, predigest—the protein in meat. The latex contains the most enzymes, followed by the leaves and then the fruits, but even the fruit has enough enzymes to enhance digestion. (Incidentally, one of those enzymes, papain, is the active ingredient in the cleaning solutions developed for soft contact lenses.)

DIGESTIVE PROBLEMS. Of all papaya's enzymes, papain may be the most important. It's similar to the human digestive enzyme pepsin, which helps break down proteins. In fact, papain is sometimes called vegetable pepsin. Papaya's other enzymes include one similar to rennin, which breaks down milk proteins, and one similar to pectase, which helps digest starches.

ULCERS. One laboratory study found that papaya exerts a direct effect on the stomach, helping to prevent ulcers. In the study, two groups of experimental animals were fed large doses of ulcer-inducing aspirin and steroids. Those that were also fed papaya for 6 days prior to receiving the drugs developed significantly fewer ulcers. This finding suggests that papaya may be of particular benefit to people with inflammatory conditions who take aspirin or steroids.

SLIPPED DISKS. In 1982, the FDA approved another papaya enzyme, chymopapain, as a treatment for herniated ("slipped") vertebral disks in the back. Injected directly into the affected area, chymopapain helps dissolve cellular debris.

Rx Recommendations

Papaya fruit is soft when ripe, and it tastes similar to cantaloupe. Have some as an appetizer before meals to stimulate digestion.

For a pleasant-tasting infusion to aid digestion, use 1 to 2 teaspoons of dried, powdered leaves per cup of boiling water. Steep for 10 minutes, then strain if you wish. Drink during or after meals, especially those high in protein (red meat and dairy products). Do not boil papaya leaves; boiling deactivates the papain.

When using commercial preparations, follow the package directions.

The Safety Factor

Pregnant and nursing women may eat ripe papaya fruit in moderation, but they should avoid papaya latex and medicinal doses of the herb's leaves. Many cultures used papaya latex and leaves as a menstruation promoter and labor inducer.

Some allergic reactions, including asthma, have been reported with papaya. The latex may cause stomach inflammation (gastritis).

Inform health care professionals of the herbs you use. Problematic herb-drug interactions are possible.

For more on herb safety, see Chapter 2.

If symptoms get worse or persist longer than 2 weeks, consult a health care professional promptly.

Growing Information

Native to the Caribbean and now naturalized throughout the tropics, papaya trees can reach 25 feet. The trunk is hollow, with spongy wood and fibrous, light-colored bark that is used to make rope. Its leaves are smooth, hand-shaped (palmate), and large, often 2 feet across.

The fruits are yellow-green, pear-shaped melons with tasty orange-yellow pulp. Papayas sold in the United States are typically about the size of large potatoes, but in the tropics, they grow to the size of large honeydews and can weigh up to 10 pounds. That's where the name melon tree comes from.

PARSLEY

More Than Just a Garnish

Family: Umbelliferae; other members include carrot, celery, fennel, dill, and angelica

Genus and species: *Petroselinum crispum, P. hortense,* and *P. sativum*

Also known as: Rock selinon

Parts used: Leaves, fruits (seeds), and roots

Few herbs are more familiar than parsley. Many recipes call for it. And its lacy sprigs typically adorn restaurant plates—where they usually remain uneaten. This is unfortunate, for parsley is nutritious and an effective after-dinner breath freshener. It has other benefits, too.

Healing History

Parsley is one of the first herbs to appear in spring. For centuries, it has been used in the Seder, the ritual Jewish Passover meal, as a symbol of new beginnings.

The ancient Greeks had a different view of the herb. In Greek mythology, parsley sprang from the blood of Opheltes, infant son of King Lycurgus of Nemea, who was killed by a serpent while his nanny directed some thirsty soldiers to a spring. For centuries, Greek soldiers believed that any contact with parsley before battle signaled impending death.

Because of its association with death, parsley was planted on Greek graves. Ironically, this custom gradually changed public perception of the herb. To honor the memory of important figures, the Greeks held athletic contests and crowned the winners with parsley wreaths. Over the course of a few centuries, the herb came to symbolize strength.

The shadow of bad luck clung to the herb well into the Middle Ages, however. Some Europeans considered parsley a "devil's herb," sure to bring disaster upon those who grew it—unless they planted it on Good Friday.

Parsley was not widely used in ancient medicine, but the Roman physician Galen prescribed it for "falling sickness" (epilepsy) and as a diuretic for water retention. The Romans also munched sprigs to freshen their breath—the beginnings of the parsley garnish on restaurant plates today.

Medieval German abbess/herbalist Hildegard of Bingen prescribed parsley compresses for arthritis and parsley boiled in wine for chest and heart pain.

Seventeenth-century English herbalist Nicholas Culpeper reiterated Galen's recommendations and added to them, prescribing parsley to "provoke urine and women's courses [menstruation] . . . to expel wind . . . to break the stone [kidney stones] and ease the pains and torments thereof . . . and against cough." Culpeper also endorsed parsley compresses for inflamed eyes and black-and-blue marks and suggested that the herb be "fried with butter and applied to [the] breasts" for nipple soreness due to nursing.

Over the centuries, herbalists recommended topical applications of parsley to treat insect bites, wounds, and lice and internal doses to treat dysentery, gallstones, and some tumors.

From the 1850s through 1926, parsley was recognized by the *U.S. Pharmacopoeia*, a standard drug reference, as a laxative, a diuretic for kidney problems and the fluid accumulation of congestive heart failure, and a substitute for quinine in treating malaria.

America's 19th-century Eclectic physicians, forerunners of today's naturopaths, echoed the *Pharmacopoeia*. Their main text, *King's American Dispensatory* (1898), chronicled the isolation of a chemical called apiol from parsley oil. It recommended apiol as a treatment for "menstrual derangements," although it also noted that high doses could cause "intoxication, giddiness, flashes of light, vertigo, and ringing in the ears [tinnitus]."

During the early 20th century, large doses of apiol were used to induce abortion, despite its considerable toxicity.

Contemporary herbalists recommend parsley in cooking as a rich source of vitamins A and C, calcium, and iron. They suggest the fresh herb as a breath freshener and an infusion or a tincture as a diuretic, digestive aid, and gas expeller.

Therapeutic Uses

Parsley roots, leaves, and fruits (seeds) all contain the plant's volatile oil, but the highest concentrations are in the seeds.

Parsley oil contains the chemicals apiol and myristicin, two significant diuretics that are also uterine stimulants and mild laxatives. Commission E, the expert panel that evaluates herbal medicines for the German counterpart of the FDA, approves parsley as a diuretic.

HIGH BLOOD PRESSURE. Physicians often prescribe diuretics to treat high blood pressure. A study published in the *American Journal of Chinese Medicine* suggests that parsley's diuretic action can also help control the condition. In Germany, where herbal medicine is more mainstream than in the United States, parsley seed tea is often prescribed for high blood pressure.

High blood pressure is a serious health problem that requires professional care. If you'd like to include parsley in your overall treatment plan, do so only with the approval of your physician.

CONGESTIVE HEART FAILURE. Physicians often prescribe diuretics to combat the fluid accumulation associated with congestive heart failure. This condition demands professional care, so if you'd like to include parsley in your overall treatment plan, do so only with the approval and supervision of your physician.

BAD BREATH. Parsley has one of the highest levels of chlorophyll of any herb. Chlorophyll is the active ingredient in many breath fresheners, such as Clorets. This supports the herb's ancient use as a breath freshener.

PREMENSTRUAL SYNDROME. As a diuretic, parsley may help relieve the bloated feeling caused by premenstrual fluid buildup. Women who are bothered by premenstrual syndrome may want to try some parsley in the days leading up to their periods.

LABOR. Both apiol and myristicin are uterine stimulants. In Russia, a preparation called Supetin, which contains 85 percent parsley juice, is used to induce uterine contractions during labor.

ALLERGIES. A study published in the *Journal of Allergy and Clinical Immunology* showed that parsley inhibits the secretion of histamine, a compound that's produced by the body and is responsible for triggering allergy symptoms. Parsley's apparent antihistamine action may help people with hay fever or hives.

FEVER. Parsley has never been proven effective against malaria, so the *Pharmacopoeia* was incorrect on that score. But apiol has some fever-reducing (antipyretic) properties. While you shouldn't count on parsley to take the place of aspirin, ibuprofen, or acetaminophen, you may want to try it in addition to mainstream medications.

Intriguing Possibilities

Animal studies suggest that parsley reduces blood sugar levels, hinting that it may help treat human diabetes.

In addition, parsley contains psoralen, a chemical that's best known for causing sun sensitivity. But psoralen shows promise in the treatment of one form of cancer, cutaneous T-cell lymphoma. Although it's premature to recommend parsley as a cancer therapy, testing the herb for this purpose is certainly warranted.

Rx Recommendations

To freshen breath, chewing on a few sprigs of fresh parsley is usually sufficient.

For a pleasant-tasting infusion that may help treat high blood pressure, congestive heart failure, allergies, or fever or induce labor, use 2 teaspoons of dried leaves or root or 1 teaspoon of crushed

seeds per cup of boiling water. Steep for 10 minutes, then strain. Drink up to 3 cups a day.

As a homemade tincture, take $\frac{1}{2}$ to 1 teaspoon up to three times a day.

When using commercial preparations, follow the package directions.

The Safety Factor

Diuretics deplete the body of potassium, an essential nutrient. If you frequently take medicinal preparations of parsley, be sure to eat potassium-rich foods such as bananas and fresh vegetables.

Although some weight-loss programs tout diuretics to eliminate water weight, weight-management experts discourage the use of diuretics for this purpose. Any pounds taken off with diuretics almost invariably return. The key to permanent weight control is a low-fat, high-fiber diet and regular aerobic exercise.

Pregnant women may eat culinary amounts of parsley, but they should not take medicinal preparations, except possibly at term and under the supervision of a physician, to help induce labor. Other women might try parsley tea to bring on their periods.

Nursing women should avoid diuretics, including parsley.

The psoralen in parsley has been known to cause skin rashes in agricultural workers who harvest large quantities. People with sensitive skin should be aware of this possible side effect.

The Eclectics were right about large doses of parsley oil causing headache, nausea, vertigo, giddiness, hives, and liver and kidney damage. Nevertheless, the medical literature contains no reports of problems from the herb itself, even when used in medicinal quantities.

Children may eat small amounts of parsley leaves. But do not give medicinal preparations of parsley to children under 2. In older children, adjust the recommended dose based on the child's weight. For example, give a 50-pound child one-third of the dose a 150-pound adult would take.

If you're over 65, start with a low dose, and increase only if necessary.

Inform health care professionals of the herbs you use. Problematic herb-drug interactions are possible.

Parsley may cause allergic reactions or other unexpected side effects. If any develop, reduce your dose or stop taking it.

For more on herb safety, see Chapter 2.

If symptoms get worse or persist longer than 2 weeks, consult a health care professional promptly.

Growing Information

Parsley is a small, bright green biennial that reaches 12 inches the first year and up to 3 feet the second year, when it flowers. The plant has a thick, carrotlike taproot and juicy stems terminating in feathery, deeply divided, curly or flat leaves, depending on the variety. Its tiny yellow-green flowers develop on the umbrella-like canopy (umbels) characteristic of the Umbelliferae family.

Although it's a biennial, parsley should be cultivated as an annual. The seeds are slow to germinate, often requiring up to 6 weeks. Sow them any time from early spring to autumn. Parsley can be sown indoors and transplanted, but most authorities recommend outdoor planting with $1/4$ inch of soil cover.

Parsley grows best in moist, sandy, well-drained loam with a neutral pH. Thin seedlings to 8-inch spacing. Late-season planting is fine. Even as a seedling, the herb usually survives one or two frosts.

You may harvest the leaves once the plants have reached about 8 inches. Harvest the fruits when they appear full-size and gray brown. Dig the roots during the autumn of the first year or the spring of the second.

Caution: Unless you are an experienced field botanist, *never* pick wild parsley. It closely resembles three potentially lethal plants: water hemlock, poison parsley (also known as poison hemlock), and fool's parsley (also known as dog parsley or small hemlock).

PASSIONFLOWER

Relieves Tension and Insomnia

Family: Passifloraceae; other members include granadilla, sweet calabash, and Jamaican honeysuckle

Genus and species: *Passiflora incarnata*

Also known as: Maypop, apricot vine, and water lemon

Parts used: Leaves and flowers

In the 1560s, 20 years after Francisco Pizarro brutally suppressed the Incas' last rebellion and forced their conversion to Christianity, Dr. Nicolas Monardes of Seville apparently developed a guilty conscience for the carnage his countrymen had wrought. An avid botanist, he searched among the plants sent back from the New World for some sign of divine approval of the Spanish conquest. He found it in a vine that had large, beautiful blossoms with parts that seemed to evoke the Passion of the Crucifixion.

To Dr. Monardes, the plant's three styles represented the three nails of the cross. Its ovary looked like a hammer. Its corona evoked the crown of thorns, and its 10 petals suggested the 10 true apostles (the original 12 minus Judas, the betrayer, and Peter, who denied Christ). Dr. Monardes christened the vine passionflower.

Healing History

The Incas brewed a tonic tea from passionflower. The herb's pleasant taste and its Christian symbolism quickly turned its leaves into a popular item in Europe, where it was used as a tranquilizer and mild sedative.

When colonists settled the American Gulf Coast, they found that the area's Native Americans used a tea made from their local passionflower to calm nervousness and applied the herb's crushed leaves as poultices on cuts and bruises.

Southerners adopted passionflower as both an ornamental and a medicinal vine. It remained a folk remedy until 1839, when two Gulf Coast Eclectic physicians touted it in the *New Orleans Medical Journal* as a non-narcotic sedative and digestive aid.

The Eclectics, forerunners of today's naturopaths, adopted passionflower as "an important remedy" for insomnia, restlessness, menstrual discomforts, diarrhea, epilepsy, and whooping cough. They also prescribed juice from the leaves externally for burns, scalds, wounds, and toothache.

Contemporary herbalists recommend passionflower primarily as a tranquilizer and sedative. They also consider it a digestive aid and pain reliever.

From 1916 to 1936, passionflower was recognized as a tranquilizer and sedative in the *National Formulary*, the pharmacists' reference. In 1978, however, the FDA banned the herb from sleep aids for lack of proven effectiveness.

Therapeutic Uses

The FDA had a reasonable argument for banning passionflower before it had been extensively studied. Unfortunately, the agency has not kept up with more recent research findings.

STRESS, ANXIETY, AND INSOMNIA. Passionflower contains compounds that are indeed tranquilizing (maltol, flavonoids, and passiflorine, which is chemically similar to morphine). It also has substances that are potentially stimulating (harmala compounds). Various researchers have concluded that the herb has complex activity in the central nervous system, with an overall mild tranquilizing-sedative effect despite the presence of stimulants.

The herb is clearly sedative in animals, and that effect has been confirmed by research in humans. French researchers gave 91 people with anxiety problems either a placebo or an herbal preparation containing passionflower and several other herbs (including hawthorn and valerian). After 28 days, those taking the herb formula reported significantly greater anxiety relief.

In Europe, passionflower is an ingredient in many tranquilizing and sedative preparations. It's non-narcotic, so no need for a prescription, and no possibility of addiction. Commission E, the expert panel that evaluates herbal medicines for the German counterpart of the FDA, approves passionflower for nervousness and restlessness.

DIGESTIVE PROBLEMS. Passionflower relaxes the smooth muscle lining the digestive tract, which means that it is an antispasmodic. This property lends credence to the herb's traditional role as a digestive aid.

WOMEN'S HEALTH CONCERNS. Antispasmodics relax not only the digestive tract but also other smooth muscles, such as the uterus. This supports passionflower's traditional use as a remedy for menstrual discomforts.

WOUNDS. One study suggests that passionflower helps relieve pain, while two others show that it kills many disease-causing molds, fungi, and bacteria. These findings support the Native American and Eclectic use of passionflower as a wound treatment.

Intriguing Possibilities

In animal studies, the harmala compounds in passionflower dilate (open) the coronary arteries. Blocked coronary arteries result in heart attack, so the herb may help prevent and treat heart disease.

One day, passionflower may also be used to ease withdrawal from narcotic addiction. Animals experimentally addicted to morphine experienced easier withdrawal when treated with passionflower.

Rx Recommendations

For first aid in the garden, crush a few passionflower leaves and flowers into minor cuts until you can wash and bandage them.

For a pleasant-tasting infusion that may help you relax, calm down, or fall asleep, use 1 teaspoon of dried leaves per cup of boiling water. Steep for 10 to 15 minutes, then strain. For insomnia, drink a cup of tea before bed. For other conditions, drink up to 3 cups a day.

As a homemade tincture, take ¼ to 1 teaspoon up to three times a day.

When using commercial preparations, follow the label directions.

The Safety Factor

Some sources warn that passionflower contains cyanide, a potent poison. This is a botanical error. Ornamental blue passionflower, *Passiflora caerulea*, contains the poison. The healing herb, *P. incarnata*, does not. When buying passionflower, check the label to be sure that the product is *P. incarnata*.

The harmala compounds in passionflower are uterine stimulants. Whole passionflower has not been associated with miscarriage, but pregnant women would be prudent to stay away from an herb with such complex effects on the central nervous system. Nursing women should also avoid it.

Do not give passionflower to children under 2. In older children, adjust the recommended dose based on the child's weight. For example, give a 50-pound child one-third of the dose a 150-pound adult would take.

If you're over 65, start with a low dose, and increase only if necessary.

Inform health care professionals of the herbs you use. Problematic herb-drug interactions are possible.

Passionflower may cause allergic reactions or other unexpected side effects. If any develop, reduce your dose or stop taking it.

For more on herb safety, see Chapter 2.

If symptoms get worse or persist longer than 2 weeks, consult a health care professional promptly.

Growing Information

Passionflower has a perennial root with fast-growing, climbing, annual tendrils that may reach 30 feet. The leaves are dull green, 4 to 6 inches long, and deeply divided into three to five lobes with serrated edges. Its sweet-scented white flowers are 3 inches across and tinged with purple. They bloom in May, hence the name maypop, and produce egg-size yellow or orange edible fruits, the source of the names apricot vine and water lemon.

Passionflower grows easily from seeds, cuttings, or root runners divided in autumn. It prefers rich, slightly acidic, well-watered, well-drained loam in locations that have plenty of light but are shaded from strong, direct summer sun.

The perennial root is hardy but may not survive temperatures below −15°F. The vine tendrils need something to climb, such as a fence or trellis.

Harvest the leaves around the time the flowers bloom. When the plant is generously watered, the fruits are edible and sweet.

PAU D'ARCO

The Bark That Treats Yeast Infections

Family: Bignoniaceae; other members include jacaranda

Genus and species: *Tabebuia impetiginosa*

Also known as: Lapacho, ipe, taheebo, trumpet tree

Part used: Inner bark

The Incas used the wood of the South American tree they called *lapacho* to make bows for hunting. The Spanish adopted this use, and called the tree *pau d'arco*, meaning "bow stick." The name stuck, and now refers to various trees of the *Tabebuia* genus that grow in the mountains of Brazil, Argentina, Bolivia, Paraguay, and Peru. But pau d'arco does more than shoot arrows. It also helps treat vaginal yeast infections—and shows promise against cancer.

Healing History

A thousand years ago, the Incas considered pau d'arco indispensable for treating fever, sore throat, dysentery, snakebite, bladder and yeast infections, and even cancer. Early explorers noticed that while most nearby trees had fungus growing on them, pau d'arco did not. As a result, the tree began to be used to treat fungal infections.

Therapeutic Uses

YEAST INFECTIONS. Speaking of fungal infections, pau d'arco is an effective treatment for *Candida albicans*, the fungus that causes vaginal yeast infections. Writing in the *British Journal of Phytotherapy*, a Dutch researcher suggests using a tampon that has been soaked in a strong pau d'arco infusion while also taking the herb orally.

ANTIBIOTIC POWER. Since the 1950s, South American researchers have shown that pau d'arco's inner bark has antibacterial action. Researchers at the University of Rio de Janeiro discovered that it helps treat staph infections that resist pharmaceutical antibiotics. Korean researchers at Seoul National University have found that it's also active against the bacteria that cause food poisoning, thus validating the herb's traditional use as a treatment for dysentery.

Brazilian researchers have found that pau d'arco treats some tropical parasites, among them, the organism that causes Chagas disease. In addition, pau d'arco has some antiviral activity, especially against herpes.

Intriguing Possibility

The most intriguing pau d'arco research has focused on the possibility that this herb might treat cancer. During the 1950s, Brazilian researchers discovered that it was effective against leukemia and other cancers. During the 1960s, our own National Cancer Institute (NCI) studied lapachol, the pau d'arco constituent with the most pronounced anti-tumor activity. But the NCI obtained disappointing results and gave up on it.

The NCI was a bit hasty. Recent studies by various Korean researchers have focused on another pau d'arco constituent, beta-lapachone. Laboratory studies show that this compound kills cancer cells in the lung, colon, and prostate. Pau d'arco is still years away from being used to treat cancer, but it appears that the Incas may have been on the right track.

Rx Recommendations

Follow package directions; when using tablets or capsules, the recommended dose is 1 to 4 grams per day in divided doses.

To use pau d'arco to treat a yeast infection, open a few capsules and make a strong infusion. Immerse a tampon in it and insert. Repeat every few hours while also taking the herb by mouth.

When using a tincture, take 1 to 2 teaspoons three times a day. A tampon may also be immersed in tincture.

The Safety Factor

Large doses may cause nausea, vomiting, diarrhea, and dizziness.

Pau d'arco has anticoagulant action. Users might notice that they bruise more easily and that cuts take longer to clot. Those with clotting disorders as well as those who are taking anticoagulant drugs or are about to have surgery should not use this herb.

Pregnant and nursing women should not use it.

Do not give pau d'arco to children under 2. In older children, adjust the recommended dose based on the child's weight. For example, give a 50-pound child one-third of the dose a 150-pound adult would take.

If you're over 65, start with a low dose, and increase only if necessary.

Inform health care professionals of the herbs you use. Problematic herb-drug interactions are possible.

Pau d'arco may cause allergic reactions or other unexpected side effects. If any develop, reduce your dose or stop taking it.

For more on herb safety, see Chapter 2.

If symptoms get worse or persist longer than 2 weeks, consult a health care professional promptly.

Growing Information

Pau d'arco grows in the Andes and in parts of Paraguay and Brazil. It is not grown in the United States. It takes 40 years for the tree to mature enough to produce medicinally valuable bark. The bark is similar to cork and can be harvested without killing the tree. The tree can live 700 years. It produces trumpet-shaped violet flowers, hence the name trumpet tree.

PELARGONIUM

For Bronchitis, Colds, and Tonsillitis

Family: Geraniaceae; other members include geranium

Genus and species: *Pelargonium sidoides*

Also known as: South African geranium, kalwerbossie, and rabassam

Part used: Root juice

Native to the grasslands of southern Africa, *P. sidoides* is a low-growing perennial that produces velvety, heart-shaped, mildly aromatic leaves and distinctive dark, reddish-purple (almost black) flowers in spring and summer. But this geranium is more than just a pretty plant. It's also a real healer.

Healing History

For centuries, the Zulu and other indigenous tribes of southern Africa used *Pelargonium sidoides* to treat respiratory conditions.

Therapeutic Uses

South African geranium has immune-stimulating action. It activates germ-devouring natural killer cells and spurs production of interferon, which helps defend cells against infection.

BRONCHITIS. In nonsmokers, bronchitis typically develops at the tail end of a cold as a dry, hacking cough that can take weeks to go away. Eventually, people get fed up and see their doctors, who typically prescribe an antibiotic. Antibiotics treat bacterial bronchitis, but only rarely is cold-related bronchitis caused by bacteria. Before you call your doctor, try *Pelargonium sidoides.* Since the turn of the 21st century, a half-dozen studies have shown that it's effective against bronchitis.

In one study, German researchers gave 468 adults with bronchitis either a placebo or 30 drops of pelargonium root juice three times a day. After 7 days, the herb provided significantly greater relief. The researchers concluded: "Treatment with pelargonium clearly reduced the severity of symptoms and allowed users to return to work 2 days faster." Similar studies have shown the herb effective against childhood bronchitis.

COLDS. Ukrainian scientists gave 103 adults with colds either a placebo or 30 drops of pelargonium three times a day. In the pelargonium group, symptoms were only half as severe. After 10 days, 31 percent of the placebo group pronounced themselves cured. In the pelargonium group, the figure was 79 percent.

TONSILLITIS. Another group of Ukrainian researchers gave 143 children with tonsillitis either a placebo or 20 drops of pelargonium twice a day. After 6 days, the herb group reported significantly reduced symptoms.

Rx Recommendations

Most studies have used 30 drops three times a day. Or follow package directions.

The Safety Factor

Pelargonium has been a popular herbal medicine in Germany since the 1980s. No serious side effects have been reported, but stomach upset and, rarely, allergic reactions are possible.

Those with kidney or liver disease should avoid this herb.

Pregnant and nursing women should not use pelargonium.

Do not give this herb to children under 2. In older children, adjust the recommended dose based on the child's weight. For example, give a 50-pound child one-third of the dose a 150-pound adult would take.

If you're over 65, start with a low dose, and increase only if necessary.

Inform health care professionals of the herbs you use. Problematic herb-drug interactions are possible.

Pelargonium may cause allergic reactions or other unexpected side effects. If any develop, reduce your dose or stop taking it.

For more on herb safety, see Chapter 2.

If symptoms get worse or persist longer than 2 weeks, consult a health care professional promptly.

Growing Information

Pelargonium can be grown indoors or outside in temperate climates from seed or cuttings treated with rooting hormone. It grows 6 to 12 inches tall. This herb prefers full sun, sandy or clay-loam soil, and generous watering in summer, but less water during winter. Once established, it's drought-tolerant. Top dressing with fertilizer in spring improves growth and flowers in summer. Remove dead leaves and old flower stalks in winter. Start outdoor plants in pots indoors, then transplant.

PENNYROYAL

A Good Herb with a Bad Reputation

Family: Labiatae; other members include mints

Genus and species: *Mentha pulegium* (European); *Hedeoma pulegioides* (American)

Also known as: Pulegium, hedeoma, fleabane, tickweed, mosquito plant, and squawmint

Parts used: Leaves and flowers

Few healing herbs have a reputation as bad—or as undeserved—as pennyroyal. Critics charge that ingesting even small amounts can be fatal. While as little as 2 tablespoons of pennyroyal *oil* can cause death, the dried herb is not dangerous. Pennyroyal's highly aromatic leaves and flowers are a safe decongestant, cough remedy, and digestive aid.

Healing History

Pennyroyal became popular during the 1st century A.D. after the Roman naturalist Pliny noted that the aromatic plant repelled fleas (hence its common name, fleabane). When crushed and rubbed on the skin or strewn, pennyroyal repels other insects as well (hence the names tickweed and mosquito plant).

Pliny also touted pennyroyal as a cough remedy and digestive aid. He recommended hanging the plant in sickrooms in the belief that its fragrance promoted healing. The Greek physician Dioscorides seconded Pliny's recommendations, adding that pennyroyal stimulates menstruation and helps expel the afterbirth.

During the early Middle Ages, pennyroyal was recommended for truly bizarre purposes. Physician-philosopher St. Albertus Magnus wrote that by covering drowning bees in the herb's warm ashes, "they shall recover their lyfe after a space of one houre."

In the 16th century, British herbalist John Gerard touted pennyroyal's ancient use as an expectorant: "Penny-royale taken with honey cleanseth the lungs and cleareth the breast from all gross and thick humors."

Seventeenth-century English herbalist Nicholas Culpeper recommended the herb for many other conditions: "Drunk with wine, it is of singular service to those stung or bit by any venomous beast . . . applied to the nostrils with vinegar, it is very reviving [for] fainting . . . being dried and burnt, it strengtheneth the gums, and is helpful for those troubled with the gout . . . being applied as a plaster, it taketh away carbuncles [boils]."

Early American colonists introduced European pennyroyal (*Mentha pulegium*) into North

America. They found, however, that Native Americans were already using the American herb (*Hedeoma pulegioides*) for similar purposes—externally to dress wounds and repel insects and internally to treat colds, flu, coughs, and congestion and to stimulate menstruation and abortion. Folk healers also recommended aromatic pennyroyal garlands for headache and dizziness.

During the early 19th century, Thomsonian herbalists packed pennyroyal leaves into the nostrils to treat nosebleeds. After the Civil War, Eclectic physicians, forerunners of today's naturopaths, adopted pennyroyal as a stimulant, fever treatment, digestive aid, and menstruation promoter. Their text *King's American Dispensatory* (1898) described the herb as "an excellent remedy for the common cold" and recommended it for arthritis, whooping cough (pertussis), "colic in children . . . and hysteria" (menstrual discomforts).

Around 1887, the Eclectics began using pennyroyal oil, which they considered more convenient than the raw herb. They also recognized its potential hazards. *King's American Dispensatory* mentioned a case of pennyroyal poisoning caused by ingesting just 1 tablespoon.

From 1831 to 1916, pennyroyal was listed in the *U.S. Pharmacopoeia*, a standard drug reference, as a stimulant, digestive aid, and menstruation promoter. From 1916 to 1931, pennyroyal oil was listed as an intestinal irritant and abortion inducer.

Contemporary herbalists advise against taking pennyroyal oil because of its toxicity, but they recommend using the whole herb externally as an insect repellent and treatment for cuts and burns. They also suggest taking the herb (not the oil) internally for colds, coughs, upset stomach, flatulence, anxiety, and menstruation promotion.

Therapeutic Uses

Pennyroyal oil contains pulegone, a compound that accounts for its actions as an insect repellent, menstruation promoter, and abortion inducer.

INSECT REPELLENT. Pliny was right: Pennyroyal oil helps repel flies, gnats, mosquitoes, fleas, and ticks. It is the active ingredient in most natural insect repellents. If you buy an herbal flea collar for your dog or cat, it's likely to contain pennyroyal oil.

CONGESTION AND COUGHS. Because pennyroyal is one of the most aromatic mints, the strong aroma of a pennyroyal infusion can serve as a decongestant and possible expectorant.

DIGESTIVE PROBLEMS. Pennyroyal contains compounds similar to the stomach-soothing menthol in its botanical relative, peppermint. While pennyroyal's stomach-settling action is not as strong as peppermint's, the herb is still an effective digestive aid.

Rx Recommendations

To repel insects, rub fresh, crushed plant material over your body, or mix pennyroyal tincture into a skin cream and apply.

To make an herbal flea collar, try hanging a pennyroyal garland or a bag of the herb from a regular collar. Do not apply pennyroyal oil to your pet's fur or skin. The animal may get a toxic dose from licking itself.

For an infusion to help treat coughs, congestion, or stomach upset, use 1 to 2 teaspoons of dried herb per cup of boiling water. Steep for 10 to 15 minutes, then strain. Drink up to 2 cups a day. Its aroma resembles spearmint's, but it's sharper and not quite as inviting. The taste is warm and pleasant, initially bitter with a cool finish.

As a homemade tincture, use $1/4$ to $1/2$ teaspoon up to twice a day.

When using commercial preparations, follow the package directions.

The Safety Factor

Ever since pennyroyal's abortion-inducing oil was first distilled more than 100 years ago, the herb has been notorious because the oil is so toxic. Pulegone does indeed stimulate uterine contractions. Unfortunately, the dose necessary for abortion is quite close to the lethal dose, a fact that many women learned the hard way. As little as $1/2$ teaspoon of pennyroyal oil can cause convulsions. Doses not much larger can be fatal.

The British medical journal *Lancet* cited a case of abortion-related pennyroyal oil poisoning as early as 1897. Since then, many similar reports have appeared in the medical literature. According to one such report in the *Journal of the American Medical Association*, a pregnant 18-year-old woman died within 2 hours after taking 2 tablespoons of the oil, despite emergency treatment. Clearly, women wishing to terminate pregnancy should not use pennyroyal oil. In fact, no one should.

Although small amounts of pennyroyal oil can be fatal, the oil is a super-concentrated extract of the herb. Drinking a few cups of infusion made from dried pennyroyal leaves poses no hazard. University of Illinois pharmacognosist Norman Farnsworth, Ph.D., estimates that it would take 75 gallons of strong pennyroyal infusion to approach the potential toxicity of a fatal dose of pennyroyal oil.

Pregnant and nursing women should not use pennyroyal.

Do not give pennyroyal to children under 2. In older children, adjust the recommended dose based on the child's weight. For example, give a 50-pound child one-third of the dose a 150-pound adult would take.

If you're over 65, start with a low dose, and increase only if necessary.

Inform health care professionals of the herbs you use. Problematic herb-drug interactions are possible.

Pennyroyal may cause allergic reactions or other unexpected side effects. If any develop, reduce your dose or stop taking it.

For more on herb safety, see Chapter 2.

If symptoms get worse or persist longer than 2 weeks, consult a health care professional promptly.

Growing Information

Despite their botanical differences, both European and American pennyroyal yield similar oils and are used interchangeably.

The European herb is a perennial that spreads by underground runners. Its square stems grow to about 12 inches, and its opposite, oval leaves are smooth or slightly hairy. Tight whorls of small lilac flowers appear in midsummer. European pennyroyal may be propagated from root runner divisions in early spring or fall or by rooting stem cuttings during summer.

American pennyroyal is an annual with

square stems that reach 15 inches. Its leaves resemble those of the European variety, but its summer-blooming flowers tend to be smaller and more bluish. It must be grown from seeds sown in spring or fall. Cover them with ¹/₄ inch of soil. Thin seedlings to about 5-inch spacing.

Both types do best in rich, well-watered, sandy, slightly acidic loam under full sun, although the European herb tolerates partial shade. It also needs room to spread. Its runners emerge after it flowers.

Harvest the leaves and flowers of both plants when they are in full bloom. In the fall, cut them back to a few inches above the ground and hang the herb to dry.

PEPPERMINT AND SPEARMINT

Marvelous Menthol

Family: Labiatae; other members include balm, basil, catnip, horehound, marjoram, and pennyroyal

Genus and species: *Mentha piperita* (peppermint); *M. spicata, M. viridis, M. aquatica, M. cardiaca* (spearmint)

Also known as: No other names, but there are hundreds of varieties of mint

Parts used: Leaves and flowers

Have you ever had an after-dinner mint? Those familiar candies evolved from the ancient custom of concluding feasts by chewing a sprig of mint to soothe the stomach. Modern research has shown the wisdom of this age-old practice and has verified other therapeutic uses of peppermint and spearmint.

Both mints are popular in herbal medicine, and they have similar effects. But of the two, peppermint is generally regarded as tastier. It's more medicinally potent, too.

Spearmint was the original medicinal mint. Peppermint appeared later, a natural hybrid of spearmint species. Authorities aren't exactly sure which species combined to form the spicier mint or when it first appeared. All of the mints were considered one plant, called mint, until 1696, when British botanist John Ray differentiated them.

Healing History

Mint was mentioned as a stomach soother in the *Ebers Papyrus*, the world's oldest surviving medical text. From Egypt, mint spread to Palestine, where it was accepted as payment for taxes. In Luke (11:39), Jesus scolds the Pharisees, "You pay tithes of mint and rue . . . but have no care for justice and the love of God."

From the Holy Land, mint spread to Greece and entered Greek mythology. It seems that Pluto, god of the dead, fell in love with the beautiful nymph Minthe. Pluto's goddess-wife, Persephone, became jealous and changed Minthe into mint. Pluto could not bring Minthe back to life, but he gave her plant form a fragrant aroma. *Minthe* evolved into the mints' genus name, *Mentha*.

Greek and Roman homemakers added mint to milk to prevent spoilage and served the herb after meals as a digestive aid. The Roman naturalist Pliny wrote that mint "reanimates the spirit" and recommended hanging it in sickrooms to assist convalescence. The Greek physician Dioscorides considered mint "heating" and therefore a promoter of lust. Other Greek and Roman herbalists prescribed mint for everything from hiccups to leprosy.

Chinese and Ayurvedic physicians have used mint for centuries as a tonic and digestive aid and as a treatment for colds, coughs, and fevers.

Twelfth-century German abbess/herbalist Hildegard of Bingen recommended mint for digestion and gout.

Seventeenth-century English herbalist Nicholas Culpeper wrote, "[Mint] is very profitable to the stomach . . . especial to dissolve wind [and] help the colic. . . . It is good to repress the milk in women's breasts . . . and a very powerful medicine to stay women's courses [stop menstrual flow]. It helpeth the biting of a mad dog . . . and is good to wash the heads of young children against all manner of breaking out, sores, and scabs. . . ."

Culpeper disagreed with Dioscorides on mint and sex, however. Instead of calling it a lust promoter, Culpeper considered it "an especial remedy for venereal [sexual] dreams and pollutions in the night [nocturnal emissions], being applied outwardly to the testicles."

Shortly after Culpeper's time, peppermint and spearmint were differentiated. Herbalists decided that the former was the better digestive aid, cough remedy, and treatment for colds and fever.

Early colonists found Native Americans using the American mints to treat coughs, chest congestion, and pneumonia. The colonists introduced peppermint and spearmint, and the plants quickly went wild.

By the late 19th century, the Eclectic physicians, forerunners of today's naturopaths, prescribed peppermint for headache, coughs, bronchitis, stomach distress, and hysteria (menstrual discomforts). They also added it to laxatives to minimize intestinal cramping and disguise their unpleasant taste.

The Eclectics also valued spearmint but considered it "somewhat inferior to peppermint" except for its superior ability to treat fever.

Chemists distilled menthol from peppermint oil in the early 1880s. The Eclectic text *King's American Dispensatory* (1898) touted menthol's "active germicidal properties," and its "considerable anesthetic power" when applied to wounds, burns, scalds, insect bites and stings, eczema, hives, and toothache. The Eclectics also used menthol vapors in inhalants and chest rubs to relieve asthma, hay fever, and morning sickness.

Contemporary herbalists recommend peppermint externally for itching and inflammations and internally as a digestive aid and treatment for menstrual cramps, motion sickness, morning sickness, colds, cough, flu, congestion, headache, heartburn, fever, and insomnia. Some herbalists consider peppermint and spearmint interchangeable, but most believe peppermint to be more potent. As they do with so many other aromatic herbs, herbalists also recommend these herbs for relaxing herbal baths.

Therapeutic Uses

Both spearmint and peppermint owe their value in healing to their aromatic oils. Peppermint oil is mostly menthol. Spearmint oil contains a similar compound, carvone. These chemicals have similar properties, but as the herbalists of old believed, menthol is the more potent and is the one more widely used in herbal medicine.

DIGESTIVE PROBLEMS. Thumbs-up for the after-dinner mint. Menthol and carvone soothe the smooth muscle lining the digestive tract, preventing muscle spasms, which means that they are antispasmodics.

In Germany, where herbal medicine is more mainstream than in the United States, an over-the-counter digestive capsule called Enteroplant

has two active ingredients: peppermint oil (90 milligrams) and caraway oil (50 milligrams). German researchers gave 45 people with chronic indigestion either a placebo or Enteroplant (one capsule three times a day) with meals. After 4 weeks, those taking the placebo reported no change in abdominal distress. In comparison, 95 percent of the peppermint-caraway group reported significant improvement, with 63 percent declaring themselves free from pain.

In another German study, a different herbal digestive aid—this one containing peppermint, caraway, fennel, and wormwood—produced similar relief from indigestion in only 2 weeks. It's no wonder that Commission E, the expert panel that evaluates herbal medicines for the German counterpart of the FDA, endorses peppermint for indigestion and abdominal distress.

IRRITABLE BOWEL SYNDROME (IBS). Also known as spastic colon and functional bowel disorder, IBS causes a variety of symptoms: abdominal cramps, bloating, flatulence, diarrhea or constipation, and possibly heartburn and queasiness.

Danish researchers reviewed 16 trials of enteric-coated peppermint oil capsules (taken in doses of 180 to 200 milligrams one to three times a day) to treat IBS. On average, 29 percent of those who took placebos reported relief. But in the peppermint oil group, the figure was 58 percent. The researchers concluded that, compared with currently available drugs, peppermint oil should be "the drug of first choice" for IBS.

PAIN. The Eclectics were on the right track about menthol's "considerable anesthetic power." It's an ingredient in many over-the-counter pain-relieving skin creams, including Absorbine and Bengay. It is also added to throat lozenges such as Cepacol. It's also an ingredient in many ointments marketed to soothe insect bites and stings as well as rashes caused by poison ivy, poison oak, and sumac. And some cigarette brands contain menthol to numb the throat irritation smoking causes.

Commission E approves peppermint oil as a treatment for muscle aches.

COLDS AND CONGESTION. Menthol vapors do indeed help relieve nasal, sinus, and chest congestion. Menthol is an ingredient in Afrin Nasal Spray, Mentholatum, and Vicks VapoRub.

Peppermint is an FDA-approved remedy for the common cold, primarily because of its decongestant action. Commission E also approves peppermint as a cold remedy.

COUGHS. Several studies show that in addition to its decongestant action, menthol is an effective cough suppressant. Researchers in England had 20 volunteers inhale citric acid, which triggers coughing. Five minutes beforehand, the participants received either one of two medically inactive placebos or menthol. For the people treated with menthol, coughing was significantly reduced. Menthol is an ingredient in Hall's, Luden's, Ricola, Robitussin, and Vicks Cough Drops.

HEADACHES. In two similar studies, German researchers gave people who had tension headaches either placebos or different combinations of peppermint and eucalyptus oils. Participants rubbed the preparations on their foreheads and temples. The herb treatments produced greater relief. The formula that was mostly eucalyptus oil provided the most muscle relaxation, while the one that was mostly peppermint oil yielded the greatest headache pain relief. The researchers suggest trying an herbal treatment instead of or in addition to over-the-counter pain relievers.

INFECTIONS. The Eclectics may have been on to something when they described menthol as being actively germicidal. In laboratory studies, peppermint oil kills many types of bacteria and fungi (including *Candida albicans*, which causes vaginal yeast infections), plus the herpes simplex virus, which causes cold sores and genital herpes. These findings seem to validate peppermint's traditional roles in treating wounds and bronchitis.

WOMEN'S HEALTH CONCERNS. Antispasmodics soothe not only the smooth muscle lining the digestive tract but also other smooth muscles, such as the uterus. Several herbals recommend peppermint as a treatment for morning sickness. *The Toxicology of Botanical Medicines*, however, suggests that medicinal concentrations of peppermint may promote menstruation and miscarriage.

LACTATION PROBLEMS. Breastfeeding often causes nipple pain and damage that forces new mothers to stop nursing before they or their doctors would like. In Iran, a traditional remedy for lactation-related nipple problems is peppermint compresses. Iranian researchers asked 196 first-time mothers to use compresses of either expressed breast milk or peppermint tea. In the breast milk group, 27 percent developed nipple problems. But in the peppermint group, the figure was just 9 percent.

Intriguing Possibility

An animal study suggests that pretreatment with peppermint protects the digestive tract from damage caused by radiation.

Rx Recommendations

For an anesthetic to treat wounds, burns, scalds, and herpes sores, apply a few drops of peppermint oil directly to the affected area.

For a decongestant, cough suppressant, or digestive infusion, use 1 to 2 teaspoons of dried peppermint or spearmint per cup of boiling water, steep for 10 minutes, and strain. Drink up to 3 cups a day. Peppermint has a sharper taste than spearmint, and it cools the mouth.

As a homemade tincture, take $1/4$ to 1 teaspoon up to three times a day.

When using commercial preparations, follow the package directions.

For an herbal bath, fill a cloth bag with a few handfuls of dried or fresh herb and let the water run over it.

The Safety Factor

As dried plant material, neither peppermint nor spearmint has been reported to cause problems, except for skin irritation in sensitive individuals.

Do not ingest pure menthol. As little as a teaspoon (about 2 grams) can be fatal.

Since pure peppermint oil has also been found to produce toxic effects, such as heart rhythm disturbances (cardiac arrhythmias), do not ingest peppermint oil, either.

Pregnant women who want to try peppermint for morning sickness should stick with dilute, beverage-tea concentrations rather than more potent medicinal infusions. Women with a history of miscarriage should not use this herb while pregnant.

You may give dilute peppermint or spearmint preparations cautiously to children under age 2, but youngsters may find the taste too pungent and may gag.

In children older than 2, adjust the recommended dose based on the child's weight. For example, give a 50-pound child one-third of the dose a 150-pound adult would take.

If you're over 65, start with a low dose, and increase only if necessary.

Inform health care professionals of the herbs you use. Problematic herb-drug interactions are possible.

Peppermint may cause allergic reactions or other unexpected side effects. If any develop, reduce your dose or stop taking it.

For more on herb safety, see Chapter 2.

If symptoms get worse or persist longer than 2 weeks, consult a health care professional promptly.

Growing Information

Spearmint is a perennial that reaches 2 feet and spreads by underground root runners. It has the mint family's characteristic square stems with wrinkled, lance-shaped, serrated, 2-inch leaves, and flower spikes with whorls of small white, pink, or lilac flowers that bloom in midsummer.

Peppermint looks like spearmint, except that it grows somewhat taller, spreads by surface runners, has stems with a purplish cast, and has longer, less wrinkled leaves.

Mints crossbreed so easily that it's often impossible to tell what's sprouting from seeds. The best way to propagate true peppermint or spearmint is to use root cuttings. Any piece of root with a joint or node can produce a plant. Contain your mint bed or plant in containers. In rich, moist, well-drained soil, under full sun or partial shade, spreading mints may become pests.

Frequent cutting encourages bushiness. You may harvest leaves as they mature. Cut the entire plant back to within a few inches of the ground when the first flowers appear. Most species become woody after a few years, so dig them out and plant new root cuttings.

POMEGRANATE

From Biblical Fruit to Modern Healer

Family: Lythraceae; other members include myrtle

Genus and species: *Punica granatum*

Also known as: No other names

Part used: Fruit juice

In the Old Testament, the Promised Land flows with milk and honey—and pomegranates. In addition, in an erotic double entendre in the Biblical Song of Songs (8:2), the bride invites the groom to "drink the juice of my pomegranate."

The name "pomegranate" derives from the Latin *pomum* (apple) and *granatus* (seeded). *Granatum* is Latin for grain, a reference to this fruit's seeds, which are so numerous they suggest a handful of grain. The generic name, *Punica*, refers to the Phoenicians, who cultivated the shrubby tree around the ancient Mediterranean and prized the sweet, tart juice contained in its seed casings.

Native to the area from northern India to eastern Iran, pomegranate and its juice have been popular in the Middle East, Iran (Persia), and India since ancient times. But until recently, the only pomegranate product popular in the West was the syrup made from its reduced juice, grenadine. Now that's changing as pomegranate juice has become a popular beverage thanks to its delicious taste and high antioxidant content.

Healing History

In the traditional medicine of the Middle East, pomegranate juice was used to treat cuts, sore throat, diarrhea, and gum disease. Hippocrates, the father of medicine, recommended the boiled juice for treating fever.

Therapeutic Uses

Like all brightly colored fruits and vegetables, the pigments that give pomegranate juice its deep red color are potent antioxidants that help prevent and heal the cell damage at the root of heart disease, most cancers, and many other conditions. However, pomegranate juice is among nature's richest sources of antioxidants, containing more than either tea or red wine. The specific antioxidant compounds in the juice are called punicalagins.

ANTIOXIDANT POWER. University of Florida researchers asked 11 adults to abstain from fruits, vegetables, and antioxidant supplements for 3 days to minimize the amounts of antioxidants in their bloodstreams. Then they were given 800 milligrams of pomegranate extract. Subsequent blood samples showed a major jump in antioxidant content.

HEART DISEASE. Noted heart disease researcher Dean Ornish, M.D., and colleagues at the Preventive Medicine Research Institute in Sausalito, California, asked 45 people with heart disease and poor bloodflow through their hearts to drink either a placebo beverage or about 1 cup of pomegranate juice a day. After 3 months, bloodflow through the heart decreased in the placebo group, but increased significantly in those who drank the pomegranate juice, thus reducing risk of heart attack.

STROKE. Israeli researchers reported similar results in a study of pomegranate juice effects on bloodflow through the carotid artery, which carries blood into the brain. After 1 year, participants drinking the placebo beverage showed carotid arteries made 9 percent narrower by the growth of the cholesterol-rich deposits that lead to heart attack and stroke. But those who drank about 3 ounces of pomegranate juice a day showed carotid arteries 30 percent more open, meaning more bloodflow into the brain and significantly less risk of stroke.

BLOOD PRESSURE. High blood pressure is a major risk factor for heart attack and the leading risk factor for stroke. The Israeli study also showed that 1 year of daily pomegranate juice consumption reduced blood pressure 21 percent, adding to protection against heart attack and stroke.

DIABETES. Diabetes is a major risk factor for heart attack and stroke. In another study, the Israeli team asked people with type 2 diabetes to drink about 2 cups of pomegranate juice daily. After 3 months, blood tests showed biochemical markers indicating improved blood-

flow and less risk of heart attack and stroke.

CANCER. Several laboratory and animal studies show that pomegranate juice and extract have anti-tumor properties. UCLA researchers gave 1 cup of pomegranate juice a day to men with prostate cancer who'd had first-line treatment (surgery, radiation, or hormones), but still had rising levels of prostate-specific antigen (PSA), suggesting that the cancer had metastasized. Controls who did not drink the juice saw their PSA double in an average of 15 months. In the pomegranate group, however, PSA doubling took 54 months.

Intriguing Possibilities

Several laboratory studies show that pomegranate juice and extract activate immune constituents that help prevent inflammatory diseases including allergies, Alzheimer's, arthritis, and Crohn's disease. The herb also boosts immune response to bacterial infection. Researchers have not yet shown clear benefit in treating these diseases, but that's a good bet.

In addition, animal studies show that pomegranate juice helps fetal brains develop normally and protects against prenatal brain injury.

Rx Recommendations

Eat pomegranates in season. Drink 1 to 2 cups per day of commercial juice.

The Safety Factor

No side effects have been reported. Allergic reactions are possible.

Because pomegranate juice is tart, commercial brands add considerable sugar. Those who must watch sugar intake—such as people with diabetes—should be careful.

Growing Information

The Spanish brought pomegranate to California and Arizona in the 16th century. They can be grown throughout the southwestern United States. Pomegranates grow on small deciduous trees that look like woody, thorny shrubs. Mature plants typically attain heights of 6 to 12 feet. They require full sun and tolerate alkaline soil, drought, desert heat, and winter lows to about 15°F. For juicy fruit, adequate watering is necessary, but overwatering rots the roots.

Plants in 5-gallon containers are available in nurseries in areas where pomegranate can grow. The Wonderful variety is the most popular in the United States. Alternately, pomegranate can be grown from seed or 6-inch cuttings treated with rooting hormone and planted vertically, with the dormant bud exposed.

PSYLLIUM
A Fiber-Rich Cholesterol Cutter

Family: Plantaginaceae; other members include about 250 *Plantago* species, including rib grass

Genus and species: *Plantago psyllium*

Also known as: Fleaseed, plantago, and plantain

Parts used: Seeds

Mention psyllium (pronounced *SILLY-um*), and most people say, "Huh?" Mention the brand-name laxative Metamucil instead, and everyone says, "Oh, yes."

The fact is, except for a little sweetener, color, and flavoring, Metamucil *is* psyllium, the seeds of a hardy plant distributed around the world. Psyllium is among the safest, gentlest laxatives, an attribute that earned it a place in herbal healing centuries ago.

In addition, modern research shows that psyllium seed has a remarkable ability to reduce cholesterol. This makes the herb beneficial in preventing heart disease and most strokes.

Healing History

Psyllium is often called plantain, but it should not be confused with the other plantain (*Muca paradisiaca*), a palmlike tree that produces fruits similar to bananas.

For centuries, traditional Chinese and Ayurvedic physicians have used the seeds and leaves of several Asian *Plantago* species to treat diarrhea, hemorrhoids, constipation, urinary problems, and, more recently, high blood pressure.

Psyllium entered European folk medicine in the 16th century as a remedy for diarrhea and constipation. Seventeenth-century English herbalist Nicholas Culpeper recommended the seeds for inflammation, gout, hemorrhoids, and sore nipples (mastitis) in nursing mothers.

European physicians eventually adopted psyllium, but it was not widely used on this side of the Atlantic until after World War I.

Therapeutic Uses

About one-third of psyllium's seed coat is a soluble fiber called mucilage. When exposed to water, psyllium seeds swell to more than 10 times their original size and become gelatinous. The herb's mucilage accounts for its medicinal action.

DIARRHEA. Psyllium absorbs excess fluid in the intestinal tract and helps restore normal bulk to stool. Commission E, the expert panel that evaluates herbal medicines for the German counterpart of the FDA, approves psyllium for the treatment of uncomplicated diarrhea.

CONSTIPATION. Israeli researchers gave 35 people with chronic constipation either a placebo or laxatives containing psyllium and aloe. After 2 weeks, those taking the placebo showed no improvement. But those taking the psyllium-aloe combination reported softer stools, more frequent bowel movements, and less use of pharmaceutical laxatives.

Psyllium's bulk-forming action increases stool volume. Larger stools press on the colon wall, triggering the wavelike contractions (peristalsis) that we recognize as "the urge." As stool gains bulk, it also becomes softer and easier to pass.

Most Americans eat a low-fiber diet, with fewer fruits, vegetables, beans, and whole grains than nutrition authorities recommend. A low-fiber diet results in hard, dense stools that are often difficult and painful to pass. Psyllium's fiber content and water-absorbing action can compensate to some extent for a deficiency of dietary fiber.

Today, psyllium is one of North America's most popular bulk-forming laxatives. It's the active ingredient in Metamucil, Fiberall, and several other products. Commission E endorses psyllium as a treatment for constipation and irritable bowel syndrome, which may involve either constipation or diarrhea.

HEMORRHOIDS. Because psyllium softens stool, it can bring some relief from the pain and bleeding of hemorrhoids, according to a report in *Diseases of the Colon and Rectum*. This supports Culpeper's recommendation. Commission E approves psyllium as a hemorrhoid treatment.

HIGH CHOLESTEROL. Oat bran has garnered much of the publicity, but the fact is, all high-fiber foods pull cholesterol out of the bloodstream so it doesn't wind up narrowing artery walls and increasing the risk of heart disease and stroke. Many studies show that as dietary fiber increases, the risk of elevated cholesterol decreases. Psyllium is high in fiber, and several studies show that it reduces cholesterol.

🍀 A study published in *Archives of Internal Medicine* showed that 1 teaspoon of psyllium taken three times a day for 8 weeks produced significant decreases in participants' cholesterol levels. The researchers concluded that many people with moderately elevated cholesterol may be able to bring it down to healthy levels with psyllium alone, without cholesterol-lowering medication.

🍀 A similar study published in the *Journal of the American Medical Association* found that 1 teaspoon of psyllium taken a few times a day reduces total cholesterol by about 5 percent in 12 weeks. Heart disease experts say that for every 1 percent decrease in total cholesterol, heart attack risk drops 2 percent, so a 5 percent cholesterol reduction means a 10 percent decrease in heart attack risk.

🍀 Mexican researchers placed 125 people with diabetes—all at high risk for heart attack—on a low-fat diet. In addition, the participants were given either a placebo or psyllium (about 2 teaspoons three times a day). After 3 months, those taking psyllium had significantly lower cholesterol levels.

In all of these trials, psyllium treatment caused no significant side effects, just some transient stomach upset, making the herb safer than prescription drugs used to reduce cholesterol. If you would like to include psyllium in a cholesterol reduction program, consult your physician.

In 1997, the FDA hopped on the psyllium bandwagon. Any food that contains at least 1.7 grams of psyllium per serving can make a claim on its label that it helps prevent heart disease. Kellogg's Bran Buds cereal contains the requisite amount of psyllium.

Intriguing Possibilities

One study showed that psyllium protects laboratory animals from intestinal damage associated with toxic food additives. The psyllium increased the bulk of the animals' stools, so the toxic chemicals had less direct contact with sensitive intestinal tissues and less opportunity to cause harm. Researchers believe that the same mechanism is the reason that a high-fiber diet is associated with reduced risk of colorectal cancer.

To date, no studies have shown that psyllium helps prevent colon cancer, the leading cause of cancer deaths among nonsmokers. Even so, the American Cancer Society recommends a diet high in fiber such as psyllium to possibly help reduce the risk of colon cancer.

Finally, like other dietary fibers, psyllium reduces blood sugar (glucose) levels in laboratory animals, suggesting a possible role in diabetes management for humans.

Rx Recommendations

Most studies show that a teaspoon or two of psyllium three times a day, along with plenty of water or fruit juice, usually produces significant relief from constipation. Psyllium is odorless and almost tasteless, but it has a gritty texture that some people find unpleasant.

If you take a commercial preparation, follow the label directions.

The Safety Factor

As a laxative and cholesterol cutter, psyllium does not work by itself. It swells only in the presence of fluid. If you take psyllium but don't drink lots of water or juice with it, you could end up like the man whose intestine became completely blocked by a large psyllium plug. He required abdominal surgery. Drink at least one tall glass of water or juice every time you take psyllium.

Inhaling dust from psyllium seeds may trigger an allergic reaction. As a result, someone who is sensitive to psyllium could later experience allergy symptoms from ingesting it. Severe allergic reactions are extremely rare, but if you have breathing difficulties after ingesting psyllium, seek emergency help immediately.

Psyllium has no history as a menstruation promoter, but other *Plantago* species do. Although constipation is a common complaint during pregnancy, pregnant women should avoid laxatives, including psyllium, and control constipation by eating high-fiber foods such as fruits, vegetables, beans, and whole-grain bread products.

Do not give psyllium to children under 2. In older children, adjust the recommended dose based on the child's weight. For example, give a 50-pound child one-third of the dose a 150-pound adult would take.

If you're over 65, start with a low dose, and increase only if necessary.

Inform health care professionals of the herbs you use. Problematic herb-drug interactions are possible.

Psyllium may cause allergic reactions or other unexpected side effects. If any develop, reduce your dose or stop taking it.

For more on herb safety, see Chapter 2.

If symptoms get worse or persist longer than 2 weeks, consult a health care professional promptly.

Growing Information

Psyllium is an annual that reaches 18 inches and produces inconspicuous white flowers in summer that soon give way to small brown seed pods.

Most of the psyllium used in this country is imported from France. Although available from specialty seed houses, psyllium is not usually grown as a garden herb. It looks like a weed, and if the seed pods are not harvested before they break open, the wind scatters the seeds. This can be a major problem when you consider that each pod contains up to 15,000 seeds and that the plant grows aggressively.

PUMPKIN

From Jack-o'-Lanterns to Benign
Prostate Enlargement

Family: Cucurbitaceae; other members
include gourds

Genus and species: *Cucurbita pepo*

Also known as: Pepo; the seeds are also
known in Spanish as *pepitas*

Parts used: Seed and seed oil

Pumpkins are native to Central America. The
oldest seeds, dated to 14,000 B.C., were found in
Mexico. But by biblical times, pumpkins were
grown throughout the world, from ancient China
to ancient Rome, where Dioscorides, the father
of botany, mentioned them as a food.

Our word *pumpkin* comes from the Greek
pepon, meaning large melon. Large is right.
Pumpkins can weigh more than 1,000 pounds.
Many areas where they are grown have giant

pumpkin contests every fall, with prizes for the
largest and heaviest.

Pumpkin pulp is very nutritious and is particularly high in vitamin A. It can be cooked as
a vegetable or made into soup, but it's of course
most popular as a Thanksgiving pie filling.

The custom of carving pumpkins to make
jack-o'-lanterns for Halloween originated in
Britain and Ireland. These countries share a
long tradition of carving lanterns from hollowed-
out vegetables, particularly turnips, and placing
candles inside for decorative use in winter. The
term *jack-o'-lantern* was coined in the 17th century and originally referred to a night watchman,
the man (or jack) with the lantern. Middle-aged
night watchmen who used pumpkin lanterns
and ate the seeds probably didn't have to get up
too often from sleep to urinate. Pumpkin seeds
help prevent benign prostate enlargement.

Healing History

Once pumpkins were introduced into Europe,
pumpkin seed oil became a culinary specialty in
eastern Europe. It also gained a folk reputation
for treating the urinary symptoms associated
with benign prostate enlargement: reduced flow,
trouble starting and stopping, and nighttime
wake-ups to urinate.

Pumpkin seeds and the seed oil have also
been used in German and eastern European folk
medicine to treat intestinal parasites.

Therapeutic Uses

BENIGN PROSTATE ENLARGEMENT. Medically, this condition is known as benign prostatic
hypertrophy (BPH). Pumpkin seed oil contains
constituents that arrest the overgrowth of prostate

tissue, the cause of BPH. Scientists remain unclear about the biochemical mechanism for this effect, however. Other herbs that help prevent BPH (see Saw Palmetto on page 422 and Pygeum on page 381) interfere with the action of 5-alpha-reductase. This enzyme converts the male sex hormone, testosterone, into dihydrotestosterone (DHT), which spurs overgrowth of prostate tissue. But pumpkin seed oil is a very weak 5-alpha-reductase inhibitor. Whatever the mechanism, pumpkin seeds and their oil have been shown to reduce risk of BPH.

German researchers assessed BPH symptoms in 2,245 middle-aged men and then had them take 500 to 1,000 milligrams of pumpkin seed oil capsules (Prosta Fink Forte) a day. After 3 months, the men's symptom scores decreased significantly.

Commission E, the expert panel that evaluates herbal medicines for the German counterpart of the FDA, approves pumpkin seed oil for treatment of benign prostate enlargement.

KIDNEY STONES. Two Thai studies show that pumpkin seeds reduce risk of kidney stones.

Intriguing Possibilities

Pumpkin seed oil is rich in the amino acid tryptophan, large amounts of which have tranquil-izing action. As a result, pumpkin seeds and their oil have been tested as treatments for insomnia and anxiety—so far with inconclusive results.

Rx Recommendations

For BPH prevention, Commission E recommends 10 grams of pumpkin seeds a day, which is about one-third of an ounce, or a handful. Or take 480 milligrams per day of seed oil in divided doses. Or follow package directions.

The Safety Factor

No significant side effects. Allergic reactions are possible.

Growing Information

Pumpkins can be grown throughout most of North America. Plant in late spring when all danger of frost has passed, and the soil has warmed. Plant seeds 1 inch deep in mounds, a half-dozen seeds per hill. Allow 5 to 6 feet between hills. When plants are established, thin to retain the best two or three plants per hill. Water and weed regularly. Harvest in October, retaining some stem. Pumpkins without stems do not keep well.

PYGEUM

African Plum Prevents Prostate Enlargement

Family: Rosaceae; other members include rose, plum, cherry, pear, and apple

Genus and species: *Pygeum africanum* or *Prunus africana*

Also known as: African plum, African prune, African cherry, iron wood, and red stinkwood

Part used: Bark

Pygeum is an evergreen tree native to the mountains of sub-Saharan Africa and Madagascar. It grows to 80 feet and thrives at altitudes ranging from 3,000 to 10,000 feet. Pygeum timber is a very hard hardwood, hence the name iron wood, which is used for firewood and furniture. When harvested, it has a pungent bitter-almond smell, hence the name stinkwood. Aged wood turns mahogany-colored and odorless. The fruits resemble plums, prunes, or cherries, hence some of the tree's common names. Fruits are too bitter for human consumption, but are a favorite food of mountain gorillas.

Healing History

Southern Africans used pygeum bark to treat urinary problems, including "old man's disease," an archaic term for benign prostate enlargement. Eighteenth-century European explorers were introduced to the bark and brought it to Europe, where it was slow to catch on. European herbalists and physicians began recommending it for prostate enlargement only in the 1960s. Today, it is a popular treatment for the condition in Europe, particularly in France.

Therapeutic Uses

BENIGN PROSTATE ENLARGEMENT. Medically, this condition is known as benign prostatic hypertrophy (BPH). Like saw palmetto (see page 422), pygeum contains constituents that interfere with the action of 5-alpha-reductase. This enzyme converts the male sex hormone, testosterone, into dihydrotestosterone (DHT), which spurs overgrowth of prostate tissue and causes BPH symptoms: reduced urine flow, trouble starting and stopping, and nighttime wake-ups to urinate.

Many studies have shown that pygeum reduces risk of BPH. For example, in a German trial, 263 men with BPH were given either a placebo or 50 milligrams of pygeum twice a day. After 2 months, one-third of the placebo group reported benefit, but among pygeum users, that figure was two-thirds.

Slovakian scientists assessed BPH symptoms in 85 men, then had them take 50 milligrams of pygeum twice a day. After 2 months, their symptoms decreased significantly—and the benefit persisted for a month after treatment was stopped.

Finally, researchers with the Minneapolis VA Hospital analyzed 18 studies and reported the following: "*Pygeum africanum* provided a moderately large improvement in urologic symptoms and flow measures. [Compared with placebo-takers], men using pygeum were more than twice as likely to report improvement in symptoms. Peak flow increased 23 percent. Nighttime wake-ups to urinate decreased 19 percent."

Rx Recommendations

Studies have used 75 to 200 milligrams per day of bark extract. Most have used 100 milligrams per day in one dose, or two daily 50-milligram doses, one taken in the morning and one at night.

The Safety Factor

Nausea and abdominal distress are possible.

Women and children have no need for pygeum and should not use it.

Inform health care professionals of the herbs you use. Problematic herb-drug interactions are possible.

Pygeum may cause allergic reactions or other unexpected side effects. If any develop, reduce your dose or stop taking it.

For more on herb safety, see Chapter 2.

If symptoms get worse, consult a health care professional promptly.

Growing Information

Pygeum is not grown in the United States. Use of pygeum bark for BPH prevention has spurred unsustainable harvesting, leaving the tree endangered. It is now being cultivated commercially, however, with the bark harvested in a sustainable manner.

RASPBERRY

A Potent Antioxidant

Family: Rosaceae; other members include rose, peach, almond, apple, and strawberry

Genus and species: *Rubus idaeus* and *R. strigosus*

Also known as: Hindberry and bramble

Parts used: Leaves and fruits

For more than 2,000 years, raspberry was considered a minor healer, a footnote under blackberry. Since the 1940s, however, it has emerged from blackberry's shadow and virtually replaced it in herbal medicine—all because it has become *the* herb for pregnant women. The latest research also shows that raspberry fruits are very high in antioxidants, the nutrients that help prevent many degenerative diseases.

Healing History

The ancient Greeks, Chinese, Ayurvedics, and Native Americans hardly distinguished raspberry from blackberry. They used the leaves of the two bushes interchangeably—externally to treat wounds and in tea to treat diarrhea.

Seventeenth-century English herbalist Nicholas Culpeper recommended raspberry leaf as "very binding" (astringent) and good for "fevers, ulcers, putrid sores of the mouth and secret parts [genitals] . . . spitting blood [tuberculosis] . . . piles [hemorrhoids], stones of the kidney . . . and too much flowing of women's courses [heavy menstrual flow]."

America's 19th-century Eclectic physicians, forerunners of today's naturopaths, continued the long tradition of considering raspberry a footnote under blackberry. The Eclectic text *King's American Dispensatory* (1898) recommended blackberry as being "of much service in dysentery . . . pleasant to the taste, mitigating suffering, and ultimately effecting a cure." Then it noted that raspberry helped, too.

Contemporary herbalists recommend raspberry to relieve diarrhea and to end nausea and vomiting, especially the morning sickness of pregnancy. One herbalist goes so far as to call raspberry a "panacea during pregnancy . . . allaying morning sickness, preventing miscarriage, [and] erasing labor pains." The berries are also increasingly touted for their antioxidant content.

Therapeutic Uses

Raspberry won't erase labor pains, and it's no panacea during pregnancy. But science has shown it to be of some value for pregnant women.

PREGNANCY COMPLAINTS. In 1941, raspberry came into its own when an animal study published in the British medical journal *Lancet* showed that the herb contains a "uterine relaxant principle." Over the next 30 years, several other studies confirmed this finding. Today, physicians in England and Europe prescribe a number of raspberry preparations for morning sickness, uterine irritability, and threatened miscarriage. The herb is also included in many herbal pregnancy blends sold in the United States.

But does it ease labor? Australian researchers asked 192 women pregnant with their first child to take either a placebo or raspberry (1.2 grams of leaf twice a day from 32 weeks gestation to delivery). The herb did not shorten the first stage of labor (contractions, cervical dilation). But it did shorten the second stage (pushing) and reduced the need for forceps delivery—30 percent in the control group, 19 percent among those taking the herb.

DIARRHEA. Raspberry leaves contain tannins, which are astringent. This helps explain the traditional use of raspberry leaf tea as a diarrhea remedy.

PREVENTION OF DEGENERATIVE DISEASES. Raspberries owe their red color to high levels of anthocyanoside pigments, compounds that are potent antioxidants. Antioxidants help prevent and reverse the harm to cells caused by highly reactive oxygen molecules called free radicals. Scientists now agree that free radical damage (oxidative damage) is the underlying cause of heart disease, many cancers, and other degenerative illnesses.

Antioxidants—among them, vitamins C and E, the mineral selenium, and anthocyanosides—are found in fruits and vegetables. Researchers at the Jean Mayer USDA Human Nutrition Research Center on Aging at Tufts University in Boston analyzed the antioxidant content of dozens of common plant foods. Those richest in antioxidants turned out to be the dark-colored fruits and berries that contain generous amounts of anthocyanosides, including raspberries, blackberries, blueberries, cherries, and red grapes.

CATARACTS. Cataracts are a major cause of vision impairment and blindness among older Americans. They occur when oxidative damage to the normally clear lens of the eye leads to the development of cloudy spots. For reasons that remain unclear, anthocyanosides have unusually powerful effects on the eyes.

In one Italian study, 50 people with early-stage cataracts were given extracts of bilberry, a fruit similar to raspberry, in combination with another antioxidant, vitamin E, three times a day. The treatment stopped cataract progression in 97 percent of the study participants. Raspberries and bilberries contain comparable amounts of anthocyanosides, so presumably, raspberries have similar effects.

MACULAR DEGENERATION. The nerve-rich retina at the back of the eye plays a key role in vision. Macular degeneration involves deterioration of the macula, the most sensitive part of the retina—the part responsible for seeing fine detail and what's directly in front of you.

In a European study, 31 people with various types of retinal eye problems, including macular degeneration, were given bilberry extract. Those with macular degeneration experienced significant vision improvement. Again, raspberries presumably produce similar benefits.

DIABETIC RETINOPATHY. Diabetes damages all of the blood vessels in the body, including the tiny capillaries in the eye that nourish the retina. When these capillaries are weakened, they leak blood into the eye, causing the blurred vision of retinopathy.

Bilberry's powerful antioxidants help strengthen retinal blood vessels, reducing that blood leakage. In the European macular degeneration study mentioned on page 384, people with diabetic retinopathy showed significant improvement when treated with bilberry. Raspberries probably produce similar benefits.

Intriguing Possibility

One animal study has found that raspberry helps reduce blood sugar (glucose) levels, suggesting the herb's possible value in diabetes management.

Rx Recommendations

For a treat rich in antioxidants, enjoy raspberries. Whether fresh, frozen, canned, or in preserves, they supply generous amounts of anthocyanosides.

For a pleasantly astringent, sweet infusion to treat diarrhea or the discomforts of pregnancy, use 1 to 2 teaspoons of dried herb per cup of boiling water. Steep for 10 to 15 minutes and strain. Drink as needed.

As a homemade tincture, take $1/2$ to 1 teaspoon up to three times a day.

When using commercial preparations, follow the package directions.

The Safety Factor

Standard medical advice warns pregnant women against taking any drugs during pregnancy because of the possibility of harming the fetus. Raspberry used medicinally is an exception to this rule, although you should use it only in consultation with a prenatal care provider.

Raspberry has been widely recommended as a uterine relaxant for decades, and there are no reports in the medical literature of any adverse effects in mothers or their babies. Women with a history of miscarriage may find it especially valuable.

You may use cool, dilute raspberry tea cautiously to treat infant diarrhea in consultation with the child's physician.

In older children, adjust the recommended dose based on the child's weight. For example, give a 50-pound child one-third of the dose a 150-pound adult would take.

If you're over 65, start with a low dose, and increase only if necessary.

Inform health care professionals of the herbs you use. Problematic herb-drug interactions are possible.

Raspberry may cause allergic reactions or other unexpected side effects. If any develop, reduce your dose or stop taking it.

For more on herb safety, see Chapter 2.

If symptoms get worse or persist longer than 2 weeks, consult a health care professional promptly.

Growing Information

Raspberry's perennial invasive roots produce a dense, spreading mass of thorny biennial stems that can grow to 10 feet. The bush has serrated, lance-shaped leaves, small white summer-blooming flowers, and hanging clusters of tart red berries that become very sweet as they ripen.

Raspberry bushes grow so vigorously and

invasively that they quickly become impenetrable pests. Rooting them out is quite difficult. Even when cleared, stray root fragments send up new shoots. Be sure that your raspberries are well contained.

Plant ¹/₂-inch root cuttings in a few inches of soil. Raspberry grows best under full sun in loose, rich, well-drained soil amended with manure or compost.

You can harvest the leaves at any time. Mature fruits appear in summer. For ease of harvesting the berries, train the branches along supports, and prune mercilessly.

RED CLOVER

A Controversial Treatment for Menopausal Discomforts

Family: Leguminosae; other members include beans and peas

Genus and species: *Trifolium pratense*

Also known as: Trifolium, purple clover, sweet clover, and cow clover

Parts used: Flowers

Red clover is one of the world's oldest agricultural crops, cultivated as forage since prehistoric times. The small, ball-shaped flowers of the three-leafed herb have been used for almost as long in herbal healing. But despite centuries of medicinal use, this herb is still controversial.

Healing History

Because of its importance in early agriculture, red clover has a long history as a religious symbol. The ancient Greeks and Romans and the Celts of pre-Christian Ireland all revered it. Early Christians linked the plant to the Trinity, and some say red clover is the model for Ireland's symbol, the shamrock. It was also the model for the suit of clubs in playing cards.

During the Middle Ages, red clover was considered a charm against witchcraft. A more potent protector was the rare four-leaf clover, which represented the cross and the four aspects of happiness: health, wealth, fame, and a faithful lover. Today, children still search for four-leaf clovers.

Traditional Chinese physicians have long used red clover blossoms in expectorant herb blends. Russian folk healers recommended the herb for asthma. Other cultures have used it externally in salves for skin sores and eye problems and internally as a diuretic to treat water retention and as a sedative, anti-inflammatory, cough medicine, and cancer treatment.

America's 19th-century Eclectic physicians, forerunners of today's naturopaths, were great promoters of red clover. Their text *King's American Dispensatory* (1898) deemed the herb "one of the few remedies which favorably influences pertussis [whooping cough] . . . possess[ing] a peculiar soothing property." The Eclectics recommended red clover for coughs, bronchitis, and tuberculosis. But they waxed truly enthusiastic about the herb as a cancer treatment: "It unquestionably retards the growth of carcinomata."

During the late 19th and early 20th centuries, red clover was the major ingredient in many patent medicines known as Trifolium Compounds. The most popular, produced by the William S. Merrell Chemical Company of Cincinnati, was a combination of red clover and several other herbs. Manufacturers claimed that Trifolium

Compounds were whole-body tonics and treatments for skin diseases, syphilis, and scrofula (tuberculosis of the lymph nodes).

In 1912, the American Medical Association's Council on Pharmacy and Chemistry attacked Trifolium Compounds, saying, "We have no information to indicate they possess medicinal properties." Nonetheless, red clover remained in the *National Formulary*, the pharmacists' reference, as a treatment for skin diseases until 1946.

Red clover was also one of the herbs in ex–coal miner Harry Hoxsey's controversial alternative cancer treatment (see page 33).

Contemporary herbalists recommend red clover externally as a treatment for eczema and psoriasis and internally to aid digestion, ease the discomforts of menopause, and relieve coughs, bronchitis, and whooping cough. Some continue to recommend it for cancer.

Therapeutic Uses

Red clover doesn't get much respect among many herbal experts. The FDA says, "There is not sufficient reason to suspect it of any medicinal value." That's a bit of an overstatement. But the research to date shows that red clover produces less benefit than its advocates claim.

MENOPAUSAL COMPLAINTS. Red clover contains plant compounds similar to estrogen (phytoestrogens), among them, isoflavones similar to those found in soybeans (see page 439). Consumption of soy foods and soy isoflavone supplements has been shown to reduce the hot flashes associated with menopause. Similar isoflavones are included in an Australian red clover supplement, Promensil, available in the United States. If soy isoflavones reduce hot flashes, red clover isoflavones should, too. Or maybe not.

A few studies have shown that red clover relieves hot flashes.

🍀 Dutch researchers gave 30 women complaining of more than five hot flashes a day either a placebo or 80 milligrams of red clover isoflavones daily. After 12 weeks, the isoflavone group experienced 44 percent fewer hot flashes.

🍀 Researchers in Gig Harbor, Washington, gave 25 women with menopausal complaints a red clover–based isoflavone supplement. After 12 weeks, they reported 46 percent fewer hot flashes.

🍀 Scientists in Ecuador gave 60 postmenopausal women either a placebo or 80 milligrams of red clover isoflavones daily. After 90 days, the researchers reported that "red clover isoflavone supplementation significantly decreased menopausal symptoms."

Makers of red clover products tout these reports. However, two analyses of multiple trials concluded that red clover is at best marginally effective or ineffective for menopausal complaints. In the first, British researchers analyzed five studies. They found "a marginally significant effect of red clover isoflavones for treating hot flashes. Whether this effect is clinically relevant [makes a real difference] remains unclear."

In the second analysis, scientists in New Zealand analyzed five studies. Their finding? "There was no significant difference in frequency of hot flashes between red clover and placebo."

For menopausal complaints, the value of red clover, if any, remains controversial. If you'd like to try it, feel free—as long as there's no medical reason to limit your exposure to phytoestrogens. It might work for you. Then again, it might not.

HEART DISEASE AND STROKE. On the other hand, a study of 27 postmenopausal women by Australian researchers showed that 40 milligrams of red clover a day significantly improves arterial elasticity. This suggests that red clover may help prevent heart disease, the leading cause of death in postmenopausal women.

Intriguing Possibilities

One laboratory study shows that red clover is effective against several kinds of bacteria, including the type that causes tuberculosis. This finding lends some credence to the Eclectics' use of the herb in treating TB.

Several studies have also investigated red clover's effects on cholesterol levels. Again, the results have been maddeningly inconsistent. Some show small decreases. Others show no effect.

Researchers from the National Cancer Institute (NCI) felt compelled to investigate the anti-tumor properties of red clover after the Institute's own Jonathan Hartwell, Ph.D., published a monograph in the *Journal of Natural Products* in which he pointed out that 33 different cultures around the world had used red clover to treat cancer. Sure enough, NCI researchers confirmed that red clover contains four anti-tumor compounds, including daidzein and genistein, which are also isoflavone phytoestrogens.

In addition, red clover contains significant amounts of vitamin E. This vitamin is a potent antioxidant that helps prevent cancer and heart disease.

Red clover is no substitute for mainstream cancer treatment, but for those with cancers not aggravated by estrogen (non-estrogen-dependent tumors), red clover may hold some promise. Ask your physician about using it in addition to your regular treatment.

Finally, pilot studies suggest that red clover may help treat benign prostatic hypertrophy (BPH) and reduce risk of prostate cancer.

Rx Recommendations

For a pleasantly sweet infusion, use 1 to 3 teaspoons of dried flowers per cup of boiling water. Steep for 10 to 15 minutes, then strain. Drink up to 3 cups a day.

As a homemade tincture, use $^1/_2$ to $1^1/_2$ teaspoons up to three times a day.

When using commercial preparations, follow the package directions.

The Safety Factor

The medical literature contains no reports of harm from red clover. But because this herb is rich in phytoestrogens, some people should avoid it. Estrogens may accelerate the growth of estrogen-dependent breast and gynecological tumors. Estrogen also increases the risk of blood clots (thromboembolisms) and inflammation of blood vessels (thrombophlebitis). People who have a history of any of these disorders or of heart disease or stroke should use red clover cautiously, if at all. And women on estrogen-based birth control pills should consult their physicians before using this herb.

Pregnant and nursing women should not use red clover.

If you're over 65, start with a low dose, and increase only if necessary.

Inform health care professionals of the herbs you use. Problematic herb-drug interactions are possible.

Red clover may cause allergic reactions or other unexpected side effects. If any develop, reduce your dose or stop taking it.

For more on herb safety, see Chapter 2.

If symptoms get worse or persist longer than 2 weeks, consult a health care professional promptly.

Growing Information

Red clover is a three-leafed perennial that grows to 2 feet. Its fragrant, edible, red or purple, ball-shaped flowers are composed of many tiny florets.

Because it's a legume, red clover adds nitrogen to the soil, and its deep roots help break up compacted soil. Plant seeds in spring or fall. In sunny conditions, this herb thrives in a variety of moist, well-drained soils but does not grow well in sand or gravel. Harvest the flowers when the tops are in full bloom.

RED PEPPER

For Pain, It's Hot!

Family: Solanaceae; other members include potato, tomato, eggplant, tobacco, and nightshade

Genus and species: *Capsicum annuum* and *C. frutescens* (green and red bell pepper, paprika, and pimiento are all milder varieties of *C. annuum*)

Also known as: Hot, African, Tabasco, Guinea, and bird pepper; Louisiana long (and short) pepper, cayenne chili pepper, and capsicum

Parts used: Fruits

The fiery taste and bright crimson color of red pepper make it one of the world's most noticeable and popular spices. Recently, the herb has become as hot in healing as it is on the tongue. Extracts of red pepper are remarkably effective in relieving certain types of severe, chronic pain. The herb can also help prevent and treat ulcers.

Red pepper has been discovered at Central American archeological sites dating to 7000 B.C. The herb has been a culinary staple in Asia since ancient times. It was unknown in Europe, however, until Columbus returned with it from his first voyage to the New World.

You may have heard red pepper referred to as cayenne, a name that comes from the Caribbean Indian word *kian*. Today, Cayenne is the capital of French Guiana. Ironically, only a tiny fraction of the U.S. red pepper supply comes from South America or the Caribbean. Most comes from India and Africa. Tabasco (Louisiana pepper) grows along the Gulf Coast of the United States.

Because so little of the herb comes from around Cayenne, the American Spice Trade Association considers the name a misnomer and urges people to call this herb red pepper.

Healing History

Seventeenth-century English herbalist Nicholas Culpeper wrote that immoderate use of red pepper "inflames the mouth and throat so extremely it is hard to endure," and warned that the herb "might prove dangerous to life." But he believed that sparing amounts were of "considerable service" to "help digestion, provoke urine, relieve toothache, preserve the teeth from rottenness, comfort a cold stomach, expel the stone from the kidney, and take away dimness of sight."

Culpeper urged women to mix red pepper, gentian, and bay laurel oil in cotton and insert it vaginally to "bring down the courses" (menstruation). He warned, though, that "if [it] be put into the womb after delivery, it will make [the woman] barren forever."

During the 18th century, red pepper was mixed with snuff to boost the inhaled tobacco's kick. Herbalist Phillip Miller warned against this, saying that the combination caused "such violent fits of sneezing as to break the blood vessels in the head."

In India, the East Indies, Africa, Mexico, and the Caribbean, red pepper enjoys a long history as a digestive aid. This use never caught on among Europeans, who have traditionally believed that hot spices cause stomach ulcers.

The first North American to advocate red pepper in healing was Samuel Thomson, creator of Thomsonian herbal medicine, which enjoyed considerable popularity before the Civil War. Thomson believed most disease was caused by cold and cured by heat, so he prescribed "warming" herbs, red pepper among them.

After the Civil War, America's Eclectic physicians, forerunners of today's naturopaths, called red pepper capsicum and recommended it externally for arthritis and muscle soreness and internally as a digestive stimulant and treatment for colds, coughs, fever, diarrhea, constipation, nausea, and toothache. The Eclectics also advised placing red pepper in socks to warm cold feet, a use echoed in some herbals today.

The Eclectics considered red pepper invaluable in the treatment of delirium tremens, the combination of hallucinations and violent tremors common among advanced alcoholics: "Capsicum is the very best agent that can be used in delirium tremens. It enables the stomach to take and retain food. The best form is in a tea or strong beef soup. There is no danger of overdose as a [large] quantity may be swallowed with evident pleasure and without ill results."

American folk healers have also recommended dusting children's hands with powdered red pepper to stop thumb sucking and nail biting.

An estimated 25 percent of the world's population uses red pepper daily as a culinary spice. Some 2.5 million acres are planted with the herb.

Contemporary herbalists prescribe capsules of cayenne powder for colds and gastrointestinal and bowel problems, and as a digestive aid. They also recommend cayenne plasters for arthritis and muscle soreness.

Therapeutic Uses

Red pepper owes its heat and its value in herbal healing to one compound found in its fruit—capsaicin. Research supports the herb's traditional uses as a digestive aid and pain reliever.

DIGESTIVE PROBLEMS. Red pepper assists digestion by stimulating secretion of saliva and stomach acids. Saliva contains enzymes that initiate the breakdown of carbohydrate, while stomach secretions (gastric juices) contain acids and enzymes that break down food even further.

In cultures with bland cuisines, such as the traditional American meat-and-potatoes fare, people often believe that highly spiced foods damage the stomach and contribute to ulcers. This is not the case. In a study published in the *Journal of the American Medical Association*, researchers used tiny video cameras to examine volunteers' stomach linings after both bland meals and meals liberally spiced with jalapeño peppers. The researchers found no difference in stomach condition, concluding, "Ingestion of highly spiced meals by normal individuals is not associated with [gastrointestinal] damage."

Speaking of ulcers, some evidence suggests that red pepper inhibits the growth of *Helicobacter pylori*, the bacteria that cause ulcers.

DIARRHEA. In addition to its action against *H. pylori*, red pepper helps combat other bacteria. This seems to validate traditional claims that the herb helps treat infectious diarrhea.

CHRONIC PAIN. For centuries, herbalists have recommended rubbing red pepper into the skin to treat muscle and joint pain. Medically, this is known as applying a counterirritant. The body can pay attention to only so many pain signals at once. The minor superficial pain caused by counterirritants such as red pepper reduces the nervous system's ability to alert the brain to deeper, more severe pain.

More recently, red pepper has been shown to possess direct pain-relieving properties for certain kinds of chronic pain. For reasons that are still not completely understood, capsaicin interferes with the action of substance P, the chemical in the peripheral nerves that sends pain messages to the brain. Since the mid-1980s, dozens of studies have found capsaicin to be remarkably effective at relieving many types of pain.

The FDA has approved capsaicin for use in many over-the-counter pain-relieving creams, including Arthricare, Capzasin, Dencorub, Icy Hot Arthritis Therapy, Pain-X, and Zostrix.

OSTEOARTHRITIS. This is the most common type of arthritis. It causes joint pain and stiffness for more than 16 million Americans, most of them older adults.

At the Veterans Affairs Hospital in Miami, researchers asked 113 people with osteoarthritis to apply either a placebo ointment or one containing capsaicin to their stiff, painful joints four times a day. After 12 weeks, those using the capsaicin ointment reported significantly greater relief.

At Rush-Presbyterian–St. Luke's Medical Center in Chicago, a similar 9-week study of 59 people with osteoarthritis produced similar results. In this trial, the participants rubbed their painful joints with capsaicin cream just twice a day.

FIBROMYALGIA. Fibromyalgia causes muscle pain and tenderness. At the Medical College of Wisconsin in Milwaukee, 45 people with fibromyalgia rubbed their painful or tender spots four times a day with either a placebo ointment or capsaicin ointment. After a month, those using the capsaicin reported significantly less pain and tenderness.

PSORIASIS. In some cases, the red, scaly patches caused by psoriasis become very itchy (pruritic). At the University of Michigan, 197 people with pruritic psoriasis treated their skin patches with either a placebo cream or capsaicin. After 6 weeks, those who applied the capsaicin reported significantly greater relief.

SHINGLES. Capsaicin ointment is the most effective treatment yet for the severe chronic pain associated with shingles, or herpes zoster. Shingles is an adult disease caused by the same virus that produces chickenpox in children. The virus remains dormant in the body until later in life when, for unknown reasons, it reappears in some people as shingles, causing a rash on one side of the body that progresses from red bumps to blisters to crusty pox resembling chickenpox.

In healthy adults, shingles clears up by itself within 3 weeks. But some people—typically the elderly or those with other illnesses, particularly Hodgkin's disease—develop severe, chronic pain, a condition that doctors call post-herpetic neuralgia. Now, thanks to capsaicin, they don't have to suffer as much.

DIABETIC NEUROPATHY. A common complication of diabetes, diabetic neuropathy causes pain in the arms, hands, legs, feet, and possibly elsewhere. Researchers at several medical centers around the United States instructed people with diabetic neuropathy to rub either a placebo cream or a capsaicin ointment on the painful parts of their bodies four times a day. After 8 weeks, the capsaicin group reported significantly less pain, improved sleep, and greater ability to walk, work, and participate in recreational activities.

CLUSTER HEADACHES. Capsaicin helps relieve cluster headaches, which cause extremely severe pain on one side of the head. At the University of Florence in Italy, researchers had 16 people with cluster headaches apply a capsaicin preparation inside their nostrils on the affected side for several days. Eleven of the participants (69 percent) experienced complete relief.

In another study, people with cluster headaches rubbed a capsaicin preparation inside their nostrils and the outside of their noses. Within 5 days, 75 percent reported less pain and fewer headaches. They also reported burning nostrils and runny noses, but these side effects subsided within a week.

SELF-DEFENSE. Capsaicin is the active ingredient in many self-defense sprays, aptly known as pepper sprays. When directed into an attacker's eyes, pepper spray causes pain and blindness that lasts up to 30 minutes, but does not damage the eye.

Intriguing Possibility

Red pepper may help cut cholesterol and prevent heart disease, according to Indian and U.S. researchers. While it is too early to recommend red pepper for these conditions, the common kitchen spice may someday play a role in heart health.

Rx Recommendations

Season food with red pepper to taste, but err on the side of caution. A little too much can set your mouth afire. If your mouth begins to burn uncomfortably, the best treatment is milk. Casein, a protein in milk, pulls capsaicin off the tastebuds.

For an infusion to aid digestion and help prevent or treat ulcers, use $1/4$ to $1/2$ teaspoon of red pepper per cup of boiling water. Drink it after meals.

For external application to help treat pain, mix $1/4$ to $1/2$ teaspoon of red pepper into a cup of warm vegetable oil and rub it on the affected area.

When using a commercial capsaicin ointment, follow the label directions.

The Safety Factor

Chopping red peppers may burn the fingertips, a condition dubbed "Hunan hand" because it was first identified in a man who was preparing a Hunan Chinese recipe that called for chopping many of the fiery fruits. He wound up in an emergency room with severe hand pain.

Red pepper does not wash off the hands easily (vinegar removes it best). Even with careful washing, the pungent herb may remain on the fingertips for hours and cause severe pain if contaminated fingers touch the eyes. Consider wearing rubber gloves when handling red peppers.

Red pepper has not been linked to menstruation promotion since the 17th century, but some research suggests that the herb's stems and leaves, not the more typically used powdered fruits, stimulate uterine contractions in animals. Women who are pregnant or trying to conceive should stick with products made from the powdered fruits.

Do not give red pepper to children under 2. In older children, adjust the recommended dose based on the child's weight. For example, give a 50-pound child one-third of the dose a 150-pound adult would take.

If you're over 65, start with a low dose, and increase only if necessary.

Inform health care professionals of the herbs you use. Problematic herb-drug interactions are possible.

Red pepper may cause allergic reactions or other unexpected side effects. If any develop, reduce your dose or stop taking it.

For more on herb safety, see Chapter 2.

If symptoms get worse or persist longer than 2 weeks, consult a health care professional promptly.

Growing Information

Red pepper is a shrubby, tropical perennial with shiny, pendulous, leathery fruits. It grows best in tropical or subtropical areas but also prospers in south-facing windows and greenhouses. The fruits' boxy shape is the source of the plant's genus name, *Capsicum*, from the Latin *capsa*, meaning "box."

In southern states, seeds may be sown after the danger of frost has passed. Farther north, sow seeds indoors in flats 8 weeks before the final frost date, then transplant. Space seedlings 12 inches apart.

Red pepper prefers rich, well-watered, sandy soil and full sun, but it tolerates some shade. When harvesting the ripened fruit, be careful not to break the stems, or the peppers may spoil. To dry red peppers, hang them in a warm, dry place. Drying takes several weeks.

REISHI

"Mushroom of Immortality" Is a Stretch—But Not by Much

Family: Polyporaceae; other members include other mushrooms

Genus and species: *Ganoderma lucidum*

Also known as: Spirit plant, ling zhi, mushroom of immortality, and mannentake

Parts used: Powdered mushroom

Reishi is a hard, woody fungus that grows on tree stumps and decaying wood in Asia, Europe, and North America. Its cap is so shiny it looks lacquered. Unlike other mushrooms, reishi caps come in six colors: blue, red, yellow, white, black, and purple.

In Japan, dried reishi was hung at home entrances to ward off evil. When they married, Japanese women carried a reishi mushroom into their new home for good luck.

Healing History

Extolled in Chinese medical texts since the 1st century A.D., reishi is prescribed by practitioners of Chinese medicine to treat fatigue, respiratory conditions, and liver ailments, and to strengthen life force (*qi*) and promote longevity. Reishi's connection to *qi* is reflected in its Chinese name, *ling zhi*, which means "spirit plant." Its connection to longevity earned it the name "mushroom of immortality." Immortality is a stretch. But this mushroom is so medically potent, it certainly might extend longevity.

Therapeutic Uses

Like ginseng and eleuthero, reishi is considered an adaptogen that strengthens the whole body.

ENHANCED IMMUNITY. Chinese researchers have shown that reishi activates many components of the immune system, among them B-cells, T-cells, natural killer cells, and interleukins.

PREVENTION OF DEGENERATIVE DISEASES. Chinese scientists have found that reishi has "substantial antioxidant activity." Antioxidants prevent and help reverse the cell damage at the root of heart disease, many cancers, and many other conditions associated with aging.

HEART DISEASE AND STROKE. Researchers in the United States, Switzerland, and China have discovered that reishi lowers cholesterol and blood pressure, thus reducing risk of heart disease and stroke. Chinese scientists have found that it also helps prevent the internal blood clots that trigger heart attacks and most strokes.

CANCER. Laboratory studies show that

reishi increases production of the body's own cancer-fighter, tumor necrosis factor. Animal studies around the world have shown that reishi helps prevent cancers of the lung, colon, breast, and prostate. In addition to its antioxidant and immune-boosting action, both of which help prevent and treat cancer, reishi also prevents new blood vessels from forming to feed growing tumors (angiogenesis inhibition), resulting in the tumors starving. In China and Japan, reishi is widely used to supplement other cancer therapies.

DIABETES. Reishi lowers blood sugar, suggesting that it can help treat diabetes. Diabetes is a major risk factor for heart disease, so reishi's effects on blood sugar also help prevent heart attack.

KIDNEY AND LIVER PROTECTION. Researchers in Taiwan have discovered that reishi's antioxidant action protects the kidneys and liver from chemical damage.

BACTERIAL INFECTIONS. Korean researchers tested reishi's action against common bacteria by giving it in combination with antibiotics. The combination of the mushroom and antibiotics killed significantly more bacteria than the antibiotics alone.

HERPES. Japanese researchers asked 15 people with recurrent herpes sores (genital herpes and cold sores) how long they typically lasted. Their answer: about 9 days. Then the researchers gave them an herb mixture containing a substantial proportion of reishi. Subsequent outbreaks cleared up in an average of 4 days, a highly significant difference.

Intriguing Possibility

Preliminary studies suggest that reishi may help treat cirrhosis.

Rx Recommendations

Recommendations vary, but most sources suggest 500 to 2,000 milligrams of powdered mushroom twice a day. Or follow your practitioner's or the package directions.

The Safety Factor

Reishi may cause dizziness, stomach upset, skin irritation, and diarrhea or constipation. It may also interfere with blood clotting. Side effects typically subside after 3 to 6 months of steady use.

Pregnant and nursing women should not use reishi.

Do not give reishi to children under 2. In older children, adjust the recommended dose based on the child's weight. For example, give a 50-pound child one-third of the dose a 150-pound adult would take.

If you're over 65, start with a low dose, and increase only if necessary.

Inform health care professionals of the herbs you use. Problematic herb-drug interactions are possible.

This mushroom may cause allergic reactions or other unexpected side effects. If any develop, reduce your dose or stop taking it.

For more on herb safety, see Chapter 2.

If symptoms get worse or persist longer than 2 weeks, consult a health care professional promptly.

Growing Information

Reishi is considered an Asian mushroom, but it also grows in woodsy areas of North America and Europe. In the wild, it grows on tree stumps or decaying wood, typically plum or oak. Reishi grows very slowly, hence its Japanese name *mannentake*, which means "10,000-year-old mushroom." Commercial cultivation began in Asia in the 1980s.

Those with patience can grow reishi indoors from kits marketed by Fungi Perfecti (www. fungi.com) or Mycosource (www.mycosource. com). Reishi tastes very bitter and is not eaten as a food.

RHODIOLA
Russia's Secret Cold War Adaptogen

Family: Crassulaceae; other members include jade plant

Genus and species: *Rhodiola rosea*

Also known as: Golden root, rose root, and arctic root

Part used: Root

Rhodiola is a perennial that grows to 30 inches, produces bushy yellow flowers, and has a thick, gold-pink rhizome, hence the names golden root and rose root. It thrives in some of the harshest conditions on Earth—high in arctic mountains from Scandinavia to Siberia. It also helps people thrive despite physical challenges, such as fatigue and many illnesses.

For centuries, rhodiola enjoyed a folk reputation in Russia as a whole-body strengthener. After World War II, Russian researchers investigated its potential for enhancing the performance of Russian soldiers and Olympic athletes. The researchers, N.V. Lazarev, Ph.D., and Israel I. Brekhman, Ph.D., were the same scientists who coined the term *adaptogen* to describe plants such as ginseng that strengthen the body and provide a large number of other health benefits. They were also the ones who discovered the adaptogenic benefits of eleuthero (Siberian ginseng) and introduced that herb to herbal medicine.

The Soviet military kept rhodiola secret, however. During the Cold War, they were convinced that the herb could give Russian soldiers and Olympic athletes a competitive edge. Soviet soldier Zahir Ramazanov drank rhodiola tea while fighting in Afghanistan in 1979. He found that it enhanced his endurance, quickened his hiking, and helped him recover faster from a variety of illnesses.

In the early 1990s, Ramazanov moved to New York and began importing rhodiola and translating then–newly declassified Russian research about its many adaptogenic benefits. Eventually the herb came to the attention of Richard Brown, M.D., a Columbia University psychiatrist. At the time, his wife, Patricia Gerbarg, M.D., was debilitated by a case of Lyme disease that had gone undiagnosed for years. Standard therapies weren't helping. She tried rhodiola. Ten days later, she felt better. After a few months, she felt cured. Since the mid-1990s, Ramazanov, Brown, and Gerbarg have been instrumental in popularizing rhodiola.

Healing History

For a plant kept secret for so long, rhodiola has a long history in herbal medicine. Since ancient times, folk healers in Scandinavia and Russia have used it to treat a broad range of conditions. Dioscorides, the Greek physician who traveled with Roman legions, mentioned it in his classic book *De Materia Medica* (written in 77 A.D.).

In traditional Tibetan medicine, it has been revered for centuries. Elsewhere in Asia, it was used to treat colds and flu. The Vikings used the herb to increase their strength and endurance. In the early 19th century, French physicians prescribed rhodiola as a "brain tonic." From 1725 well into the 1960s, rhodiola was touted in medical journals in Sweden, Norway, Russia, France, Germany, and Iceland. But at the time, American researchers had little interest in medicinal herbs, and rhodiola remained largely unknown in the United States until the mid-1990s.

Therapeutic Uses

STAMINA. In animal studies, treatment with rhodiola improves physical endurance substantially. Belgian researchers gave competitive cyclists either a placebo or 200 milligrams of rhodiola. An hour later, the herb group showed significantly greater stamina and aerobic capacity.

In another study, Russian scientists gave 161 military cadets either a placebo or rhodiola. The herb produced "a pronounced anti-fatigue effect."

STRESS. Chinese researchers measured standard biomarkers of stress in laboratory animals and then gave some of the animals rhodiola while subjecting all of them to very loud noise. Untreated animals showed clear signs of emotional stress. The rhodiola group showed significantly less stress.

COGNITIVE ABILITY. In maze studies, rhodiola improves animals' learning speed and memory.

In hospitals, medical mistakes are most likely to occur late at night when physicians are fatigued and drowsy. Armenian researchers gave 56 medical residents on overnight duty either a placebo or rhodiola, and shortly after, gave them a battery of mental acuity tests. The herb group fared significantly better. A similar Russian experiment tested rhodiola in students preparing for exams. Those who took the herb showed significantly less mental fatigue.

HEART DISEASE AND STROKE. High blood pressure is a key risk factor for heart attack and the leading risk factor for stroke. A Chinese study shows that rhodiola lowers blood pressure.

Heart rhythm disturbances (arrhythmia) are potentially serious. A Russian study shows that rhodiola produces "a pronounced anti-arrhythmic effect."

DEPRESSION. Scandinavian researchers gave 89 people with depression either a placebo or 340 milligrams of rhodiola daily. After 6 weeks, standard tests of mood and depression showed that the herb group was significantly more improved.

INSOMNIA. The depression study just mentioned also showed that rhodiola improved users' sleep quality.

LIVER PROTECTION. Korean researchers treated laboratory animals with a chemical that injures the liver. During this treatment, some animals were also given rhodiola. The untreated animals experienced serious liver damage, but the animals given rhodiola suffered significantly less liver damage.

CANCER PREVENTION AND TREAT-MENT. Russian studies show that rhodiola reduces risk of cancer-causing DNA mutations. The herb also helps treat cancer. Russian researchers gave it to people with bladder cancer, a disease that typically recurs. Compared with people with bladder cancer who didn't take the herb, those who took rhodiola had significantly less frequent recurrences.

Intriguing Possibility

Pilot research suggests that rhodiola may help normalize irregular menstrual periods.

Rx Recommendations

Standard rhodiola dosage is 5 to 10 drops of tincture two or three times a day, taken 15 to 30 minutes before eating. Or you can take 200 to 450 milligrams daily of extract. Or follow package directions.

The Safety Factor

Caffeinelike jitters are possible. People with bipolar disorder should not use rhodiola.

Pregnant and nursing women should not use rhodiola.

Do not give rhodiola to children under 2. In older children, adjust the recommended dose based on the child's weight. For example, give a 50-pound child one-third of the dose a 150-pound adult would take.

If you're over 65, start with a low dose, and increase only if necessary.

Inform health care professionals of the herbs you use. Problematic herb-drug interactions are possible.

Rhodiola may cause allergic reactions or

other unexpected side effects. If any develop, reduce your dose or stop taking it.

For more on herb safety, see Chapter 2.

If symptoms get worse or persist longer than 2 weeks, consult a health care professional promptly.

Growing Information

Except for Alaska, rhodiola is not grown in the United States. Those interested in purchasing rhodiola products may contact the Alberta (Canada) Rhodiola Rosea Growers Organization at www.arrgo.ca.

RHUBARB
More Than Pie Filling

Family: Polygonaceae; other members include buckwheat

Genus and species: *Rheum officinale* and *R. palmatum* (garden rhubarb, *R. rhaponticurn*, has similar but less powerful action)

Also known as: Rheum, or Chinese, Himalayan, Turkish, or medicinal rhubarb

Parts used: Roots

Rhubarb is an odd plant. Its roots are medicinal. Its stems make tasty pies. And its leaves are poisonous.

Healing History

Chinese physicians have used rhubarb root since ancient times. They prescribed it externally as a treatment for cuts and burns, and internally in small amounts to treat dysentery. They also discovered that large amounts have powerful laxative action and promote menstruation. In the 13th century, China traveler Marco Polo wrote in his journal about rhubarb's use as a medicine in Asia.

Over the centuries, the Indians, Russians, and Europeans adopted rhubarb as a healing herb and discovered that their own native species have similar, though less powerful, effects.

Seventeenth-century English herbalist Nicholas Culpeper endorsed rhubarb's laxative action: "This herb purges downward." He also recommended it externally as "a most effectual remedy to heal scabs and running sores." In addition, Culpeper claimed that rhubarb "heals jaundice . . . provokes urine . . . is very effectual for reins [gonorrhea] . . . and helps gout, sciatica . . . toothache . . . the stone [kidney stones] . . . and dimness of sight."

Later herbalists repudiated most of Culpeper's recommendations. They returned to prescribing small doses of rhubarb root for diarrhea and larger doses as a laxative.

America's 19th-century Eclectic physicians, forerunners of today's naturopaths, used rhubarb primarily to treat diarrhea and dysentery. The Eclectic text *King's American Dispensatory* (1898) noted the herb's effectiveness for constipation but said "it sometimes produces griping [cramping]." The Eclectics also considered the herb helpful in treating "hepatic derangement" (liver problems) and delirium tremens.

Bacterial dysentery was a common—and often fatal—disease in British East Africa between World Wars I and II. In 1921, Nairobi-based physician R. W. Burkitt wrote in the British medical journal *Lancet* that he'd treated

it with rhubarb almost exclusively for 3 years: "I know of no remedy in medicine which has such a magical effect. No one who has ever used rhubarb would dream of using anything else . . . in this dreadful tropical scourge."

Contemporary herbalists are divided on rhubarb. Some recommend low doses for diarrhea and large doses for constipation. Others simply recommend it as a laxative.

Therapeutic Uses

The ancient Chinese appear to have been right about rhubarb's dual effects.

DIARRHEA. Studies show that small amounts of rhubarb help relieve diarrhea.

CONSTIPATION. Large amounts of rhubarb have powerful laxative action. The herb contains anthraquinones, compounds similar to those found in other laxative herbs such as buckthorn, cascara sagrada, and senna.

Anthraquinone laxatives should be used only as a last resort to treat constipation. First, eat more fresh fruits and vegetables, drink plenty of water, and get more exercise. If that doesn't work, try a bulk-forming laxative such as psyllium (see page 375). If you still need help, try cascara sagrada (see page 132), generally regarded as the gentlest anthraquinone. Finally, if you're still having difficulty, try rhubarb, buckthorn (see page 119), or senna (see page 429) in consultation with your physician.

Commission E, the expert panel that evaluates herbal medicines for the German counterpart of the FDA, approves rhubarb root as a laxative.

WOMEN'S HEALTH CONCERNS. Some animal studies suggest that rhubarb stimulates uterine contractions, lending some credence to the herb's use in China as a menstruation promoter. Women who are pregnant or trying to conceive should avoid rhubarb. Other women might try it to start their periods.

Intriguing Possibility

Chinese researchers have reported that rhubarb root helps prevent the progression of kidney failure.

Rx Recommendations

For diarrhea, make a decoction by gently boiling $1/2$ teaspoon of powdered root per cup of water for 10 minutes, then strain if you wish. Take 1 tablespoon at a time periodically, up to 1 cup a day. Rhubarb tastes bitter and unpleasant.

For constipation, make a decoction by boiling 1 to 2 teaspoons of powdered root per cup of water for 10 minutes, then strain if you wish. Take 1 tablespoon at a time, up to 1 cup a day.

If you're using a homemade tincture, take $1/4$ teaspoon daily for diarrhea and $1/2$ to 1 teaspoon daily for constipation.

When using commercial preparations, follow the package directions.

The Safety Factor

Rhubarb may color the urine bright yellow or red, which is harmless.

Rhubarb stems are used in pie fillings, but the plant's leaf blades contain oxalic acid, which is poisonous. Ingesting the leaves can cause burning in the mouth and throat, nausea, vomiting, weakness, and other symptoms. Deaths have occurred.

Because of rhubarb's powerful action, laxative amounts should not be used by people with chronic intestinal problems such as ulcers or colitis.

Do not use laxative amounts of rhubarb for more than 2 weeks. Over time, it causes lazy bowel syndrome, an inability to have bowel movements without chemical stimulation.

Pregnant and nursing women should not use anthraquinone laxatives.

Do not give rhubarb to children for medicinal purposes.

If you're over 65, start with a low dose, and increase only if necessary.

Inform health care professionals of the herbs you use. Problematic herb-drug interactions are possible.

Rhubarb may cause allergic reactions or other unexpected side effects. If any develop, reduce your dose or stop taking it.

For more on herb safety, see Chapter 2.

If symptoms get worse or persist longer than 2 weeks, consult a health care professional promptly.

Growing Information

Medicinal rhubarb is a large, leafy perennial that reaches 10 feet. Its root is thick and branching, brown on the outside and yellow inside. Its round, hollow stems are jointed and terminate in branching spikes of numerous small flowers. The medicinal species are not garden herbs.

Garden rhubarb reaches only 3 feet. It has thick roots—reddish outside and yellow inside—and purple stems. Garden rhubarb is considered less potent in herbal healing. If you use it medicinally, start with the amounts recommended above, but be prepared to adjust them upward.

Garden rhubarb requires a dormant period in winter and does not do well in the South, where winters are warm. Sow seeds or root cuttings 4 feet apart in late spring in deeply dug, well-watered beds under full sun or partial shade. Add compost and mulch in winter. Harvest stems for pies the second year and roots the fourth.

ROSE
Rose Is a Rose Is a Medicine

Family: Rosaceae; other members include peach, apple, almond, and strawberry

Genus and species: *Rosa canina, R. rugosa,* and *R. centifolia*

Also known as: Hipberry

Parts used: Fruits (hips) and petals

Prized since the dawn of history, the rose is the queen of flowers. In herbal healing, however, this plant becomes noteworthy only after the velvety petals have fallen away, revealing its cherry-size fruits, or "hips."

Rose hips contain vitamin C, but authorities disagree on how much. Some herbalists call rose hips one of the best natural sources of vitamin C. Scientific sources scoff at this claim, asserting that it would take more than a dozen cups of rose hip tea to help treat colds and flu.

While herbalists have generally overstated the herb's vitamin C content, it may still be of some benefit for colds and flu.

Healing History

Roses were a favorite of the ancient Egyptians, who used the fragrant petals as air fresheners and rose water as a perfume. During the 1st century A.D., when Marc Antony wooed Cleopatra, legend has it that the Egyptian queen ordered the floors of her palace covered knee deep in rose petals to welcome her lover.

In Greece, Hippocrates recommended rose flowers mixed with oil for diseases of the uterus. India's traditional Ayurvedic physicians have long considered rose petals cooling and astringent, leading to their application as poultices to treat skin wounds and inflammations. The Ayurvedics also used rose petals and rose water as laxatives.

Western herbalists mirrored the Ayurvedic uses of the herb. The 12th-century German abbess/herbalist Hildegard of Bingen recommended rose hip tea as the initial treatment for just about every illness.

Seventeenth-century English herbalist Nicholas Culpeper called the herb "binding and restringent [astringent]." He wrote that it "strengthens the stomach, prevents vomiting, stops tickling coughs . . . [is] good against all kinds of fluxes [diarrhea] . . . [and is] of great service in consumptions [tuberculosis]."

As the centuries passed, European herbalists recommended dried rose petal tea for headache, dizziness, mouth sores, and menstrual cramps.

Americans have always loved roses. The flowers were among the first planted around the White House, which now boasts an enormous rose garden. American herbalists considered the rose only a minor healing herb, however. The 19th-century Eclectic physicians, forerunners of today's naturopaths, did not use rose petals at all. They beat the hips into a pulp and used it as a base for making pills that contained other medicines.

Roses almost disappeared from early 20th-century herbals. Then came the discovery of vitamin C in the 1930s and the finding that rose hips may contain appreciable amounts.

Contemporary herbalists are almost unanimous in their praise of rose hips as a source of vitamin C. One best-selling herbal claims, "Rose hips are rich in vitamin C, richer by far ounce for ounce than oranges. Some people say we should make rose hip tea a part of our daily diet."

Because of rose hips' vitamin C content, herbalists tout them for colds and flu. Some also recommend the herb as a mild laxative.

Therapeutic Uses

There's nothing wrong with making rose hips a part of your daily diet, but don't count on them—or the prepackaged teas containing them—to supply all the vitamin C you need. This is especially true if you're using the vitamin to treat the common cold and flu.

While rose hips contain a significant amount of vitamin C, the drying process destroys from 45 to 90 percent of it, and infusions extract only about 40 percent of what's left. That still leaves a fair amount of vitamin C, but it's considerably less than most herbals promise.

Many companies that manufacture vitamin C supplements claim that their products are made from rose hips. In fact, no product is made exclusively from rose hips. In commercial "rose hip" vitamin C preparations, the hips are combined with ascorbic acid from other sources.

COLDS AND FLU. The weight of the scientific evidence shows that vitamin C is of only marginal benefit in cold prevention. Once you've caught one, though, the nutrient helps reduce the severity and duration of the illness, provided that you take at least 2,000 milligrams per day from the moment you feel the telltale scratchy throat until you feel that you're well again.

It's not easy to obtain 2,000 milligrams of vitamin C exclusively from rose hips, but there's no harm in combining the herb with other sources.

Another argument in favor of rose hip infusion is that hot liquids help relieve the sore throat, nasal congestion, and cough associated with colds. They also warm the throat, which helps impair viral replication (cold viruses reproduce best at around 95°F).

MOUTH SORES. Commission E, the expert panel that evaluates herbal medicines for the German counterpart of the FDA, approves rose petal infusion for one of its many traditional uses: treating sores in the mouth, such as canker sores.

Rx Recommendations

For a pleasant-tasting, mildly astringent infusion that may help treat colds, flu, and mouth sores, use 2 to 3 teaspoons of dried chopped hips or dried powdered petals per cup of boiling water. Steep for 10 minutes and strain if you wish. Drink as needed.

As a homemade tincture, use $1/2$ to 1 teaspoon as needed.

When using commercial preparations, follow the package directions.

The Safety Factor

High doses of vitamin C cause diarrhea in some people. If you develop diarrhea, reduce your intake of the nutrient.

High doses of vitamin C may also strain the kidneys. This is not a problem for people with healthy kidneys, but those with kidney disease should consult their physicians before using large amounts of rose hips.

Do not give rose hips to children under 2. In older children, adjust the recommended dose based on the child's weight. For example, give a 50-pound child one-third of the dose a 150-pound adult would take.

If you're over 65, start with a low dose, and increase only if necessary.

Inform health care professionals of the herbs you use. Problematic herb-drug interactions are possible.

Rose hips may cause allergic reactions or other unexpected side effects. If any develop, reduce your dose or stop taking it.

For more on herb safety, see Chapter 2.

If symptoms get worse or persist longer than 2 weeks, consult a health care professional promptly.

Growing Information

Roses have been bred for every climate. "Old roses" are generally more fragrant than newer hybrids, but they have less showy, faster-wilting flowers. Consult a nursery for the variety best suited to your conditions and desires. Enjoy the flowers, then, when the petals fall, harvest and dry the hips.

ROSEMARY
The Tasty Natural Preservative

Family: Labiatae; other members include
mints

Genus and species: *Rosmarinus officinalis*
and *R. prostratus*

Also known as: Rosemarine and incensier
(French)

Parts used: Leaves

Thousands of years before refrigeration, ancient
people noticed that wrapping meats in crushed
rosemary leaves preserved them and imparted a
fresh fragrance and pleasing flavor. To this day,
the herb remains a favorite in meat dishes.

Rosemary's ability to preserve food also led
to the belief that it helped preserve memory.
Greek students wore rosemary garlands to assist
their powers of recall. As the centuries passed,
the herb was incorporated into wedding ceremonies as a symbol of spousal fidelity and into
funerals to help survivors to remember the dead.
In *Hamlet*, Ophelia gives Hamlet a sprig, saying,
"There's rosemary . . . for remembrance."

Healing History

The ancients used rosemary as they used all
aromatic, preservative herbs—for respiratory
and gastrointestinal problems. Traditional Chinese physicians mixed it with ginger as a treatment for headache, indigestion, insomnia, and
malaria.

During the Middle Ages, rosemary's association with weddings evolved into its use as a love
charm. If a young person tapped another with a
rosemary twig containing an open blossom, the
couple would supposedly fall in love.

Placed under a pillow, the aromatic herb was
believed to repel bad dreams. Planted around a
home, it was reputed to ward off witches. By the
16th century, this practice became a bone of contention in England, where it was believed to
signify a household where the woman ruled.
Men were known to rip out rosemary plants as
evidence that they, not their wives, ruled the
roost.

In 1235, Queen Elizabeth of Hungary became
paralyzed. According to legend, a hermit soaked
a pound of rosemary in a gallon of wine for several days, then rubbed it on her limbs, curing
her. Rosemary-wine combinations became
known as Queen of Hungary's Water and were
used externally for centuries for gout, dandruff,
baldness prevention, and skin problems. As the
centuries passed, pennyroyal and marjoram
were incorporated into what became known as
Hungary Water.

The French hung rosemary around sickrooms and in hospitals as a kind of healing incense, calling it *incensier*. As recently as World War II, French nurses burned a mixture of rosemary leaves and juniper berries in hospital rooms as an antiseptic.

Colonists brought rosemary to North America. An early medical guide, *The American New Dispensatory*, recommended the herb's leaves and flowers and Hungary Water for use "in nervous and menstrual affections, for strokes, paralysis, and dizziness."

Oddly, those great proponents of botanical medicine, the Eclectics, forerunners of today's naturopaths, had little use for rosemary. Their text *King's American Dispensatory* (1898) noted its use as a digestive aid and menstruation promoter but declared that it was "seldom used except as a perfume."

Central American folk healers use rosemary oil as an insect repellent and menstruation promoter.

Contemporary American herbalists say that rosemary stimulates the circulatory, digestive, and nervous systems. They recommend it as a treatment for headache, indigestion, and depression and as a gargle for bad breath. They also advocate its external use for muscle aches and in baths for relaxation.

Therapeutic Uses

Rosemary may not guarantee A's on exams, marital fidelity, or vivid memories of the dear departed—but the ancients were right about the herb's ability to preserve meats.

FOOD POISONING. Meats spoil in part because their fats oxidize and turn rancid. Rosemary and its oil contain compounds that are potent antioxidants. In fact, rosemary's preservative power compares favorably with the commercial food preservatives BHA and BHT.

Rosemary's preservative action may help prevent food poisoning on your next picnic. Mix the crushed leaves generously into hamburger meat and tuna, pasta, and potato salads.

INFECTIONS. The same compounds that retard spoilage also inhibit the action of many microorganisms that can cause infection. For a minor cut in the garden, press some fresh, crushed rosemary leaves into the wound on the way to wash and bandage it.

DIGESTIVE PROBLEMS. Like most culinary herbs, rosemary may help relax the smooth muscle lining the digestive tract, an action that makes it an antispasmodic. The ancients appear to have been on the right track when they used it as a digestive aid. Commission E, the expert panel that evaluates herbal medicines for the German counterpart of the FDA, approves rosemary as a treatment for indigestion.

CONGESTION. Like other aromatic herbs, rosemary may help relieve nasal and chest congestion caused by colds, flu, and allergies.

WOMEN'S HEALTH CONCERNS. Antispasmodics soothe not only the digestive tract but other smooth muscles as well, such as the uterus. As an antispasmodic, rosemary should theoretically calm the uterus, but Italian researchers have discovered that it does exactly the opposite. Pregnant women should steer clear of medicinal preparations of rosemary. Other women might try the herb to bring on their periods.

Intriguing Possibilities

Antioxidants help prevent cancer. The high levels in rosemary led researchers at Pennsylvania

State University to add powdered leaves to the food of some laboratory animals. Then all of the animals were injected with chemicals known to cause cancer. Compared with the animals that ate plain food, those that consumed rosemary enjoyed significant protection from cancer.

Rosemary may also have potential in the future for treating Alzheimer's disease. The drugs used to slow the progression of dementia inhibit the action of an enzyme, acetylcholinesterase. Several compounds in rosemary oil are also acetylcholinesterase inhibitors. To date, no studies have been published showing that rosemary helps treat dementia. But it's possible that the "herb of remembrance" just might help preserve cognitive function.

Rx Recommendations

For a pleasantly aromatic infusion to settle the stomach or clear a stuffy nose, use 1 teaspoon of crushed herb per cup of boiling water. Steep for 10 to 15 minutes, then strain. Drink up to 3 cups a day.

As a homemade tincture, use $1/4$ to $1/2$ teaspoon up to three times a day.

When using commercial preparations, follow the package directions.

The Safety Factor

In culinary amounts, rosemary poses no hazards. But even small amounts of rosemary oil may cause stomach, kidney, and intestinal irritation. Larger doses may cause poisoning. Do not ingest more than a drop or two of concentrated rosemary oil.

Pregnant and nursing women should not use medicinal preparations of rosemary or its oil.

Do not give rosemary to children under 2. In older children, adjust the recommended dose based on the child's weight. For example, give a 50-pound child one-third of the dose a 150-pound adult would take.

If you're over 65, start with a low dose, and increase only if necessary.

Inform health care professionals of the herbs you use. Problematic herb-drug interactions are possible.

Rosemary may cause allergic reactions or other unexpected side effects. If any develop, reduce your dose or stop taking it.

For more on herb safety, see Chapter 2.

If symptoms get worse or persist longer than 2 weeks, consult a health care professional promptly.

Growing Information

Rosemary is a woody, pine-scented, evergreen perennial with needlelike leaves. It reaches 3 feet in the United States and produces small, pale blue flowers in summer. Creeping rosemary (*Rosmarinus prostratus*) is widely used in the western United States as a ground cover and cascade over garden walls.

Rosemary can be grown from seeds, but germination can be a problem and seedlings are slow to develop, which is why most herb growers prefer to start with cuttings. If you sow seeds, plant them in the spring, 6 inches apart. Plant cuttings in sandy soil, leaving only one-third of each twig showing.

Rosemary prefers light, sandy, well-drained soil and full sun. Overwatering may cause root rot. It usually survives frigid winter temperatures without special care. If you live where temperatures dip below zero, mulch plants each autumn or grow the herb in pots, bring them indoors each winter, and keep them in a south-facing window.

Cut twigs and strip the leaves any time after the plants have become established.

SAGE

An Herb for the Wise

Family: Labiatae; other members include mints

Genus and species: *Salvia officinalis*

Also known as: Garden, meadow, Spanish, Greek, and Dalmatian sage

Parts used: Leaves

Close your eyes and imagine Thanksgiving turkey stuffing. Smell that warm, rich aroma? Chances are, it comes from sage.

Thousands of years before the Pilgrims stuffed the first Thanksgiving turkey, people all over the world were celebrating the healing powers of this aromatic herb. The genus name for sage, *Salvia*, comes from the Latin word meaning "to heal."

Down through history, sage has been used to

treat so many maladies that it gained a reputation as a panacea, prompting the late herb expert Varro E. Tyler, Ph.D., to write, "If one consults enough herbals . . . every sickness known to humanity will be listed as being cured by sage." Sage is no cure-all, but research shows that this herb has some value as an antiperspirant, preservative, wound treatment, and digestive aid. It might even help treat dementia.

Healing History

The ancient Greeks and Romans first used sage as a meat preservative. They also believed that like another powerful preservative, rosemary, it could enhance memory.

Sage gained a much broader medicinal reputation than rosemary did, however. The Roman naturalist Pliny prescribed it for snakebite, epilepsy, intestinal worms, chest ailments, and menstruation promotion. The Greek physician Dioscorides considered it a diuretic and menstruation promoter and recommended sage leaves as bandages for wounds.

Around the 10th century, Arab physicians believed that sage extended life to the point of immortality. After the Crusades, this belief showed up in Europe, where students at the medieval world's most prestigious medical school in Salerno, Italy, recited, "Why should a man die who grows sage in his garden?" The same thought evolved into a medieval English proverb: "He that would live foraye [forever] / Must eat sage in May."

The French called the herb *toute bonne*, meaning "all's well," and had their own adage: "Sage helps the nerves, and by its powerful might / Palsy is cured and fever put to flight." Charlemagne ordered sage grown in the medicinal herb gardens on his imperial farms.

"The Knight's Tale" in Chaucer's *Canterbury Tales* echoed the ancient use of sage as a treatment for wounds: "To use on . . . wounds and broken arms . . . sage they drank. . . ."

Around the year 1000, an Icelandic herbal recommended sage for bladder infections and kidney stones. The 12th-century German abbess/herbalist Hildegard of Bingen prescribed sage for headache and gastrointestinal and respiratory ailments, from the common cold to tuberculosis.

During the 16th century, Dutch explorers introduced sage to the Chinese, who prized the herb so highly that they gladly traded 3 pounds of their own tea for each pound of the new European healer. Chinese physicians used sage to treat insomnia, depression, gastrointestinal distress, mental illness, menstrual complaints, and nipple inflammation (mastitis) in nursing mothers.

India's traditional Ayurvedic physicians used Indian sage similarly. They also prescribed it for hemorrhoids, gonorrhea, vaginitis, and eye disorders.

Sixteenth-century British herbalist John Gerard called sage "singularly good for the head and brain. It quickeneth the senses and memory, strengtheneth the sinews, restoreth health to those that have palsy, and taketh away shaky trembling of the members."

In the 17th century, English herbalist Nicholas Culpeper seconded Gerard, and recommended sage "boiled in water or wine to wash sore mouths and throats, cankers, or the secret parts [genitals] of man or woman."

Colonists introduced sage into North America, where it was widely used by folk healers to treat insomnia, epilepsy, measles, seasickness, and intestinal worms.

America's 19th-century Eclectic physicians, forerunners of today's naturopaths, used sage primarily to treat fever. They also prescribed sage poultices for arthritis and the tea as "a valuable anaphrodisiac [sexual depressant] to check excessive venereal desires . . . used in connection with moral . . . and other aids, if necessary."

As late as the 1920s, U.S. medical texts recommended sage tea as a gargle for sore throat and sage leaf poultices for sprains and swellings.

Modern herbalists recommend sage as an external treatment for wounds and insect bites; as a gargle for bleeding gums, sore throat, laryngitis, and tonsillitis; and as an infusion to reduce perspiration, terminate milk production, and relieve dizziness, depression, menstrual irregularity, and intestinal upsets.

Therapeutic Uses

The name *toute bonne* overstates sage's healing potential a bit, but the herb does contain an aromatic oil with some therapeutic value. The oil has one unique property that sets sage apart from all other healing herbs: It reduces perspiration.

EXCESSIVE PERSPIRATION. Several studies show that sage cuts perspiration by as much as 50 percent, with the maximum effect occurring 2 hours after ingestion. This effect helps explain how sage developed a reputation for treating fever, which causes profuse sweating, and for drying up mothers' milk.

Today, a sage-based antiperspirant (Salysat) is marketed in Germany. In addition, Commission E, the expert panel that evaluates herbal medicines for the German counterpart of the FDA, approves sage infusion as a treatment for "excessive perspiration."

WOUNDS. In laboratory studies, sage is active against several infection-causing bacteria. This finding lends some credence to the herb's age-old use in treating wounds. Modern physicians would not recommend bandaging wounds with sage leaves as Dioscorides did, but you can use fresh leaves as garden first aid for minor wounds.

FOOD POISONING. Meats spoil in part because their fats turn rancid (oxidize). Like rosemary, sage contains powerful antioxidants, which slow spoilage. The antioxidants are comparable to the commercial preservatives BHA and BHT, supporting sage's traditional use as a preservative. Sage's preservative action may help prevent food poisoning on your next picnic. Mix it generously into hamburger meat and tuna, pasta, and potato salads.

DIGESTIVE PROBLEMS. Like most culinary spices, sage helps relax the smooth muscle lining the digestive tract, an action that makes it an antispasmodic. This property lends support to the herb's traditional role in relieving gastrointestinal complaints. Commission E approves sage as a treatment for indigestion.

SORE THROATS. Sage contains astringent tannins, which account for its traditional use in treating canker sores, bleeding gums, and sore throat. In Germany, where herbal healing is more mainstream than in the United States, physicians recommend a hot sage gargle for sore throat and tonsillitis.

WOMEN'S HEALTH CONCERNS. As an antispasmodic, sage should theoretically calm the uterus. Some studies suggest, however, that sage oil may stimulate it instead, possibly explaining its traditional role in menstruation promotion. Pregnant women should not take medicinal doses of sage, but other women might try it to bring on their periods.

Intriguing Possibilities

John Gerard may have been on to something when he wrote that sage "quickeneth the memory." A pilot study in Iran suggests that the herb (taken in doses of 60 drops of tincture per day for 4 months) slows the progression of Alzheimer's disease.

Additionally, a German study has found that sage reduces blood sugar (glucose) levels in people with diabetes who drink the infusion on an empty stomach. Diabetes is a serious condition requiring professional care. If you'd like to include sage in your overall management plan, discuss it with your physician.

Rx Recommendations

For garden first aid, crush some fresh leaves into a cut or scrape until you can thoroughly wash and bandage it.

For an infusion to settle the stomach or possibly to help manage diabetes, use 1 to 2 teaspoons of dried leaves per cup of boiling water. Steep for 10 minutes, then strain. Drink up to 3 cups a day. The infusion may also be used as a gargle. Sage tastes warm, pleasantly aromatic, and somewhat pungent.

As a homemade tincture, take $1/2$ to 1 teaspoon up to three times a day. This may help reduce wetness if you perspire a lot.

When using commercial preparations, follow the package directions.

The Safety Factor

The medical literature contains a few reports of inflammation of the lips and lining of the mouth associated with ingestion of sage tea.

Concentrated sage oil is toxic and should not be ingested.

Sage contains relatively high levels of a toxic chemical called thujone. In large amounts, thujone causes a variety of symptoms that culminate in convulsions. As a result, some sources call sage potentially toxic. However, the heat used in preparing a sage infusion eliminates much of the thujone, so the risk from recommended medicinal amounts is negligible.

Pregnant and nursing women should not use sage beyond culinary amounts.

Do not give sage to children under 2. In older children, adjust the recommended dose based on the child's weight. For example, give a 50-pound child one-third of the dose a 150-pound adult would take.

If you're over 65, start with a low dose, and increase only if necessary.

Inform health care professionals of the herbs you use. Problematic herb-drug interactions are possible.

Sage may cause allergic reactions or other unexpected side effects. If any develop, reduce your dose or stop taking it.

For more on herb safety, see Chapter 2.

If symptoms get worse or persist longer than 2 weeks, consult a health care professional promptly.

Note: When smoked, one species of sage, *Salvia divinorum*, has intoxicant/hallucinogenic action. It has become a recreational drug. At this writing, *S. divinorum* is still legal. Intoxicating substances should never be mixed with driving or operating machinery. Beyond intoxication, *S. divinorum*'s effects are currently unknown.

Growing Information

Sage is a perennial, branching, evergreen shrub that reaches about 3 feet. It has square, woolly, woody stems near its base, which become herbaceous toward the top. Its 2-inch leaves are oval, velvety, and gray green, with long stalks. Depending on the species, sage's small, summer-blooming flowers are pink, white, blue, or purple.

Sage is not related to the West's sagebrush, so named because of its vaguely sagelike aroma.

Sage may be propagated from seeds or cuttings. Germination takes a few weeks. Sow seeds $1/2$ inch deep in spring. It takes about 2 years to grow good-size plants from seeds, which is why many authorities recommend planting 4-inch cuttings taken in the fall for use the following spring.

Sage grows well in almost any soil, but it requires good drainage and full sun. Water well until the plants have become established, after which they require less water. Sage should be replaced every 3 or 4 years because the plants become woody and less productive. If your winter temperatures fall below zero, mulch your sage in fall.

Harvest leaves before the flower buds open by cutting the plant back to 4 inches above ground. Discard the stems and leaf stalks. Dry the herb, then store it in airtight containers.

ST. JOHN'S WORT

The Premier Herbal Antidepressant

Family: Hypericaceae; other members include rose of Sharon

Genus and species: *Hypericum perforatum*

Also known as: Hypericum

Parts used: Leaves and flowers

St. John's wort has been used in herbal healing for more than 2,000 years, most notably as a treatment for wounds. Today, the herb is more popular than ever—in fact, it's one of the nation's top-selling herbal medicines. The reason? In the 1980s, scientists discovered that St. John's wort is as potent an antidepressant as prescription pharmaceuticals.

Before the herb became known as an antidepressant, its annual sales worldwide totaled around $10 million. Now they top $500 million.

Healing History

The word *wort* is Old English for "plant." The leaves and flowers of St. John's wort contain special glands that release a red oil when pinched. Early Christians named the plant in honor of John the Baptist, because they believed it released its blood-red oil on August 29, the anniversary of the saint's beheading.

In the 1st century A.D., the Roman naturalist Pliny prescribed St. John's wort steeped in wine as a cure for the bites of poisonous snakes. The Greek physician Dioscorides recommended it externally for burns and internally as a diuretic, menstruation promoter, and treatment for sciatica and recurring fevers (malaria).

The Greeks and Romans also believed that St. John's wort protected against witches' spells. Christians adopted this pagan belief, burning the herb in bonfires on St. John's Eve, June 23, to purify the air, drive away evil spirits, and ensure healthy crops. This poem from around 1400 summed up the popular view.

St. John's wort doth charm all witches away
If gathered at midnight on the saint's holy day.
Any devils and witches have no power to harm
Those that gather the plant for a charm.
Rub the lintels with that red juicy flower;
No thunder nor tempest will then have the power
To hurt or hinder your house; and bind
Round your neck a charm of a similar kind.

Under the Doctrine of Signatures, the medieval belief that an herb's physical appearance revealed its healing value, red plants were believed to be good treatments for bleeding wounds. "The red juicy flower" of St. John's wort was no exception. In the 16th century, herbalist John Gerard recommended it as a "most precious remedy for deepe wounds," and wrote that the herb "provoketh urine and is right good against stone in the bladder."

In 1618, the first *London Pharmacopoeia* advised chopping St. John's wort flowers, immersing them in oil, and placing the mixture in the sun for 3 weeks. The resulting tincture was a standard treatment for wounds and bruises for several hundred years.

Seventeenth-century English herbalist Nicholas Culpeper called St. John's wort "a singular wound herb; boiled in wine and drank, it healeth inward hurts or bruises; made into an ointment, it opens obstructions, dissolves swellings, and closes up the lips of wounds. . . . [It] helpeth all manner of vomiting and spitting blood [tuberculosis]."

Early colonists introduced St. John's wort into North America, but they found Native Americans using the American form of the herb in much the same way Europeans used the Old World plant—as a tonic and treatment for diarrhea, fever, snakebite, wounds, and skin problems.

Nineteenth-century botanical medicine authority Charles Millspaugh, M.D., touted St. John's wort's value as a wound treatment during the Civil War: "Lacerations of parts rich in nerves yield nicely to this drug." Dr. Millspaugh railed against the orthodox physicians of his day ("regulars"), who dismissed the herb as obsolete, saying, "Any homeopathic physician of at least 3 months practice can attest to its merits."

Throughout the 19th century, homeopathy was as popular as orthodox medicine. Homeopaths prescribed St. John's wort for a variety of ailments, including wounds, asthma, bites, sciatica, diarrhea, hemorrhoids, and certain forms of paralysis. Contemporary homeopaths continue this tradition.

America's 19th-century Eclectic physicians, forerunners of today's naturopaths, also considered St. John's wort an effective wound healer and tetanus preventive. They advocated the whole herb as a treatment for "hysteria" (menstrual discomforts) because of its "undoubted power over the nervous system and spinal cord."

Contemporary herbalists generally recommend St. John's wort only as an antidepressant, but for this indication they are enthusiastic. Some also suggest it for treating viral illnesses, notably HIV and herpes.

Therapeutic Uses

St. John's wort contains hypericin, the source of its antidepressant action. It also contains antiviral compounds and immune-boosting chemicals known as flavonoids, which explain its action against viral, bacterial, and fungal infections.

DEPRESSION. In the early 1980s, German researchers discovered that hypericin interferes with the activity of a compound in the body known as monoamine oxidase (MAO). MAO inhibitors are an important class of antidepressant drugs. In small pilot studies in Germany, people with mild to moderate depression obtained significant relief after taking St. John's wort, including mood elevation, improved self-esteem, greater interest in life, increased appetite, and more normal sleep patterns.

Herbalists began recommending the herb for depression, but it did not rocket to prominence until 1996. That year, German researchers published a meta-analysis of human studies (clinical trials) in the prestigious *British Medical Journal*, now called *BMJ*. (Meta-analysis is a statistical technique that allows the results of small studies to be combined as if they'd all been part of one large study. In medical research, one large study is more compelling than several small ones.)

The meta-analysis included 23 trials involving a total of 1,757 adults with mild to moderate depression. Combining the results of the trials, the researchers found that 22 percent of the people who took placebos experienced significant mood elevation. But among those using St. John's wort, 55 percent reported similar results.

Since then, many more studies have shown that St. John's wort is an effective antidepressant. In 1999, researchers at the University of Hawaii School of Medicine performed another meta-analysis of six rigorously scientific trials that had been conducted since the earlier report. Again, St. John's wort provided significant benefit.

How beneficial is the herb? As effective as the most popular class of pharmaceutical antidepressants, the selective serotonin reuptake inhibitors (SSRIs), including Prozac, Paxil, and Zoloft.

🌿 German researchers gave 161 people with mild to moderate depression either Prozac (fluoxetine) or 400 milligrams of St. John's wort twice a day. After 6 weeks, the two treatments produced comparable results—72 percent of those taking Prozac and 71 percent of those taking St. John's wort experienced significant mood elevation. But the herb produced fewer side effects.

🌿 Harvard researchers conducted a similar trial, comparing Prozac and St. John's wort in 135 people with mild to moderate depression. In this study, researchers reported that "St. John's wort was significantly more effective than Prozac."

✣German scientists gave 251 clinically depressed adults either Paxil (paroxetine) or 300 milligrams of St. John's wort three times a day. After 6 weeks, the Paxil group improved 45 percent on standard mood scales. But the St. John's wort group improved 57 percent, and the herb caused fewer side effects. The researchers concluded that St. John's wort "is at least as effective as Paxil, and is better tolerated."

✣Researchers at St. John's Episcopal Hospital in New York City gave 30 depressed adults either Zoloft (sertraline HCl) or 900 milligrams of St. John's wort daily. After 6 weeks, 40 percent of the Zoloft group showed significant improvement. But in the herb group, the figure was 47 percent. The scientists noted that St. John's wort "is at least as effective" as Zoloft.

✣Finally, German researchers analyzed 29 trials that compared St. John's wort to placebos and to pharmaceutical antidepressants. Their conclusion: For mild to moderate depression, St. John's wort "is superior to placebo, and similarly effective to standard antidepressants."

St. John's wort is generally recommended for mild to moderate depression, but at least one study suggests that it also helps relieve severe depression.

The herb also helps prevent recurrent episodes of depression. German researchers gave either a placebo or St. John's wort to 703 adults, ages 18 to 65, who had experienced two or three episodes of major depression. After 18 months, those taking the herb were significantly less likely to have another recurrence.

Like pharmaceutical antidepressants, St. John's wort requires some patience. According to German medical herbalist Rudolph Fritz Weiss, M.D., the benefit "does not develop quickly . . . [and may take as long as] 2 or 3 months."

Commission E, the expert panel that evaluates herbal medicines for the German counterpart of the FDA, approves St. John's wort as a treatment for depression.

SEASONAL AFFECTIVE DISORDER (SAD). SAD is winter depression caused by short day length and lack of exposure to sunlight. British researchers gave 301 people with SAD either standard light therapy (exposure to ultrabright light) or light therapy plus St. John's wort. Both treatments produced significant mood elevation, but those who also took the herb reported much more restful and refreshing sleep.

MENOPAUSAL COMPLAINTS. Beyond hot flashes, many menopausal women also experience mood changes and depression. Korean researchers gave 77 menopausal women either a placebo or a combination of black cohosh and St. John's wort. Black cohosh provides effective relief of hot flashes (see page 102) but does not treat the psychological challenges of menopause. After 3 months, the herb group reported fewer hot flashes and less depression, strongly suggesting that St. John's wort can help women with menopausal depression. Two similar German studies showed similar results.

INFECTIONS. Hypericin is active against a broad range of viral infections, including influenza, herpes, polio, hepatitis C, and HIV, the virus that causes AIDS. It also helps combat several types of bacteria.

Hypericin's "dramatic" activity against HIV, discovered in 1988 by researchers at New York University and the Weizmann Institute in Israel, sent many people with AIDS rushing to health food stores to stock up on St. John's wort. Some have reported benefits from taking the herb, including increased immune function.

Since the introduction in the late 1990s of the powerful AIDS drugs known as protease inhibitors, enthusiasm for hypericin has waned. Ironically, people who take protease inhibitors should not use St. John's wort because the herb interferes with the action of these drugs.

WOUNDS. Several studies support St. John's wort's traditional use as a treatment for wounds. Hypericin and other antibiotic and anti-inflammatory compounds in the herb's red oil help prevent infection and speed healing.

One German study showed that compared with conventional treatment, a St. John's wort ointment substantially cut the healing time of burns and caused less scarring. (This product is not available in the United States.) Commission E approves topical application of St. John's wort preparations for the treatment of minor wounds and burns.

Rx Recommendations

To treat depression, buy a standardized extract and use it according to the label directions, in consultation with a physician. (Most studies have used 300 milligrams three times a day.)

To heal wounds, apply crushed leaves and flowers to the affected area after you have cleaned it with soap and water. Or you can apply a tincture.

To use St. John's wort as part of a treatment plan for AIDS, consult a physician.

The Safety Factor

In livestock fed large amounts of St. John's wort, the hypericin concentrates near the skin and causes sun sensitivity (photosensitization) and blistering sunburn. Laboratory animals injected with large doses of hypericin have died after exposure to sunlight.

As a result of these findings, in 1977, the FDA declared St. John's wort unsafe. The agency presumed that humans would develop the same reactions, but time has proven the FDA's concerns to be unfounded.

Millions of people use St. John's wort to treat depression, but the medical literature contains very few reports of photosensitization and none of serious sun-related harm. On the other hand, if you have fair, sensitive skin or have become photosensitive when using other medications, take extra precautions when out in the sun.

Initially, hypericin was dubbed an antidepressant because it appeared to be an MAO inhibitor. People who take pharmaceutical MAO inhibitors must refrain from eating a large number of foods to avoid unpleasant side effects. Many people taking St. John's wort did not observe these food restrictions but did not develop MAO side effects. German researchers have discovered why: Although hypericin resembles an MAO inhibitor, it is more complicated chemically and more similar to an SSRI, the Prozac family of antidepressants. No food restrictions are necessary when taking St. John's wort.

AIDS patients report that the herb is relatively nontoxic, but some have experienced sun sensitivity, drowsiness, nausea, and diarrhea.

St. John's wort oil may irritate sensitive skin.

Do not take St. John's wort in combination with any other antidepressant medication without first consulting your physician. Likewise, don't take the herb if you have HIV and are already taking any of the protease inhibitor medications. It impedes the action of those drugs.

Also, do not take St. John's wort if you are taking cyclosporine to control organ transplant rejection. The herb may interfere with the drug.

Pregnant and nursing women should not use St. John's wort unless advised to do so by a physician, for example, for postpartum depression.

Do not give St. John's wort to children under 2. In older children, adjust the recommended dose based on the child's weight. For example, give a 50-pound child one-third of the dose a 150-pound adult would take.

If you're over 65, start with a low dose, and increase only if necessary.

Inform health care professionals of the herbs you use. Problematic herb-drug interactions are possible.

St. John's wort may cause allergic reactions or other unexpected side effects. If any develop, reduce your dose or stop taking it.

For more on herb safety, see Chapter 2.

If symptoms get worse or persist longer than 2 weeks, consult a health care professional promptly.

Growing Information

St. John's wort is a woody, invasively spreading perennial that reaches 2 feet and has an aroma reminiscent of turpentine. Its leaves are dotted with glands that produce red oil. Its striking star-shaped flowers bloom bright yellow in summer. They also contain the leaf oil and turn red when pinched.

The herb is best propagated from root divisions in spring or fall. It grows in almost any well-drained soil under full sun or partial shade. Contain the herb to control its spread.

Although it is a perennial, St. John's wort is not particularly long-lived. Replant it every few years. Harvest the leaves and flowers as the plants bloom. Dry them and store in airtight containers.

SARSAPARILLA

A Sexy Reputation

Family: Liliaceae; other members include lily, tulip, garlic, and onion

Genus and species: *Smilax officinalis,* *S. febrifuga,* and other *Smilax* species

Also known as: Mexican, Vera Cruz, Honduran, Jamaican, American, and Ecuadoran sarsaparilla

Parts used: Rhizomes and roots

In old Western movies, the cowboy who didn't want whiskey told the saloon keeper, "Give me a sarsaparilla." Chances are the bartender gave him a bottle of Ayer's Sarsaparilla, a popular beverage back in the days before modern soft drinks.

Cowboys who ordered sarsaparilla usually had more than refreshment in mind. The herb was among the most widely used 19th-century treatments for syphilis, and men often ordered it after visiting the local brothel.

Scientists say sarsaparilla has no effect against syphilis, but modern studies suggest this herb does have some intriguing benefits.

Healing History

The ancient Greeks and Romans considered European sarsaparilla an antidote to poisons. But the herb was not popular in herbal healing until the 16th century, when Spanish explorers discovered the Caribbean species, a prickly (*zarza*) vine (*parra*) that was small (*illa*). That description became our word *sarsaparilla.*

Caribbean Indians and Native Americans used sarsaparilla to treat skin conditions and urinary complaints. They also viewed the herb as a tonic for preserving youth and vigor, both physically and sexually.

In 1494, an epidemic of unusually virulent syphilis swept Europe, killing thousands, rather like the AIDS epidemic today. Europeans considered the disease an import from the New World, and they looked to herbs from across the Atlantic to treat it. They focused on sarsaparilla.

The conquistadors began shipping Mexican sarsaparilla back to Spain around 1530, and by 1600, it was widely used throughout Europe as a strengthening tonic and treatment for syphilis. Sarsaparilla and syphilis have been entwined ever since.

Sarsaparilla enjoyed a meteoric rise in popularity. Seventeenth-century English herbalist Nicholas Culpeper called it the treatment of choice for "the French disease," the British term for syphilis. Echoing the ancients, he wrote, "If the juice of the berries be given to a newborn child, it shall never be hurt by poison." Culpeper also recommended sarsaparilla for eye problems, head colds, gas pains, pimples, and "all manner of aches in the sinews or joints."

By 1800, many physicians denounced sarsaparilla as completely ineffective against syphilis, but their words fell on deaf ears. Mid-19th-century trade records indicate that Britain imported upward of 150,000 pounds a year, much of it for the treatment of syphilis.

In 19th-century America, sexually transmitted infections were never mentioned in polite conversation. Nonetheless, syphilis was quite prevalent, and physicians experimented with many herbs and patent medicines to treat it. These remedies were known euphemistically as blood purifiers. One of the most popular was Ayer's Sarsaparilla, marketed for blood purification and "disorders of the liver, stomach, and kidneys, as well as tuberculosis, tumors, rheumatism, female weakness, sterility, and pimples."

Sarsaparilla was listed as a syphilis treatment in the *U.S. Pharmacopoeia*, a standard drug reference, from 1820 to 1882. After the Civil War, the anti-sarsaparilla bandwagon gained momentum, and by the late 19th century, most physicians dismissed it as worthless.

Therapeutic Uses

Sarsaparilla may be a minor medicinal herb, but it's by no means worthless. Research shows that it has some benefits, although not as a treatment for syphilis. Sarsaparilla contains saponins, compounds that have diuretic action. This property may explain the herb's long association with the genitals. In addition, the herb binds certain toxins produced by bacteria (endotoxins) and speeds their elimination, which makes it a blood purifier, although not in the historical sense. Sarsaparilla also has anti-inflammatory action.

HIGH BLOOD PRESSURE. Physicians often prescribe diuretics for high blood pressure. Since high blood pressure is a serious condition that requires professional care, if you'd like to include sarsaparilla in your overall treatment plan, discuss it with your physician.

Diuretics deplete the body of potassium, an essential nutrient. If you use sarsaparilla frequently, be sure to eat potassium-rich foods such as bananas and fresh vegetables.

CONGESTIVE HEART FAILURE. Physicians often prescribe diuretics to combat the fluid accumulation associated with congestive heart failure. This condition requires professional care. If you'd like to include sarsaparilla in your overall treatment plan, discuss it with your physician.

PREMENSTRUAL SYNDROME (PMS). Sarsaparilla's diuretic action may benefit women bothered by premenstrual fluid retention.

Intriguing Possibilities

Preliminary studies from around the world suggest that sarsaparilla helps treat psoriasis and leprosy. Some animal studies indicate that the herb may also have liver-protective effects.

Medicinal Myths

Sarsaparilla contains a compound, sarsapogenin, that can be chemically converted to the male sex hormone testosterone. Some writers have claimed that sarsaparilla contains testosterone. It does not, and ingesting the herb does not raise testosterone levels.

Sarsaparilla has also enjoyed some popularity among bodybuilders who believe that the herb contains anabolic steroids, chemical relatives of testosterone that are taken, against medical advice, to increase muscle mass. For the record, sarsaparilla contains no anabolic steroids.

Rx Recommendations

For a diuretic decoction, use 1 to 2 teaspoons of powdered root per cup of water. Bring to a boil, simmer for 10 to 15 minutes, then strain if you wish. Drink up to 3 cups a day. Sarsaparilla tastes initially sweetish, then unpleasant.

As a homemade tincture, take $1/4$ to $1/2$ teaspoon up to three times a day.

When using commercial preparations, follow the package directions.

The Safety Factor

No significant side effects from using sarsaparilla have ever been reported.

Some weight-loss programs tout diuretics to eliminate water weight, but weight-loss experts advise against taking diuretics. Any pounds lost with help from diuretics almost invariably return. The key to permanent weight control is a low-fat, high-fiber diet and regular aerobic exercise.

Ingesting large amounts of sarsaparilla's saponins may cause a transient burning sensation in the mouth and throat as well as stomach and intestinal irritation.

Pregnant and nursing women should not use sarsaparilla.

Do not give sarsaparilla to children under 2. In older children, adjust the recommended dose based on the child's weight. For example, give a 50-pound child one-third of the dose a 150-pound adult would take.

If you're over 65, start with a low dose, and increase only if necessary.

Inform health care professionals of the herbs you use. Problematic herb-drug interactions are possible.

Sarsaparilla may cause allergic reactions or other unexpected side effects. If any develop, reduce your dose or stop taking it.

For more on herb safety, see Chapter 2.

If symptoms get worse or persist longer than 2 weeks, consult a health care professional promptly.

Growing Information

Sarsaparilla is not a garden herb in the United States. It's a perennial, climbing, woody, prickly-stemmed vine with pointed, generally oval-shaped leaves. Its small flowers are dioecious (male and female on different plants) and green, yellow, or bronze. The medicinal parts, the rhizome and long, slender roots, are underground.

SAW PALMETTO

The Top Choice for Prostate Enlargement

Family: Palmae; other members include the various palms

Genus and species: *Serenoa repens*

Also known as: Sabal and American dwarf palm

Parts used: Fruits (berries)

Saw palmetto is a small palm tree native to Florida and the Gulf Coast that produces a brownish berry. Centuries ago, Native Americans discovered that its berries have diuretic action and began using them to treat urinary problems. Today, saw palmetto is the premier herbal treatment for benign prostate enlargement (known medically as benign prostatic hypertrophy, or BPH).

Healing History

Native Americans had many uses for the saw palmetto. They harvested the plant's leaves for mattress stuffing and thatched roofing and to weave into hats and baskets.

White settlers adopted the plant, and during the 19th century, physicians throughout the South recommended berry preparations to treat coughs and bronchitis.

Saw palmetto was used primarily for two other purposes, however—to enlarge women's breasts, and to treat BPH in men. *King's American Dispensatory* (1898), the standard text for Eclectic physicians, who were forerunners of today's naturopaths, said: "Long continued use is said to slowly and surely cause the mammary glands to enlarge. Paradoxically, it also reduces hypertrophy of the prostate. [Saw palmetto] has been lauded as 'the old man's friend,' giving relief to the many annoyances commonly attributed to the enlarged prostate." The text went on to note that saw palmetto "is reputed to strengthen the sexual appetite and restore sexual activity after exhaustive excesses."

By the early 20th century, as herbal medicine fell from favor among mainstream American doctors, saw palmetto was abandoned. Fortunately, European researchers remained interested in the plant. During the 1960s, they discovered that the Eclectics were right: Saw palmetto fruits contain fatty acids called sitosterols that help prevent and treat BPH.

Therapeutic Uses

Saw palmetto is no aphrodisiac, nor does it enlarge the breasts. But since the early 1990s, the herb's berry extract has become a widely accepted treatment for BPH.

BENIGN PROSTATIC HYPERTROPHY. After age 40, men's levels of testosterone decline, while levels of other hormones, notably prolactin, increase. This results in an elevation of the male sex hormone dihydrotestosterone, which is responsible for the overgrowth of prostate tissue that is characteristic of BPH. An enzyme, 5-alpha-reductase, converts testosterone to dihydrotestosterone. Pharmaceutical BPH treatments work by interfering with the action of 5-alpha-reductase. Saw palmetto has the same biochemical action, thanks to its sitosterol compounds.

Many studies have shown that saw palmetto shrinks enlarged prostates and relieves BPH symptoms, including the need to urinate immediately (urgency), difficulty getting started (hesitancy), decreased flow, difficulty finishing (dribbling), and perhaps most annoying, the need to get up at night to urinate (nocturia).

- European researchers gave 1,098 men with BPH either Proscar (finasteride), which is a standard drug used to treat prostate enlargement, or 160 milligrams of saw palmetto twice a day. After 26 weeks, both treatments showed about equal effectiveness. Proscar decreased BPH symptoms by 39 percent, compared with 37 percent for saw palmetto. Urine flow improved by 30 percent in the men taking the drug, compared with 25 percent in those taking the herb. But saw palmetto caused fewer side effects, namely, less risk of erection problems and loss of libido.

- Turkish researchers gave 60 men with BPH one of three treatments: Flomax (tamsulosin), a popular pharmaceutical; 320 milligrams of saw palmetto per day; or a combination of the two. The herb worked as well as the drug. (The combination provided no additional benefit.)

- Researchers at the Veterans Affairs Hospital in Minneapolis analyzed 21 studies of saw palmetto for BPH. The trials involved a total of 3,319 men and lasted up to 48 weeks. Their conclusion: It works.

Every now and then, a study shows no benefit; for example, this was the case with a report published in the *New England Journal of Medicine* in 2006. But the clear weight of the evidence favors saw palmetto. Commission E, the expert panel that evaluates herbal medicines for the German counterpart of the FDA, approves saw palmetto as a treatment for BPH. In the United States, prescription medications are generally used to treat BPH, but in Europe, saw palmetto is more popular.

Note: Neither saw palmetto nor pharmaceutical treatments cure BPH. They reduce prostate size and relieve symptoms. Continued enlargement may get the better of either herbal or pharmaceutical treatment, and surgery may become necessary.

Intriguing Possibility

Chinese physicians prescribe an herbal formula whose main ingredient is saw palmetto as a treatment for prostate cancer. At the University of California, San Francisco, Medical Center, researchers gave the Chinese formula to 61 men with advanced prostate cancer whose tumors no longer responded to mainstream medication.

Levels of prostate-specific antigen, a standard indicator of tumor activity, declined by at least 50 percent in three-quarters of the men. It's too early to call saw palmetto a treatment for prostate cancer, but that day may come.

Rx Recommendations

Studies showing that saw palmetto reduces the symptoms of prostate enlargement have used 320 milligrams of a standardized extract a day, split into two or three doses. Unfortunately, however, the more doses per day, the less likely people are to take their medicine as they should.

Researchers in Brussels, Belgium, conducted a 1-year study of 132 men with enlarged prostates to compare two different saw palmetto regimens: the standard two doses (160 milligrams each) daily versus one large dose (320 milligrams) a day. The single large dose produced the same symptom improvement as the two smaller doses.

To use saw palmetto, look for a standardized extract and take 320 milligrams a day, as either one or two doses.

The Safety Factor

If saw palmetto causes any side effects, they're mild—stomach upset and headache. Allergic reactions are also possible in some people.

Because saw palmetto has hormonal action, men with hormone disorders should consult a physician before taking it.

If you are already using another BPH medication, do not take saw palmetto without consulting your physician.

If you are having trouble urinating or if you pass blood in your urine, talk to your doctor.

Growing Information

When early explorers sailed along the coast of the United States from the Carolinas to Texas, they saw small palm trees that they called scrub palms, now known as saw palmettos. Saw palmetto grows easily to about 10 feet in sandy soil, and it is used as an ornamental in the Southeast. The plant produces edible brown-black fruits (berries), an extract of which is the herbal medicine.

SCHISANDRA

Five Tastes for Healing

Family: Schisandraceae; other members include magnolia vine

Genus and species: *Schisandra chinensis*

Also known as: Schizandra, five-taste berry, wu-wei-zi (Chinese), gomishi, hoku-gomishi (Japanese)

Parts used: Dried berries

Schisandra is a woody, deciduous vine native to northeastern and north central China. It grows to 20 feet and produces clusters of small, bright red fruits (berries). Its Chinese name, *wu-wei-zi*, means five-taste berry. Taste is an important attribute of Chinese medicinal herbs, and schisandra is notable because it's one of the few herbs that incorporate all five: sweet, sour, bitter, salty, and spicy (pungent).

Healing History

Most Chinese herbal medicines have one taste that, according to Chinese medical philosophy, plays a key role in its action. Schisandra is unusual because it contains all five tastes. As a result, in traditional Chinese medicine, it was used to "balance" multi-herb medicinal formulas. In addition, practitioners of traditional Chinese medicine used it to treat fatigue and respiratory problems including cough, asthma, and shortness of breath. It was also used to treat night sweats and insomnia.

Therapeutic Uses

For an herb used so widely for so long, it's surprising how little is known about how it works, and how few human studies of its effects have been conducted. Most studies have been conducted using cell cultures or animals. Nonetheless, results have been intriguing.

ADAPTOGEN POWER. Schisandra is most widely used as an adaptogen, an herb that strengthens the whole body, counteracts fatigue, and improves overall health and well-being. However, it is not as potent an adaptogen as ginseng, eleuthero, or rhodiola.

Intriguing Possibilities

Korean researchers have discovered that schisandra inhibits the release of mast cells and pro-inflammatory compounds in the respiratory tract. Mast cells and inflammatory compounds play key roles in triggering allergies and asthma attacks, validating the herb's traditional use to treat respiratory problems.

In addition, some studies suggest that schisandra can counteract the stimulant action of caffeine. If confirmed, this finding would validate the traditional practice of using the herb to treat insomnia.

Laboratory studies show that schisandra kills cancer cells. It's too soon to call it a cancer treatment, but one day, it might be.

In animal studies, schisandra improves memory and learning.

Animal studies also show that this herb reduces the neurological damage caused by amyloid-beta peptide, a protein involved in the development of Alzheimer's disease.

Finally, when animals are treated with chemicals that cause liver damage, schisandra spurs regeneration of liver cells.

Rx Recommendations

Take 1.5 to 6 grams of dried berries per day (1 to 4 teaspoons). Or try 500 milligrams to 2 grams per day of extract.

The Safety Factor

Few side effects have been reported, but heartburn, stomach upset, loss of appetite, rashes, and hives are possible.

Pregnant and nursing women should not use schisandra.

Do not give this herb to children under 2. In older children, adjust the recommended dose based on the child's weight. For example, give a 50-pound child one-third of the dose a 150-pound adult would take.

If you're over 65, start with a low dose, and increase only if necessary.

Inform health care professionals of the herbs you use. Problematic herb-drug interactions are possible.

Schisandra may cause allergic reactions or other unexpected side effects. If any develop, reduce your dose or stop taking it.

For more on herb safety, see Chapter 2.

If symptoms get worse or persist longer than 2 weeks, consult a health care professional promptly.

Growing Information

Schisandra thrives in most soils. It likes shade and grows best up shaded walls. In China, it is grown from seeds sown in spring. It blooms from April to May, with flowers about 1 inch in diameter. The berries are harvested in autumn and sun-dried. Schisandra may also be propagated from cuttings of shoots taken in late summer. It is not widely grown in the United States, but American gardeners should be able to grow it. To purchase seeds, visit www.botanical.com/products/seeds/seeds.html.

SCULLCAP

An All-American Tranquilizer

Family: Labiatae; other members include mints

Genus and species: *Scutellaria lateriflora*

Also known as: Skullcap, Virginia scullcap, Quaker bonnet, hoodwort, helmet flower, and mad dog weed

Parts used: Leaves

For an herb reputed to have calming effects, scullcap has caused considerable controversy. One respected herbalist calls the blue-flowered North American native "perhaps the most widely relevant tranquilizer" in medicine. On the other hand, skeptics have dismissed it as "nearly worthless and essentially inactive." The truth is, scullcap's traditional use as a tranquilizer appears to have scientific support.

Healing History

For centuries, Chinese physicians have used Asian scullcap (*Scutellaria baicalensis*) as a tranquilizer-sedative and to treat many other conditions.

Writing in 1892, medical herbalist Charles F. Millspaugh, M.D., recounted the herb's odd history of use in the United States: "The first introduction of this plant into medicine was the experiments of Dr. Vandesveer [of Roysfield, New Jersey], in 1772, who claimed it curative and prophylactic [preventive] in hydrophobia [rabies], his reported cases being 1,400. This seems a large number to fall to one physician. His son after him claimed to cure 40 cases more in 3 years. [But] its worthiness was greatly doubted, and the plant much railed against. Many regulars [orthodox physicians] and empirics [folk herbalists] used the remedy with success, while many others wrote essays against it. . . . The plant has also proved itself a useful nervine [tranquilizer], antispasmodic [digestive aid], and tonic in wakefulness, convulsions, and delirium tremens."

America's 19th-century Eclectic physicians, forerunners of today's naturopaths, recommended scullcap primarily as a tranquilizer-sedative for insomnia and nervousness and as a treatment for "intermittent fever" (malaria), convulsions, and the delirium tremens of advanced alcoholism.

Nineteenth-century patent medicine makers used scullcap extensively in tonics for "female weakness" (menstrual discomforts).

Scullcap entered the *U.S. Pharmacopoeia*, a standard drug reference, as a tranquilizer in 1863. It remained there until 1916, when it moved to the *National Formulary*, the pharmacists' reference. It stayed there until 1947.

Contemporary herbalists recommend scullcap as a tranquilizer for insomnia, nervous tension, premenstrual syndrome, and drug and alcohol withdrawal. Some say the herb treats fever and convulsions.

Asian scullcap is one of the most widely used plants in Chinese herbal medicine. Practitioners prescribe it for viral infections (including flu and hepatitis), bacterial infections, fever, and high blood pressure.

Therapeutic Uses

American scientists are almost unanimous in their condemnation of scullcap. They've never gotten over those old, mistaken claims that it treats rabies. They should.

INSOMNIA, STRESS, AND ANXIETY. European and Russian studies have lent support to scullcap's traditional role as a tranquilizer. European medical experts now accept its potential usefulness as a tranquilizer and sedative. The herb is an ingredient in many European over-the-counter sleep preparations.

Intriguing Possibilities

Japanese researchers have discovered that the Asian species of scullcap has anti-inflammatory properties.

Two other Japanese studies, both involving animals, have shown that scullcap increases levels of "good" cholesterol (high-density lipoprotein, or HDL). As HDL levels increase, the risk of heart attack decreases. These findings suggest that the herb may help prevent heart disease and some strokes in humans.

Chinese physicians claim to have treated hepatitis successfully with the herb. It's too early to tout scullcap for this potentially serious liver disease, but the herb deserves further research.

Rx Recommendations

For a tranquilizing infusion, use 1 to 2 teaspoons of dried herb per cup of boiling water. Steep for 10 to 15 minutes, then strain. Drink up to 3 cups a day. Scullcap tastes bitter; adding honey, sugar, and lemon or mixing it with an herbal beverage blend will improve the flavor.

When using commercial preparations, follow the package directions.

The Safety Factor

There are no reports of toxicity from scullcap infusions, but unusually large amounts of tincture can cause confusion, giddiness, twitching, and possibly convulsions.

Pregnant and nursing women should not use scullcap.

Do not give scullcap to children under 2. In older children, adjust the recommended dose based on the child's weight. For example, give a 50-pound child one-third of the dose a 150-pound adult would take.

If you're over 65, start with a low dose, and increase only if necessary.

Inform health care professionals of the herbs you use. Problematic herb-drug interactions are possible.

Scullcap may cause allergic reactions or other unexpected side effects. If any develop, reduce your dose or stop taking it.

For more on herb safety, see Chapter 2.

If symptoms get worse or persist longer

than 2 weeks, consult a health care professional promptly.

Growing Information

Many scullcap species grow in Europe, but the American herb is the one used in herbal healing. It's sometimes called Virginia scullcap, but it grows all over the United States and southern Canada.

The plant is a 2-foot, slender, branching, square-stemmed perennial with opposite, serrated leaves. The flowers have two lips. The upper lip includes an elongated caplike appendage, which is the source of most of the herb's popular names.

Scullcap may be propagated from seeds or root divisions planted in early spring. Thin seedlings to 6-inch spacing. It grows in any well-drained soil under full sun and requires little care. Although it is a perennial, scullcap rarely lives longer than 3 years.

Harvest the leaves in midsummer.

SENNA
A Powerful Laxative

Family: Caesalpinaceae; other members include brazilwood

Genus and species: *Cassia senna,* *C. acutifolia* (Alexandrian and Khartoum), *C. angustifolia* (Indian or Tennevelly), and *C. marilandica* (American)

Also known as: Cassia

Parts used: Leaflets and seed pods

Senna is a powerful laxative—so powerful, in fact, that many authorities call it a cathartic. Arab physicians first wrote of its action as a bowel stimulant in the 9th century, but their descriptions suggest that it had been widely used for centuries from the Middle East to India. Senna was introduced into European herbal healing before the Crusades and has played a prominent role ever since.

Both senna and cinnamon come from woody plants—senna is a shrub, cinnamon a tree—with peelable bark. Hence the Arabic name *quetsiah*, meaning "to cut," as in removing the bark. *Quetsiah* evolved into senna's genus name, *Cassia*. Although both senna and cinnamon are sometimes called cassia today, these two herbs have very different actions and should not be confused.

Healing History

Seventeenth-century English herbalist Nicholas Culpeper, who came close to prescribing every herb for every ill, could not resist claiming that senna "cleanses the stomach, purges melancholy and phlegm from the head, brain, lungs, heart, liver, and spleen, cleansing those parts of evil humour; strengthens the senses, procures mirth, purifies the blood [treats venereal disease], and is also good in chronic agues [fevers]." Other herbalists generally recommended senna only as a laxative.

Native Americans recognized the laxative action of the American form of senna but used the herb primarily to treat fever. The Eclectics, 19th-century forerunners of today's naturopaths, were influenced by Native American medicine and called senna "very useful in all forms of febrile [fever-producing] diseases in which laxative action is desired."

Contemporary herbalists tout senna's laxative action but warn of its terrible taste and side effects, primarily intestinal cramps.

Therapeutic Uses

Senna does not treat fever, nor does it "purge melancholy and procure mirth." Quite the contrary. If you're not careful with this herb, you'll live to regret using it.

CONSTIPATION. Like aloe, buckthorn, and cascara sagrada, senna contains anthraquinones, chemicals that stimulate the colon. The herb is an ingredient in many over-the-counter laxatives, including Correctol, Ex-Lax, Fletcher's Castoria, and Perdiem.

Senna and the other anthraquinone laxatives should be considered last resorts for constipation. First, increase your fiber intake, drink more fluids, and exercise more often. If that doesn't work, try the bulk-forming laxative psyllium (see page 375). If that's not successful, try cascara sagrada, a gentler anthraquinone (see page 132). Finally, if you still need relief, try senna in consultation with your physician.

Commission E, the expert panel that evaluates herbal medicines for the German counterpart of the FDA, approves senna as a laxative.

Rx Recommendations

Because of senna's disgusting taste, herbalists generally discourage using the plant material. Instead, they recommend over-the-counter products containing it. Follow the package directions.

Those game enough to try the unprocessed herb can brew an infusion from 1 to 2 teaspoons of dried leaves per cup of boiling water. Steep for 10 minutes, then strain. Drink up to 1 cup a day in the morning or before bed for no more than a few days.

The taste of senna is nauseating. To make it more palatable, add sugar, honey, and lemon and mix senna with taste-masking herbs such as anise, fennel, peppermint, chamomile, ginger, coriander, cardamom, or licorice.

Some sources say the pods have milder action. To use them, steep four pods in a cup of warm water for 6 to 12 hours. Drink up to 1 cup a day in the morning or before bed for no more than a few days.

As a tincture, use $1/2$ to 1 teaspoon in the morning or before bed for no more than a few days.

The Safety Factor

Senna's powerful action means that it should not be used by those with chronic gastrointestinal conditions such as ulcers, colitis, or hemorrhoids.

Do not take senna for more than 2 weeks. Over time, it causes lazy bowel syndrome, an inability to have bowel movements without chemical stimulation.

Large amounts of senna cause diarrhea, nausea, and severe cramps with possible dehydration. Long-term use may cause enlargement of the fingertips (clubbing). An article in *Lancet* described this effect in a woman who had taken up to 40 senna laxative tablets a day for 15 years. Her fingers returned to normal when she stopped using the herb.

Senna leaves may cause a skin rash in people who are sensitive to the plant.

Pregnant and nursing women and children should not use senna.

If you're over 65, start with a low dose, and increase only if necessary.

Inform health care professionals of the herbs you use. Problematic herb-drug interactions are possible.

Senna may cause allergic reactions or other unexpected side effects. If any develop, reduce your dose or stop taking it.

For more on herb safety, see Chapter 2.

If symptoms get worse or persist longer than 2 weeks, consult a health care professional promptly.

Growing Information

Senna is not a garden herb in the United States. Native to Egypt and Sudan, it's a small, woody shrub that reaches 3 feet and has branching stems, pointed leaves, and seeds encased in a leathery pod. The species generally used in herbal medicine is grown in the Tennevelly region of India, near the subcontinent's southern tip. One species grows in the eastern United States.

SHEPHERD'S PURSE

Stops Bleeding Naturally

Family: Cruciferae; other members include cabbage, broccoli, and cauliflower

Genus and species: *Capsella bursa-pastoris*

Also known as: Lady's purse, rattle pouches, and rattle weed

Parts used: Leaves and flowers

Shepherds never get much respect. In the ancient world, theirs was a humble calling. And in the Old West, cattle ranchers looked down on "sheep herders." So perhaps we should not be surprised that the herb named for shepherds has shared a similar fate.

More than 300 years ago, Nicholas Culpeper wrote, "Few plants possess greater virtues than this, and yet it is utterly disregarded." No one is interested, some authorities say, because shep-herd's purse is a common weed that's medicinally worthless. But the few scientific studies done to date have revealed some intriguing possibilities for treating bleeding and inducing labor.

Healing History

Ancient Greek and Roman physicians recommended shepherd's purse seeds as a laxative. It was not widely used until the 16th century, however, when an Italian physician promoted it to stop bleeding, particularly to eliminate blood in the urine. Some physicians adopted the plant, but most dismissed it as worthless.

The Pilgrims introduced shepherd's purse into North America, where it quickly became a weed. Folk herbalists used it to stop bleeding, while physicians generally regarded it as useless.

America's 19th-century Eclectic physicians, forerunners of today's naturopaths, prescribed shepherd's purse to stop bleeding. Their text *King's American Dispensatory* (1898) attempted to explain the controversy over the herb's effectiveness by observing that "the fresh herb is decidedly more active than the dried." *King's* called shepherd's purse very efficient for treating bloody urine and recommended it to stop excessive menstrual flow and to relieve diarrhea, dysentery, and bleeding hemorrhoids.

During World War I, when other coagulants were in short supply, wounded soldiers were given shepherd's purse tea.

Contemporary herbalists recommend the internal use of dried shepherd's purse, not the fresh herb, for bloody urine, nosebleeds, heavy menstrual flow, and bleeding after childbirth. They also support the herb's external use as an astringent to treat wounds and hemorrhoids.

Therapeutic Uses

Shepherd's purse won't set the world of herbal medicine on fire, but it may help some women with heavy menstrual flow or pregnant women waiting to go into labor—if they can stomach its taste.

BLEEDING. Shepherd's purse contains substances that hasten the coagulation (clotting) of blood, according to an article in the British scientific journal *Nature*. German medical herbalist Rudolph Fritz Weiss, M.D., writes that the herb "definitely has haemostatic [blood-stopping] properties . . . [but they are] not very great."

First-aid experts recommend treating bleeding with sustained pressure on the wound. Blood in phlegm, urine, or stool requires prompt professional treatment.

Although shepherd's purse is no substitute for standard medical care, people with ulcers, colitis, Crohn's disease, or bleeding disorders or women with heavy menstrual flow might try it in consultation with their physicians.

Commission E, the expert panel that evaluates herbal medicines for the German counterpart of the FDA, approves shepherd's purse as a treatment for persistent nosebleeds and menorrhagia (heavy menstrual flow).

LABOR INDUCEMENT. Shepherd's purse contains some substances that may help stimulate uterine contractions as effectively as the drug oxytocin (Pitocin), which is often given to trigger labor. Women who are trying to conceive or are pregnant should not use shepherd's purse, except at term and in consultation with their physicians.

WOUNDS. Shepherd's purse has some mild anti-inflammatory astringent action, lending some support to its traditional role as a treatment for wounds and hemorrhoids.

Rx Recommendations

To help stop bleeding or to hasten labor, use 1 teaspoon of dried herb per cup of boiling water. Steep for 10 minutes, then strain. Drink up to 2 cups a day. Shepherd's purse has a biting, unpleasant taste. To make it more palatable, add sugar, honey, and lemon or mix it with an herbal beverage blend.

As a homemade tincture, use $1/4$ to $1/2$ teaspoon up to twice a day.

When using commercial preparations, follow the package directions.

To use shepherd's purse externally on wounds or hemorrhoids, soak a clean cloth in either an infusion or a tincture.

The Safety Factor

Those with heart disease or a history of stroke or mini-strokes (TIAs) should not use shepherd's purse. Its pro-clotting action may cause the internal blood clots that trigger heart attacks or strokes.

Anyone taking anticoagulant (blood-thinning) medication, including low-dose aspirin, should not use shepherd's purse.

The medical literature contains no reports of harm from this herb.

Pregnant and nursing women should not use shepherd's purse.

Do not give shepherd's purse to children under 2. In older children, adjust the recommended dose based on the child's weight. For example, give a 50-pound child one-third of the dose a 150-pound adult would take.

If you're over 65, start with a low dose, and increase only if necessary.

Inform health care professionals of the herbs you use. Problematic herb-drug interactions are possible.

Shepherd's purse may cause allergic reactions or other unexpected side effects. If any develop, reduce your dose or stop taking it.

For more on herb safety, see Chapter 2.

If symptoms get worse or persist longer than 2 weeks, consult a health care professional promptly.

Growing Information

Shepherd's purse is a foul-smelling annual that reaches 18 inches. Its slender stem rises from a rosette of deeply toothed leaves similar to dandelion. The stem bears a few small leaves and terminates in small white flowers. The fruits are wedge-shaped seed pods containing literally thousands of yellow seeds, hence the herb's common names.

Shepherd's purse grows easily from seeds planted in spring under full sun. It prefers well-drained sandy loam but tolerates most North American soils.

If unchecked, shepherd's purse can become a garden and lawn pest. To avoid this, clip the seed pods before they open. The young leaves have a peppery taste and may be added to soups and stews or eaten like spinach. Harvest the leaves and flowers as the flowers open.

SHIITAKE

This Tasty Mushroom Boosts Immune Function

Family: Polyporaceae; other members include other mushrooms

Genus and species: *Lentinula edodes*

Also known as: Chinese black mushroom and fragrant mushroom

Parts used: Stem and cap, and cultured mycelial extract

The English word *shiitake* (*shih-TAH-kay*) comes from the Japanese for "mushroom of the *shii* tree," on whose decaying logs it grows. Native to East Asia, shiitakes have been cultivated in China, Japan, Korea, and Southeast Asia since ancient times, and are widely used in those cuisines. In these areas of the world, they are often known as Chinese black mushrooms, because of their dark color, or fragrant mushrooms, because of their distinctive aroma.

Wild shiitakes were eaten as long ago as A.D. 200. Cultivation began around 1000. The first documented medicinal use of shiitakes dates from around 1400. Today, shiitake mushrooms are Japan's leading agricultural export.

Healing History

In traditional Japanese medicine, shiitakes were used to treat fatigue, muscle aches, intestinal parasites, poor circulation, and heart disease. In traditional Chinese medicine, the mushroom was used to treat colds, flu, weakness, fatigue, and liver problems, and to invigorate *qi*, life energy.

Therapeutic Uses

Westerners first learned of shiitakes' medicinal benefits in 1974 when Japanese mycologist Kisaku Mori's book, *Mushrooms as Health Foods*, was published in English. The medicinal constituent of shiitake is the compound lentinan, though a slightly different compound, *Lentinula edodes* mycelial extract (LEM), cultured from the mushroom, is also used.

ENHANCED IMMUNITY. Many laboratory and animal studies show that lentinan and LEM activate many components of the immune system, notably natural killer cells, T-helper cells, interleukin-1 and -2, and germ-eating white blood cells known as macrophages. These actions help treat all manner of illness, particularly viral infections and cancer.

HEPATITIS. Shiitake's immune-boosting action helps treat chronic hepatitis B, an infection that can lead to liver failure or liver cancer. Chinese researchers gave lentinan to 44 people with chronic hepatitis B. Two months later, their immune systems were more active, and the researchers noted "therapeutic effectiveness" in treating the infection.

GENITAL WARTS. Chinese scientists treated 36 people with genital warts with either laser therapy, which is a standard approach, or laser plus 12.5 milligrams of lentinan twice a day. After 2 months, 47 percent of the laser-only group experienced a recurrence. But in the laser-lentinan group, the figure was just 11 percent.

HIV/AIDS. University of California researchers gave lentinan to 98 people with AIDS. They showed improved immune function. In another study, Japanese researchers gave people with AIDS 9 grams of LEM a day. After 2 years, symptoms subsided in every one of them.

CANCER. Several studies show that lentinan inhibits reproduction of various cancer cells, including breast cancer cells, and boosts the immune function of cancer patients. Japanese researchers gave standard care or that plus lentinan to a group of people with various advanced cancers. After 10 days, the lentinan group showed improved immune function and survived longer. Another Japanese team gave standard chemotherapy or that plus lentinan to people with advanced stomach cancer. In the standard care group, not one person survived for a year. In the lentinan group, half did. Different Japanese scientists gave men with advanced prostate cancer either standard hormone therapy and chemotherapy or that plus lentinan. In the standard-care group, 29 percent survived 5 years. But among those who took lentinan, the figure was 43 percent.

HIGH CHOLESTEROL. Japanese scientists encouraged 90 women with high cholesterol to add shiitakes to their diets (one-third of an ounce to 3 ounces per day). In just 7 days, their total cholesterol fell 7 to 14 percent.

VITAMIN D. Shiitake is one of the few plant sources of vitamin D.

Intriguing Possibility

A pilot study suggests shiitake may help treat tuberculosis.

Rx Recommendations

Enjoy shiitake mushrooms in food—soups, stir-fries, or anywhere you would use other mushrooms. Fresh and dried shiitakes can be found at many health food stores and some supermarkets. Studies have shown medical benefits from eating eight whole mushrooms a day, or taking LEM in doses of 9 to 25 grams per day.

The Safety Factor

In healthy people, side effects are uncommon, but stomach upset is possible. If any develop, reduce your dose or stop taking it. In people with AIDS or cancer, more side effects have been reported, including fever, allergic reactions, and back and leg pain.

Pregnant and nursing women should not consume more than typical food amounts.

Do not give shiitake to children under 2. In older children, the mushroom may be eaten as a food.

For more on herb safety, see Chapter 2.

If symptoms get worse or persist longer than 2 weeks, consult a health care professional promptly.

Growing Information

Shiitake mushrooms can be grown indoors from kits sold by Fungi Perfecti. Visit www.fungi.com.

SLIPPERY ELM

An Early American Favorite

Family: Ulmaceae; other members include the elms

Genus and species: *Ulmus rubra* and *U. fulva*

Also known as: Red elm and Indian elm

Part used: Inner bark

No food or drug of today comes close to matching the place of honor that slippery elm held in 18th- and 19th-century America. Great elm forests covered the East, and even in cities, the versatile bark was always close at hand.

Soaked in water and wrapped around meats, slippery elm bark retarded spoilage in the days before refrigeration. Coarsely ground and mixed with water, it turned into a spongy mass and was molded into bandages to cover wounds and made into pill-like coverings for unpleasant-tasting medicines. Ground and mixed with water

or milk, slippery elm bark turned into a soothing, nutritious gruel similar to oatmeal that was used to treat sore throats, coughs, colds, and gastrointestinal ailments and to feed infants and hospital patients. Slippery elm sore throat lozenges were a fixture in home medicine cabinets. The herb was the nation's leading home remedy for anything in need of soothing.

Slippery elm is still listed in the *National Formulary*, the pharmacists' reference, and health food stores still sell throat lozenges containing the herb. But our once-great elm forests have been decimated by Dutch elm disease, and both our landscapes and our herbal healing heritage are poorer as a result.

Healing History

The 1st-century Greek physician Dioscorides prescribed soaking in a European elm bath to speed the healing of broken bones. His prescription survived for more than 1,500 years.

In the 17th century, English herbalist Nicholas Culpeper wrote, "The decoction being bathed in, heals broken bones . . . [and] is excellent [for] places . . . burnt with fire. The leaves bruised, applied, and being bound thereon with its own bark heal wounds." Culpeper also claimed that elm root decoction restored hair on bald scalps.

Colonists found the Native Americans using American slippery elm bark as a food and treatment for wounds, sore throats, coughs, inflamed nipples (mastitis), and many other ailments. The colonists adopted these uses and developed many more, including applying slippery elm poultices to bring boils to a head.

Native American women inserted slippery elm sticks to induce abortion, and white women adopted the practice, which caused many deaths from uterine infection and hemorrhage. As a result, several state legislatures passed laws forbidding the sale of slippery elm bark in pieces longer than $1^1/_2$ inches.

America's early 19th-century Thomsonian herbalists recommended slippery elm tea as a laxative gentle enough for children. Thomsonian midwives lubricated their hands with the slippery bark before performing internal examinations.

By the time of the Civil War, slippery elm was being used to treat syphilis, gonorrhea, and hemorrhoids. America's 19th-century Eclectic physicians, forerunners of today's naturopaths, deemed the herb very valuable and suggested that "a tablespoon of the powder boiled in milk affords a nourishing diet for infants newly weaned, preventing the bowel complaints to which they are subject. Some physicians consider the constant use of it, during and after the seventh month of gestation, as advantageous in facilitating an easy delivery."

Contemporary herbalists recommend slippery elm bark externally to cover wounds and soothe skin problems and internally as a tea to treat sore throats and coughs as well as diarrhea, ulcers, colitis, and other gastrointestinal complaints.

Therapeutic Uses

Even the FDA, which is usually critical of herbal medicines, calls slippery elm "an excellent demulcent" (soothing agent). The herb's bark is rich in a soluble fiber called mucilage that swells and becomes spongy and gelatinous when mixed with water.

WOUNDS. When applied to thoroughly washed wounds, slippery elm bark mucilage dries to form an herbal bandage.

COUGHS, SORE THROATS, AND DIGESTIVE PROBLEMS. Slippery elm decoction helps soothe the throat and digestive tract. Besides providing mucilage, the herb stimulates production of digestive tract mucus, which also acts as a soother.

WOMEN'S HEALTH CONCERNS. Slippery elm decoction has a long history of use as a laxative by pregnant women, and the medical literature contains no reports of problems. The active constituent, mucilage, should not harm the fetus. If you have a history of problematic pregnancy, however, consult your physician before trying a slippery elm preparation.

Medicinal Myth

Slippery elm has never been shown to speed the healing of broken bones.

Rx Recommendations

For a poultice to bandage wounds, stir enough water into powdered bark to make a paste and apply to the affected area.

For a soothing decoction, use 1 to 3 teaspoons of powdered herb per cup of water. Blend a little water in with the powder first to prevent lumpiness. Bring to a boil and simmer for 15 minutes, then strain if you wish. Drink up to 3 cups a day. Slippery elm has only a slight taste and a mild aroma reminiscent of maple.

When using commercial preparations, follow the package directions.

You may give slippery elm cautiously to children under age 2.

The Safety Factor

Allergic reactions are possible. Otherwise, the medical literature contains no reports of slippery elm causing harm.

Growing Information

Slippery elm is a stately tree that reaches 60 feet. Its trunk bark is brown, but its branch bark is whitish. Its leaves are broad, rough, hairy, and toothed. Check local nurseries to see if this tree can be grown in your area.

SOYBEAN

FDA-Approved
for Cholesterol Control

Family: Leguminosae; other members include beans and peas

Genus and species: *Glycine max*

Also known as: Soya

Parts used: Beans

Soybeans are the United States' fourth leading legal agricultural product, surpassed only by cattle, dairy products, and corn. An astonishing 70 million acres of American farmland are planted with soybeans, largely for cattle feed and export to Asia. The U.S. soybean crop accounts for almost half of the world production and generates $14.6 billion a year in revenues.

Healing History

Soybeans were cultivated in China as early as 1200 B.C. They were that country's second most important crop, after rice. Soybeans served as a key source of protein for a culture that was largely vegetarian. The Chinese developed tofu around 200 B.C.

The ancient Japanese adopted soybeans and tofu enthusiastically. During the 18th century, soybeans were introduced into Europe, but they didn't arrive in the United States until Chinese immigrants brought them in the 1880s. Soybeans quickly became a major U.S. crop, raised almost entirely as cattle feed and for export to Asia. Tofu did not become a food in this country until health foods became popular in the late 1960s.

From the 1970s through the 1980s, tofu was the food Americans loved to hate. The water-packed, spongy white blocks, resembling pressed cottage cheese, were the butt of countless put-downs by the hosts of late-night TV shows and others who considered health foods as bland and tasteless as, well, plain tofu.

During the 1990s, public opinion began to shift. Tofu and other soy foods have still not become national favorites, but the jokes have largely ceased, for two reasons. First, soy foods—in particular, soy-based textured vegetable protein—have become more familiar. Soy protein is now added to a large number of supermarket items, including soy dogs (a substitute for beef and pork franks), soy burgers (a substitute for hamburgers), and soy crumbles (a substitute for chopped meat).

Second, studies have now shown that tofu and other soy foods offer a remarkable number of health benefits—so many that the FDA allows soy products to carry a health claim on their labels. Supplement companies have even packaged the bean's health-promoting compounds, isoflavones, into pills and capsules that have become popular.

Therapeutic Uses

The key isoflavones in soybeans are genistein and daidzein. The following chart shows how the various types of soy foods stack up in terms of their isoflavone content. (Incidentally, soy sauce is *not* a source of isoflavones.)

SOY PRODUCT	PORTION	ISOFLAVONES (MG)
Raw soybeans	½ cup (34 g)	176
Roasted soybeans	½ cup (30 g)	167
Tempeh	4 oz. (19 g)	61
Soy protein	1 oz. (26 g)	57
Soy flour	¼ cup (8 g)	44
Tofu	4 oz. (18 g)	38
Textured soy protein	¼ cup (18 g)	28
Soy milk	8 oz. (10 g)	20

Soy and soy products have a remarkable number of health benefits.

HIGH CHOLESTEROL. While a smattering of studies show that soy has little or no effect on cholesterol, the great majority of trials show that it reduces cholesterol significantly, and with it, risk of heart attack and most strokes.

☘ Wake Forest University researchers placed 156 men and women with high cholesterol on the low-fat diet recommended by the American Heart Association. In addition, the study participants were given one of five supplement drinks: a placebo or four beverages containing varying amounts of soy isoflavones. After 9 weeks, those who received the placebo drink showed no reduction in cholesterol, but all of those who received the soy drinks showed reductions, with the greatest decrease occurring in the group whose beverage contained the most isoflavones.

❧ Researchers at the Veterans Affairs Medical Center in Lexington, Kentucky, analyzed 38 studies of soy protein's effect on cholesterol. They found that soy lowered cholesterol significantly. Study participants who consumed 47 grams (1.7 ounces) of soy protein a day saw their total cholesterol decline by 23 milligrams per deciliter of blood (mg/dl). The researchers concluded that substituting soy protein for animal protein significantly decreases cholesterol.

❧ English researchers analyzed 39 studies of soy's effects on cholesterol. The herb reduced cholesterol significantly.

Because of all the research showing that soy protein helps cut cholesterol, in 1999, the FDA ruled that foods containing at least 6.25 grams of soy protein per serving may state on their labels that they reduce cholesterol and the risk of heart disease.

Commission E, the expert panel that evaluates herbal medicines for the German counterpart of the FDA, approves soy foods as a treatment for elevated cholesterol.

HOT FLASHES. At menopause, women produce less estrogen and many experience resulting menopausal discomforts, notably, hot flashes. Soy isoflavones are plant estrogens (phytoestrogens). They're similar to the human hormone, but chemically weaker. Soy phytoestrogens are strong enough to prevent and relieve hot flashes but not so strong that they cause estrogen's downsides, one of which is the stimulation of breast tumors. In fact, mounting evidence suggests that soy foods help prevent breast cancer (see below).

In one study, Italian researchers gave 104 women with severe hot flashes either a placebo or 76 milligrams of soy isoflavones a day. After 1 month, the women taking the soy reported significantly fewer hot flashes.

In another study, Harvard researchers gave 147 menopausal women either a placebo or a soy supplement. After 12 weeks, the soy group reported a 52 percent decrease in hot flashes.

HIGH BLOOD PRESSURE. As people eat fewer animal foods and more plant foods, including beans, blood pressure tends to decrease. In a Chinese study of 302 adults with high blood pressure, researchers gave participants biscuits either with or without soy. The soy biscuits contained about 2 ounces of soy. After 12 weeks, the soy group showed significantly lower blood pressure.

English researchers analyzed nine studies and concluded that soy "significantly reduces blood pressure."

BREAST CANCER. Many studies have shown that compared with Americans, Asian women are substantially less likely to develop breast cancer. Epidemiologists used to believe that Asian women's lower-fat diet accounted for the difference. Now, many scientists believe that what makes the difference is less fat and more soy.

Human estrogen stimulates the growth of

breast tumors. Weaker soy phytoestrogens attach to estrogen receptors on breast cells, effectively locking out the body's own estrogen and reducing its stimulating effect. In laboratory studies, breast cancer cells exposed to soy isoflavones had their growth reduced by 30 percent.

Australian researchers conducted diet surveys of 144 women newly diagnosed with breast cancer and 144 demographically similar women who were cancer free. After accounting for other known risk factors (such as family history), the researchers determined that the women who were cancer free consumed significantly more soy isoflavones than those with breast cancer.

University of Arkansas researchers analyzed 14 studies on soy and breast cancer risk. They concluded that compared with women who eat little or no soy, those who eat it a few times a week have 22 percent less risk of breast cancer.

OTHER CANCERS. The same researchers also analyzed 15 studies of soy and colon cancer and 6 studies of soy and prostate cancer. They found that a high-soy diet reduces risk of colon cancer by 30 percent and prostate cancer by 34 percent.

OSTEOPOROSIS. Estrogen replacement reduces risk of osteoporosis, suggesting that soy might do the same. Thirty-one clinical trials have been published on the effects of soy foods on bone mineral density. Twenty-two (71 percent) show that the herb increases bone density. One of them, a study of 24,403 postmenopausal women followed for $4^{1}/_{2}$ years, shows that a high-soy diet also reduces risk of fractures.

Researchers at the University of Illinois gave three groups of postmenopausal women 40 grams of protein a day. In one group, the protein came from non-soy sources (meat and dairy products). In another group, the protein included moderate levels of soy isoflavones, and in the third group, the protein included high levels of soy isoflavones. After 6 months, the women consuming the non-soy protein showed bone loss, while those eating the most soy isoflavones showed significantly increased bone mineral density.

Rx Recommendations

If you get your soy from foods, most experts recommend consuming about 5 ounces of tofu (about 1.5 servings) containing approximately 50 to 70 grams of soy protein weekly. If you have any of the conditions that may be prevented by soy, feel free to eat more.

Soy isoflavones are also available as supplements. Follow the label directions.

Because soybeans are such a major crop in the United States, the soy trade organizations have had the financial resources to fund the studies showing soy's benefits. These results have not been duplicated for other beans, but according to research at the USDA, all edible beans contain isoflavones.

Soy contains the most isoflavones per serving, but it wouldn't take too many dishes made with other beans (burritos, baked beans, bean soups, or salads) to consume significant amounts of isoflavones. The chart on the next page shows how various legumes compare in terms of isoflavone content (the figures are in parts per million).

LEGUME	GENISTEIN (PPM)	DAIDZEIN (PPM)	TOTAL (PPM)
Soybeans	24	38	62
Black beans	45	0	45
Pinto beans	22	23	45
Lima beans	40	0	40
Kidney beans	29	3	32
Red lentils	25	5	30
Fava beans	20	5	25
Great Northern beans	17	7	24
Black-eyed peas	23	0	23
Mung beans	22	0	22

The Safety Factor

Estrogen counteracts the effects of male sex hormones. Phytoestrogens have similar action. Men with suppressed male sex hormones often have low sperm counts, so Harvard researchers investigated the effects, if any, of dietary soy on the sperm counts of 99 men at an infertility clinic. Those who ate the most soy had the lowest sperm counts. Men in couples trying to get pregnant should avoid soy.

Soy is safe for the vast majority of people, but allergies and other sensitivities are possible.

Growing Information

The soybean plant is an annual that grows from 1 to 5 feet tall. Its stems, leaves, and bean pods are covered with fine hairs that give the plant a fuzzy appearance and feel. The pods contain up to four seeds (beans).

Soybean is not a garden herb, but if you grow peas, you might grow soybeans. The beans can be roasted and eaten.

TARRAGON
Good for an Aching Tooth

Family: Compositae; other members
include daisy, dandelion, and marigold

Genus and species: *Artemisia
dracunculus*

Also known as: French or Russian tarragon,
estragon, and dragon herb

Parts used: Leaves

Tarragon is best known as the main seasoning
in béarnaise sauce. Like all aromatic herbs, it
also has a long history in herbal healing.

Unlike most other aromatics, however, tarragon fell from healing fashion in the 17th
century. Only recently has the herb been rediscovered as an oral anesthetic with some potential for treating diabetes and preventing varicose
veins.

Healing History

After discovering that chewing tarragon numbs
the mouth, the ancient Greeks used the herb to
treat toothache. They also decided that its
anesthetic power and its wide-ranging root runners meant that it could help relieve the discomforts of traveling. The 1st-century Roman
naturalist Pliny wrote that tarragon prevented
fatigue on long journeys. During the Middle
Ages, pilgrims placed tarragon sprigs in their
shoes.

Oddly enough for an herb that numbs the
mouth, around the 10th century, Arab physicians recommended tarragon as an appetite
stimulant.

Under the Doctrine of Signatures, the medieval belief that an herb's appearance revealed its
medicinal value, tarragon's serpentine roots
were considered a sign that it could cure snakebite. Over the centuries, the belief expanded to
include the bites of rabid dogs. But by the 17th
century, this belief had faded. Nicholas Culpeper, who recommended dozens of herbs for the
bites of "venomous creatures," did not mention
tarragon in this regard. In fact, he hardly mentioned it at all.

After Culpeper, herbalists virtually abandoned tarragon because it loses most of its aromatic healing oil as it dries. Even America's
19th-century Eclectic physicians, forerunners of
today's naturopaths, prized medicinal herbs but
had no use for tarragon.

Few contemporary herbalists value tarragon
except in French cooking. Those who do recognize it reiterate its traditional uses as a diuretic,
appetite stimulant, digestive aid, and toothache
treatment.

Therapeutic Uses

While tarragon is no wonder herb, it deserves a place in herbal healing. Its active component is its oil, but drying largely destroys it. Either fresh or frozen leaves or generous amounts of dried leaves must be used.

TOOTHACHE. Tarragon oil contains the same anesthetic compound, eugenol, as clove oil. This supports its age-old use for toothache. Tarragon provides only temporary relief of oral pain, however. If toothache persists, consult a dentist.

INFECTIONS. Like many culinary herbs, tarragon oil fights disease-causing bacteria in laboratory studies. You can use fresh leaves as garden first aid for minor wounds.

Intriguing Possibilities

Animal studies by Rutgers University researchers show that tarragon lowers blood sugar, suggesting that it might help manage diabetes.

In addition, tarragon oil contains rutin, a compound that strengthens blood vessel walls. Herbalists often recommend other herbs rich in rutin, notably violet and onion, for the treatment of varicose veins in the legs. These herbs may also help hemorrhoids, which are varicose veins in the anal area.

An animal study published in the *Journal of the National Cancer Institute* suggests that rutin has some anti-tumor activity.

Rx Recommendations

For temporary relief of oral pain, chew fresh leaves as needed.

For garden first aid, apply fresh, crushed leaves to a cut or scrape until you can wash and bandage it.

For a pleasant, licorice-flavored infusion that may help prevent varicose veins and hemorrhoids, use 1 to 2 teaspoons of fresh or frozen herb per cup of boiling water. Steep for 10 to 15 minutes, then strain. Drink up to 3 cups a day.

As a homemade tincture, use $1/2$ to 1 teaspoon up to three times a day.

When using commercial preparations, follow the package directions.

The Safety Factor

Large amounts of estragole, a compound in tarragon, produce tumors in mice. Tarragon has never been associated with human cancer, but until its effects are clarified, people with a history of cancer should probably not use the herb in medicinal amounts.

Otherwise, the medical literature contains no reports of tarragon causing harm.

Pregnant and nursing women should not use medicinal amounts of tarragon.

Do not give tarragon to children under 2. In older children, adjust the recommended dose based on the child's weight. For example, give a 50-pound child one-third of the dose a 150-pound adult would take.

If you're over 65, start with a low dose, and increase only if necessary.

Inform health care professionals of the herbs you use. Problematic herb-drug interactions are possible.

Tarragon may cause allergic reactions or other unexpected side effects. If any develop, reduce your dose or stop taking it.

For more on herb safety, see Chapter 2.

If symptoms get worse or persist longer than 2 weeks, consult a health care professional promptly.

Growing Information

Tarragon comes in two varieties, Russian and French. The former has less oil—and therefore, less flavor and medicinal value—so a mention of tarragon almost always refers to the French plant.

Russian tarragon may be grown from seeds, but the more desirable French variety must be propagated from cuttings or root divisions. Divide the roots in spring and plant 1-inch pieces of their tips, or take cuttings in summer. Thin plants to 2-foot spacing.

French tarragon is a perennial with a creeping, serpentine root and stems that reach 2 feet. Its leaves look like a larger version of rosemary. This herb rarely flowers, and if it does, the fruits are sterile.

Tarragon grows best in rich, well-drained soil under full sun. Make sure the roots do not become waterlogged. If your winter temperatures drop below the teens, mulch well each fall. Divide tarragon roots every few years to retain the plants' vigor.

Tarragon leaves bruise easily. Harvest them carefully in early summer. Because it loses medicinal value when dried, freeze the fresh herb or preserve it in vinegar.

TEA
A Longer, Healthier Life in Every Cup

Family: Theaceae; other members include camellia

Genus and species: *Camellia sinensis*

Also known as: White, green, oolong, and black tea

Parts used: Leaves

Tea is the world's second most popular beverage (after water). Until recently, most Americans and Europeans drank it only as a tasty, mildly stimulating alternative to coffee. But that's been changing as the research on tea's many health benefits becomes more widely known. The fact is, drinking a few cups of tea every day—especially green tea—substantially reduces the risk of a remarkably large number of serious conditions, notably heart disease and cancer.

But first, let's clear up some confusion: Many people use the term *tea* to describe any herbal beverage made by steeping plant material in boiled water, such as chamomile tea and mint tea. This works colloquially, but in herbal medicine, it becomes confusing. Using the colloquial definition, coffee is a tea because it's a hot-water extract of plant material. Technically, however, hot-water extracts are not teas, but infusions. In herbal medicine, *tea* is an infusion made with tea leaves (*Camellia sinensis*).

Few traditional herbals mention tea. In fact, many people don't even consider tea an herb. They typically ask, "Would you like coffee, tea, or herb tea?" Of course, coffee and tea are both herbs, so all of these beverages are herb teas. However, in common parlance, "herb tea" typically means a noncaffeinated herbal beverage.

There are four basic types of tea: white, green, oolong, and black. They all begin as leaves of *Camellia sinensis*. Soon after harvesting, unless the leaves are dried, they wilt and oxidize, turning progressively darker as their chlorophyll breaks down and combines with oxygen in the air. Chemically, this is oxidation, but the tea industry calls it fermentation.

- White tea is picked and dried immediately. It is unwilted and unoxidized.
- Green tea is wilted but unoxidized.
- Oolong tea is wilted and partially oxidized.
- Black tea is wilted and fully oxidized.

Black tea accounts for an estimated 78 percent of worldwide tea consumption. Green tea accounts for about 20 percent. White and oolong together account for only around 2 percent.

In addition, many teas have been named for the region where the leaves were grown, for example, Darjeeling (in India) or Ceylon (now Sri Lanka).

Teas have also been named for other reasons:

- The Chinese called black tea *pek-ho*. The British heard the term as *pekoe*, which came to mean any black tea. The English considered tea so divine that they gave it the name tea from the Greek *thea*, meaning "goddess."
- English Breakfast is a blend of various black teas.
- Earl Grey is named for the second Earl Grey, a British prime minister in the 1830s who reputedly received a gift of black tea flavored with oil of bergamot, an orangelike citrus fruit. Traditionally, Earl Grey meant citrus-flavored black tea. But today Earl Grey white, green, and oolong teas are available.
- Pu-er tea is a large-leaf tea from Yunnan, China.
- Lapsang souchong is a smoked black tea originally from the Wuyi region of Fujian Province, China. Today other teas are also smoked.
- Chai is an Indian combination of tea (usually black) with a blend of spices, including cardamom, cinnamon, clove, and pepper.

Note: African red bush tea, sometimes called red tea, is not tea. It's rooibos (*Aspalathus linearis*), a plant native to South Africa.

Note: Tea tree is not tea. It's an Australian herb (*Melaleuca alternifolia*) whose oil is a powerful topical antiseptic.

A Brief History of Tea

Legend has it that 5,000 years ago, the mythical Chinese emperor Shen Nung asked a servant for a cup of boiled water. A few leaves from a nearby tree accidentally fell into it, giving the water a golden color and pleasant flavor. Shen Nung pronounced it refreshing. The Chinese have been drinking tea ever since.

As time passed, tea spread throughout Asia. It became particularly popular in Japan, where its preparation was elevated to an art form, the Japanese tea ceremony.

The first European to mention tea was Portuguese Jesuit Father Jasper de Cruz, who visited China in 1560. But it was Dutch traders who first brought tea to Europe, where it became an immediate hit—but only with the wealthy because tea was rare and coveted and, therefore, costly.

Tea arrived in England in 1652. By then, increased importation from China had reduced the price to the point where all but the poor could afford a few cups a day. Tea quickly replaced ale as England's national beverage.

In 1618, the Chinese ambassador to Russia presented Czar Alexis with some tea. Tea quickly became popular throughout Russia. So did the Tibetan method of brewing it in a large pot, which the Russians transformed into the samovar.

Around 1800 in England, Anna, the Duchess of Bedford, began serving tea with a light snack in the late afternoon. She invented "tea time."

Tea first arrived in the Western Hemisphere in 1650 when Peter Stuyvesant introduced it to New Amsterdam, later New York. But it did not catch on until importation increased and the price dropped around 1700. By 1720, tea was a beloved staple in colonial America.

From 1754 to 1763, during what we call the French and Indian War, England fought the French for control of North America. It was an expensive war, and because it safeguarded the colonies, England decided that her American colonists should pay for it through taxes, including a tax on tea. The colonists hated the tea tax and boycotted English tea, buying smuggled Dutch tea instead. Then on December 16, 1773, Samuel Adams, John Hancock, and other disgruntled colonists stormed a British merchant ship and threw hundreds of pounds of tea into Boston Harbor—the Boston Tea Party. In retaliation, the British closed the port of Boston and sent troops to occupy the city. One could argue that Americans' love of tea sparked the American Revolution.

Despite the Boston Tea Party, by the 19th century, Americans preferred coffee. But tea remained popular. In 1904, one tea merchant, Richard Blechynden, planned to give away cups of hot tea at the St. Louis World's Fair. But a heat wave struck and no one wanted a hot drink. Blechynden served his tea over ice—the birth of iced tea. It was the hit of the fair, and quickly became a national craze.

In 1908, tea merchant Thomas Sullivan packaged individual cup-size portions of tea in porous paper wrappers. The idea went nowhere until some restaurants began serving tea "in the bag" to save waiters the time of handling loose tea. Tea bags have been with us ever since.

For most of the 20th century, "tea" meant Lipton orange pekoe. But starting in the 1970s, as Americans developed a taste for exotic coffees, they also became more interested in other teas, including green, white, oolong, Pu-er, and Darjeeling. Today, tea is more popular than ever in the United States, thanks, ironically, to coffee shops such as Starbucks that also serve tea.

Healing History

Tea has been used in Chinese medicine for at least 3,000 years to treat headache, diarrhea, dysentery, colds, coughs, asthma, and other respiratory problems. The Chinese also view tea as a grease cutter and recommend drinking it with fatty meals.

Seventeenth-century English herbalist Nicholas Culpeper called tea "more used for pleasure than as a medicine," but suggested it as a digestive aid and "for all inward decays." He also recommended it for "violent headaches and sickness occasioned by inebriation." But he warned that it should be avoided by those with "weak nerves."

America's 19th-century Eclectic physicians, forerunners of today's naturopaths, called tea "a harmless and refreshing beverage . . . unless taken very strong or in large quantities." They called it "very agreeable to the invalid," and recommended it for fever, colds, muscle aches, headache, and stomach distress. But they warned that its stimulant action might interfere with sleep.

In the 1930s, Maude Grieve, a prominent British herbalist, noted "tea is rarely used as a medicine, but the infusion is useful to relieve headaches."

Until the 1990s, Americans drank tea primarily as a stimulant beverage, but also to treat diarrhea, colds, and other respiratory problems. It was a minor player in herbal medicine. But since the 1990s, and especially since the turn of the century, tea has suddenly become a major herbal medicine. Thanks to the antioxidants it contains, tea substantially reduces risk of heart disease, stroke, all major cancers, diabetes, osteoporosis, rheumatoid arthritis, dementia, and other conditions.

Therapeutic Uses

Tea contains three stimulant compounds: caffeine, theobromine, and theophylline, which account for its stimulant effect.

STIMULANT ACTION. Cup for cup, tea has about half the caffeine of brewed coffee. But if you drink 2 cups of tea, you don't get the same buzz as you would from 1 cup of coffee. The reason is that tea also contains a compound (L-theanine) with tranquilizing action. The Chinese say that tea produces "relaxed alertness."

COLDS AND ASTHMA. Like coffee, the stimulants in tea also open the bronchial tubes (act as a bronchodilator). This action helps treat the chest congestion of colds and may help control asthma.

PAIN RELIEF. The combination of caffeine and pain relievers treats a headache better than pain relievers by themselves. Wash down aspirin, ibuprofen, or acetaminophen with a cup of tea, and the pain reliever works better. For more on this, see Coffee on page 164.

ANTIOXIDANT POWER. Beyond its stimulant action, tea contains powerful antioxidant polyphenols that, over the past 20 years, have rocketed this herb into medicinal prominence. Antioxidants help prevent and repair the cell damage at the root of heart disease, most strokes and cancers, and many other degenerative conditions associated with aging.

In traditional Chinese medicine, tea is considered a "grease cutter" that prevents diseases associated with fatty foods, such as heart disease. Japanese researchers wondered if this traditional belief might be scientifically verified. In the 1980s, they found potent antioxidant compounds in tea, notably epigallocatechin-3-gallate (EGCG), thus validating traditional Chinese medicine's claim.

However, the oxidation process that turns tea from white to green to oolong to black destroys some of the EGCG. As a result, white and green teas have greater antioxidant content than oolong teas, which contain more antioxidants than black teas. In laboratory studies, black tea has been shown to have only $1/10$ to $1/100$ of green tea's antioxidant punch. Black teas still contain significant amounts of antioxidants, which is why they reduce risk of heart disease and stroke (more on that below). But black teas have not shown much ability to reduce cancer risk. For cancer prevention, green tea is the way to go because it retains the most EGCG. (Currently, scientists can't explain why black tea reduces risk of heart disease and stroke, but not cancer.)

HEART DISEASE. In the West, tea began its transformation from a beverage into a health food in 1993, when Dutch researchers published a study in the British medical journal *Lancet* on the effects of dietary antioxidants on heart attack risk among residents of Zutphen, a city in the Netherlands. Men who consumed the most fruits and vegetables—all rich in antioxidants—had the lowest heart attack risk. But tea was also very protective, a finding that surprised Western scientists—and sent them scurrying to the earlier Japanese EGCG research.

How do the antioxidants in tea reduce risk of heart disease? Several ways: They lower cholesterol. They improve arterial function. And they reduce atherosclerosis, the formation of fatty deposits in the arteries that clog them, and in heart attacks, block them.

Since then, dozens of studies have shown that tea—both black and green—helps prevent heart disease.

- In a different Dutch study, researchers followed 4,807 men for 5 years. Compared with those who drank no tea, men who drank a cup or two a day had 43 percent fewer heart attacks—and 70 percent fewer heart attack deaths.

- Saudi Arabian scientists surveyed 3,430 adults ages 30 to 70. As tea consumption increased, their risk of heart disease decreased significantly.

- Harvard researchers surveyed 340 people who had suffered heart attacks and a similar number of healthy controls. Drinking more than 1 cup of tea a day reduced heart attack risk by 44 percent.

If tea really helps the heart, it should exhibit a "dose-response" effect—as tea consumption increases, heart disease risk should decline. That is the case. In the Harvard study, moderate tea drinkers were 31 percent less likely to have a heart attack. The figure for heavy tea drinkers was 39 percent. The Saudi study also showed a dose-response effect.

Warning: If you drink tea for heart benefits, don't add milk. A German study suggests that milk neutralizes the EGCG, counteracting tea's heart-helping actions.

STROKE. Most strokes (ischemic strokes) are biologically similar to heart attacks. Instead of a blockage in one of the coronary arteries, though, ischemic strokes involve blockage of an artery in the brain. Antioxidants reduce risk of ischemic stroke. Dutch researchers followed 552 men for 15 years. Compared with those who drank less than 2 cups of tea a day, men who drank more than 4 cups daily saw their stroke risk plummet by 69 percent.

CANCER. Green tea was shown to have cancer-preventive value in laboratory animals in the early 1980s. The first study to find the same benefit in humans was published in 1988. For that study, researchers in Kyushu, Japan, compared the diets and lifestyles of 139 people with stomach cancer and 2,852 people who were cancer free. After accounting for other variables, the researchers determined that as green tea consumption increased, stomach cancer risk decreased significantly.

Since then, an occasional report has shown no cancer-protective benefits for green tea, but these few negative findings are vastly outnumbered by dozens of trials showing that as green tea consumption increases, risk of *all* major cancers decreases: lung, colon, breast, prostate, ovarian, esophageal, pancreatic, malignant melanoma, and stomach cancers, plus leukemia.

- Lung cancer. Japanese scientists analyzed the effect of drinking green tea on lung cancer risk in 333 Okinawans with the disease and 666 who were cancer free. Among women, tea drinking reduced cancer risk from 23 to 62 percent, with increasing amounts of tea producing greater risk reductions. Among men, risk reductions ranged from 15 to 43 percent.

- Colon cancer. University of Minnesota researchers analyzed 25 studies of tea's impact on risk of colon cancer. Black tea had no effect. Compared with those who drank no green tea, however, regular green tea drinkers were significantly less likely to develop colon cancer.

- Breast cancer. Another group of University of Minnesota scientists analyzed 13 studies of green tea's effect on breast cancer risk. Compared with women who did not drink it, those who drank the most green tea had 22 percent less risk of breast cancer.

- Prostate cancer. Australian researchers asked 130 men with prostate cancer and 274 men who were cancer free about their green tea drinking. Among those with cancer, 55 percent drank green tea. Among those free of prostate cancer, the figure was 80 percent. And as green tea consumption increased, cancer risk decreased.

- Ovarian cancer. Swedish scientists followed 61,057 women for 15 years. Compared with those who drank tea (green or black) less than once a month, women who drank more than 2 cups a day were 46 percent less likely to develop ovarian cancer.

- Esophageal cancer. Chinese researchers compared green tea consumption among 902 people ages 30 to 74 who had esophageal cancer and 1,552 people who were cancer free. For women, regular green tea drinking cut esophageal cancer risk by 50 percent. For men who did not smoke or drink alcohol, green tea cut esophageal cancer risk by 57 percent.

- Pancreatic cancer. Columbia University scientists documented green tea consumption among 451 Chinese in Shanghai with pancreatic cancer and 1,552 healthy controls. Regular green tea drinking reduced pancreatic cancer risk by 47 percent.

❧Malignant melanoma. Italian researchers tracked tea drinking in 542 people with malignant melanoma and 538 healthy matched controls. Compared with those who did not drink tea, those who drank the most had 29 percent less risk of melanoma.

❧Stomach cancer. Chinese scientists surveyed green tea drinking in 711 people with stomach cancer and 711 healthy matched controls. Compared with nondrinkers, those who drank green tea regularly had 29 percent less risk of stomach cancer.

❧Leukemia. Harvard researchers surveyed green tea consumption in 252 people with leukemia and 637 healthy controls. As tea consumption increased, leukemia risk decreased.

Green tea shows a clear dose-response effect for cancer prevention. Consider breast cancer: Australian researchers categorized green tea consumption in 2,018 Chinese women as low, moderate, or high. Low intake reduced breast cancer risk by 13 percent; moderate, by 32 percent; high, by 41 percent. A study at the University of Southern California showed a similar dose-response effect.

Of course, some green tea drinkers still develop cancer. If green tea has cancer-preventive benefits, then compared with those who do not drink it, we would expect green tea drinkers to get cancer later in life. That's precisely what Japanese researchers showed in a study correlating tea drinking in Japan with people's age at cancer diagnosis. Compared with Japanese who drank less than 3 cups of green tea a day, women who drank 10 or more cups developed all cancers an average of 8.7 years later. The figure for men was 3.0 years later.

If tea protects against cancer, we would also expect milder cancers in those who drink it. Another Japanese study confirms this. Compared with Japanese breast cancer patients who drank little or no green tea, those who regularly drank it (8 to 10 cups a day) had milder cases at diagnosis (fewer positive lymph nodes), a greater likelihood of estrogen-positive disease (which correlates with improved prognosis), less risk of metastasis (spread), less risk of recurrence, and a better rate of survival.

Finally, if tea protects against cancer, we would expect tea drinkers to have less chance of recurrence. Again, this is the case. Japanese researchers analyzed the breast cancers of 472 women. Those who drank the most green tea had the lowest likelihood of recurrences.

DIABETES. Japanese researchers followed 17,413 adults ages 40 to 65 for 5 years. Compared with those who drank little green tea (less than 1 cup per week), participants who drank 6 cups or more a day were 33 percent less likely to develop type 2 diabetes. Another Japanese research team came up with similar results using oolong tea.

WEIGHT CONTROL. Caffeine increases basal metabolic rate, the rate at which the body burns calories while at rest. Several studies show that in physician-supervised weight-loss programs, coffee drinking modestly increases weight loss (see Coffee on page 164). French and Japanese studies show that tea also contributes to weight loss.

COGNITIVE FUNCTION. The risk factors for heart disease and stroke—high cholesterol, high blood pressure, sedentary lifestyle, high-fat diet, smoking, and diabetes—also increase risk for dementia. Tea helps prevent heart disease, so researchers have begun to study its impact on cognition. Animal studies suggest that tea's antioxidant constituents improve cognition. In addition, Japanese researchers surveyed 1,003 elderly Japanese about their tea consumption, and then gave them standard cognitive function tests. As green tea drinking increased, cognitive impairment decreased. One cup a day cut cognitive impairment in half.

OSTEOPOROSIS. Fluoride plays a role in bone strength, and tea contains it. Japanese researchers surveyed the diets and lifestyles of 632 women and then tested their bone mineral density (BMD), a measure of bone strength. Compared with those who drank green tea infrequently, women who drank it regularly had significantly greater BMD. Studies in Australia and Iran agree that habitual tea drinking improves BMD and reduces risk of osteoporosis.

RHEUMATOID ARTHRITIS (RA). University of Alabama researchers followed 31,336 women ages 55 to 69 for 9 years. At the start of the study, none had RA, but by the end, 158 had been diagnosed. They drank less tea than those who remained free of RA. In fact, drinking more than 3 cups of tea a day reduced RA risk by 61 percent.

ECZEMA. In addition to its potent antioxidant action, the EGCG in tea is also anti-inflammatory, and several studies have shown that it helps manage eczema. In one study, Japanese scientists asked 118 people with severe eczema to add 3 cups of oolong tea a day to their treatment regimens. After 1 month, 63 percent showed "moderate to marked improvement."

DIARRHEA. Tea contains astringent tannins, whose binding action helps treat diarrhea. Tea is one component of the BRATT diet, a popular home remedy for diarrhea that consists of bananas, rice, applesauce, tea, and toast.

TOOTH DECAY. Tea is a good source of fluoride, which helps prevent tooth decay. Both green and black teas contain more fluoride than fluoridated water. The tannins in tea may also help fight the bacteria that cause tooth decay. A Japanese study shows that tea inhibits the bacteria that cause tooth decay and produce dental plaque.

DEATH FROM ALL CAUSES. With tea reducing the risk of so many serious conditions, Japanese researchers wondered if it might be literally a lifesaver. To find out, they followed 40,530 healthy Japanese adults for 11 years. Drinking tea decreased risk of death from *all causes*. Compared with those drinking less than 1 cup a day, people who drank tea regularly had reduced risk of death, with greater tea consumption corresponding to greater benefit. Drinking 5 or more cups a day cut death risk by 12 percent in men and by 23 percent in women.

Different Teas, Different Amounts of Caffeine

Tea leaves contain caffeine. But as the leaves dry, wilt, and oxidize, they lose water and become more compressed—and the caffeine they contain becomes more concentrated. As a result, white tea contains the least caffeine (less than 30 milligrams per 5-ounce cup). Green tea contains more (about 30 milligrams). Oolong has even more (about 50 milligrams), and black tea contains the most (about 100 milligrams per cup).

Intriguing Possibilities

In a pilot study in Japan, people with genital warts treated them with either a skin cream or a cream infused with extracts of green tea. In the tea group, the warts cleared up significantly faster.

A Chinese report claims that tea helps treat hepatitis. Hepatitis is a serious disease that requires professional care, but during convalescence, tea does no harm, and it may do some good.

Rx Recommendations

Based on current research, green tea is the variety with the most beneficial health effects. If you're used to the rich, full-bodied flavor of black tea, green tea may taste thin and watery at first. But over time, you may come to appreciate its delicate flavor.

How strong a brew is necessary to maximize green tea's antioxidant benefits? University of Hawaii researchers steeped batches of green tea for 3, 5, and 10 minutes, then ran laboratory tests to determine each brew's antioxidant activity. They all packed about the same antioxidant punch. Apparently, the antioxidant compounds in green tea are released quickly, and steeping longer than 3 minutes does not appreciably increase their concentration.

For a pleasantly bitter infusion, use 1 tea bag or 1 to 2 teaspoons of dried herb per cup of boiling water. Steep for 10 to 15 minutes and strain (if you use loose tea).

In many of the studies showing that tea reduces risk of cancer and heart disease, participants drank more than 5 cups a day. That might expose you to more caffeine than you can comfortably tolerate. Decaffeinated tea retains its antioxidants.

The Safety Factor

Caffeine is a classically addictive drug that causes nervousness, restlessness, insomnia, and many other potentially problematic effects. (For more information, see Coffee on page 164.)

Caffeine has been linked to an increased risk of birth defects, so pregnant women should not consume it.

Brewing the Perfect Cup of Tea

It starts with the water. Nonchlorinated is best, according to Lori Glenn of the American Botanical Council (ABC), because chlorination interferes with tea's flavor.

Tea connoisseurs advise against boiling the water. They say tea tastes best when made with water that's not quite boiled, or that has boiled and cooled a bit. The optimal steeping temperature for oolong and black teas is approximately 175°F, for white and green teas, around 140°F.

Tea strength depends on the amount of leaves used and steeping time. The amount typically recommended is 3 grams per cup, or about a rounded teaspoon. Steeping time is a matter of personal preference, but ABC recommends 2 to 3 minutes for green tea, longer for oolong and black teas. If you enjoy strong tea, keep the leaves in the water as you drink.

Large amounts of tea may cause gastrointestinal upset.

Do not give tea to children under 2. Young children may drink weak tea. Kids over 12 can drink adult-strength tea.

Inform health care professionals of the herbs you use. Problematic herb-drug interactions are possible.

Tea may cause allergic reactions or other unexpected side effects. If any develop, reduce your dose or stop taking it.

For more on herb safety, see Chapter 2.

If symptoms get worse or persist longer than 2 weeks, consult a health care professional promptly.

Growing Information

Tea is not grown in the United States. It's native to the area where southwest China meets northwest India.

Tea leaves grow on a subtropical evergreen tree that can reach 30 feet, but growers prune it into a waist-high bush for easy leaf harvesting. China and India each produce about one-quarter of the world's production, with most of the rest grown in Sri Lanka, Kenya, Turkey, Indonesia, and Vietnam.

TEA TREE
The Antiseptic from Down Under

Family: Myrtaceae; other members include eucalyptus, myrtle, and clove

Genus and species: *Melaleuca alternifolia*

Also known as: Tea tree oil and Australian tea tree

Part used: Leaf oil

Don't confuse tea tree with *Camellia sinensis*, the plant whose leaves give us the tasty, mildly stimulating beverage—and powerful medicine—known as tea (see page 446). Tea tree, *Melaleuca alternifolia*, has some impressive therapeutic powers of its own.

Healing History

When the British explorer Captain James Cook first arrived in Australia in 1777, he found the indigenous people treating skin infections with crushed tea tree leaves. White settlers adopted the plant and used its leaves to make a tealike beverage, hence the name tea tree. They also used the leaves to flavor beer. Australian physicians introduced tea tree's medicinal benefits to Europe and the United States.

During the 1920s, tea tree oil was used as an antiseptic in surgery and dentistry. During World War II, it was used to disinfect wounds.

Today, tea tree oil is an ingredient in some antiseptic soaps, creams, acne products, deodorants, toothpastes, mouthwashes, and antifungal creams and vaginal suppositories.

Therapeutic Uses

Modern science has discovered that the essential oil liberated by crushing tea tree leaves is a powerful antiseptic.

WOUNDS. A study at the University of Western Australia found that tea tree oil kills many microorganisms that can cause infection, including the yeast fungus *Candida albicans* and several bacteria—*Escherichia coli, Staphylococcus aureus,* and *Pseudomonas aeruginosa.* Another study at the same university showed that even when *Staphylococcus* bacteria are resistant to pharmaceutical antibiotics, tea tree oil often kills them.

Tea tree oil can also be used to treat insect bites and stings. It even has a reputation for relieving the pain of fire ant bites.

ATHLETE'S FOOT. Australian researchers gave people with athlete's foot one of the following treatments: a medically inactive placebo cream; a cream containing 1 percent tolnaftate, a standard pharmaceutical (used in Desenex and Tinactin); or a cream containing 10 percent tea tree oil. The herb was as effective as the tolnaftate.

ACNE. At Royal Prince Alfred Hospital in Australia, researchers gave 124 people with mild to moderate acne either an over-the-counter 5 percent benzoyl peroxide lotion or a lotion containing tea tree oil. The benzoyl peroxide lotion worked faster, but by the end of the study, both treatments were equally effective. Tea tree oil caused fewer side effects such as skin irritation.

FUNGAL TOENAIL INFECTIONS. Stubborn, hard-to-treat fungal toenail infections discolor and thicken toenails. At the University of Rochester School of Medicine, researchers had 117 people with fungal toenail infections apply either a standard pharmaceutical (1 percent clotrimazole) or tea tree oil (100 percent) twice a day for 6 months. Both treatments produced the same results. Sixty percent of the people in each group experienced improvements or cure.

YEAST INFECTIONS. Tea tree oil's activity against the yeast fungus has led to its use in treating vaginal yeast infections.

Intriguing Possibilities

Added to baths or vaporizers, tea tree oil may help treat respiratory infections.

Australians also use tea tree oil to treat scabies and head lice.

Rx Recommendations

Use a cotton ball or cotton swab to apply 100 percent tea tree oil to affected skin or toenails twice a day.

If you've been diagnosed with a vaginal yeast infection, try placing a few drops of tea tree oil on a tampon and inserting it. Leave it in place for 24 hours, then remove it. If continued treatment is necessary, use a new tampon.

The Safety Factor

Do not ingest tea tree oil. Swallowing as little as a few teaspoons can be fatal.

Anyone may use tea tree oil topically, including children, the elderly, and pregnant or nursing women (who should use it in consultation with their physicians). For those with sensitive skin (particularly children and people with fair complexions), dilute the oil in vegetable oil before applying.

A report in the *New England Journal of Medicine* describes three boys who developed enlarged breasts (gynecomastia) after applying tea tree oil to their skin. Their breasts returned to normal when the oil treatment was discontinued. Evidently, tea tree oil has estrogenic action that in rare cases causes breast tissue overgrowth. Oddly, however, there are no reports of women using tea tree oil for breast augmentation.

Inform health care professionals of the herbs you use. Problematic herb-drug interactions are possible.

Tea tree oil may cause allergic reactions or other unexpected side effects. If any develop, reduce your dose or stop taking it.

For more on herb safety, see Chapter 2.

If symptoms get worse or persist longer than 2 weeks, consult a health care professional promptly.

Growing Information

Native to the swampy lowlands of New South Wales, Australia, tea tree is an evergreen that can reach 40 feet. It has narrow, needlelike leaves that release the plant's antiseptic, aromatic oil when crushed. Its white flowers bloom in summer. The tree is not grown in the United States.

THYME

The Power behind Listerine

Family: Labiatae; other members include mints

Genus and species: *Thymus vulgaris* and
  T. serpyllum

Also known as: Common or garden thyme
  (*T. vulgaris*); wild thyme, creeping thyme,
  mother thyme, and mother of thyme
  (*T. serpyllum*)

Parts used: Leaves and flowers

Parsley, sage, rosemary, and . . . Listerine? Or
perhaps Vicks VapoRub?

Thyme is commonly found in kitchen spice
racks, but without realizing it, millions of Americans stock the herb's oil in their medicine chests
as well. Its inclusion in mouthwashes and decongestants is no coincidence. Thyme has a long
history of use as an antiseptic, cough remedy,
and digestive aid.

Healing History

Both the Roman poet Virgil and his naturalist
countryman Pliny mention thyme as a meat preservative. The herb was sprinkled on sacrificial
animals to make them more acceptable to the
gods.

Like so many other aromatic herbs, thyme
was introduced into cooking as an offshoot of its
meat-preserving action. The Romans also used
it medicinally as a cough remedy, digestive aid,
and treatment for intestinal worms.

The emperor Charlemagne ordered thyme
grown in all of his imperial gardens for both its
culinary and medicinal value. The 12th-century
German abbess/herbalist Hildegard of Bingen
considered it the herb of choice for skin problems, anticipating its later use as an antiseptic.

During the Middle Ages, thyme became
linked to courage. It was fashionable for noble-
women to embroider sprigs of thyme on scarves
and give them to favorite knights departing for
the Crusades.

As the centuries passed, thyme was used as
an antiseptic during plagues. Those troubled by
"melancholia" (depression) were advised to sleep
on thyme-stuffed pillows.

Medieval anatomists named the lymph gland
in the chest the thymus because it reminded
them of a thyme flower.

Sixteenth-century British herbalist John
Gerard recommended thyme for leprosy and to
"cure sciatica . . . pains in the head . . . [and]
falling sickness [epilepsy]."

In the 17th century, Nicholas Culpeper called
thyme "excellent for nervous disorders . . . headaches . . . and a certain remedy for that troublesome complaint, the nightmare." He claimed
that the herb "provokes the terms [menstrua-

tion], gives safe and speedy delivery to women in travail [labor], and brings away the after-birth." Culpepper also recommended thyme as "a noble strengthener of the lungs . . . an excellent remedy for shortness of breath. . . . It purges the body of phlegm . . . comforts the stomach much and expels wind."

By the late 17th century, apothecary shops were selling thyme oil as a topical antiseptic under the name "oil of origanum." In 1719, German chemist Caspar Neumann extracted thyme oil's active constituent, which he called "camphor of thyme." In 1853, French chemist M. Lallemand named it thymol.

From the mid-19th century through World War I, thymol enjoyed great popularity as an antiseptic. America's Eclectic physicians, forerunners of today's naturopaths, extolled it in their textbook *King's American Dispensatory* (1898): "Thymol is considered by many to be superior to carbolic acid [the antiseptic made famous in 1867 by the father of antiseptic surgery, Joseph Lister]. It prevents putrefaction and arrests it when it has commenced. . . . Dissolved in water, it forms an invaluable disinfectant [for] sick rooms." The Eclectics also prescribed thyme infusion for headache, gastrointestinal upsets, "hysteria" (menstrual cramps), and as a menstruation promoter.

World War I caused a major thymol crisis. Most of the world's supply was distilled in Germany. When the British and French declared war on Germany, they had to scramble to overcome a terrible shortage of the suddenly vital battlefield antiseptic.

Although thymol has since been replaced by more potent germ fighters, it remains an ingredient in several antiseptic mouthwashes, including Listerine.

Contemporary herbalists recommend thyme externally for disinfecting wounds and internally for indigestion, sore throats, laryngitis, coughs, whooping cough, and nervousness.

Therapeutic Uses

Thyme's aromatic oil contains two compounds, thymol and carvacol, that account for its medicinal value. Both chemicals have preservative, antibacterial, and antifungal properties. They also have expectorant properties and may be useful as digestive aids.

INFECTIONS. In laboratory studies, thyme fights several disease-causing bacteria and fungi, supporting the herb's traditional role as an antiseptic. Infusions of the dried herb are nowhere near as powerful as the oil or distilled thymol, but you can use fresh leaves as garden first aid for minor wounds.

COUGHS. German researchers have lent support to thyme's traditional role as a phlegm loosener (expectorant). In Germany, where herbal medicine is considerably more mainstream than in the United States, thyme preparations are frequently prescribed to relax the respiratory tract and treat coughs, whooping cough, and emphysema.

German medical herbalist Rudolph Fritz Weiss, M.D., writes, "Thyme is to the trachea [windpipe] and the bronchi what peppermint is to the stomach and intestines." Commission E, the expert panel that evaluates herbal medicines for the German counterpart of the FDA, approves thyme as a treatment for cold-related coughs, bronchitis, and whooping cough.

DIGESTIVE PROBLEMS. Thymol and carvacol relax the smooth muscle tissue of the gastrointestinal tract, making thyme an antispasmodic. The action of these chemical constituents lends support to its traditional role as a digestive aid.

WOMEN'S HEALTH CONCERNS. Antispasmodics relax not only the digestive tract but also other smooth muscles, such as the uterus. Tincture of thyme may help relieve menstrual cramps, lending credence to the Eclectic physicians' use of this herb.

In large amounts, thyme oil and thymol are considered uterine stimulants.

Intriguing Possibility

In a laboratory study, Israeli scientists have found that thyme infusion inhibits the growth of *Helicobacter pylori*, the bacteria that cause most gastrointestinal ulcers. It's too early to call thyme an ulcer treatment, but if you have ulcers, you may want to try drinking thyme tea.

Rx Recommendations

For garden accidents, crush fresh leaves into minor wounds until you can wash and bandage them. After you have thoroughly washed them, apply a few drops of thyme tincture as an antiseptic.

For an infusion to help settle the stomach, soothe a cough, or possibly help relieve menstrual symptoms, use 2 teaspoons of dried herb per cup of boiling water. Steep for 10 minutes, then strain. Drink up to 3 cups a day. Thyme tastes pleasantly aromatic, with a faint clovelike aftertaste.

As a homemade tincture, take $1/2$ to 1 teaspoon up to three times a day.

When using commercial preparations, follow the package directions.

The Safety Factor

Use the herb, not its oil. Even a few teaspoons of thyme oil can be toxic, causing headache, nausea, vomiting, weakness, thyroid impairment, and heart and respiratory depression.

One animal study showed that thyme suppresses thyroid activity in rats. People with thyroid conditions should consult their physicians before taking medicinal doses.

Pregnant women may use thyme as a culinary spice, but they should avoid large amounts and not ingest the oil. Nursing women should also avoid thyme oil.

Do not give medicinal preparations of thyme to children under 2. In older children, adjust the recommended dose based on the child's weight. For example, give a 50-pound child one-third of the dose a 150-pound adult would take.

If you're over 65, start with a low dose, and increase only if necessary.

Inform health care professionals of the herbs you use. Problematic herb-drug interactions are possible.

Thyme or thyme oil may cause a rash in sensitive individuals. It may also cause allergic reactions or other unexpected side effects. If any develop, reduce your dose or stop taking it.

For more on herb safety, see Chapter 2.

If symptoms get worse or persist longer than 2 weeks, consult a health care professional promptly.

Growing Information

Thyme is an aromatic, perennial, many-branched, ground-cover shrub that reaches about 12 inches. It has small, opposite, virtually stalkless leaves and lilac or pink flowers that bloom in midsummer.

This hardy herb can be propagated from seeds, cuttings, and root divisions. Seeds require a temperature around 70°F to germinate and often do best when started indoors. For cuttings, snip 3-inch pieces from stems with new growth and place them in wet sand. Roots should appear in about 2 weeks.

The best time for root division is in spring. Uproot a plant carefully, preserving as much of its root soil as possible. Divide it in half or thirds and replant the divisions 12 inches apart in moist soil.

Once established, thyme requires little care. It prefers well-drained, slightly dry soil. Wetting thyme leaves during watering reduces their fragrance.

Clumps tend to become woody after a few years. To prevent this, roots should be divided periodically.

Thyme survives frost, but in areas with cold winters, use mulch. Thyme may be killed if winter temperatures drop below 10°F.

Harvest the leaves and flowers just before the flowers bloom. Dry and store them in airtight containers to preserve the herb's oil.

TURMERIC

Yellow Curry Is Loaded with Healing Potential

Family: Zingiberaceae; other members include ginger

Genus and species: *Curcuma longa*

Also known as: Curcumin

Parts used: Rhizomes and roots

Turmeric is a fairly recent addition to most American spice racks, but it's been a mainstay in Indian curries for thousands of years. Its arrival here is good news for both our palates and our health. The culinary herb is called turmeric, but in herbal medicine, this herb is usually called curcumin, the name of the pigment that gives the rhizome its yellowish color.

To date, there have been more than 1,000 laboratory and animal studies of curcumin. The weight of the available evidence suggests that curcumin is a powerfully medicinal herb that stimulates the immune system and reduces risk of heart disease, cancer, dementia, ulcers, colitis, arthritis, cataracts, scabies, liver damage, food poisoning, and irritable bowel syndrome.

Unfortunately, curcumin has not been well researched in humans. However, the clinical trials that have been published corroborate the laboratory and animal findings. At this point, we can say with confidence that curcumin is loaded with healing potential. And because it's been a food for thousands of years, it's not necessary to wait for definitive evidence to incorporate more curry dishes into your diet or take a curcumin supplement.

Healing History

In Indian cooking, the term *curry* means any multispice blend. But in the United States, most curry comes prepackaged and has a yellow cast because it contains turmeric.

In addition to its role in cooking, the herb holds a place of honor in India's traditional Ayurvedic medicine. A symbol of prosperity, it was considered a cleanser for the whole body. Medically, it was used as a digestive aid and as a treatment for fever, infections, dysentery, arthritis, and jaundice and other liver problems.

Traditional Chinese physicians prescribed turmeric to treat liver and gallbladder problems, stop bleeding, and relieve chest congestion and menstrual discomforts.

The ancient Greeks were well aware of turmeric, but unlike its close botanical relative, ginger, it never caught on in the West as either a culinary or a medicinal herb. It was, however, used to make orange-yellow dyes.

In the 1870s, chemists noticed that turmeric's orange-yellow root powder turned reddish brown when exposed to alkaline chemicals. This discovery led to the development of "turmeric paper," thin strips of tissue brushed with a decoction of turmeric, then dried. During the late 19th century, turmeric paper was used in laboratories around the world to test for alkalinity. Eventually, it was replaced by litmus paper, which is still used today.

American chemists used turmeric paper, but not even the botanically oriented 19th-century Eclectic physicians, forerunners of today's naturopaths, had much use for turmeric itself, except to add color to medicinal ointments.

In the 1930s, Maude Grieve's influential *Modern Herbal* said that turmeric was "once a cure for jaundice," then dismissed it as "seldom used in medicine except as a coloring."

Today's naturopaths may be the intellectual heirs of Eclectic medicine, but they've parted company with their predecessors when it comes to turmeric. They extol the herb as an anti-inflammatory. "Turmeric is one of nature's most potent anti-inflammatory agents," says Joseph Pizzorno, N.D., coauthor of *The Textbook of Natural Medicine* and former president of Bastyr University, the naturopathic medical school near Seattle.

Naturopaths also recommend turmeric for the prevention and treatment of degenerative conditions that respond to antioxidants, including cancer and heart disease.

Therapeutic Uses

Curcumin has a remarkable number of healing actions.

ENHANCED IMMUNITY. Indian researchers tested the immune function of laboratory animals, then fed them a curcumin-enriched diet for 5 weeks. Subsequent retesting showed significant improvement in immune function.

FOOD POISONING. Because it stimulates the immune system, curcumin is effective against a number of disease-causing microorganisms, including salmonella bacteria, a frequent cause of food poisoning (also called gastroenteritis and stomach flu).

PREVENTION OF DEGENERATIVE DISEASES. Curcumin is a rich source of antioxidants that help prevent and reverse the cell damage (oxidative damage) at the root of heart disease, cancer, and many other conditions associated with aging.

CANCER. Curcumin helps prevent cancer in two ways. Its immune-boosting action has a cancer-preventive effect, and its high antioxidant content helps prevent the cell damage that sets the stage for cancer. Many laboratory and animal studies show that curcumin has anti-cancer activity. Reports published in journals such as *Cancer Letters, Cancer Research,* and *Carcinogenesis* say that the compound inhibits the growth of several cancers, among them colon cancer and lymphoma.

Indian researchers tested smokers' urine for compounds that cause genetic mutations (mutagens), a marker for cancer-causing biochemical activity. Then they were given 1.5 grams of turmeric (about a teaspoon) for 30 days. Even though they didn't change their smoking habits, the number of mutagens in their urine decreased significantly.

Another Indian clinical trial shows that as curcumin consumption increases, risk of colon cancer decreases.

HEART DISEASE. Turmeric's close botanical relative, ginger, reduces cholesterol, lowers blood pressure, and helps prevent the blood clots that trigger heart attacks and most strokes. Animal studies show that curcumin offers similar benefits.

In a pilot study, Indian researchers measured the cholesterol levels of 10 adults, then asked them to take 500 milligrams of curcumin. After 10 days, their cholesterol levels had fallen significantly.

COGNITIVE FUNCTION. Oxidative damage plays a substantial role in age-related loss of cognitive function, and the development of dementia. Antioxidants such as curcumin help prevent cognitive impairment.

Researchers in Singapore surveyed the curry/curcumin consumption of 1,010 elderly Asians, and then gave them a battery of cognitive function tests. Compared with those who ate curries with curcumin rarely, those who enjoyed curries frequently had significantly better cognitive function, with function improving as curcumin intake increased.

CATARACTS. Cataracts are caused by oxidative damage to the lens of the eye, the type of damage that antioxidants help prevent. In one study, animals were fed a diet enriched with either corn oil or turmeric for 14 days, then exposed to conditions that produce cataracts. The animals that were fed turmeric developed significantly fewer cataracts.

ARTHRITIS. Joint pain and stiffness often respond to aspirin or ibuprofen. Chemically, these familiar pain relievers are nonsteroidal anti-inflammatory drugs (NSAIDs). However, aspirin and ibuprofen are not powerful enough to relieve chronic arthritis and conditions such as rheumatoid arthritis, which is why doctors often prescribe more powerful prescription NSAIDs. Unfortunately, these drugs may cause potentially severe stomach distress. Curcumin is a natural member of a non-NSAID class of anti-inflammatory agents, the COX-2 inhibitors, that pose much less risk of stomach upset. (While turmeric's COX-2 action can help treat inflammatory conditions, it is not as potent as COX-2 pharmaceuticals. This has one key benefit—unlike the pharmaceuticals, which have been linked with increased risk of stroke and heart attack, there are no such documented side effects with turmeric. In fact, the herb's antioxidant action helps prevent stroke and heart attack.)

Several Indian studies have tested curcumin as a treatment for osteoarthritis and rheumatoid arthritis, with positive results. In one study, the herb relieved the morning stiffness and joint swelling of rheumatoid arthritis as well as a prescription NSAID, but caused no significant abdominal distress.

LIVER DAMAGE. Several animal studies suggest that turmeric protects the liver from the damaging effects of many toxic compounds, including alcohol, aflatoxin, and carbon tetrachloride.

The drugs used to treat tuberculosis often cause liver damage. Indian researchers gave 508 people being treated for tuberculosis either standard medications or those drugs plus curcumin (1 gram twice a day) and another herb, guduchi (1 gram twice a day). In the drugs-only group, 14 percent developed signs of liver damage. But in the herb group, the figure was less than 1 percent. These findings lend credence to the herb's traditional use in liver ailments.

If you regularly drink alcohol and/or regularly take certain pharmaceuticals, including large doses of the common pain reliever acetaminophen, you may be at risk for liver damage. Curcumin might help protect your liver.

IRRITABLE BOWEL SYNDROME. British researchers surveyed the symptoms of 207 people with irritable bowel syndrome, then gave them turmeric. After 8 weeks, their symptom scores declined significantly.

ULCERS. Thai scientists gave 45 people with ulcers large amounts of curcumin (600 milligrams five times a day). Within 2 weeks, many reported fewer symptoms using standard measures of ulcer severity. After 12 weeks, 76 percent reported improvement.

ULCERATIVE COLITIS. Japanese gastroenterologists gave either standard drugs or the drugs plus 1 gram of curcumin twice a day to 45 people with ulcerative colitis who were not having significant symptoms. After 6 months, 21 percent of the drugs-only group relapsed. But among those who took curcumin, the figure was only 5 percent.

DIGESTIVE PROBLEMS. Turmeric stimulates the flow of bile, which helps digest fats. This validates the herb's traditional role as a digestive aid. Commission E, the expert panel that evaluates herbal medicines for the German counterpart of the FDA, approves turmeric for indigestion.

SCABIES. In an Indian study, 814 people infested with tiny, itchy scabies mites were treated with a combination of curcumin and another Indian herb, neem (see page 345). Almost all of the study participants (97 percent) reported that the infestation disappeared in 3 to 15 days. The treatment was cheaper than standard medical scabicides and caused no adverse reactions.

Intriguing Possibilities

In laboratory studies, curcumin shows potent action against disease-causing protozoa, lending some credence to its traditional use in treating amoebic dysentery. One of the world's pernicious protozoa is the one-celled animal that causes malaria. Indian researchers infected mice with the disease, and then gave them curcumin. After herb treatment, blood levels of the protozoa dropped by 80 percent.

Indian animal studies also suggest that curcumin might have a mood-elevating effect.

At the cellular level, curcumin has effects that inhibit the cascade of biochemical reactions involved in cystic fibrosis (CF). Studies of laboratory animals bred to develop CF suggest that curcumin extends their lives. It's too early to call the herb a treatment for CF, but in the future, it might be. Meanwhile, for those with CF, there's no harm in eating turmeric-rich curries and taking curcumin supplements.

Other laboratory and animal studies suggest that turmeric may help prevent ulcers, gallstones, and Parkinson's disease. Studies also show that it may lower blood sugar, suggesting that it could help control diabetes.

Medicinal Myth

The Chinese used turmeric to stimulate menstruation. To date, no research has confirmed that the herb has any effect on the uterus.

Rx Recommendations

For an infusion to help aid digestion, use 1 teaspoon of turmeric powder per cup of warm milk.

Drink up to 3 cups a day. Turmeric tastes pleasantly aromatic, but in large amounts, it becomes somewhat bitter.

Another option is to buy curcumin supplements. Dr. Pizzorno recommends 400 milligrams of curcumin three times a day, or you can follow the package directions on the product you choose.

The Safety Factor

Unusually large amounts of turmeric may cause stomach upset.

Inform health care professionals of the herbs you use. Problematic herb-drug interactions are possible.

Turmeric and curcumin may cause allergic reactions or other unexpected side effects. If any develop, reduce your dose or stop taking it.

For more on herb safety, see Chapter 2.

If symptoms get worse or persist longer than 2 weeks, consult a health care professional promptly.

Growing Information

Turmeric is not a garden herb in North America. Grown from India to Indonesia, it's a perennial with a pulpy, orange, tuberous rhizome (underground stem) that grows to about 2 feet in length. The aerial parts, which reach 3 feet, include large, lily-like leaves; a thick, squat, central flower spike; and funnel-shaped yellow flowers.

UVA-URSI

The Urinary Antiseptic

Family: Ericaceae; other members include azalea, blueberry, and cranberry

Genus and species: *Arctostaphylos uva-ursi*

Also known as: Bearberry, bear's grape, upland cranberry, and arbutus

Parts used: Leaves

Ancient Mediterranean bears must have loved the bright red, mealy, currant-size berries of this delicate, branching, perennial ground cover. Both its Greek genus name, *Arctostaphylos*, and its Latin-rooted species name, *uva-ursi*, mean bear's berry. The plant is often called bearberry in English. It's the leaves, however, not the berries, that are used in herbal healing.

Uva-ursi has been used as a diuretic and urinary antiseptic for more than 1,000 years by cultures as widely separated as the Chinese and Native Americans. Today, it is an ingredient in many herbal diuretics, urinary remedies, and weight-loss formulas. Even the late herbal conservative Varro E. Tyler, Ph.D., described uva-ursi as "a modestly effective urinary antiseptic and diuretic."

Uva-ursi may not be effective if it's taken in combination with certain foods, however. This is important information that some herbals fail to mention.

Healing History

The Roman physician Galen used uva-ursi's astringent leaves to treat wounds and stop bleeding, but the herb was largely ignored by Western herbalists until the 13th century. Then, Marco Polo reported that Chinese physicians prescribed it as a diuretic to treat kidney and urinary problems. Polo's famous travelogue popularized uva-ursi in Europe as a urinary and kidney remedy.

Uva-ursi's association with the kidney was strengthened by the medieval Doctrine of Signatures, the belief, once widely held, that a plant's physical attributes revealed its healing virtues. The herb grew in rocky, gravelly places, and at the time, kidney stones were called "gravel."

North American colonists found that Native Americans had independently discovered uva-ursi's urinary benefits. They also mixed its leathery leaves with tobacco and created the smoking mixture kinnikinnik.

Uva-ursi was incorporated into the *U.S. Pharmacopoeia*, a standard drug reference, as a urinary antiseptic in 1820 and remained there until 1936. Chemists isolated the herb's major active compound, arbutin, in 1852.

America's 19th-century Eclectics, forerunners of today's naturopaths, recommended uva-ursi for diarrhea, dysentery, gonorrhea, bed-wetting, and "chronic affections of the kidneys and urinary passages."

Today, homeopaths recommend a microdose of uva-ursi for incontinence, blood in the urine, and kidney and urinary tract infections.

Contemporary herbalists continue to recommend uva-ursi for kidney and urinary problems.

Therapeutic Uses

According to several studies, the arbutin in uva-ursi is chemically transformed into an antimicrobial antiseptic, hydroquinone, in the urinary tract. In addition, the herb contains several diuretic chemicals (including ursolic acid), powerful astringents (tannins), and allantoin, a chemical that helps promote the growth of healthy new cells.

URINARY TRACT INFECTIONS. The actions of uva-ursi's active compounds support its age-old use in treating urinary tract infections (UTIs) and other urinary ailments. The herb is notably effective against *Escherichia coli*, the most frequent cause of UTIs. Some herbalists report that uva-ursi has cured UTIs that were unresponsive to pharmaceutical antibiotics. This is certainly possible, but scientific sources say that pharmaceutical antibiotics are generally more effective.

For mild urinary symptoms, try uva-ursi as herbal first aid. For urinary problems that require professional care, use the herb in addition to standard therapies. Commission E, the expert panel that evaluates herbal medicines for the German counterpart of the FDA, approves uva-ursi for urinary tract ailments.

There's an important catch to using uva-ursi, however. To receive the greatest antiseptic benefit, the urine must be alkaline. This means that you must avoid acidic foods and supplements, such as sauerkraut, citrus fruits and their juices, and vitamin C, while taking the herb. You must also cut down on protein (meats, poultry, fish, and dairy foods) because proteins are composed of amino acids that also turn the urine acidic.

PREMENSTRUAL SYNDROME. Diuretics may provide relief from the premenstrual bloating that bothers many women. Pregnant and nursing women should not take diuretics, however. Uva-ursi also stimulates uterine contractions in animal studies, making it even more off-limits to women who are pregnant or trying to conceive.

HIGH BLOOD PRESSURE. Physicians often prescribe diuretics to treat high blood pressure. High blood pressure is a serious condition that requires professional care, so if you have it and would like to include uva-ursi in your overall treatment plan, discuss it with your physician.

Diuretics deplete the body of potassium, an essential nutrient. If you use uva-ursi regularly, be sure to eat more potassium-rich foods such as bananas and fresh vegetables.

CONGESTIVE HEART FAILURE. Physicians often prescribe diuretics to treat congestive heart failure, which involves serious fatigue of the heart. This condition requires professional care. If you would like to include uva-ursi in your overall treatment plan, discuss using it with your physician.

WOUNDS. When applied topically, uva-ursi's allantoin may help spur wound healing. Allantoin is the active ingredient in Derma-Heal, an over-the-counter skin cream.

DIARRHEA. The astringent tannins in uva-ursi are binding and help relieve diarrhea.

Intriguing Possibilities

Uva-ursi appears to have some anti-inflammatory action and may help heal dermatitis. In animal studies, the herb has helped treat hepatitis.

Rx Recommendations

To treat wounds, apply fresh, crushed leaves to minor cuts and scrapes after thoroughly washing them with soap and water. You can also dip a clean cloth in a decoction and apply the compress to the affected area.

To minimize the unpleasantly astringent taste of this high-tannin herb, soak the leaves in cold water overnight. Then, to prepare a decoction for relief from urinary symptoms or diarrhea, simmer 1 teaspoon per cup of boiling water for 10 minutes, then strain. Drink up to 3 cups a day.

As a homemade tincture, use $1/4$ to 1 teaspoon up to three times a day.

When using commercial preparations, follow the package directions.

The Safety Factor

Uva-ursi often turns urine a dark green. This is harmless and should be no cause for alarm.

Herbal weight-loss formulas typically contain diuretics, with uva-ursi being among the common ingredients. Because diuretics boost urine production, they temporarily eliminate some water weight. Any pounds lost with help from diuretics almost invariably return, however, and weight-loss experts advise against using diuretics. The keys to permanent weight control include a low-fat, high-fiber diet and regular aerobic exercise.

Because uva-ursi is astringent, it can help treat diarrhea. The main medical hazard of diarrhea is dehydration, and because uva-ursi is a diuretic, it may contribute to dehydration. If you use uva-ursi to treat diarrhea, be sure to drink plenty of water and other nonalcoholic fluids.

Uva-ursi has such high levels of tannins that it has been used to tan leather. Large doses of tannins may cause stomach upset.

Tannins also have both pro- and anti-cancer action. Some authorities warn against their use, but tannins' role in human cancers, if any, remains unclear. That said, people who have a history of cancer should either add milk, which appears to neutralize tannins, or not use uva-ursi in large amounts.

Pregnant and nursing women should not use uva-ursi.

Do not give uva-ursi to children under 2. In older children, adjust the recommended dose based on the child's weight. For example, give a 50-pound child one-third of the dose a 150-pound adult would take.

If you're over 65, start with a low dose, and increase only if necessary.

Inform health care professionals of the herbs you use. Problematic herb-drug interactions are possible.

Uva-ursi may cause allergic reactions or other unexpected side effects. If any develop, reduce your dose or stop taking it.

For more on herb safety, see Chapter 2.

If symptoms get worse or persist longer than 2 weeks, consult a health care professional promptly.

Growing Information

Uva-ursi grows throughout the temperate world. It has a long, fibrous root; woody stems and branches; inch-long, leathery, evergreen, paddle-shaped leaves; and tiny white flowers tinged with red. The plant rarely grows taller than a few inches and prefers a dry, rocky, or sandy habitat.

Uva-ursi is typically propagated from cuttings. Be patient. This plant takes an unusually long time to root. It's more convenient simply to buy small plants from a specialty herb nursery.

Uva-ursi does poorly in rich soil. It prefers poor, gravelly, acidic soil, under full sun or partial shade. Keep your uva-ursi patch well weeded until the plants have become established. It does not transplant well. Once established, uva-ursi spreads to become a hearty, attractive ground cover that can survive temperatures of −50°F.

Harvest leaves in autumn before the first frost. Because of their leathery texture, they are difficult to air-dry. Spread them in a single layer and dry them in the oven.

VALERIAN
You're Getting Sleepy . . .

Family: Valerianaceae; other members include spikenard and Jacob's ladder

Genus and species: *Valeriana officinalis*

Also known as: Garden valerian, phu, and all-heal

Parts used: Rhizomes and roots

Back in the 13th century, the elders of Hamelin, Germany, decided to rid their town of rats. They contracted with an itinerant flute player, one Pied Piper, whose music attracted the rodents, allowing him to lead them out of town. But when the Pied Piper returned for his fee, the elders of Hamelin refused to pay him. In revenge, he used his flute to charm Hamelin's children away forever.

In modern versions of this story, the Pied Piper's powers are entirely musical, but early

German folklore also credits him with being an accomplished herbalist. In addition to his hypnotic flute playing, the Pied Piper charmed both the rats and the children with hypnotic valerian root.

Valerian can, indeed, charm rats—and cats. The herb contains chemicals similar to those in catnip.

Healing History

Valerian has such a disagreeable odor that ancient Greek and Roman authorities, including Dioscorides, Pliny, and Galen, all called it *fu*. The term *Valeriana* first appeared around the 10th century, derived from the Latin *valere*, to be strong.

Dioscorides recommended valerian as a diuretic and antidote to poisons. Pliny considered it a pain reliever. Galen prescribed it as a decongestant and sleep aid.

By the time the plant's name became valerian, early European herbalists considered it a panacea and also called it all-heal. The 12th-century German abbess/herbalist Hildegard of Bingen recommended the herb as a tranquilizer and sleep aid about 100 years before the Pied Piper used it as a hypnotic.

During the late 1500s, valerian's popularity grew after an Italian physician claimed that the herb had cured him of epilepsy. In 1597, British herbalist John Gerard wrote that in Scotland "no broth or physic [medicine] . . . be worth anything" if it did not include valerian. Gerard recommended the herb enthusiastically for chest congestion, convulsions, bruises, and falls.

Seventeenth-century English herbalist Nicholas Culpeper added several of his own recommendations: "The decoction of the root . . . is of special virtue against the plague. . . . [It] provokes women's courses [menstruation] . . . is singularly good for those troubled with cough . . . is excellent [for] any sores, hurts, or wounds. . . . " Later, European herbalists considered the herb a digestive aid and treatment for "hysteria" (menstrual discomforts).

Early colonists discovered several Native American tribes using the pulverized roots of American valerian to treat wounds. This use of the herb brought it to the attention of Samuel Thomson, the founder of Thomsonian herbal medicine, which was popular before the Civil War. Thomson called valerian "the best nervine [tranquilizer] known."

Valerian entered the *U.S. Pharmacopoeia*, a standard drug reference, as a tranquilizer in 1820 and remained there until 1942. It was listed in the *National Formulary*, the pharmacists' guide, until 1950.

America's 19th-century Eclectic physicians, forerunners of today's naturopaths, prescribed valerian as a "calmative . . . for epilepsy . . . mild spasmodic affections . . . [and] hypochondria." But the Eclectic text *King's American Dispensatory* (1898) warned against using large doses because they caused "restlessness, agitation, giddiness, nausea, and visual illusions."

During World War I, Europeans afflicted with "overwrought nerves" from artillery bombardment frequently took valerian.

Contemporary herbalists generally agree with David Hoffmann's *Holistic Herbal*, which deems valerian "one of the most useful relaxing herbs." Today's herbalists recommend it for nervousness, anxiety, insomnia, headache, and intestinal cramps.

In Germany, where herbal medicine is considerably more mainstream than in the United

States, valerian is the active ingredient in more than 100 over-the-counter tranquilizers and sleep aids. Some are specially formulated for children, a use the Pied Piper would probably endorse.

Therapeutic Uses

All parts of valerian contain valepotriates, compounds with sedative properties. They occur in highest concentration in the roots.

INSOMNIA. Many studies have found valerian to be an effective sedative.

In one study, German researchers gave 128 people with insomnia either medically inactive placebos or 400 milligrams of valerian root daily. Those who took the herb showed significant improvement in sleep quality without morning grogginess or other significant side effects.

Another team of German scientists gave 68 adults with chronic insomnia either a placebo or a sleep aid containing 320 milligrams of valerian and 160 milligrams of lemon balm, also an herbal tranquilizer (see page 305). Those taking the herbal medicine fell asleep significantly faster, enjoyed significantly longer periods of sleep, and reported significantly greater overall feelings of well-being. The herbal preparation caused no morning hangover.

Swiss researchers repeated this study using a slightly different formula: 360 milligrams of valerian and 240 milligrams of lemon balm once a day, 30 minutes before bedtime. Once again, those who took the herbal combination reported significantly better sleep quality with no side effects.

A third German study used standard physiological tests to measure the depth of sleep in 14 elderly people with insomnia. Compared with those who took placebos, the study participants who took valerian passed more quickly from light stage 1 sleep into deeper sleep. Other studies have reported similar results.

Another German trial tested valerian as a treatment for 918 children with insomnia. Eighty-one percent showed significant improvement in sleep duration and quality.

Some researchers have compared valerian with benzodiazepines such as diazepam (Valium) and triazolam (Halcion). Valerian is a much milder and safer sedative, for the following reasons:

- The benzodiazepines can cause dependence and addiction. Regular users may develop a tolerance and require increasing amounts to obtain the desired effect. When the drug is stopped, they may develop withdrawal symptoms, including restlessness, insomnia, headache, nausea, and vomiting. Although a psychological dependence may develop, valerian is not addictive and discontinuation rarely produces Valium-withdrawal symptoms, but withdrawal reactions, including anxiety, are possible.

- The benzodiazepines' sedative effects increase substantially with simultaneous use of alcohol or barbiturates. The combination is often used in suicide attempts. Valerian's sedative effect increases less with alcohol or barbiturates.

- The benzodiazepines often cause morning grogginess. Unusually large amounts of valerian may cause morning grogginess, but recommended amounts do not.

- Children born to women who used Valium while pregnant are at increased risk for cleft palate. Valerian has not been linked to birth defects.

Commission E, the expert panel that evaluates herbal medicines for the German counterpart of the FDA, endorses valerian for sleep problems.

Intriguing Possibilities

Animal studies suggest that valerian has anticonvulsant effects, lending some credence to its traditional use in treating epilepsy.

Animal studies have also found that valerian reduces blood pressure. Of course, what occurs in animals does not necessarily apply to people, but if you have high blood pressure and want to incorporate valerian into your overall treatment plan, discuss it with your physician.

Finally, valerian may have anti-tumor effects.

Rx Recommendations

As a sleep aid, buy a commercial valerian root extract or tincture and follow the label directions. Herbalists discourage using valerian infusions because they taste foul.

The Safety Factor

Unusually large amounts of valerian may cause headache, giddiness, blurred vision, restlessness, nausea, and morning grogginess.

In 1998, a case report in the *Journal of the American Medical Association* suggested that withdrawal from valerian might have contributed to serious complications in one man who was hospitalized for congestive heart failure. It's possible—but this man was taking almost a dozen pharmaceutical drugs, had undergone two invasive procedures (lung

biopsy and cardiac catheterization) under anesthesia, and had taken up to 2 grams of valerian a day for several years, many times the recommended dose.

The Duke University physicians who reported the case concluded: "Valerian root may be associated with serious withdrawal symptoms following abrupt discontinuation." Given this man's precarious medical situation, this seems extremely unlikely for healthy people who take valerian in the recommended amounts.

Harm from valerian overdose seems unlikely. The journal *Veterinary and Human Toxicology* reported the case of a woman who tried to commit suicide by taking 40 capsules of valerian root extract, each containing 470 milligrams of the herb. She experienced fatigue, abdominal cramps, chest tightness, light-headedness, dilated pupils, and hand tremors, all of which cleared up without medical treatment in 24 hours. Medical tests, including liver function tests, were all normal.

Pregnant and nursing women should not use valerian.

Do not give valerian to children under 2. In older children, adjust the recommended dose based on the child's weight. For example, give a 50-pound child one-third of the dose a 150-pound adult would take.

If you're over 65, start with a low dose, and increase only if necessary.

Inform health care professionals of the herbs you use. Problematic herb-drug interactions are possible.

Valerian may cause allergic reactions or other unexpected side effects. If any develop, reduce your dose or stop taking it.

For more on herb safety, see Chapter 2.

If symptoms get worse or persist longer

than 2 weeks, consult a health care professional promptly.

Growing Information

Medicinal valerian is a hardy perennial that reaches about 5 feet. Its medicinal roots consist of long, cylindrical fibers issuing from its rhizome. Its stem is erect, grooved, and hollow. Valerian leaves are fernlike. Tiny white, pink, or lavender flowers develop in umbrella-like clusters and bloom from late spring through summer. When dried, valerian roots have an unpleasant odor, once described by American herbalist Michael Moore as the smell of dirty socks.

Valerian may be propagated from seeds or root divisions. Seeds have limited viability. When viable, they germinate in about 20 days. Roots may be divided in spring or fall. Thin plants to 12-inch spacing. Valerian grows in many soils but does best in rich, moist, well-drained loam under full sun or partial shade. Once established, the plants self-sow and spread by root runners. Older plants become weedy and overcrowded and lose vitality. Thin them when harvesting their roots.

Valerian has an effect on cats similar to that of catnip. Intoxicated felines have been known to destroy plants; use chicken-wire fencing if necessary. Harvest roots in the fall of their 2nd year, and split thick roots to speed drying.

VERVAIN
A Joy of a Healer

Family: Verbenaceae; other members include teak and many other tropical trees and shrubs

Genus and species: *Verbena officinalis* (European); *V. hastata* (American)

Also known as: Simpler's joy, blue vervain, verbena, herb-of-the-cross, enchanter's herb, and Indian hyssop

Parts used: Leaves, flowers, and roots

During the Middle Ages, healing herbs were often called simples, and herbalists were known as simplers. Vervain was prescribed so frequently for so many conditions that it became known as simpler's joy.

The name has some basis in fact. Vervain appears to act like mild aspirin, helping to relieve minor pain and inflammation.

Healing History

In Egyptian mythology, vervain grew from the tears of Isis, goddess of fertility, as she grieved for her murdered brother-husband, Osiris. A thousand years later, vervain entered Christian mythology as the herb pressed into Christ's wounds to stanch his bleeding, hence its name herb-of-the-cross.

Hippocrates recommended vervain for fever and plague. The court physician to Roman emperor Theodosius the Great prescribed it for tumors of the throat (probably goiters). His fanciful prescription advised cutting vervain root into two pieces, then tying one around the patient's throat and hanging the other over a fire. As the heat and smoke shriveled the hanging root, the tumor was supposed to shrink.

The Romans spread vervain throughout Europe, where it became especially popular among the Druids of pre-Christian England. They used the herb in magic spells, hence its name enchanter's herb.

The 12th-century German abbess/herbalist Hildegard of Bingen prescribed a decoction of vervain and vermouth for "toxic blood [infections], toothache, [and] discharges from the brain to the teeth."

Our word *vervain* comes from the Celtic *fer-faen*, from *fer*, to drive away, and *faen*, a stone. This is a reference to the herb's traditional role in treating kidney stones.

During the Middle Ages, vervain became a popular acne remedy. People who had pimples stood outside at night holding a handful of the herb wrapped in a cloth. When a shooting star passed, they rubbed the cloth over their pimples and the blemishes were supposed to disappear.

From a remedy for acne, vervain evolved into a treatment for other skin problems. Seventeenth-century herbalist Nicholas Culpeper wrote, "The leaves bruised, or the juice mixed with vinegar, does wonderfully cleanse the skin, and take away morphew [dandruff]." Culpeper recommended vervain to treat jaundice, gout, cough, wheezing, bleeding gums, shortness of breath, fever, plague, gravel (kidney stones), and dropsy (congestive heart failure). He also said that "used with hog grease, it helps with swellings and pains of the secret parts [genitals]."

Colonists introduced European vervain into North America, and it quickly went wild. They also found Native Americans using the American form of vervain, also known as Indian hyssop, to treat fever and gastrointestinal complaints and to clear cloudy urine.

During the Revolutionary War, military physicians relied on vervain to relieve pain, loosen bronchial mucus, and induce vomiting. More than a century later, the Eclectics, forerunners of today's naturopaths, recommended it as a treatment for fever, colds, coughs, intestinal worms, menstrual irregularity, and bruises, and as a tonic "during convalescence from acute diseases."

Contemporary herbalists recommend vervain as a tranquilizer, expectorant, menstruation promoter, and treatment for headache, fever, depression, seizures, wounds, dental cavities, and gum disease.

Therapeutic Uses

The standard prescription to "take two aspirin and call me in the morning" has long been attributed to physicians. But an herbalist might say the same thing, substituting vervain for aspirin. No wonder they called this herb simpler's joy.

PAIN AND INFLAMMATION. Chemically, vervain is quite different from aspirin, but German and Japanese studies suggest that it has similar effects, combining mild pain relief with some ability to reduce inflammation. These findings support vervain's traditional use in treating headache, toothache, wounds, and kidney stones.

CONSTIPATION. One study suggests that vervain has a mild laxative effect.

Medicinal Myth

Vervain has never been shown to treat dandruff, induce vomiting, promote menstruation, or expel kidney stones. Its primary benefit is its ability to provide mild pain relief.

Rx Recommendations

For a very bitter infusion to help treat headache, mild arthritis, and other minor pains, use 2 teaspoons of dried herb per cup of boiling water. Steep for 10 to 15 minutes, then strain. Drink up to 3 cups a day. Mask vervain's bitterness with sugar, honey, and lemon or mix the herb with an herbal beverage tea.

As a homemade tincture, use $1/2$ to 1 teaspoon up to three times a day.

When using commercial preparations, follow the package directions.

The Safety Factor

European animal studies have found that vervain depresses the heart rate, constricts the bronchial passages, and stimulates the intes-

tines and uterus. Because it may slow heart rate, it should not be used by anyone with congestive heart failure or a history of heart disease. The possibility of bronchial constriction may cause problems for people with asthma and other respiratory conditions. Intestinal stimulation may aggravate chronic gastrointestinal conditions, such as colitis or Crohn's disease.

Because of vervain's potential stimulating effect on the uterus, pregnant women should steer clear of the herb, except possibly at term and under the supervision of a physician to help induce labor.

Nursing women should not use vervain.

Do not give vervain to children under 2. In older children, adjust the recommended dose based on the child's weight. For example, give a 50-pound child one-third of the dose a 150-pound adult would take.

If you're over 65, start with a low dose, and increase only if necessary.

Inform health care professionals of the herbs you use. Problematic herb-drug interactions are possible.

Vervain may cause allergic reactions or other unexpected side effects. If any develop, reduce your dose or stop taking it.

For more on herb safety, see Chapter 2.

If symptoms get worse or persist longer than 2 weeks, consult a health care professional promptly.

Growing Information

Vervain is a 3-foot perennial with thin, erect, stiff stems. Its opposite leaves are oblong and toothed near the ground and lance-shaped and deeply lobed higher up. The plant develops slender flower spikes that bear small blue or lilac flowers from early summer through mid-fall. The herb's bluish flowers gave it the name blue vervain.

Vervain grows easily from seeds planted in spring after the danger of frost has passed. Although it's a perennial, the herb is rather short-lived, but it does self-sow. Vervain prefers rich, moist loam under full sun. Harvest the leaves and flowers as the plants flower.

WHITE WILLOW

Potent against Pain

Family: Salicaceae; other members include poplar

Genus and species: *Salix alba*

Also known as: Salicin willow and weeping willow

Part used: Bark

Look at a white willow, and what do you see? Most people see only a stately shade tree—but herbalists also see the potent pain reliever aspirin.

In fact, aspirin was originally created from a compound in white willow bark, salicin, whose name comes from the herb's genus, *Salix*.

White willow grew on the banks of the Nile, and the ancient Egyptians considered it a symbol of joy. The Hebrews adopted the beautiful tree. In Leviticus (23:40), God commands them to celebrate the autumn harvest festival by setting up temporary shelters covered with willow boughs: "Take . . . boughs of willow . . . and rejoice seven days."

The willow became a symbol of sorrow, however, after the destruction of the first Temple in Jerusalem, which began the Jews' Babylonian exile. Consider the willow's transformation in Psalm 137: "By the rivers of Babylon, where we sat down, and there we wept, when we remembered Zion. Upon the willows, we hanged up our harps, for they that led us there captive asked of us . . . song." Since that time, the graceful tree has been known as weeping willow.

Healing History

Chinese physicians have used white willow bark to relieve pain since 500 B.C. That application took 5 centuries to find its way to Europe. The 1st-century Greek physician Dioscorides was the first Westerner to recommend willow bark for pain and inflammation, but his prescription did not catch on. A century later, the Roman doctor Galen recommended the herb only for the vague purpose of "drying up humors."

As the centuries passed, herbalists prescribed white willow bark for many ailments, including suppressing sexual desire. Seventeenth-century English herbalist Nicholas Culpeper noted, "The leaves, bark, and seed are used to stanch bleeding . . . stay vomiting . . . provoke urine . . . take away warts . . . and clear the face and skin from spots and discolourings. . . . The leaves bruised and boiled in wine stays the heat of lust in man or woman, and quite extinguishes it if it be long used."

White willow was a minor medicinal herb during Culpeper's time. But 50 years after his death, it became a sensation, thanks to the work of Rev. Edmund Stone. He was looking for a substitute for cinchona, the bark of the South American cinchona tree, which had been brought to Europe from the New World a century earlier. Cinchona was the first effective treatment for malaria, a scourge throughout Europe since ancient times, but it was extremely expensive.

In 1757, Stone collected some white willow bark for the medicinal uses that Culpeper had described, and he happened to taste it. He was surprised at its bitterness, which reminded him of cinchona. Stone wondered if willow bark might be a poor person's cinchona for fever and chills.

From the perspective of the Doctrine of Signatures, the medieval belief that a plant's physical appearance pointed to its medicinal uses, the signs looked promising. Willows grew along cool, damp riverbanks and in swampy lowlands, exactly the environments that physicians of Stone's era (wrongly) believed produced malaria and other illnesses marked by fever, or "ague."

For 6 years, Stone pulverized white willow bark, brewed a bitter tea with the powder, and gave his experimental medicine to 50 people with fevers. According to Stone, most of his patients' agues and chills disappeared shortly after drinking his concoction.

Stone wrote a report, "An Account of the Success of the Bark of the Willow in the Cure of Agues," in which he touted white willow bark as a cheap substitute for cinchona: "As this tree delights in a moist or wet soil where agues chiefly abound, the general maxim that many natural maladies carry their cures along with them, or that their remedies lie not far from the cause was so very [appropriate] to this particular case that I could not help applying it."

On April 25, 1763, Stone sent his report to the Royal Society, England's most prestigious scientific organization. Its publication in the society's journal, *Philosophical Transactions*, later that year finally popularized white willow bark in the West as a treatment for fever—more than 2,000 years after the Chinese had first touted it for that purpose.

Alas, white willow was no cinchona. It contains no quinine, the drug that treats malaria. Nonetheless, it brought down other fevers and quickly became Europe's drug of choice for fever, pain, and inflammation.

Early colonists introduced the tree into North America and found many Native American tribes using the bark of native willows to treat pain, chills, and fever.

From Salicin to Aspirin

Around 1828, French and German chemists extracted white willow bark's active compound, salicin. Ten years later, an Italian chemist isolated salicin's aspirin precursor, salicylic acid. Although this potent pain reliever was first discovered in white willow, chemists made the first aspirin from another herb that contains the same chemical, meadowsweet (see page 323). Salicin was discovered in meadowsweet in 1839.

During the mid-19th century, researchers showed that both salicin and salicylic acid reduce fever and relieve pain and inflammation. Unfortunately, they also have unpleasant—and potentially hazardous—side effects: nausea, diarrhea, bleeding, stomach ulceration, ringing in the ears (tinnitus), and at high doses, respiratory paralysis and death.

Chemists began tinkering with salicylic acid, hoping to preserve its benefits while minimizing its side effects. In 1853, German chemists added a molecular acetyl group to an extract of meadowsweet to create acetylsalicylic acid. The new compound was as effective as salicylic acid. It still had some of salicylic acid's side effects, but its action was more benign.

"Acetylsalicylic acid" was quite a mouthful, so the scientists who synthesized it took the "a" from *acetyl* and "spirin" from meadowsweet's genus name, *Spirea*, to create the word *aspirin*.

News of aspirin's synthesis was published in an obscure German medical journal—and forgotten for 50 years. Then in the late 1890s, a German drug chemist, Felix Hoffman, got upset that his father's rheumatoid arthritis medications brought him so little relief. Hoffman was an employee of Fredrich Bayer and Company. He began looking for a better pain reliever. He delved into the journals and found the old reports of aspirin. Hoffman prepared the drug, and his father's condition improved significantly.

At first, Hoffman's superiors at Bayer were not interested in aspirin, but eventually, they got behind it. In 1899, they released it in Europe and North America under the brand name Aspirin.

Aspirin quickly became the household drug of choice for a broad range of everyday ailments. Then, in a landmark trademark-protection battle, Bayer lost its trademark on Aspirin. The court ruled that the term had already passed into general usage.

Contemporary herbalists recommend white willow bark for headache, fever, arthritis, and other pain and inflammation, plus prevention of heart attack.

Therapeutic Uses

Contrary to Culpeper's opinion, white willow bark won't cure malaria. But it is indeed herbal aspirin.

It contains more salicylates than meadowsweet, making it a more potent natural healer.

FEVER, PAIN, AND INFLAMMATION. Try white willow any time that you think you need aspirin. Aspirin is a more concentrated source of salicylates, the active chemicals in white willow, so don't expect the herb to be as potent. On the other hand, compared with the little white pills, white willow bark causes fewer side effects.

Commission E, the expert panel that evaluates herbal medicines for the German counterpart of the FDA, approves white willow bark for the treatment of fever, headaches, and muscle and joint pain.

OSTEOARTHRITIS. German researchers gave 59 people with osteoarthritis of the hip and/or knee either a standard nonsteroidal anti-inflammatory drug, or NSAID (diclofenac) or 180 milligrams of white willow bark (salicin) per day. The NSAID worked better, but the high-dose herb worked almost as well. Using standard tests of arthritis, 48 percent of people given the drug reported significant improvement, while the figure for those given white willow was 40 percent.

LOWER BACK PAIN. German scientists gave 210 people with back pain either a placebo or white willow bark (in doses of either 120 milligrams or 240 milligrams salicin). In the placebo group, 6 percent reported significant pain relief. In the low-dose herb group, the figure was 21 percent, and in the high-dose group, 39 percent.

HEART ATTACK AND STROKE. Low-dose aspirin, one-half to one standard tablet a day, has become a standard preventive and first aid for heart attack. Aspirin helps prevent and dissolve the blood clots that trigger heart attack and most strokes. A cup of willow bark tea contains a similar low dose of aspirin-like salicin.

There have been no studies on willow bark as an aspirin substitute for heart attack prevention, but biochemically, the herb should be expected to have similar value. If you've been advised to take low-dose aspirin regularly, ask your physician about including willow bark in your regimen.

WOMEN'S HEALTH CONCERNS. Like aspirin, white willow contains enough salicylates to suppress the action of compounds called prostaglandins that are involved in menstrual cramps. If you have mild cramps, the herb may help.

Pregnant women should not use white willow. In animal studies, aspirin is associated with an increased risk of birth defects. The herb is not as powerful, but better safe than sorry.

Intriguing Possibilities

One laboratory study suggested that white willow may reduce blood sugar (glucose) levels. The herb's effect on diabetes in humans, if any, remains unclear.

Regular aspirin use has also been associated with reduced risk of digestive tract cancers, including colon cancer. White willow bark may provide similar preventive benefits.

Rx Recommendations

For a decoction to relieve pain, fever, and inflammation, use 1 teaspoon of powdered bark per cup of cold water and soak for 8 hours, then strain if you wish. Drink up to 3 cups a day. White willow tastes bitter and astringent. You can add honey and lemon or mix the herb with an herbal beverage tea.

To help prevent heart attack and stroke, drink 1 or 2 cups a day.

When using commercial preparations, follow the package directions.

The Safety Factor

Do not give white willow bark to children under age 16 with fevers related to colds, flu, or chickenpox. It may cause Reye's syndrome, a rare but potentially fatal condition. Aspirin clearly causes Reye's. White willow has never been linked to this syndrome, but because of its aspirin-like action, do not give this herb to children with colds, flu, or chickenpox.

Aspirin upsets some people's stomachs. White willow bark is less potent and rarely causes this problem, but stomach upset is still possible in those who are sensitive to aspirin. If stomach upset, nausea, or tinnitus develops, reduce your dose or stop using the herb.

People with chronic gastrointestinal conditions, such as ulcers and gastritis, should not use the herb.

Aspirin also triggers asthma attacks in some people. If you are aspirin-sensitive, do not use white willow bark.

Pregnant and nursing women should not use white willow bark.

Do not give white willow to children under 2. In older children who do not have colds, flu, or chickenpox, adjust the recommended dose based on the child's weight. For example, give a 50-pound child one-third of the dose a 150-pound adult would take.

If you're over 65, start with a low dose, and increase only if necessary.

Inform health care professionals of the herbs you use. Problematic herb-drug interactions are possible.

White willow may cause allergic reactions or other unexpected side effects. If any develop, reduce your dose or stop taking it.

For more on herb safety, see Chapter 2.

If symptoms get worse or persist longer than 2 weeks, consult a health care professional promptly.

Growing Information

Throughout history, many of the 500 willow species have been used in herbal healing. For the last 200 years, however, only white willow has been commonly used. It reaches 75 feet and has rough, grayish brown bark and long, thin leaves on flexible branches, which give the tree a graceful beauty.

White willows grow in almost any moist garden soil under full sun. Buy saplings at nurseries or propagate them from first-year branches several feet in length rooted in water or from foot-long hardwood cuttings taken in spring or fall and rooted the same way. Do not transplant willows.

Willows grow quickly and must be pruned regularly. Harvest the bark from older branches during pruning and dry it.

WITCH HAZEL

A Cooling, Soothing Astringent

Family: Hamamelidaceae; no other members

Genus and species: *Hamamelis virginiana*

Also known as: Winterbloom, snapping hazelnut, and hamamelis

Parts used: Leaves and bark

The next time someone you know pooh-poohs herbal healing, ask what the person thinks of witch hazel. The clear, pungent liquid extract of this bushy herb is a standard home remedy for cuts, bruises, hemorrhoids, and other minor skin conditions. More than 1 million gallons of witch hazel are sold each year in the United States, making it one of the nation's most widely used healing herbs.

The "hazel" in the herb's name comes from its similarity to the common hazelnut. As for the "witch," some say that early colonists used the shrub to make brooms, witches' favorite form of transportation. Others trace it to witch hazel's winter flowering and the loud "pop" when it disperses its seeds, supposedly evidence of occult influence. Still others claim that the shrub's forked branches were used by dousers looking for water and that dousing was once associated with witchcraft.

For the record, the herb's name has nothing to do with witchcraft. In medieval Middle English, "witch" was spelled *wych* and meant pliant or flexible. Witch hazel's branches are, indeed, flexible—so springy, in fact, that Native Americans used them to make bows.

Healing History

Witch hazel was highly valued in Native American medicine. Many tribes rubbed a decoction of the herb on cuts, bruises, insect bites, aching joints, sore muscles, and sore backs. They also drank witch hazel tea to stop internal bleeding, prevent miscarriage, and treat colds, fevers, sore throats, and menstrual pain.

The colonists adopted witch hazel, but the herb was not very popular until the 1840s, when a medicine man of the Oneida tribe reportedly introduced the plant to Theron T. Pond of Utica, New York. Pond was impressed with the plant's astringent properties and its ability to treat burns, boils, wounds, and hemorrhoids. In 1848, he began marketing witch hazel extract as Pond's Golden Treasure. Later, the name was changed to Pond's Extract, and the product became a big hit. Witch hazel water has been with us ever since.

Early witch hazel water was simply a strained decoction of the shrub's leaves and twigs that contained tannins, which made the extract highly astringent. By the late 19th century, manufacturers switched to steam distillation, a simpler process but one that left the resulting water with little if any of the plant's astringent tannins. That's when the controversy erupted.

King's American Dispensatory (1898), the text used by Eclectic physicians, forerunners of today's naturopaths, asserted: "The decoction is very useful in hemorrhage, diarrhea, dysentery, swellings, inflammations, tumors, hemorrhoids, epistaxis [nosebleed], and uterine hemorrhage following delivery. . . . [However] since the introduction of the distilled extract [witch hazel] has been largely abandoned. . . . The fluid extract has little to recommend it."

Nonetheless, witch hazel was listed as an astringent and anti-inflammatory in the *U.S. Pharmacopoeia*, a standard drug reference, from 1862 through 1916 and in the *National Formulary*, the pharmacists' reference, from 1916 to 1955. The *National Formulary* finally dropped it because in 1947, the 24th edition of *The Dispensatory of the United States* stated that witch hazel "is so nearly destitute of medicinal virtues, it scarcely deserves official recognition. . . . [Its continued use serves only to fill] the need in American families for an embrocation [liniment] which appeals to the psychic influence of faith."

Yet today, witch hazel can be found on the shelves of every pharmacy. Contemporary herbalists sidestep the controversy by recommending only the decoction of witch hazel bark, which contains astringent tannins. They are unanimous in their praise of the herb's cooling, astringent action when used externally for cuts, burns, scalds, bruises, inflammation, and hemorrhoids. They recommend it as a gargle for sore throat and sores in the mouth and internally to treat diarrhea.

Therapeutic Uses

While it's true that steam-distilled witch hazel water contains no astringent tannins, several studies show that it still retains astringent action, presumably from other compounds in the plant.

HEMORRHOIDS AND SKIN PROBLEMS. Commercial witch hazel water may lack tannins, but it contains other compounds with reported antiseptic, anesthetic, astringent, and anti-inflammatory action. Witch hazel water is an ingredient in Fleet Medicated Wipes for hemorrhoids, Tucks pads, and several over-the-counter treatments for poison ivy, oak, and sumac.

Commission E, the expert panel that evaluates herbal medicines for the German counterpart of the FDA, approves witch hazel for hemorrhoids and skin inflammations.

SUNBURN. German researchers gave 30 people with sunburn one of three treatments: a medically inactive placebo cream, a skin cream containing aloe gel and vitamin E (both recommended for skin problems), or a lotion containing 10 percent witch hazel distillate. Participants applied their treatments three times over a 48-hour period. Although differences in redness were not clearly visible to the naked eye, they were to an instrument called a chromameter—and the witch hazel lotion reduced redness best.

Another German study compared witch hazel with a chamomile preparation and hydrocortisone, an over-the-counter anti-inflammatory drug, in 24 people with sunburn. The hydrocortisone worked best, but witch hazel was almost as effective and "clearly superior" to the chamomile lotion.

Rx Recommendations

It's most convenient to use commercial witch hazel water, which is available in pharmacies.

If you'd like to make an extra-astringent decoction, boil 1 teaspoon of powdered leaves or twigs per cup of water for 10 minutes. Strain and cool. Apply the liquid directly or mix it into a skin lotion.

For a bitter, astringent gargle, use 1 teaspoon of bark per cup of boiling water. Steep for 10 minutes, then strain.

The Safety Factor

The medical literature contains no reports of harm from using witch hazel externally or as a gargle, but most experts advise against ingesting this herb.

You may use witch hazel externally on anyone, but dilute it for use on children under age 2.

Witch hazel may cause allergic reactions or other unexpected side effects. If any develop, reduce your dose or stop taking it.

For more on herb safety, see Chapter 2.

If symptoms get worse or persist longer than 2 weeks, consult a health care professional promptly.

Growing Information

Witch hazel's Latin name refers to Virginia, but the shrub grows all over the eastern United States. Most commercial witch hazel is grown in the Carolinas and Tennessee.

Witch hazel is a perennial that drops its leaves each autumn. Its single root sends up several twisting stems that fork into many flexible, hairy branches. It blooms long after most other flowers have disappeared—from September to December, depending on location. This is how it got one of its common names, winterbloom. As a late bloomer, it makes a colorful addition to any garden.

The shrub's spidery yellow flowers appear at the same time that its previous year's fruits mature. Its woody seed pods burst open with an audible pop and propel their two hard black seeds up to 25 feet. The seeds are edible and have been compared with hazelnuts, hence the name snapping hazelnut.

Witch hazel grows from seeds or twig cuttings. Refrigerate seeds at around 40°F for several months before planting to encourage germination. Cuttings generally produce roots in about 10 weeks.

Witch hazel grows best in moist, rich, sandy or peaty soil under partial shade, but it tolerates poorer soil and full sun. Harvest the leaves and twigs at any time and dry them.

YARROW

The Herbal Bandage

Family: Compositae; other members include daisy, dandelion, and marigold

Genus and species: *Achillea millefolium*

Also known as: Thousand weed, milfoil, soldier's woundwort, herbe militaire, nosebleed wort, bloodwort, and bad man's plaything

Parts used: Leaves, stems, and flowers

Legend has it that during the Trojan War, Achilles stopped the bleeding of his fellow soldiers' wounds by applying yarrow's fernlike leaves. Scientists have discovered that the mythological hero may have been on to something.

Yarrow contains substances that may stop bleeding and may have pain-relieving and anti-inflammatory properties helpful in wound treatment. Yarrow also appears to have potential as a digestive aid, menstrual remedy, and mild sedative.

Healing History

Achilles defined yarrow's use in herbal healing for more than 2,500 years. Dioscorides, a 1st-century physician attached to Roman legions, recommended rubbing the crushed plant on wounds.

The herb's many popular names—herbe militaire, nosebleed wort, soldier's woundwort, and bloodwort—attest to its use as a blood stopper during the Middle Ages. (The word *wort* is Old English for "plant.") Perhaps from an association with brawling, yarrow also became linked to ruffians, earning the name bad man's plaything.

Around Achilles' time, ancient Chinese physicians were prescribing Asian yarrow to treat inflammations, bleeding, heavy menstrual flow, dog bites, and snakebites. The Chinese also used yarrow in the ritual of the I Ching, the oracle consulted to predict the future. Coins are typically used today, but the traditional way to cast the I Ching involved dried yarrow stems.

India's Ayurvedic physicians recommended yarrow to treat fevers.

Sixteenth-century British herbalist John Gerard suggested yarrow for "swellings . . . of the privie parts." In the 17th century, John Parkinson advised, "If it be put into the nose, assuredly it will stop the bleeding of it." And his contemporary Nicholas Culpeper wrote, "An ointment of the leaves cures wounds . . . restrains violent bleedings . . . is good for inflammations and ulcers . . . and is excellent for the piles [hemorrhoids]."

Colonists introduced yarrow into North America. Native Americans adopted it enthusiastically as an external treatment for wounds and burns and as an internal treatment for colds, sore throats, arthritis, toothaches, insomnia, and indigestion.

America's 19th-century Eclectic physicians, forerunners of today's naturopaths, considered yarrow a "tonic upon the venous system" but downplayed its age-old role in wound treatment. Their text *King's American Dispensatory* (1898) recommended the herb for bloody urine, incontinence, hemorrhoids, menstrual cramps, diarrhea, dysentery, and "hemorrhage where the bleeding is small in amount."

Contemporary herbalists recommend yarrow as an "herbal Band-Aid." They also prescribe it for fevers and urinary tract infections and as a digestive aid.

Therapeutic Uses

If Achilles had had some yarrow on hand when his vulnerable heel was wounded, he might have survived the Trojan War.

WOUNDS. Yarrow contains many chemicals that support its traditional use as a wound treatment. Two of them, achilletin and achilleine, spur blood coagulation. Several more—azulene, camphor, chamazulene, eugenol, menthol, quercetin, rutin, and salicylic acid—have anti-inflammatory and pain-relieving action. Several others—tannins, terpeniol, and cineol—are antiseptic.

DIGESTIVE PROBLEMS. Chamazulene, one of the compounds in yarrow (and chamomile), helps relax the smooth muscle tissue of the digestive tract. This makes the herb an antispasmodic.

Commission E, the expert panel that evaluates herbal medicines for the German counterpart of the FDA, endorses yarrow as a digestive aid.

WOMEN'S HEALTH CONCERNS. Antispasmodics relax not only the digestive tract but also other smooth muscles, such as the uterus. This lends some credence to yarrow's use in treating menstrual cramps.

STRESS, ANXIETY, AND INSOMNIA. Yarrow contains a small amount of a hypnotic chemical called thujone, the effects of which have been compared to marijuana. The thujone in yarrow may account for the herb's traditional use as a sedative. In large amounts, thujone is poisonous, but the recommended amounts of yarrow do not supply enough of the compound to cause harm.

Intriguing Possibility

Two animal studies have shown that yarrow protects the liver from toxic chemical damage, and a scientifically conducted trial in India found that yarrow helps treat hepatitis.

Rx Recommendations

To treat wounds, press fresh leaves and flowers into cuts and scrapes until you can wash and bandage them. To help promote healing, apply the herb externally to clean wounds and inflamed skin.

For an infusion to soothe digestive upset and possibly act as a tranquilizer, use 1 to 2 teaspoons of dried herb per cup of boiling water.

Steep for 10 to 15 minutes, then strain. Drink up to 3 cups a day. Yarrow tastes tangy and bitter, with some astringency. To improve the flavor, add honey, sugar, or lemon or mix the herb with an herbal beverage blend.

As a homemade tincture, use $1/2$ to 1 teaspoon up to three times a day.

When using commercial preparations, follow the package directions.

The Safety Factor

Anyone may use yarrow externally, but it may cause allergic reactions or other unexpected side effects. If any develop, reduce your dose or stop taking it.

High doses of yarrow may turn urine dark brown. This is harmless and should not cause alarm.

The medical literature contains no reports of toxicity from yarrow, but people who are allergic to ragweed may develop a rash from contact with the plant.

For more on herb safety, see Chapter 2.

If symptoms get worse or persist longer than 2 weeks, consult a health care professional promptly.

Growing Information

Yarrow is an attractive 3-foot perennial covered with delicate hairs. Its feathery leaves are divided into what seem like thousands of tiny leaflets; hence its names thousand weed and milfoil (a corruption of *mille feuille*, the French term for "1,000 leaves"). Yarrow's numerous tiny white flowers develop in dense clusters on flat-topped, umbrella-like stalks in summer.

Yarrow grows easily from seeds or root divisions planted in spring or fall. Sow seeds just under the surface of fine soil and keep them moist until they germinate, usually within 2 weeks. Thin seedlings to 12-inch spacing. Yarrow adapts to many soil types but needs good drainage and does best in moderately rich soil under full sun. Divide plants every few years to keep them growing vigorously.

Harvest yarrow when the plants are in bloom and hang them to dry.

YOHIMBE

This Age-Old African Aphrodisiac Treats Erectile Dysfunction

Family: Rubiaceae; other members include coffee, gardenia, and madder

Genus and species: *Pausinystalia yohimbe*

Also known as: No other common names

Part used: Bark extract

Yohimbe is a prime example of the disdain Western science has shown toward traditional approaches to sex problems. Granted, many traditional aphrodisiacs—oysters, rhino tusk, tiger testicles—are worthless. But for 80 years after a compound in yohimbe bark, yohimbine, was first shown to have erection-boosting effects, Western researchers dismissed it. More than a decade before Viagra took the world by storm, the news that the FDA had approved yohimbine for erection difficulties was greeted by thundering silence.

Yohimbine still gets little respect. But for erectile dysfunction (ED), it works about as well as Viagra. It also shows promise for problems Viagra can't treat.

Healing History

For centuries, yohimbe bark was reputed to be an aphrodisiac that restored faltering erections. Scientists scoffed. Then in 1896, a compound isolated from the bark, yohimbine, was shown to stimulate erection in both animals and humans. Scientists ignored this report.

Fast-forward to the 1980s, when several studies showed that yohimbine increases blood-flow into the penis and helps treat ED. A dozen years before Viagra, the FDA approved yohimbine for treatment of ED. It was—and still is—marketed by prescription under three brand names: Yohimbine, Yocon, and Aphrodyne. But few people know of the natural, herbal alternative to Viagra.

Therapeutic Uses

ERECTILE DYSFUNCTION. First, let's define the term *aphrodisiac*. It refers to herbs, foods, and drugs that stimulate sexual arousal. Traditionally, a man with an erection was assumed to be sexually aroused, so the term was also applied to anything that enhanced erection. But today we know that it's possible for a man to have an erection but not feel sexually aroused and vice versa. As a result, modern sex researchers draw a distinction between things that stimulate sexual desire and arousal on the one hand, and things that stimulate erection on the other. Yohimbine (and Viagra and the other erection medications) improve erection, but they do not enhance libido.

Since the late 1980s, more than a dozen studies have shown that yohimbine treats ED. In 1997, British researchers analyzed seven studies and concluded that compared with placebo treatment, yohimbine users were almost four times more likely to raise erections.

Since then, several other studies have shown the benefit of this herb. German researchers gave 85 men with ED either a placebo or 10 milligrams of yohimbine three times a day. After 8 weeks, 45 percent of the placebo group reported erection improvement. In the yohimbine group, the figure was 71 percent.

Intriguing Possibilities

Some men can raise an erection, but can't ejaculate. British researchers gave 20 milligrams of yohimbine to 29 men with ejaculatory dysfunction. With the herb's help, 16 of the men (55 percent) were able to ejaculate.

In a study at the University of Texas, researchers gave 25 women complaining of arousal difficulties either a placebo or a combination of yohimbine and L-arginine, an amino acid precursor to nitric oxide, a compound crucial to sexual arousal. The women then viewed erotic videos. Compared with those taking the placebo, the women who took the herb/amino acid product reported greater sexual arousal.

Yohimbine may also help treat depression. Yale researchers gave 50 people with depression either Prozac plus a placebo or the drug plus yohimbine. The drug/herb group reported significantly faster mood elevation.

Rx Recommendations

Most studies have used 15 to 30 milligrams per day. Yohimbe products are widely available over the counter at health food stores and supplement shops. Unfortunately, according to an analysis by FDA chemists, many over-the-counter products contain only trace amounts of yohimbine. If you're interested in using this herb to treat ED, ask your doctor for a prescription and follow the label directions.

The Safety Factor

Possible side effects include increased heart rate and blood pressure, nervousness, irritability, headache, dizziness, tremor, and flushing. Very large doses may cause paralysis and psychosis. Do not exceed the recommended dose.

Do not mix yohimbine-based drugs with Viagra or other erection medications.

Children should not use yohimbe. If you're over 65, start with a low dose, and increase only if necessary.

Inform health care professionals of the herbs you use. Problematic herb-drug interactions are possible.

Yohimbe may cause allergic reactions or other unexpected side effects. If any develop, reduce your dose or stop taking it.

For more on herb safety, see Chapter 2.

If symptoms get worse, consult a health care professional promptly.

Growing Information

Yohimbe is an evergreen tree native to Cameroon, Gabon, and the Republic of the Congo. It is not grown in the United States.

Chapter 6

USING THE HEALING HERBS

A Quick Reference Guide

W hen you have a cold, which herbs should you reach for? How about when you have a headache? Anxiety? Indigestion?

This quick reference guide can help you make the right choice. It organizes the herbs discussed throughout the book into three categories: (1) conditions; (2) healing actions, such as antibiotic, decongestant, and so on; and (3) other uses, such as insect repellent and weight control.

Consumer Precautions

Before using any herb medicinally, read its profile in Chapter 5, especially the information on safety and side effects. Also read Chapter 2, which contains some general safe-use guidelines. Follow all of the recommendations in both chapters.

The following charts list only the most potentially hazardous herb side effects. Other side effects are possible. In addition, any herb may cause an allergic reaction.

Healing herbs are best used in consultation with a physician. This is especially true if you have a chronic condition such as asthma, arthritis, cancer, diabetes, heart disease, or high blood pressure.

Herbal oils are highly concentrated and should not be ingested unless you're under the care of a naturopath or professional herbalist. Even a small amount—a teaspoon—can be toxic, even fatal. Never allow children to ingest herbal oils.

A Special Note to Women

With few exceptions, pregnant and nursing women should not ingest medicinal amounts of healing herbs because of the possibility of harming the fetus or infant.

Most herbal digestive aids have antispasmodic action, that is, they help to relax the smooth muscle lining the digestive tract. The uterus is also a smooth muscle, so it may be affected by antispasmodic herbs. But many of these herbal digestive aids have traditionally been used to stimulate the uterus and promote menstruation, so it's possible that taking large amounts of these herbs may, over time, increase the risk of miscarriage.

This contradiction appears to be dose-related. Made with a dose of 1 to 2 teaspoons of freshly grated root, ginger tea is a safe, effective treatment for the morning sickness of pregnancy. In extremely large doses, however—20 to 40 teaspoons of root—it may induce uterine contractions.

The antispasmodic herbs are popular ingredients in cooking. Pregnant and nursing women may feel free to use culinary amounts of these herbs.

It's by no means clear from the research to date that all herbal digestive aids stimulate the uterus when taken in large doses, but given the traditional uses of antispasmodic herbs, pregnant women—and women who are trying to conceive—are best advised not to use medicinal amounts.

Conditions and Their Herbal Remedies

CONDITION	HERB(S)	SPECIAL PRECAUTION(S)
Acne	Aloe	
	Tea tree	For external use only. As little as a teaspoon of tea tree oil can be toxic. Do not ingest it, and keep it out of the reach of children.
AIDS	Garlic	Garlic is an anticoagulant and may cause bruising or delay blood clotting.
	St. John's wort	If you are taking antidepressant medication or a protease inhibitor, consult a physician before using St. John's wort.
Alzheimer's disease, Dementia	Ginkgo	None
Antidepressant-induced sexual problems	Ginkgo	None
Anxiety	Bacopa	
	Catnip	
	Celery	Long-term use of celery may deplete potassium stores.
	Chamomile	
	Ginkgo	
	Gotu kola	
	Hop	
	Kava	
	Lavender	
	Lemon balm	Lemon balm interferes with thyroid-stimulating hormone. If you have an underactive thyroid (hypothyroidism), consult a physician before using it.
	Motherwort	
	Passionflower	
	Rhodiola	
	Scullcap	
	Yarrow	

CONDITION	HERB(S)	SPECIAL PRECAUTION(S)
Aphrodisiac	Maca	None
	Muira puama	
Arthritis	Angelica	Angelica may cause a rash in sensitive people who are exposed to direct sunlight.
	Black haw	
	Boneset	
	Boswellia	
	Cat's claw	
	Chamomile	
	Chaparral	
	Comfrey	Comfrey should not be ingested.
	Devil's claw	
	Echinacea	
	Evening primrose	
	Fenugreek	Fenugreek has estrogenic action. People who have a history of blood clots (thromboembolisms), inflammation of blood vessels (thrombophlebitis), heart disease, or stroke should consult their physicians before using it.
	Gentian	
	Ginger	
	Horsetail	Long-term use of horsetail, juniper, nettle, and vervain may deplete potassium stores.
	Juniper	
	Licorice	Long-term use of licorice may cause water retention, elevated blood pressure, and a hormone imbalance (pseudoaldosteronism).
	Meadowsweet	Meadowsweet and white willow contain aspirin-like compounds. If you are aspirin-sensitive, consult a physician before using these herbs.
	Nettle	
	Red pepper	
	St. John's wort	If you are taking antidepressant medication, consult a physician before using St. John's wort.
	Turmeric	
	Vervain	Vervain may depress heart rate and constrict bronchial passages. If you have heart disease, high blood pressure, diabetes, or asthma, consult a physician before using it.
	White willow	

CONDITION	HERB(S)	SPECIAL PRECAUTION(S)
Asthma	Angelica	Angelica may cause a rash in sensitive people who are exposed to direct sunlight.
	Borage	
	Boswellia	
	Cocoa (dark chocolate)	Cocoa (chocolate), coffee, kola, maté, and tea all contain caffeine, which may cause jitters, irritability, insomnia, and addiction.
	Coffee	
	Cordyceps	
	Ephedra	Ephedra may raise blood pressure and cause jitters, irritability, and insomnia. People with high blood pressure, heart or kidney disease, or a history of stroke should not use it. In very large doses, ephedra may cause potentially fatal heart problems.
	Kola	
	Maté	
	Tea	
Athlete's foot	Tea tree	As little as a teaspoon of tea tree oil can be toxic. Do not ingest it, and keep it out of the reach of children.
Attention Deficit/Hyper-activity Disorder (ADHD)	Bacopa	None
Bad breath	Alfalfa	
	Parsley	Long-term use of large amounts of parsley may deplete potassium stores.
Benign prostate enlargement	Nettle	Long-term use of nettle may deplete potassium stores.
	Pumpkin seed	
	Pygeum	
	Saw palmetto	
Bleeding	Blackberry	
	Shepherd's purse	Shepherd's purse may cause powerful uterine contractions.
	Witch hazel	
	Yarrow	
Breast tenderness	Evening primrose	None

CONDITION	HERB(S)	SPECIAL PRECAUTION(S)
Bronchitis (see also Cough)	Angelica	
	Barberry	
	Cordyceps	
	Echinacea	
	Garlic	Garlic is an anticoagulant and may cause bruising or delay blood clotting.
	Marshmallow	
	Pelargonium	
Burns (see also Pain)	For external use:	
	Aloe	Flush burns with cold water before applying herbal medicines.
	Chamomile	Extensive burns that raise blisters or char the skin require professional attention.
	Comfrey	
	Echinacea	
	Gotu kola	
	Marshmallow	
	Passionflower	
	St. John's wort	
	Witch hazel	
	Yarrow	
Cancer prevention	Alfalfa	
	Apple	
	Ashwagandha	
	Bilberry	
	Blackberry	
	Black cohosh	
	Cat's claw	
	Cocoa (dark chocolate)	
	Cranberry	
	Dandelion	
	Flax	
	Garlic	Garlic is an anticoagulant and may cause bruising or delay blood clotting.

CONDITION	HERB(S)	SPECIAL PRECAUTION(S)
Cancer prevention (cont.)	Ginseng	
	Maitake	
	Pomegranate	
	Raspberry	
	Reishi	
	Rhodiola	
	Shiitake	
	Soybean	Soybean may suppress sperm count. Soybean also has estrogenic action. Women with hormonal conditions who have been advised to avoid birth control pills or hormone replacement therapy should consult their physicians before taking soy in amounts greater than a few servings of tofu per week.
	Tea (green)	Tea contains caffeine, which may cause jitters, irritability, insomnia, and addiction.
	Turmeric	
Cancer treatment	Borage	
	Echinacea	
	Maitake	
	Mistletoe	Mistletoe may slow heart rate and affect blood pressure. If you have heart disease, diabetes, high blood pressure, or a history of stroke, consult your physician before using it.
	Reishi	
	Rhodiola	
	Shiitake	
	Tea (green)	Tea contains caffeine, which may cause jitters, irritability, insomnia, and addiction.
Canker sores	Licorice	Long-term use of licorice may cause water retention, elevated blood pressure, and a hormone imbalance (pseudoaldosteronism).
Cataracts	Bilberry	None
	Blackberry	
	Cranberry	
	Raspberry	
	Turmeric	
Childbirth recovery	Lavender	None

CONDITION	HERB(S)	SPECIAL PRECAUTION(S)
Cholera	Barberry	Use herbs in conjunction with professional medical care.
	Goldenseal	
Cirrhosis	Ginseng	
	Licorice	Long-term use of licorice may cause water retention, elevated blood pressure, and a hormone imbalance (pseudoaldosteronism).
	Milk thistle	
Cluster headache	Red pepper	None
Colds and flu (see also Cough)	Angelica	
	Boneset	
	Cocoa (dark chocolate)	Cocoa (chocolate), coffee, and tea all contain caffeine, which may cause jitters, irritability, insomnia, and addiction.
	Coffee	
	Echinacea	
	Elderberry	
	Eleutherococcus	
	Ephedra	Ephedra may raise blood pressure and cause jitters, irritability, and insomnia. People with high blood pressure, heart or kidney disease, or a history of stroke should not use it. In very large doses, ephedra may cause potentially fatal heart problems.
	Eucalyptus	
	Garlic	
	Ginger	
	Ginseng	
	Hyssop	
	Licorice	
	Marshmallow	
	Meadowsweet	Meadowsweet contains aspirin-like compounds. If you are aspirin-sensitive, consult a physician before using it.
	Mullein	
	Pelargonium	
	Peppermint	
	Rose	
	Slippery elm	
	Tea	

CONDITION	HERB(S)	SPECIAL PRECAUTION(S)
Cold sores (see Herpes and cold sores)		
Colic	Dill	None
	Fennel	
	Slippery elm	
Congestive heart failure (see also Diuretic in "Healing Actions" table)	Buchu	All of these herbs are diuretic and may cause potassium depletion.
	Celery	
	Dandelion	
	Hawthorn	
	Juniper	
	Nettle	
	Parsley	
	Sarsaparilla	
	Uva-ursi	
Conjunctivitis	Barberry	None
Constipation	Apple	
	Buckthorn	Buckthorn, cascara sagrada, rhubarb, and senna may cause abdominal distress.
	Cascara sagrada	
	Psyllium	
	Rhubarb	
	Senna	
	Vervain	Vervain may depress heart rate and constrict bronchial passages. If you have heart disease, high blood pressure, diabetes, or asthma, consult a physician before using it.
Cough	Angelica	Angelica may cause a rash in sensitive people who are exposed to direct sunlight.
	Cocoa (chocolate)	Cocoa (chocolate), coffee, kola, maté, and tea all contain caffeine, which may cause jitters, irritability, insomnia, and addiction.
	Coffee	
	Ephedra	Ephedra may raise blood pressure and cause jitters, irritability, and insomnia. People with high blood pressure, heart or kidney disease, or a history of stroke should not use it. In very large doses, ephedra may cause potentially fatal heart problems.

CONDITION	HERB(S)	SPECIAL PRECAUTION(S)
	Eucalyptus	
	Fenugreek	Fenugreek has estrogenic action. People who have a history of blood clots (thromboembolisms), inflammation of blood vessels (thrombophlebitis), heart disease, or stroke should consult their physicians before using it.
	Horehound	
	Hyssop	
	Kola	
	Licorice	Long-term use of licorice may cause water retention, elevated blood pressure, and a hormone imbalance (pseudoaldosteronism).
	Marshmallow	
	Maté	
	Mullein	
	Pennyroyal	
	Peppermint	
	Slippery elm	
	Tea	
	Thyme	
Depression	Chamomile	
	Coffee	
	Rhodiola	
	St. John's wort	If you are already taking antidepressant medication, consult a physician before using St. John's wort.
	Tea	
Diabetes	Aloe	
	Apple	
	Ashwagandha	
	Bitter melon	
	Celery	Long-term use of celery may deplete potassium stores.
	Cinnamon	
	Eleuthero	
	Evening primrose	
	Fenugreek	Fenugreek has estrogenic action. People who have a history of blood clots (thromboembolisms), inflammation of blood vessels (thrombophlebitis), heart disease, or stroke should consult their physicians before using it.

CONDITION	HERB(S)	SPECIAL PRECAUTION(S)
Diabetes (cont.)	Flax	
	Garlic	Garlic is an anticoagulant and may cause bruising or delay blood clotting.
	Ginseng	
	Gotu kola	
	Milk thistle	
	Pomegranate	
	Red pepper	
	Reishi	
	Sage	
	Tea	Tea contains caffeine, which may cause jitters, irritability, insomnia, and addiction.
Diabetic neuropathy	Red pepper	None
Diabetic retinopathy	Bilberry	None
	Blackberry	
	Cranberry	
	Ginkgo	
	Raspberry	
Diarrhea	Apple	
	Barberry	
	Bayberry	Bayberry may change the body's sodium-potassium balance. If you have high blood pressure, heart disease, diabetes, kidney disease, or a history of stroke, consult a physician before using it.
	Bilberry	
	Blackberry	
	Chamomile	
	Dill	
	Goldenseal	
	Meadowsweet	Meadowsweet contains aspirin-like compounds. If you are aspirin-sensitive, consult a physician before using it.
	Mullein	
	Psyllium	
	Raspberry	
	Red pepper	
	Rhubarb	Large doses of rhubarb have a laxative effect and may cause abdominal distress.

CONDITION	HERB(S)	SPECIAL PRECAUTION(S)
	Slippery elm	
	Tea	Tea contains caffeine, which may cause jitters, irritability, insomnia, and addiction.
	Uva-ursi	Long-term use of uva-ursi may deplete potassium stores.
Dizziness	Ginger	None
	Ginkgo	
Dry skin	Borage	None
Ear infection	Echinacea	
	Garlic	Garlic is an anticoagulant and may cause bruising or delay blood clotting.
Eczema	Borage	
	Evening primrose	
	Tea	Tea contains caffeine, which may cause jitters, irritability, insomnia, and addiction.
Emphysema	Eucalyptus	None
	Ginseng	
	Peppermint	
Erectile dysfunction (due to poor bloodflow)	Ginkgo	None
	Ginseng	
	Yohimbe	
Fatigue	Ashwagandha	
	Cocoa (chocolate)	Cocoa (chocolate), coffee, kola, maté, and tea all contain caffeine, which may cause jitters, irritability, insomnia, and addiction.
	Coffee	
	Eleuthero	
	Ephedra	Ephedra may raise blood pressure and cause jitters, irritability, and insomnia. People with high blood pressure, heart or kidney disease, or a history of stroke should not use it. In very large doses, ephedra may cause potentially fatal heart problems.
	Ginseng	
	Kola	
	Maté	
	Rhodiola	
	Tea	

CONDITION	HERB(S)	SPECIAL PRECAUTION(S)
Fever	Andrographis	Andrographis is an anticoagulant and may cause bruising and delay blood clotting.
	Bayberry	Bayberry may change the body's sodium-potassium balance. If you have high blood pressure, heart disease, diabetes, kidney disease, or a history of stroke, consult a physician before using it.
	Black haw	
	Meadowsweet	Meadowsweet and white willow contain aspirin-like compounds. If you are aspirin-sensitive, consult a physician before using these herbs.
	White willow	
Fibromyalgia	Red pepper	None
Flu (see Colds and flu)		
Food poisoning prevention	Echinacea	None
	Rosemary	
	Sage	
	Thyme	
	Turmeric	
Food poisoning treatment	Angelica	Angelica may cause a rash in sensitive people who are exposed to direct sunlight.
	Apple	
	Barberry	
	Bayberry	Bayberry may change the body's sodium-potassium balance. If you have high blood pressure, heart disease, diabetes, kidney disease, or a history of stroke, consult a physician before using it.
	Burdock	
	Catnip	
	Chamomile	
	Cinnamon	
	Clove	
	Dill	
	Echinacea	
	Garlic	Garlic is anticoagulant and may cause bruising or delay blood clotting.
	Ginseng	

CONDITION	HERB(S)	SPECIAL PRECAUTION(S)
	Goldenseal	
	Meadowsweet	Meadowsweet contains aspirin-like compounds. If you are aspirin-sensitive, consult a physician before using it.
	Mullein	
	Peppermint	
Gallstone prevention	Coffee	Coffee contains caffeine, which may cause jitters, irritability, insomnia, and addiction.
	Dandelion	Long-term use of dandelion may deplete potassium stores.
Gas	Dill	None
Genital warts	Shiitake	None
Giardiasis	Barberry	None
	Elecampane	
	Goldenseal	
Glaucoma	Bilberry	None
	Blackberry	
	Cranberry	
	Raspberry	
Gout (see also Pain)	Celery	Long-term use of celery and nettle may deplete potassium stores.
	Coffee	
	Nettle	
Gum disease prevention	Chaparral	
	Cinnamon	
	Elderberry	
	Eucalyptus	
	Goldenseal	
	Myrrh	
	Neem	Neem oil is toxic. Use it only in commercial toothpastes.
Hay fever	Butterbur	
	Clove	
	Nettle	Long-term use of nettle and parsley may deplete potassium stores.
	Parsley	

CONDITION	HERB(S)	SPECIAL PRECAUTION(S)
Headache	Black haw	
	Eucalyptus	
	Feverfew (migraine)	
	Meadowsweet	Meadowsweet and white willow contain aspirin-like compounds. If you are aspirin-sensitive, consult a physician before using these herbs.
	Peppermint	
	Red pepper (cluster headache)	
	White willow	
Hearing loss	Gingko	None
Heart disease (see also High blood pressure and High cholesterol)	Alfalfa	
	Angelica	
	Apple	
	Ashwagandha	
	Astragalus	
	Bilberry	
	Blackberry	
	Cat's claw	
	Celery	
	Cocoa (dark chocolate)	
	Cordyceps	
	Cranberry	
	Elderberry	
	Eleuthero	
	Evening primrose	
	Flax	
	Garlic	Garlic and shepherd's purse are anticoagulants and may cause bruising and delay blood clotting.
	Ginger	
	Ginkgo	
	Ginseng	
	Hawthorn	

CONDITION	HERB(S)	SPECIAL PRECAUTION(S)
	Meadowsweet	Meadowsweet and white willow contain aspirin-like compounds. If you are aspirin-sensitive, consult a physician before using these herbs.
	Motherwort	
	Pomegranate	
	Raspberry	
	Red clover	
	Reishi	
	Rhodiola	
	Shepherd's purse	
	Soybean	Soybean may suppress sperm count. It also has estrogenic action. Women with hormonal conditions who have been advised to avoid birth control pills or hormone replacement therapy should consult their physicians before taking soy in amounts greater than a few servings of tofu per week.
	Tea (green)	Tea contains caffeine, which may cause jitters, irritability, insomnia, and addiction.
	Turmeric	
	White willow	
Heart rhythm normalization	Rhodiola	None
Hemorrhoids	*For external use:*	
	Blackberry	
	Mullein	
	Psyllium	
	Shepherd's purse	Shepherd's purse may cause powerful uterine contractions.
	Slippery elm	
	Tarragon	
	Witch hazel	
	For internal use:	
	Butcher's broom	
	Horse chestnut	

CONDITION	HERB(S)	SPECIAL PRECAUTION(S)
Hepatitis	Licorice	Long-term use of licorice may cause water retention, elevated blood pressure, and a hormone imbalance (pseudoaldosteronism).
	Maitake	
	Milk thistle	
	Shiitake	
Herpes and cold sores	*For external use:*	
	Comfrey	
	Hyssop	
	Lemon balm	Lemon balm interferes with thyroid-stimulating hormone. If you have an underactive thyroid (hypothyroidism), consult a physician before using it.
	Licorice	Long-term use of licorice may cause water retention, elevated blood pressure, and a hormone imbalance (pseudoaldosteronism).
	Peppermint	
	Uva-ursi	Long-term use of uva-ursi may deplete potassium stores.
	For internal use:	
	Echinacea	
	Garlic	
	Ginseng	
	Lemon balm	
	Reishi	
High blood pressure (see also Diuretic in "Healing Actions" table)	Barberry	
	Black cohosh	Black cohosh has estrogenic action. People who have a history of blood clots (thromboembolisms), inflammation of blood vessels (thrombophlebitis), heart disease, or stroke should consult their physicians before using it.
	Buchu	
	Cat's claw	
	Celery	Long-term use of celery may deplete potassium stores.
	Cocoa (dark chocolate)	
	Dandelion	

CONDITION	HERB(S)	SPECIAL PRECAUTION(S)
	Evening primrose	
	Garlic	Garlic is an anticoagulant and may cause bruising or delay blood clotting.
	Ginger	
	Ginseng	
	Gotu kola	
	Hawthorn	
	Hibiscus	
	Juniper	
	Mistletoe	Mistletoe may slow heart rate and affect blood pressure. If you have heart disease, diabetes, high blood pressure, or a history of stroke, consult your physician before using it.
	Motherwort	
	Nettle	
	Parsley	
	Pomegranate	
	Rhodiola	
	Sarsaparilla	
	Soybean	Soybean may suppress sperm count. It also has estrogenic action. Women with hormonal conditions who have been advised to avoid birth control pills or hormone replacement therapy should consult their physicians before taking soy in amounts greater than a few servings of tofu per week.
	Turmeric	
	Uva-ursi	
	Valerian	
High cholesterol	Alfalfa	
	Apple	
	Artichoke	
	Ashwagandha	
	Cat's claw	
	Celery	Long-term use of celery may deplete potassium stores.
	Cinnamon	

CONDITION	HERB(S)	SPECIAL PRECAUTION(S)
High cholesterol (cont.)	Cocoa (dark chocolate)	
	Evening primrose	
	Fenugreek	Fenugreek and soybean have estrogenic action. Soybean may suppress sperm count. People who have a history of blood clots (thromboembolisms), inflammation of blood vessels (thrombophlebitis), heart disease, or stroke should consult their physicians before using them.
	Flax	
	Garlic	Garlic is an anticoagulant and may cause bruising or delay blood clotting.
	Ginger	
	Ginseng	
	Hawthorn	
	Psyllium	
	Red pepper	
	Scullcap	
	Shiitake	
	Soybean	Women with hormonal conditions who have been advised to avoid birth control pills or hormone replacement therapy should consult their physicians before taking soy in amounts greater than a few servings of tofu per week.
	Tea	Tea contains caffeine, which may cause jitters, irritability, insomnia, and addiction.
	Turmeric	
HIV/AIDS	Shiitake	None
Hives	Nettle	Long-term use of nettle and parsley may deplete potassium stores.
	Parsley	
Hypothyroidism	Bacopa	None
Infertility, male	Ginseng	None
Insomnia	Catnip	
	Celery	Long-term use of celery may deplete potassium stores.
	Hop	
	Lavender	

CONDITION	HERB(S)	SPECIAL PRECAUTION(S)
	Lemon balm	Lemon balm interferes with thyroid-stimulating hormone. If you have an underactive thyroid (hypothyroidism), consult a physician before using it.
	Motherwort	
	Passionflower	
	Rhodiola	
	Scullcap	
	Valerian	
	Yarrow	
Intermittent claudication	Ginkgo	None
Irritable bowel syndrome	Artichoke	None
	Peppermint	
	Turmeric	
Jet lag	Cocoa (chocolate)	Cocoa (chocolate), coffee, kola, maté, and tea all contain caffeine, which may cause jitters, irritability, insomnia, and addiction.
	Coffee	
	Ephedra	Ephedra may raise blood pressure and cause jitters, irritability, and insomnia. People with high blood pressure, heart or kidney disease, or a history of stroke should not use it. In very large doses, ephedra may cause potentially fatal heart problems.
	Ginseng	
	Kola	
	Maté	
	Tea	
Kidney disease	Cordyceps	None
Kidney stone prevention	Coffee	Coffee contains caffeine, which may cause jitters, irritability, insomnia, and addiction.
	Horsetail	Long-term use of horsetail may deplete potassium stores.
	Pumpkin seed	
	Tea	
Lead poisoning	Apple	
	Garlic	Garlic is an anticoagulant and may cause bruising or delay blood clotting.

CONDITION	HERB(S)	SPECIAL PRECAUTION(S)
Leprosy (Hansen's disease)	Garlic	Garlic is an anticoagulant and may cause bruising or delay blood clotting.
	Gotu kola	
Lymphedema	Butcher's broom	None
Macular degeneration	Bilberry	None
	Blackberry	
	Cranberry	
	Ginkgo	
	Raspberry	
Menopausal discomforts	Angelica	All of these herbs have estrogenic action. Women who have been advised not to take birth control pills or hormone replacement therapy should consult their physicians before using them.
	Black cohosh	
	Fennel	
	Fenugreek	
	Flax	
	Ginseng	
	Licorice	Long-term use of licorice may cause water retention, elevated blood pressure, and a hormone imbalance (pseudoaldosteronism).
	Maca	
	Red clover	
	St. John's wort	
	Soybean	
Menstrual cramps (see also Pain)	Black cohosh	
	Black haw	
	Chaste tree	
	Fennel	Fennel, fenugreek, and red clover have estrogenic action. Women who have been advised not to take birth control pills or hormone replacement therapy should consult their physicians before using these herbs.
	Fenugreek	
	Feverfew	
	Lavender	
	Red clover	
	Yarrow	

CONDITION	HERB(S)	SPECIAL PRECAUTION(S)
Menstruation, delayed	Celery	Long-term use of celery or parsley may deplete potassium stores.
	Chaste tree	
	Fenugreek	Fenugreek has estrogenic action. Women who have been advised not to take birth control pills or hormone replacement therapy should consult their physicians before using it.
	Motherwort	
	Parsley	
	Pennyroyal	
	Rhubarb	Large doses of rhubarb have a laxative effect and may cause abdominal distress.
	Shepherd's purse	Shepherd's purse may cause powerful uterine contractions.
Menstruation, heavy	Chaste tree	
	Coffee	
	Shepherd's purse	Shepherd's purse may cause powerful uterine contractions.
Migraine	Butterbur	None
	Feverfew	
Morning sickness	Ginger	None
	Raspberry	
Motion sickness	Ginger	None
Mouth sores	Blackberry	None
Muscle soreness	Arnica	Arnica is toxic. Ingest only homeopathic doses.
Mushroom poisoning	Milk thistle	None
Nausea	Ginger	None
Obesity	Bitter melon	
	Coffee	Coffee and tea contain caffeine, which may cause jitters, irritability, insomnia, and addiction.
	Ephedra	Ephedra may raise blood pressure and cause jitters, irritability, and insomnia. People with high blood pressure, heart or kidney disease, or a history of stroke should not use it. In very large doses, ephedra may cause potentially fatal heart problems. Coffee and other herbs containing caffeine increase ephedra's effects and side effects. Ephedra and coffee should be used for weight control only under medical supervision.
	Maitake	
	Tea	

CONDITION	HERB(S)	SPECIAL PRECAUTION(S)
Osteoporosis prevention	Eleuthero	
	Soybean	Soybean may suppress sperm count. It also has estrogenic action. Women with hormonal conditions who have been advised to avoid birth control pills or hormone replacement therapy should consult their physicians before taking soy in amounts greater than a few servings of tofu per week.
	Tea	Tea contains caffeine, which may cause jitters, irritability, insomnia, and addiction.
Pain (see also Anesthetic in "Healing Actions" table)	Andrographis	Andrographis is an anticoagulant and may cause bruising and delay blood clotting.
	Arnica	Arnica is toxic. Ingest only homeopathic doses.
	Black haw	
	Boswellia	
	Coffee	Coffee and maté contain caffeine, which may cause jitters, irritability, insomnia, and addiction.
	Devil's claw	
	Maté	
	Meadowsweet	Meadowsweet and white willow contain aspirin-like compounds. If you are aspirin-sensitive, consult a physician before using these herbs.
	Passionflower	
	Peppermint	
	Red pepper	
	Tea	
	Vervain	Vervain may depress heart rate and constrict bronchial passages. If you have heart disease, high blood pressure, diabetes, or asthma, consult a physician before using it.
	White willow	
Pinkeye	Barberry	None
Poison ivy, oak, and sumac	Aloe	None
Postpartum hemorrhage	Shepherd's purse	Shepherd's purse may cause powerful uterine contractions.

CONDITION	HERB(S)	SPECIAL PRECAUTION(S)
Premenstrual syndrome (PMS)	Black cohosh	
	Buchu	Buchu, celery, dandelion, horsetail, juniper, nettle, parsley, sarsaparilla, and uva-ursi are diuretics and may deplete potassium stores.
	Celery	
	Chaste tree	
	Dandelion	
	Evening primrose	
	Fennel	Fennel has estrogenic action. People who have a history of blood clots (thromboembolisms), inflammation of blood vessels (thrombophlebitis), heart disease, or stroke should consult their physicians before using it.
	Horsetail	
	Juniper	
	Nettle	
	Parsley	
	Sarsaparilla	
	Uva-ursi	
Prostate cancer	Fennel	None
	Red clover	
	Saw palmetto	
Psoriasis	Aloe	None
	Barberry	
	Gotu kola	
	Red pepper	
Radiation exposure	Eleuthero	None
Rheumatoid arthritis	Borage	
	Boswellia	
	Cat's claw	
	Evening primrose	
	Tea	Tea contains caffeine, which may cause jitters, irritability, insomnia, and addiction.
Scabies	Turmeric	None
Scalds (see Burns)		
Scurvy	Nettle	None

CONDITION	HERB(S)	SPECIAL PRECAUTION(S)
Seasonal affective disorder (SAD)	St. John's wort	None
Shingles	Red pepper	None
Sinus infection	Andrographis	Andrographis is an anticoagulant and may cause bruising and delay blood clotting.
Sore throat	Fenugreek	Fenugreek has estrogenic action. People who have a history of blood clots (thromboembolisms), inflammation of blood vessels (thrombophlebitis), heart disease, or stroke should consult their physicians before using it.
	Licorice	Long-term use of licorice may cause water retention, elevated blood pressure, and a hormone imbalance (pseudoaldosteronism).
	Marshmallow	
	Mullein	
	Sage	
	Slippery elm	
Stress	Catnip	
	Celery	Long-term use of celery can deplete potassium stores.
	Chamomile	
	Ginseng	
	Hop	
	Kava	
	Lavender	
	Lemon balm	Lemon balm interferes with thyroid-stimulating hormone. If you have an underactive thyroid (hypothyroidism), consult a physician before using it.
	Motherwort	
	Passionflower	
	Rhodiola	
	Scullcap	
	Yarrow	
Stretch marks	Gotu kola	None

CONDITION	HERB(S)	SPECIAL PRECAUTION(S)
Stroke	Alfalfa	
	Angelica	
	Apple	
	Astragalus	
	Bilberry	
	Blackberry	
	Cat's claw	
	Celery	
	Cocoa (dark chocolate)	
	Cordyceps	
	Cranberry	
	Elderberry	
	Evening primrose	
	Garlic	
	Ginger	
	Ginkgo	
	Ginseng	
	Hawthorn	
	Meadowsweet	Meadowsweet and white willow contain aspirin-like compounds. If you are aspirin-sensitive, consult a physician before using these herbs.
	Motherwort	
	Pomegranate	
	Raspberry	
	Reishi	
	Rhodiola	
	Soybean	Soybean may suppress sperm count. It also has estrogenic action. Women with hormonal conditions who have been advised to avoid birth control pills or hormone replacement therapy should consult their physicians before taking soy in amounts greater than a few servings of tofu per week.
	Tea (green)	Tea contains caffeine, which may cause jitters, irritability, insomnia, and addiction.
	Turmeric	
	White willow	

CONDITION	HERB(S)	SPECIAL PRECAUTION(S)
Sunburn (see Burns)		
Tinnitus (ringing in the ears)	Ginkgo	None
	Horse chestnut	
Tonsillitis	Pelargonium	None
Toothache	*For external use, on gums only:*	Herbal oils are highly concentrated. As little as a teaspoon may be toxic if ingested. Keep herbal oils away from children.
	Clove oil	
	Tarragon oil	
Tooth decay prevention	Chaparral	
	Cinnamon	
	Neem	Neem oil is toxic. Use it only in commercial toothpastes.
	Peppermint	
	Tea	Tea contains caffeine, which may cause jitters, irritability, insomnia, and addiction.
Ulcerative colitis	Boswellia	None
	Turmeric	
Ulcers	Chamomile	
	Garlic	Garlic is an anticoagulant and may cause bruising or delay blood clotting.
	Ginger	
	Licorice	Long-term use of licorice may cause water retention, elevated blood pressure, and a hormone imbalance (pseudoaldosteronism).
	Neem	Neem oil is toxic. Use it only under a physician's supervision.
	Turmeric	
Urinary incontinence	Cranberry	None
Urinary tract infection prevention	Andrographis	Andrographis is an anticoagulant and may cause bruising and delay blood clotting.
	Cranberry	
	Dill	
	Horsetail	Long-term use of horsetail may deplete potassium stores.
	Nettle	

CONDITION	HERB(S)	SPECIAL PRECAUTION(S)
Urinary tract infection treatment	Barberry	
	Garlic	Garlic is an anticoagulant and may cause bruising or delay blood clotting.
	Meadowsweet	Meadowsweet contains aspirin-like compounds. If you are aspirin-sensitive, consult a physician before using it.
	Uva-ursi	Long-term use of uva-ursi may deplete potassium stores.
Varicose veins	Bilberry	None
	Blackberry	
	Butcher's broom	
	Cranberry	
	Gotu kola	
	Horse chestnut	
	Hyssop	
	Raspberry	
	Tarragon	
Vertigo	Ginkgo	None
Wounds	*For external use:*	
	Aloe	
	Barberry	
	Blackberry	
	Burdock	
	Chamomile	
	Comfrey	
	Echinacea	
	Eucalyptus	
	Fenugreek	
	Garlic	Garlic is an anticoagulant and may cause bruising or delay blood clotting.
	Gotu kola	
	Horsetail	Long-term use of horsetail and uva-ursi may deplete potassium stores.
	Lavender	
	Lemon balm	
	Marshmallow	

CONDITION	HERB(S)	SPECIAL PRECAUTION(S)
Wounds (cont.)	Passionflower	
	Rosemary	
	Sage	
	St. John's wort	If you are taking antidepressant medication, consult a physician before using St. John's wort.
	Shepherd's purse	Shepherd's purse may cause powerful uterine contractions.
	Slippery elm	
	Tarragon	
	Tea tree	As little as a teaspoon of tea tree oil can be toxic. Do not ingest it, and keep it out of the reach of children.
	Thyme	
	Uva-ursi	
	Witch hazel	
	Yarrow	
	For internal use:	
	Echinacea	
	Garlic	
Yeast infection (candidiasis)	Barberry	
	Chamomile	
	Cinnamon	
	Dandelion	Long-term use of dandelion may deplete potassium stores.
	Echinacea	
	Garlic	Garlic is an anticoagulant and may cause bruising or delay blood clotting.
	Pau d'arco	Pau d'arco is an anticoagulant and may cause bruising and delay blood clotting.
	Tea tree	As little as a teaspoon of tea tree oil can be toxic. Do not ingest it, and keep it out of the reach of children.

Healing Actions of Herbs

USE	HERB(S)	SPECIAL PRECAUTION(S)
Adaptogen	Ashwagandha	None
	Eleuthero	
	Ginseng	
	Reishi	
	Rhodiola	
	Schisandra	
Anesthetic	*For external use:*	Never ingest herbal oils. As little as a teaspoon can be toxic.
	Cinnamon	
	Clove	
	Peppermint	
Antibiotic (antibacterial)	Apple	
	Artichoke	
	Barberry	
	Bayberry	*Bayberry* may change the body's sodium-potassium balance. If you have high blood pressure, heart disease, diabetes, kidney disease, or a history of stroke, consult a physician before using it.
	Boneset	
	Burdock	
	Catnip	
	Chamomile	
	Cinnamon	
	Clove	
	Dill	
	Echinacea	
	Garlic	*Garlic* is an anticoagulant and may cause bruising or delay blood clotting.
	Ginseng	
	Goldenseal	
	Licorice	Long-term use of licorice may cause water retention, elevated blood pressure, and a hormone imbalance (pseudoaldosteronism).

USE	HERB(S)	SPECIAL PRECAUTION(S)
Antibiotic (antibacterial) (cont.)	Meadowsweet	*Meadowsweet* contains aspirin-like compounds. If you are aspirin-sensitive, consult a physician before using it.
	Myrrh	
	Pau d'arco	Pau d'arco is an anticoagulant and may cause bruising and delay blood clotting.
	Peppermint	
	Reishi	
	St. John's wort	If you are taking antidepressant medication, consult a physician before using *St. John's wort*.
	Tea tree	As little as a teaspoon of *tea tree* oil can be toxic. Do not ingest it, and keep it out of the reach of children.
	Thyme	
Antibiotic (antifungal)	Aloe	
	Artichoke	
	Barberry	
	Burdock	
	Chamomile	
	Cinnamon	
	Clove	
	Dandelion	Long-term use of *dandelion* may deplete potassium stores.
	Echinacea	
	Garlic	Garlic is an anticoagulant and may cause bruising or delay blood clotting.
	Goldenseal	
	Licorice	Long-term use of licorice may cause water retention, elevated blood pressure, and a hormone imbalance (pseudoaldosteronism).
	St. John's wort	If you are taking antidepressant medication, consult a physician before using St. John's wort.
	Tea tree	As little as a teaspoon of tea tree oil can be toxic. Do not ingest it, and keep it out of the reach of children.

USE	HERB(S)	SPECIAL PRECAUTION(S)
Antibiotic (antiparasitic, antiprotozoan)	Barberry	
	Bayberry	Bayberry may change the body's sodium-potassium balance. If you have high blood pressure, heart disease, diabetes, kidney disease, or a history of stroke, consult a physician before using it.
	Clove	
	Echinacea	
	Elecampane	
	Garlic	Garlic is an anticoagulant and may cause bruising or delay blood clotting.
	Goldenseal	
	Myrrh	
	Turmeric	
Anticoagulant	Garlic	Garlic and shepherd's purse may cause bruising.
	Shepherd's purse	
Antidepressant	Coffee	Coffee contains caffeine, which may cause jitters, irritability, insomnia, and addiction.
	St. John's wort	If you are already taking antidepressant medication, consult a physician before using St. John's wort.
Antihistamine	Clove	
	Nettle	Long-term use of *nettle* may deplete potassium stores.
Anti-inflammatory	Andrographis	Andrographis is anticoagulant and may cause bruising and delay blood clotting.
	Angelica	Angelica may cause a rash in sensitive people who are exposed to direct sunlight.
	Bacopa	
	Black haw	
	Boneset	
	Cat's claw	
	Chamomile	
	Chaparral	
	Echinacea	
	Fenugreek	
	Gentian	

USE	HERB(S)	SPECIAL PRECAUTION(S)
Anti-inflammatory (cont.)	Ginger	
	Horsetail	Long-term use of horsetail, juniper, and vervain may deplete potassium stores.
	Juniper	
	Licorice	Long-term use of licorice may cause water retention, elevated blood pressure, and a hormone imbalance (pseudoaldosteronism).
	Meadowsweet	Meadowsweet and white willow contain aspirin-like compounds. If you are aspirin-sensitive, consult a physician before using these herbs.
	St. John's wort	If you are taking antidepressant medication, consult a physician before using St. John's wort.
	Turmeric	
	Vervain	Vervain may depress heart rate and constrict bronchial passages. If you have heart disease, high blood pressure, diabetes, or asthma, consult a physician before using it.
	White willow	
Antioxidant	Ashwagandha	
	Bacopa	
	Bilberry	
	Blackberry	
	Cat's claw	
	Chaparral	
	Cocoa (dark chocolate)	
	Coffee	Coffee and tea contain caffeine, which may cause jitters, irritability, insomnia, and addiction.
	Cordyceps	
	Cranberry	
	Elderberry	
	Eleuthero	
	Muira puama	
	Pomegranate	
	Raspberry	
	Reishi	

USE	HERB(S)	SPECIAL PRECAUTION(S)
	Tea	
	Turmeric	
Antiperspirant	Sage	None
Antiseptic	*For external use in treating minor burns and wounds:*	None
	Aloe	
	Apple	
	Blackberry	
	Catnip	
	Chamomile	
	Chaparral	
	Cinnamon	
	Clove	
	Eucalyptus	
	Garlic	
	Hop	
	Lemon balm	
	Licorice	
	Myrrh	
	Passionflower	
	Peppermint	
	Rosemary	
	Sage	
	St. John's wort	
	Slippery elm	
	Tarragon	
	Tea tree	
	Thyme	
	Turmeric	
	Yarrow	
	For internal use:	
	Echinacea	
	Ginseng	

USE	HERB(S)	SPECIAL PRECAUTION(S)
Antiviral	Boneset	
	Cat's claw	
	Chamomile	
	Cinnamon	
	Echinacea	
	Ginger	
	Ginseng	
	Lemon balm	Lemon balm interferes with thyroid-stimulating hormone. If you have an underactive thyroid (hypothyroidism), consult a physician before using it.
	Pau d'arco	Pau d'arco is an anticoagulant and may cause bruising and delay blood clotting.
	St. John's wort	If you are taking antidepressant medication, consult a physician before using *St. John's wort*.
Decongestant	Angelica	Angelica may cause a rash in sensitive people who are exposed to direct sunlight.
	Cocoa (chocolate)	Cocoa (chocolate), coffee, kola, maté, and tea all contain caffeine, which may cause jitters, irritability, insomnia, and addiction.
	Coffee	
	Ephedra	Ephedra may raise blood pressure and cause jitters, irritability, and insomnia. People with high blood pressure, heart or kidney disease, or a history of stroke should not use it. In very large doses, ephedra may cause potentially fatal heart problems.
	Eucalyptus	
	Kola	
	Maté	
	Pennyroyal	
	Peppermint	
	Rosemary	
	Tea	
Digestive support	Angelica	Angelica may cause a rash in sensitive people who are exposed to direct sunlight.
	Artichoke	
	Caraway	

USE	HERB(S)	SPECIAL PRECAUTION(S)
	Catnip	
	Chamomile	
	Cinnamon	
	Clove	
	Cocoa (chocolate)	Cocoa (chocolate) contains caffeine, which may cause jitters, irritability, insomnia, and addiction.
	Dandelion	Long-term use of *dandelion* may deplete potassium stores.
	Dill	
	Fennel	Fennel has estrogenic action. People who have a history of blood clots (thromboembolisms), inflammation of blood vessels (thrombophlebitis), heart disease, or stroke should consult their physicians before using it.
	Feverfew	
	Gentian	
	Ginger	
	Goldenseal	
	Hop	
	Horehound	
	Lavender	
	Lemon balm	Lemon balm interferes with thyroid-stimulating hormone. If you have an underactive thyroid (hypothyroidism), consult a physician before using it.
	Marshmallow	
	Papaya	
	Passionflower	
	Pennyroyal	
	Peppermint	
	Red pepper	
	Rosemary	
	Sage	
	Slippery elm	
	Thyme	
	Turmeric	
	Yarrow	

USE	HERB(S)	SPECIAL PRECAUTION(S)
Diuretic	Buchu	Long-term use of diuretic herbs may deplete potassium stores. Do not use diuretics for weight loss.
	Celery	
	Dandelion	
	Fennel	
	Horsetail	
	Juniper	
	Nettle	
	Parsley	
	Sarsaparilla	
	Uva-ursi	
Immune stimulation	*For external use:*	
	Aloe	
	For internal use:	
	Andrographis	Andrographis and garlic are anticoagulants and may cause bruising and delay blood clotting.
	Ashwagandha	
	Astragalus	
	Barberry	
	Bitter melon	
	Boneset	
	Cat's claw	
	Chamomile	
	Cordyceps	
	Echinacea	
	Eleuthero	
	Garlic	
	Ginger	
	Ginseng	
	Goldenseal	
	Gotu kola	

USE	HERB(S)	SPECIAL PRECAUTION(S)
	Licorice	Long-term use of licorice may cause water retention, elevated blood pressure, and a hormone imbalance (pseudoaldosteronism).
	Maitake	
	Marshmallow	
	Mistletoe	Mistletoe may slow heart rate and affect blood pressure. If you have heart disease, diabetes, high blood pressure, or a history of stroke, consult your physician before using it.
	Reishi	
	St. John's wort	If you are taking antidepressant medication, consult a physician before using St. John's wort.
	Shiitake	
	Turmeric	
Kidney protection	Reishi	None
Labor stimulation	Shepherd's purse	Using herbs to induce labor requires medical supervision.
Labor support	Raspberry	None
Lactation support	Chaste tree	None
	Peppermint	
Laxative	Apple	
	Buckthorn	Buckthorn, cascara sagrada, rhubarb, and senna may cause abdominal distress. If you find yourself using these herbs more than twice a month, consult a physician.
	Cascara sagrada	
	Coffee	Coffee contains caffeine, which may cause jitters, irritability, insomnia, and addiction.
	Psyllium	
	Rhubarb	
	Senna	
	Vervain	Vervain may depress heart rate and constrict bronchial passages. If you have heart disease, high blood pressure, diabetes, or asthma, consult a physician before using it.

USE	HERB(S)	SPECIAL PRECAUTION(S)
Liver protection	Andrographis	Andrographis is anticoagulant and may cause bruising and delay blood clotting.
	Artichoke	
	Astragalus	
	Bacopa	
	Barberry	
	Cordyceps	
	Ginseng	
	Licorice	Long-term use of licorice may cause water retention, elevated blood pressure, and a hormone imbalance (pseudoaldosteronism).
	Maitake	
	Milk thistle	
	Reishi	
	Rhodiola	
	Turmeric	
Pregnancy support	Raspberry	None
Sedative	Celery	Long-term use of celery may deplete potassium stores.
	Hop	
	Lavender	
	Lemon balm	Lemon balm interferes with thyroid-stimulating hormone. If you have an underactive thyroid (hypothyroidism), consult a physician before using it.
	Motherwort	
	Passionflower	
	Scullcap	
	Valerian	
	Yarrow	
Stimulant	Cocoa (chocolate)	Cocoa (chocolate), coffee, kola, maté, and tea all contain caffeine, which may cause jitters, irritability, insomnia, and addiction.
	Coffee	

USE	HERB(S)	SPECIAL PRECAUTION(S)
Tranquilizer	Ephedra	Ephedra may raise blood pressure and cause jitters, irritability, and insomnia. People with high blood pressure, heart or kidney disease, or a history of stroke should not use it. In very large doses, ephedra may cause potentially fatal heart problems.
	Ginseng	
	Kola	
	Maté	
	Tea	
	Catnip	
	Celery	Long-term use of celery may deplete potassium stores.
	Chamomile	
	Hop	
	Lavender	
	Lemon balm	Lemon balm interferes with thyroid-stimulating hormone. If you have an underactive thyroid (hypothyroidism), consult a physician before using it.
	Motherwort	
	Passionflower	
	Scullcap	
	Yarrow	

Other Uses of Herbs

USE	HERB(S)	SPECIAL PRECAUTION(S)
Appetite loss	Ginseng	None
Athletic performance enhancement	Coffee	Coffee contains caffeine, which may cause jitters, irritability, insomnia, and addiction.
	Ginseng	
Cognitive function	Bacopa	
	Ginkgo	
	Ginseng	
	Rhodiola	
	Tea	Tea contains caffeine, which may cause jitters, irritability, insomnia, and addiction.
	Turmeric	

USE	HERB(S)	SPECIAL PRECAUTION(S)
Insect repellent	Eucalyptus	
	Lavender	
	Neem	Neem oil and pennyroyal oil are toxic. Do not ingest, and keep them out of the reach of children.
	Pennyroyal	
Memory improvement	Bacopa	None
	Eleuthero	
	Ginkgo	
	Ginseng	
Self-defense	Red pepper	None

References

Because of space limitations, only the books used as sources for *The New Healing Herbs* are listed here. Much of the information in the book comes directly from the world medical literature, which can be accessed for free at www.pubmed.gov.

American Pharmaceutical Association. *Handbook of Nonprescription Drugs.* Washington, D.C.: American Pharmaceutical Association, 1996.

Bassman, L. *The Whole Mind: The Definitive Guide to Complementary Treatments for Mind, Mood, and Emotion.* Novato, Calif.: New World Library, 1998.

Beinfield, H., and E. Korngold. *Between Heaven and Earth: A Guide to Chinese Medicine.* New York: Ballantine, 1991.

Blumenthal, M. *The ABC Clinical Guide to Herbs.* Austin, Tex.: American Botanical Council, 2003.

Blumenthal, M., et al. *The Complete German Commission E Monographs: Therapeutic Guide to Herbal Medicines.* Austin, Tex.: American Botanical Council and Integrative Medicine Communications, 1998.

———. *Herbal Medicine: Expanded Commission E Monographs.* Austin, Tex.: American Botanical Council, 2000.

Boyle, W. *Herb Doctors: Pioneers in 19th-Century American Botanical Medicine.* East Palestine, Ohio: Buckeye Naturopathic Press, 1988.

Brinker, F. J. *The Toxicology of Botanical Medicines.* 2nd ed. Portland, Ore.: Eclectic Medical Institute, 1987.

Brown, D. *Herbal Prescriptions for Better Health.* Rocklin, Calif.: Prima Publishing, 1996.

Burton Goldberg Group. *Alternative Medicine: The Definitive Guide.* Fife, Wash.: Future Medicine, 1994.

Castleman, M. *Nature's Cures.* Emmaus, Pa.: Rodale Press, 1996.

Chin, W. Y., and H. Keng. *An Illustrated Dictionary of Chinese Medicinal Herbs.* Sebastopol, Calif.: CRCS Publications, 1992.

Cichoke, A.J. *Secrets of Native American Herbal Remedies.* New York: Avery/Penguin Putnam, 2001.

Collinge, W. *The American Holistic Health Association Complete Guide to Alternative Medicine.* New York: Warner Books, 1996.

Conrow, R., and A. Hecksel. *Herbal Pathfinders: Voices of the Herb Renaissance.* Santa Barbara, Calif.: Woodbridge Press, 1983.

Coulter, H. L. *Divided Legacy.* Berkeley, Calif.: Homeopathic Educational Services, 1982.

Crenshaw, T. *The Alchemy of Love and Lust.* New York: Putnam, 1996.

Culpeper, N. *Culpeper's Complete Herbal and English Physician.* 1826 ed. Avon, England: Pitman Press, 1981.

Cummings, S., and D. Ullman. *Everybody's Guide to Homeopathic Medicines.* New York: Tarcher-Putnam, 1997.

Cumston, C. G. *An Introduction to the History of Medicine.* New York: Dorset Press, 1987.

Der Marderosian, A., and L. Liberti. *Natural Product Medicine.* Philadelphia: George F. Stickley, 1988.

DeSmet, P. A., ed. *Adverse Effects of Herbal Drugs.* Berlin: Springer-Verlag, 1993.

De Waal, M. *Medicinal Herbs in the Bible.* York Beach, Maine: Samuel Weiser, 1984.

Dobelis, I. N., ed. *Magic and Medicine of Plants.* Pleasantville, N.Y.: Reader's Digest, 1986.

Duke, J. A. *Handbook of Medicinal Herbs.* Boca Raton, Fla.: CRC Press, 1985.

———. *Ginseng: A Concise Handbook.* Algonac, Mich.: Reference Publications, 1989.

———. *The Green Pharmacy.* Emmaus, Pa.: Rodale Press, 1997.

Editors of Pharmacist's Letter. *Natural Medicines Comprehensive Database, 2008.* Stockton, Calif.: Therapeutic Research Faculty Press, 2008.

Ehrenreich, B. and D. English. *Witches, Midwives, and Nurses: A History of Women Healers.* Detroit: Black and Red, 1973.

Eskinazi, D., et al., eds. *Botanical Medicine: Efficacy, Quality Assurance, and Regulation.* Larchmont, N.Y.: Mary Ann Liebert, 1999.

Facts and Comparisons. *Drug Facts and Comparisons, 1999 and 2000.* St. Louis, Mo.: Facts and Comparisons Publishing Group, 1999 and 2000.

Felter, H. W., and J. U. Lloyd. *King's American Dispensatory.* 18th ed., 1898. Portland, Ore.: Eclectic Medical Publications, 1983.

Foster, S. *Herbal Bounty.* Salt Lake City: Peregrine Smith Books, 1984.

———. *Echinacea Exalted!* Brixley, Mo.: Ozark Beneficial Plant Project, 1985.

Foster, S., and J. A. Duke. *A Field Guide to Medicinal Plants: Eastern and Central North America* (Peterson Field Guide #40). Boston: Houghton Mifflin, 1990.

Foster, S., and V. E. Tyler. *Tyler's Honest Herbal.* 4th ed. New York and London: Haworth Herbal Press, 1999.

Fratkin, J. *Chinese Herbal Patent Formulas.* Boulder, Colo.: Shya Publications, 1986.

Fugh-Berman, A. *Alternative Medicine: What Works.* Tucson: Odonian Press, 1996.

Fulder, S. *Ginseng: Magical Herb of the East.* Northamptonshire, England: Thorsons Publishing, 1988.

Funfgeld, E. W., ed. *Rokan (Ginkgo Biloba): Recent Results in Pharmacology and Clinic.* Berlin: Springer-Verlag, 1988.

Gilman, A. G., et al., eds. *Goodman and Gilman's The Pharmacological Basis of Therapeutics.* 7th ed. New York: Macmillan, 1985.

Graedon, J., and T. Graedon. *Graedon's Best Medicine: From Herbal Remedies to High-Tech Rx Breakthroughs.* New York: Bantam Books, 1991.

Grieve, M. *A Modern Herbal.* New York: Dover, 1971.

Griffith, H. W. *The Complete Guide to Vitamins, Minerals, Supplements, and Herbs.* Tucson: Fisher Books, 1988.

Hallowell, M. *Herbal Healing: A Practical Introduction.* Bath, England: Ashgrove Press, 1985.

Harris, B. C. *Comfrey: What You Need to Know.* New Canaan, Conn.: Keats Publishing, 1982.

Harris, L. J. *The Book of Garlic.* Berkeley, Calif.: Aris Books, 1979.

Herbrandson, D. *Shaker Herbs and Their Medicinal Uses.* New Gloucester, Maine: Shaker Heritage Society, Sabbathday Lake, 1985.

Heyn, B. *Ayurvedic Medicine.* Northamptonshire, England: Thorsons Publishing, 1987.

Hobbs, C. *Medicinal Mushrooms: An Exploration of Tradition, Healing, and Culture.* Santa Cruz, Calif.: Botanica Press, 1986.

———. *The Ginsengs: A Users Guide.* Santa Cruz, Calif.: Botanica Press, 1996.

———. *Herbal Remedies for Dummies.* Foster City, Calif.: IDG Books, 1998.

Hoffman, D. *The Holistic Herbal.* Dorset, England: Element Books, 1983.

Hou, J. P. *Ginseng: The Myth and the Truth.* North Hollywood, Calif.: Wilshire Book Co., 1978.

Keville, K., and M. Green. *Aromatherapy: A Complete Guide to the Healing Art.* Freedom, Calif.: Crossing Press, 1995.

Kiangsu Institute of Modern Medicine. *Encyclopedia of Chinese Drugs,* vol. 2. Shanghai: Shanghai Scientific and Technical Publications, 1977.

Kloss, J. *Back to Eden.* Loma Linda, Calif.: Back to Eden Books, 1988.

Koch, H. P., and L. D. Lawson, eds. *Garlic: The Science and Therapeutic Application of Allium Sativum and Related Species.* Baltimore: Williams and Wilkins, 1996.

Kowalchik, C., and W. H. Hylton, eds. *Rodale's Illustrated Encyclopedia of Herbs.* Emmaus, Pa.: Rodale Press, 1987.

Kreig, M. B. *Green Medicine: The Search for Plants That Heal.* Chicago: Rand McNally, 1964.

Lad, V., and D. Frawley. *The Yoga of Herbs.* Santa Fe: Lotus Press, 1986.

Law, D. *The Concise Herbal Encyclopedia.* New York: St. Martin's Press, 1973.

Leung, A. Y. *Encyclopedia of Common Natural Ingredients Used in Food, Drugs, and Cosmetics.* New York: John Wiley & Sons, 1980.

Lewis, W., and M. P. F. Elvin-Lewis. *Medical Botany.* New York: John Wiley & Sons, 1974.

Lust, J. *The Herb Book.* New York: Bantam, 1974.

Marti-Ibaez, F. *The Epic of Medicine.* New York: Bramhall House, 1962.

McCaleb, R., et al. *The Herb Research Foundation's Encyclopedia of Popular Herbs.* Roseville, Calif.: Prima Publishing, 2000.

McGuffin, M., et al., eds. *American Herbal Products Association Botanical Safety Handbook.* Boca Raton, Fla.: CRC Press, 1997.

McIntyre, M. *Herbal Medicine for Everyone.* London: Penguin, 1988.

Medical Economics. *PDR for Herbal Medicines.* Montvale, N.J.: Medical Economics, 1998.

Micozzi, M. S. *Fundamentals of Complementary and Alternative Medicine.* New York: Churchill Livingstone, 1996.

Millspaugh, C. F. *American Medicinal Plants.* 1892 ed. New York: Dover, 1974.

Morse, F. *The Story of the Shakers.* Woodstock, Vt.: Countryman Press, 1986.

Mowrey, D. B. *The Scientific Validation of Herbal Medicine.* Lehi, Utah: Cormorant Books, 1986.

———. *Next Generation Herbal Medicine.* Lehi, Utah: Cormorant Books, 1988.

Murray, M. *The 21st Century Herbal*. Bellevue, Wash.: Vita-Line, 1987.

———. *Natural Alternatives to Over-the-Counter and Prescription Drugs*. New York: William Morrow, 1994.

Murray, M., and J. Pizzorno. *Encyclopedia of Natural Medicine*. Rocklin, Calif.: Prima Publishing, 1991.

Olsen, C. *Australian Teatree Oil Guide*. Pagosa Springs, Colo.: Kali Press, 1997.

Pendergrast, M. *Uncommon Grounds: The History of Coffee and How It Transformed Our World*. New York: Basic Books, 1999.

Pizzorno, J., and M. Murray. *A Textbook of Natural Medicine*. Kenmore, Wash.: Bastyr University Publications, 1996.

Reid, D. P. *Chinese Herbal Medicine*. Boston: Shambhala, 1987.

Riddle, J. M. *Eve's Herbs: A History of Contraception and Abortion in the West*. Cambridge, Mass.: Harvard University Press, 1997.

Schechter, S. *Fighting Radiation with Foods, Herbs, and Vitamins*. Brookline, Mass.: East West Health Books, 1988.

Simon, J. E., and L. Grant, eds. *Proceedings of the First National Herb Growing and Marketing Conference*. West Lafayette, Ind.: Purdue University Cooperative Extension Service, 1986.

———. *Proceedings of the Second National Herb Growing and Marketing Conference*. West Lafayette, Ind.: Purdue University Cooperative Extension Service, 1987.

Simon, J. E., et al. *Proceedings of the Fourth National Herb Growing and Marketing Conference*. Silver Spring, Pa.: International Herb Growers and Marketers Association, 1989.

Spencer, J. W., and J. J. Jacobs. *Complementary/Alternative Medicine: An Evidence-Based Approach*. St. Louis: Mosby, 1999.

Spoerke, D. *Herbal Medications*. Santa Barbara, Calif.: Woodbridge Press, 1980.

Starr, P. *The Social Transformation of American Medicine*. New York: Basic Books, 1982.

Strehlow, W., and G. Hertzka. *Hildegard of Bingen's Medicine*. Santa Fe: Bear, 1988.

Stuart, M., ed. *The Encyclopedia of Herbs and Herbalism*. New York: Grosset & Dunlap, 1979.

Tannahill, R. *Food in History*. New York: Stein & Day, 1973.

Therapeutic Research Faculty. *Natural Medicines Comprehensive Database, 2006*. Stockton, Calif. 2006.

Tierra, M. *The Way of Herbs*. New York: Pocket Books, 1983.

Tyler, V. *Herbs of Choice: The Therapeutic Use of Phytomedicinals*. New York: Hawthorn Press, 1994.

Tyler, V. E., et al. *Pharmacognosy*. 9th ed. Philadelphia: Lea and Febiger, 1988.

Ullman, D. *The Consumer's Guide to Homeopathy*. New York: G. P. Putnam's Sons, 1995.

Ulrich, L.T. *A Midwife's Tale: The Life of Martha Ballard, Based on Her Diary, 1785–1812*. New York: Random House, 1990.

Weed, S. S. *Wise Woman Herbal for the Childbearing Years*. Woodstock, N.Y.: Ash Tree Publishing, 1985.

Weil, A. *Natural Health, Natural Medicine*. Boston: Houghton Mifflin, 1990.

Weiner, M., and J. A. Weiner. *Herbs That Heal*. Mill Valley, Calif.: Quantum Books, 1994.

Weiner, M. A. *Earth Medicine, Earth Food*. New York: Macmillan, 1980.

———. *The People's Herbal*. New York: Perigee/Putnam, 1984.

———. *Weiner's Herbal*. New York: Stein & Day, 1980.

Weiss, G., and S. Weiss. *Growing and Using the Healing Herbs*. Emmaus, Pa.: Rodale Press, 1985.

Weiss, R. F. *Herbal Medicine*. Beaconsfield, England: Beaconsfield Publishers, 1988.

Werbach, M., and M. Murray. *Botanical Influences on Illness*. Tarzana, Calif.: Third Line Press, 1994.

Wheelwright, E. G. *Medicinal Plants and Their History*. New York: Dover, 1974.

White, L., and S. Mavor. *Kids, Herbs, and Health*. Loveland, Colo.: Interweave Press, 1998.

White, L.B., and S. Foster. *The Herbal Drugstore*. Emmaus, Pa.: Rodale, 2000.

Willard, T. *Textbook of Modern Herbology*. Calgary, Alberta: Progressive Publishing, 1988.

Wren, R. C. *Potter's New Cyclopaedia of Botanical Drugs and Preparations*. Essex, England: C. W. Daniel, 1988.

Zhu, C-H. *Clinical Handbook of Chinese Prepared Medicines*. Brookline, Mass.: Paradigm Publications, 1989.

Index

L

Labor, premature, chamomile preventing, 146

Labor aids, <u>525</u>
parsley, 355–56
raspberry, 384
shepherd's purse, 433

Lactation problems, healing herbs for
chaste tree, 152–53
dill, 188
peppermint, 371

Lactation support, healing herbs for, <u>525</u>

Lallemand, M., 459

Latin binomial names of herbs, 42

Lavender, 300–304, **300**
growing information, 304
healing history, 301–2
possible uses, 303
Rx recommendations, 303
safety, 303–4
therapeutic uses, 302–3

Law of Potentization, in homeopathy, 29

Laxative herbs, 5, <u>525</u>
aloe, 59, 61–62
avoiding problems from, 44–45
buckthorn, 119–21
cascara sagrada, 132–34
problems from, 39–40
psyllium, 376
rhubarb, 401
senna, 429–31
slippery elm, 438
vervain, 475

Lazarev, N.V., 202, 252, 398

Lead poisoning, healing herbs for, <u>507</u>
garlic, 234

Learning improvement, herbs for
gotu kola, 266
muira puama, 338
schisandra, 426

Lee, Ann, 26, 27

Leech Book of Bald, 17

Lemon balm, 305–8, **305**

Leprosy (Hansen's disease)
healing herbs for, <u>508</u>
garlic, 230
gotu kola, 264, 266
possible healing herbs for
garlic, 234
sarsaparilla, 420

Lethargy, healing herbs for
cocoa, 162
coffee, 166

Leukemia
aloe and, 61
tea preventing, 452

Leyel, C. F. (Hilda), 33

Libido improvement, herbs for
maca, 314–15
muira puama, 338

Libido reduction, chaste tree for, 151, 153

Lice, head, tea tree for, 456

Licorice, 6, 308–13, **308**
growing information, 313
healing history, 309–10
possible uses, 312
Rx recommendations, 312
safety, 312–13
therapeutic uses, 310–12

Life span extension, chaparral and, 149

Linne, Carl, 22

Liqueurs, invention of, 16

Li-Shih-Chen, 8

Liver damage
astragalus preventing, 82
drug-induced, milk thistle for, 329
healing herbs for
barberry, 87–88
evening primrose oil, 214
schisandra, 426
turmeric, 464
kava and, x, 39, 289–90, 291–94
toxin-induced, milk thistle for, 329

Liver disease. *See also* Cirrhosis, healing herbs for
healing herbs for
cordyceps, 177
maitake, 317
possible healing herbs for
ginseng, 257
licorice, 311

Liver function, eleuthero for, 203

Liver problems
healing herbs for
artichoke, 75, 76
milk thistle, 75, 76
possible healing herbs for
angelica, 67
bayberry, 90

Liver protection
healing herbs for, <u>526</u>
andrographis, 64
bacopa, 85
ginseng, 256
reishi, 396
rhodiola, 399
possible healing herbs for
sarsaparilla, 420
yarrow, 485

Lloyd, Curtis, 31

Lloyd, John Uri, 31, 191

Lloyd, Nelson, 31

Lloyd Library, 31

Lobelia, 28

About the Author

Library Journal has called Michael Castleman "one of the nation's top health writers." He has been the herbal medicine columnist for *Herb Quarterly* magazine since 1988. His articles on herbal medicine have appeared in many publications and online services, including *Prevention, Reader's Digest, Redbook, Family Circle, AARP Magazine, Natural Health, Herb Companion,* and Salon.com.

Castleman is the author of 12 consumer medical books with a combined total of more than 2 million copies in print. They include: *Blended Medicine*, a home medical guide that combines the best of mainstream and alternative medicine for 100 common conditions; *Nature's Cures*, an exploration of the science behind 30 alternative therapies; *Before You Call the Doctor*, a self-care home medical guide; and *Building Bone Vitality* (with coauthor Amy Lanou, Ph.D.), a guide to osteoporosis prevention and treatment. Castleman has also written three mystery novels.

A former adjunct professor at the University of California, Berkeley, Graduate School of Journalism, where he taught medical writing, Castleman has won numerous awards for excellence in journalism.

He and his wife live in San Francisco. They have two adult children.